HEALTH PROMOTION AND AGING

Steven M. Albert, PhD, FGSA, FAAN, is a professor in the Department of Behavioral and Community Health Sciences at the University of Pittsburgh's School of Public Health. He has 35 years of research experience in aging, neurologic disease, and interventions to change health behavior.

I took on the challenge of updating *Health Promotion and Aging* as part of a long career in aging research, which saw me move from a focus on the pathologies of aging to prevention of disease and disability and the public health goal of extending opportunities for optimal aging. This career has allowed me to move between National Institutes of Health research (three NIH R01 efforts: "Cognitive and Physical Basis of Disablement," "Depression and End of Life Care in Amyotrophic Lateral Sclerosis," and "End of Life in the Very Old"), and programmatic efforts to harness the aging services network for public health efforts. I have led a number of health promotion efforts through the Centers for Disease Control and Prevention (CDC; University of Pittsburgh Prevention Research Center), Health Resources and Services Administration (HRSA; Public Health Social Work Leadership), and National Institute of Mental Health (NIMH; Advanced Center for Intervention Services Research for Late Life Depression Prevention). I am most proud of a CDC-funded evaluation of the Pennsylvania Department of Aging's statewide falls prevention program ("Comparative Effectiveness of Community-Based Falls Prevention in Pennsylvania"). We established the evidence base for the program, which led to the program's certification and eligibility for Title III-D Older Americans Act funding. More recently, I helped develop the evaluation plan for the Pennsylvania Department of Aging 10 Year Master Plan for Aging (Aging Our Way, 2024–2034, https://www.pa.gov/agencies/aging/aging-our-way-pa.html). I also helped revise the Pennsylvania Department of Human Services screening for eligibility determination for long-term care services.

My early research examined the functional significance of mild cognitive impairment in old age and neurologic consequences of HIV infection. Since then I have been fortunate to develop a number of international research efforts, including partnerships with colleagues in Israel, Germany, Sri Lanka, and Japan (site of a Fulbright sabbatical). My ongoing research includes a study of home environmental health hazards (indoor air quality and mold) funded through the U.S. Department of Housing and Urban Development (HUD). I continue to collaborate with colleagues in Japan on deprescribing and with colleagues in medical informatics to examine inappropriate prescribing. I recently completed a term as Editor-in-Chief of *Innovation in Aging* (Gerontological Society of America, Oxford University Press) and have published four books and over 300 peer-reviewed papers.

This background helped me in updating *Health Promotion and Aging* for its ninth edition. What a pleasure it has been to build on the work of my colleague, David Haber, PhD, who has carefully nurtured this important book over its many editions. The book is Dr. Haber's lifetime project and I am but an interloper. The book's evolution is really the evolution of the field over the prior three decades and Dr. Haber has put the field on the map. I am standing on his shoulders and would not attempt such an effort from scratch!

This update extends the eighth edition to cover new advances in prevention science relevant to aging, changes in the policy landscape, and the impact of the emerging field of geroscience on prospects for optimal aging. I apologize in advance for not matching Dr. Haber's wonderful voice and personal experience with delivery of health promotion programming.

Advances in geroscience may make the 10th edition of *Health Promotion and Aging* look very different from this edition. As we better understand the molecular hallmarks of aging, we may be able to slow the rate of aging, with great consequences for health promotion in old age. Already the new generations of GLP-1 therapies have shown benefit far beyond weight management. As we move from the "spare parts" approach to geriatric medicine and clinical management (moving from hip replacements and cardiac stents to stem cell therapies and lifelong control of physiologic stress), we may need to rethink health promotion. How might this look? For example, we may need to think about falls prevention differently if people ski or snowboard at age 80. More falls at very old age could become an indicator of greater physical activity and engagement, rather than a sign of sarcopenia and debility alone. Longer periods of employment and increased take up of encore careers could mean changes in worksite health promotion. Long-term use of anti-aging therapies could mean new risks for adverse health events and tough decisions about tradeoffs for function and well-being. The shadow of quack therapies accompanying the anti-aging therapy boom will likely also grow. Health promotion in old age may become more challenging, not less.

HEALTH PROMOTION AND AGING

Practical Applications for Health Professionals

Ninth Edition

Steven M. Albert, PhD, FGSA, FAAN

SPRINGER PUBLISHING

First Springer Publishing edition 978-0-8261-8460-3 © 1995; subsequent editions © 2000, © 2004, © 2007, © 2010, © 2013, © 2016, © 2019.

Springer Publishing Company, LLC
902 Carnegie Center/Suite 140, Princeton, NJ 08540
www.springerpub.com
connect.springerpub.com

Acquisitions Editor: Mindy Okura-Marszycki
Production Editor: Joseph Stubenrauch
Compositor: S4Carlisle Publishing Services

ISBN: 978-0-8261-8385-9
e-book ISBN: 978-0-8261-8386-6
DOI: 10.1891/9780826183866

SUPPLEMENTS:

SPRINGER PUBLISHING CONNECT™ | **A robust set of instructor resources designed to supplement this text is located at http://connect.springerpub.com/content/book/978-0-8261-8386-6. Qualifying instructors may request access by emailing textbook@springerpub.com.**

Instructor Materials:
LMS Common Cartridge—With All Instructor Resources
Instructor Manual
Instructor Sample Syllabus
Instructor Test Bank
Instructor Chapter PowerPoints
Transition Guide From Eighth to Ninth Edition

25 26 27 28 / 5 4 3 2 1

Library of Congress Control Number: 2025007136

CONTENTS

PREFACE

A book about health promotion should begin by asking why we need to promote health. Doesn't everybody want it? Does it really need promoting? The question is simple but the answer complex.

While people want health, many forces conspire to make it difficult to get and maintain. Lack of opportunities to exercise or eat healthy food, threats to personal security, economic shocks, short time horizons in evaluating consequences of behavior, false or misleading advice on what is good for us, uncertainty in seeking medical care or screening for health risks, addiction and poor mental health, cognitive disorders, and health risks due to environmental exposures all challenge our ability to make healthy choices. We may all want to be healthy, but it is not easy. We need guidance.

The need for guidance may be especially important in old age. Aging is a major challenge to health. With age we face a growing cumulative risk of disease and disability. By their 40s Americans already see increases in chronic disease, the first major wave of cancer and cardiovascular deaths, and declines in many biological parameters. By age 65, musculoskeletal disorders and hypertension already affect about half the population. Ninety percent take a prescription medication. Half are obese. The effect on daily life is profound. A *New York Times* article asked, only half tongue in cheek, why middle-aged and older people groan so much (https://www.nytimes.com/2023/03/24/well/middle-aged-groan.html).

If we need guidance in securing health, we certainly need it as we age and when we are old. Medical science can help, but studies are often inconclusive or frankly disappointing. Consider the Women's Health Initiative (WHI). This large study began in 1991 as a proposed 15-year study. Women in menopause without hysterectomy (mean age 63) were randomized to take a placebo or combination estrogen-progesterone oral therapy. Women with hysterectomies took estrogen alone. The scientific premise was reasonable: With age and menopause, estrogen declines. Restoring levels to that of younger ages should improve bone health and reduce cardiovascular events, such as strokes and heart attacks. After about 10 years, however, the study was terminated early because of an increase in breast cancer and stroke and no reduction in cardiovascular events. Publication of the study led to a severe decline in estrogen supplementation. But commentators noted many uncertainties: (a) Perhaps an earlier start of estrogen would have had benefit for these older women, whose vascular health for the most part had already declined (the average age of menopause is 51). (b) Women with hysterectomies who took estrogen alone saw a decrease in breast cancer. (c) The number of events that tilted the trial in the wrong direction was actually small (seven more cardiac events, eight more strokes, eight more pulmonary emboli, and eight more breast cancers per 10,000 person-years of follow-up). The decision to end the trial was certainly appropriate, but the negative results do not suggest clear guidance beyond the limited endpoints of the trial and its particular sample.

Findings for other proposed therapies have also been equivocal. In ASPREE, a large international randomized controlled trial of daily use of aspirin, disability-free survival was lower, and mortality higher, in the intervention arm, counter to expectations and prior smaller trials. By contrast, the SPRINT trial of intensive blood pressure control in people over age 75 (lowering systolic blood pressure to 120 mmHg instead of the standard goal of 140) was terminated early because of clear benefit in reducing cardiovascular events and mortality, a win for prevention. Still, the trial excluded important subgroups (older adults residing in nursing homes and people with type 2 diabetes, stroke, or heart failure), required additional hypertension medication and monitoring, and raised the risk of potential kidney injury.

The situation is similar for behavioral interventions. The LIFE trial showed that supervised exercise could reduce the risk of mobility disability, as measured by completing a 400-meter walk in 15 minutes without stopping or sitting. However, people randomized to the intervention also faced a higher risk of hospitalization over the course of the trial.

These few examples show the complexity of promoting health in aging. Our interventions come with restrictions on who is likely to benefit and sometimes force us to trade unwelcome side effects for limited or unproven protection from threats to health. Navigating this complex literature is not easy for professional arbiters, such as the U.S. Preventive Services Task Force, let alone a lay person trying to age well and avoid preventable morbidity.

Hence the need for a book on health promotion and aging. But why a new edition? Here the answer is simpler. Our understanding of aging, health, and health promotion continues to evolve. In the 5 years since the eighth edition of *Health Promotion and Aging* much has changed. As the preface of the eighth edition noted, "major, and sometimes dramatic, research results" and promising initiatives require rethinking of many previous recommendations.

Apart from updates on health promotion, the ninth edition has a number of new sections. These include:

- older adults and clinical trials,
- prospects for geroscience,
- medicare and prevention,
- therapies for obesity,
- digital literacy and use of patient portals,
- wearable technologies for monitoring activity,
- mobility planning,
- calorie restriction,
- vitamin D trials for preventing falls and fractures,
- hormone supplementation,
- inappropriate prescription use,
- brain games and prevention of Alzheimer disease,
- model health promotion programs, and
- aging services network.

As in prior editions, this revision includes Key Terms and Learning Objectives at the start of each chapter; questions to ponder within each chapter; boxes throughout containing information to reflect upon; and new chapter-ending summaries that synthesize overarching themes in each chapter.

Steven M. Albert

LIST OF FIGURES

CHAPTER 1

CHAPTER 2

CHAPTER 3

LIST OF TABLES

ACKNOWLEDGMENT

I want to acknowledge the support of my wife, Robin Karlin, who has traveled with me in every academic and career effort even when it has required us to move and negotiate other cultures. My children Eli and Charna have patiently listened to me work through many of the topics discussed here. I have tried many of these ideas out on Ruthe and Renee, mothers and 90-year-olds, who are living labs of health promotion.

In preparing this edition, I would like to thank Xinran Liu, PhD, and Elizabeth McDermott, students in my doctoral program, for going through chapters to identify topics in need of updates. They checked every internet link, searched new literature and identified key findings, and tracked down the latest numbers for every figure reported in this edition. I am pleased to say that Dr. Haber's original numbers and conclusions stood the test of this very careful review. If readers catch errors, I take the blame.

I thank my colleagues at the University of Pittsburgh in Behavioral and Community Health Sciences (Ed Ricci, PhD), Health Policy and Management (Howard Degenholtz, PhD), Epidemiology (Anne Newman, MD, MPH), the Health Policy Institute (Everette James, JD), the Division of Geriatrics (Susan Greenspan, MD, and David Nace, MD), Neurology (Oscar Lopez, MD), and Psychiatry (Charles Reynolds, MD) for productive discussions over the years. I appreciate partners in the Pennsylvania Department of Aging, especially Tom Snedden, as well for their support.

I also had the benefit of becoming a grandfather while completing this book and continuing to learn from very active 90-year-old mothers and mothers-in-law. I am humbled to think how health promotion may differ over nine decades of life and how it may change over the next 90 years.

INSTRUCTOR RESOURCES

SPRINGER PUBLISHING CONNECT™ | A robust set of instructor resources designed to supplement this text is located at http://connect.springerpub.com/content/book/978-0-8261-8386-6. Qualifying instructors may request access by emailing textbook@springerpub.com.

- LMS Common Cartridge—With All Instructor Resources
- Instructor Manual:
  - Chapter Summaries
  - Discussion Questions and Answers
  - Examinations
  - Additional Readings and Videos
- Instructor Sample Syllabus containing a sample course syllabus with course description, course objectives, student responsibilities, course schedule, and more
- Instructor Test Bank with more than 150 multiple-choice questions (including full rationales)
- Instructor Chapter PowerPoints
- Transition Guide From Eighth to Ninth Edition

SPRINGER PUBLISHING

Visit https://www.springerpub.com/courseconnect. See inside front cover and tear-out card for CourseConnect details.

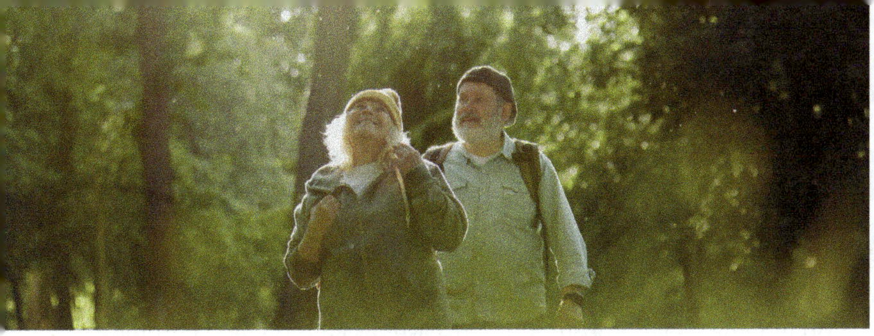

1

INTRODUCTION TO HEALTH PROMOTION AND AGING

KEY TERMS

acculturation
activities of daily living (ADLs) and instrumental activities of daily living (IADLs)
age rectangle
antiaging versus proaging
baby boomers versus the older old
cause of death
centenarian and supercentenarian
chronic conditions and disability
compression of morbidity
health expectancy versus life expectancy
health promotion and disease prevention
health-promoting initiatives
intergenerational conflict
labor force participation rate
libertarian paternalist
medical care and healthcare
Medicare, Medicaid, and Social Security
primary, secondary, and tertiary prevention
racial and ethnic composition
seven dimensions of wellness
sociodemographic trends: marital status, poverty, internet access

LEARNING OBJECTIVES

- Critically evaluate the role of the federal government in promoting health.
- Create your own hypothetical example of *libertarian paternalism.*
- Explain *your* opinion on whether health promotion, disease prevention, and chronic disease management save money.
- Describe the impact of ***sociodemographic trends*** on healthy aging.
- Contrast the baby boomers and the older old.
- Differentiate chronic disease and disability.
- Examine the pros and cons of becoming a centenarian.
- Review trends in life expectancy.
- Identify leading *causes of death.*
- Examine hospital, physician, and medication trends.
- Identify labor force participation rates among older adults.
- Contrast internet use of baby boomers versus that of older adults.
- Examine the consequences of rising educational levels on older adults.
- Describe older adult poverty.
- Identify trends in older adult racial/ethnic composition.
- Contrast definitions of healthy aging and construct your own definition.
- Identify an *extraordinary accomplishment* of an older adult that appeals to you.
- Distinguish among ***primary, secondary,*** and ***tertiary prevention.***
- Evaluate the antiaging movement.
- Define *compression of morbidity* and analyze its likely future course.
- Contrast health expectancy with life expectancy.
- Contrast physical versus emotional aspects of aging.
- Explore the potential for ***intergenerational conflict*** over healthcare.
- Describe the *Medicare,* ***Medicaid,*** *and Social Security* programs.
- Explain why medical care and healthcare are not synonymous.

Youth, large, lusty, loving—youth full of grace, force, fascination. Do you know that Old Age may come after you with equal grace, force, fascination?

—Walt Whitman

INTRODUCTION

Did you know that the federal government establishes goals for healthy aging? As far back as 1990, the U.S. Public Health Service (USPHS) established the goal of increasing the number of years of healthy life remaining at age 65 from 11.8 years, as it was in 1990, to 14 years by 2000. It turned out, however, that this goal for the decade was not close to being met—it was extended by only 4 months. Undeterred, many more goals were set during this and subsequent decades. This raises some interesting questions: Why is the federal government doing this? Should it be doing this? Is it helping to promote healthy aging?

HEALTHY PEOPLE 2010, 2020, 2030: INITIATIVES

In 1979, one of the most influential documents in the field of health promotion, *Healthy People: The Surgeon General's Report on Health Promotion and Disease Prevention*, was published (U.S. Department of Health and Human Services [USDHHS], 1979). Over the years this report was widely cited by the popular media as well as in professional journals and at health conferences. Many attribute to it a seminal role in fostering ***health-promoting initiatives*** throughout the nation.

It was closely followed by another report, and a call to action, by the USPHS in 1980, *Promoting Health/Preventing Disease: Objectives for the Nation*, which outlined health objectives for this country to achieve over the following 10 years. A decade later, in 1990, another national effort, *Healthy People 2000*, was initiated by the USPHS in an effort to reduce preventable death and ***disability*** for Americans by the year 2000. This was followed by *Healthy People 2010, 2020,* and *2030*. Healthy aging is central to the *Healthy People* vision. For example, the 2020 overarching goal is "a society in which all people live long, healthy lives."

The Midcourse Report summarizing progress toward *Healthy People 2030* objectives is not yet available. The *Healthy People 2020: An End of Decade Snapshot*, however, provides important benchmarks for the current state of health promotion among older people and expected progress in the next decade. *Healthy People 2020* identified four priorities: "(i) Attain high-quality, longer lives free of preventable disease; (ii) Achieve health equity; eliminate disparities; (iii) Create social and physical environments that promote good health; and (iv) Promote quality of life, healthy development, healthy behaviors across life stages." The four priorities involved 42 topic areas and about 1,300 different objectives. How well did we do? Table 1.1 shows some key prevention indicators relevant for older people drawn from *An End of Decade Snapshot*.

Surveillance for tracking progress for these measures comes from a variety of national, longitudinal probability samples, such as the National Health Interview Survey (NHIS) and the National Health and Nutrition Examination Survey (NHANES). Aging-specific surveys, such as the National Health and Aging Trends Survey (NHATS), provide more granular information about older adults, including long-term care populations. Other surveys focus on different components of health, such as health behavior (Behavioral Risk Factors Surveillance System [BRFSS]) or expenditures (Medical Expenditures Panel Survey [MEPS]; Medicare Current Beneficiary Survey [MCBS]). Targets for objectives are set by intergovernmental agencies and taskforces using a well-defined strategy. For example, a 10% or 20% improvement from baseline values is typically proposed for measures involving rates. Percentage improvement is calculated using prespecified small effect sizes corresponding to a 5% to 10% change. Alternatively, historical data can be used to fit a trend line for continuing progress toward meeting a goal (Hubbard et al., 2020).

As Table 1.1 shows, progress in reaching prevention targets over the prior decade is uneven. In fact, America has lost ground in addressing diabetes, suicide, and obesity. Other prevention targets have fared better. Control of hypertension and colorectal cancer screening, for example, saw substantial improvements, though neither met specified national goals. Behavioral targets, such as promoting exercise and reducing tobacco use, were more easily reached. The picture overall is mixed, suggesting variation in the difficulty of changing particular health behaviors, heterogeneity in response to public health

TABLE 1.1 *HEALTHY PEOPLE 2020*—PROGRESS IN SELECTED PREVENTION TARGETS RELEVANT TO OLDER ADULTS

	2010 BASELINE VALUE	2020 FINAL VALUE	TARGET	PROGRESS
1. Colorectal cancer screening, age 50–74, %	52.1 (2008)	65.2 (2018)	70.5	Statistically significantly improved
2. Effective control of hypertension, age 18+, %	43.7 (2005–2008)	47.8 (2013–2016)	61.2	Statistically significantly improved
3. Uncontrolled diabetes (hemoglobin A1c > 9%), age 18+, %	18.0 (2005–2008)	18.7 (2013–2016)	16.2	
4. Suicide, cases per 100,000	11.3 (2007)	14.0 (2017)	10.2	
5. Obesity, age 20+, %	33.9 (2005–2008)	38.6 (2013–2016)	30.5	
6. Aerobic or muscle strengthening exercise, age 18+, %	18.2 (2008)	24.0 (2018)	20.1	Goal achieved
7. Cigarette use, age 18+, %	20.6 (2008)	13.9 (2018)	12.0	Statistically significantly improved

Source: Office of the Assistant Secretary for Health. (2021). *Healthy People 2020: An end of decade snapshot* (pp. 10–12). U.S. Department of Health and Human Services. https://health.gov/sites/default/files/2021-03/21%20HP2020EndofDecadeSnapshot2.pdf

messaging, differences in receptivity to change, and the effect of disparities across populations that may affect access to preventive services.

Objectives for *Healthy People 2030* involving older people are shown in Table 1.2. Overall, the 2030 objectives have been scaled back to include only domains with widely accepted, measurable indicators. Unfortunately, many of these indicators still do not have strong longitudinal assessments that would allow a clear view of progress. Newly introduced measures are "developmental" and currently lack valid estimates of prevalence or incidence.

In addition to these population-specific objectives, *Healthy People 2030* also includes leading health indicators (LHI; https://health.gov/healthypeople/objectives-and-data/leading-health-indicators). They focus on risk factors and behaviors that are considered modifiable in the short term through evidence-based interventions. LHI relevant to older people include reductions in binge drinking, meeting current guidelines for physical activity, completing colorectal cancer screening, maintaining adequate blood pressure control, and reducing incident diabetes.

The midcourse review of *Healthy People 2030* goals suggests that data resources for tracking progress toward objectives are still inadequate. Fifteen of the 20 indicators for older adults listed in Table 1.2 lack multiple timepoints for measurement. On the positive side, the *Healthy People* initiatives are focused on documenting baselines, setting

TABLE 1.2 *HEALTHY PEOPLE 2030*—PREVENTION TARGETS SPECIFIC TO OLDER ADULTS

INDICATOR	CURRENT	OBJECTIVE
1. Increase the proportion of older adults with physical or cognitive health problems who get physical activity	41.3%	51.0%
2. Reduce the rate of pressure ulcer–related hospital admissions among older adults (cases per 100,000 per year)	836.9	753.2
3. Reduce the rate of hospital admissions for diabetes among older adults (cases per 100,000 per year)	293.3	264
4. Increase the proportion of older adults with dementia, or their caregivers, who know they have it	59.7%	65.1%
5. Reduce the proportion of preventable hospitalizations in older adults with dementia	23.5%	19.1%
6. Increase the proportion of adults with subjective cognitive decline who have discussed their symptoms with a provider	45.4%	50.4%
7. Reduce infections caused by *Listeria* (cases per 100,000 per year)	0.31	0.22
8. Reduce the rate of hospital admissions for urinary tract infections among older adults (cases per 100,000 per year)	551.3	496.2
9. Reduce fall-related deaths among older adults (cases per 100,000 per year)	78.0	63.4
10. Reduce the proportion of older adults who use inappropriate medications	15.9%	11.2%
11. Reduce the rate of emergency department visits due to falls among older adults (cases per 100,000 per year)	6,052.2	5,447.0
12. Reduce the proportion of older adults with untreated (tooth) root surface decay	29.1%	20.1%
13. Reduce the proportion of adults age 45+ years who have lost all their teeth	7.9%	5.4%
14. Reduce the proportion of adults age 45+ years with moderate and severe periodontitis	44.5%	39.3%
15. Reduce hip fractures among older adults (cases per 1,000 per year)	5.7	4.6
16. Increase the proportion of older adults who get screened for osteoporosis	Developmental	
17. Increase the proportion of older adults who get treated for osteoporosis after a fracture	Developmental	
18. Reduce the rate of hospital admissions for pneumonia among older adults (cases per 100,000 per year)	713.9	642.5
19. Reduce hospitalizations for asthma in adults age 65+ years (cases per 100,000 per year)	Developmental	
20. Reduce vision loss from age-related macular degeneration (cases per 1,000 per year)	15.6	12.5

Source: Office of Disease Prevention and Health Promotion. (n.d.). *Older Adults—Healthy People 2023*. U.S. Department of Health and Human Services. https://health.gov/healthypeople/objectives-and-data/browse-objectives/older-adults

objectives, and monitoring progress. This at least identifies relevant health problems and whether they are getting better or worse.

Changes in objectives between *Healthy People 2020* and *2030* are also important to note. As mentioned, some objectives have been dropped because of difficulty tracking outcomes, such as measures of unmet need. Others are now more general; for example, "reduce the proportion of older adults with disabilities who use inappropriate medications" has been replaced with "reduce the proportion of older adults who use inappropriate medications" (https://health.gov/healthypeople/about/how-has-healthy-people-changed). Another important change between the 2020 and 2030 objectives is a greater focus on social determinants of health, such as economic stability, social and community context, educational access and quality, healthcare access and quality, and neighborhood and built environment. These rightly stress the many nonmedical factors relevant for health and the need to consider the lifespan as a whole when promoting healthy aging, as highlighted in the leading health indicators across life stages.

Setting healthcare priorities is no longer a matter of tabulating the number of deaths from a few diseases and then organizing a campaign against the most prevalent ones, like a "war on heart disease" or a "war on cancer." The *Healthy People* initiatives are health oriented, not disease oriented, and are not as simple as lobbying for more research money to cure a disease. Instead, ***health-promoting initiatives*** involve the complexity of the socioeconomic, lifestyle, and other nonmedical influences that impact our ability to attain and maintain health. The emerging field of geroscience, which aims to slow the rate of aging, offers promise for promoting health in old age but will undoubtedly face the same challenges given the complex nonmedical influences that affect health over the lifespan.

POPULATION OBJECTIVES AND INDIVIDUAL PREFERENCES

With all the attention given to these population metrics and target objectives, one might say: "Mind your own business, government. I am responsible for my lifestyle and whether I want to improve my health." This raises questions in the minds of those on the right of the political spectrum: conservatives and libertarians (Box 1.1). Why should the federal government be involved at all? Isn't health promotion an individual's responsibility?

The basic premise of ***libertarian paternalism*** is that people are busy, lives are complicated, and even intelligent people can make foolish health or retirement choices. *Healthy People* initiatives should just *nudge*—Thaler and Sunstein's term—people and organizations in the right direction without excessive intrusion and cost.

QUESTION: What do *you* think is the most important health objective to set for older adults for the *Healthy People 2030* initiative? Why? What should the federal and state governments, health professionals, and laypersons do, if anything, to help achieve this objective?

If you are interested in the *Healthy People* initiatives, you can access information by going to https://health.gov/healthypeople/tools-action. One last comment. Let's return to the question raised at the beginning of this chapter: Does establishing federal goals help to promote healthy aging? and give a succinct answer: Not if the government is only setting goals and monitoring. Implementation and dissemination are critical challenges even when we have evidence of benefit for an intervention.

BOX 1.1 Libertarian Paternalism

The author is not thrilled with the effectiveness of *Healthy People* initiatives, but libertarian paternalists may be more sympathetic toward a government intervention if a compromise method for achieving specific health goals is used. What is a libertarian paternalist, you ask?

A ***libertarian paternalist*** tries to appeal to both the libertarian who believes that the less government intervention, the better off society will be, and the paternalist, a liberal who believes there is a paternal role for government to play, particularly in healthcare.

Two former colleagues at the University of Chicago, Richard Thaler of the Graduate School of Business and Cass Sunstein of the Law School, proposed the idea of libertarian paternalism—a compromise between a conservative and liberal perspective. *Perhaps you can call this a paternal nudge in the healthy direction, while leaving ultimate responsibility to the individual.*

An example to demonstrate this strategy is focused on middle-aged adults, though given the topic it is also quite relevant to older adults. Researchers targeted a group of 480 university employees prior to the annual influenza vaccination season (Lehman et al., 2016). Participants were randomly assigned to a control group that received an e-mail message that free flu shots were available at the campus health center with a link for making an appointment; or to a treatment group that received an e-mail that they had been scheduled for a flu shot at a specified time with a link for canceling or changing the appointment.

The control group had to take the initiative to opt in for a flu shot, and 33% did. *The treatment group was already opted in and* had to take the initiative to opt out. In this group, 45% received a flu shot.

The libertarian is pleased because in both instances the initiative remains with the individual. The paternal liberal is pleased because the default position, where one does not have to go to the trouble of opting out, is the healthier alternative and likely to produce the higher participation rate.

Another example? Automatic enrollment in an *employer retirement plan that requires the employee to opt out*, versus *the more typical policy to opt into a retirement plan*. This policy change increased participation rates from 50% in the traditional must-opt-in plan, to 90%—do nothing and you have opted in (Pew's 2017 Survey of Workers, September 20, 2017; Pew Charitable Trusts, 2017).

Or how about an example from life insurance? Libertarian economists argue that an older person with a terminal condition should have the option to take a one-time immediate lump sum payment of, say, 75%, of what would otherwise cover medical expenses until death. The person would be able to spend the money as they see fit, including donations to family, and perhaps forego end-of-life hospital care. Such an option, libertarians argue, would produce greater utility for society while allowing greater autonomy for the older person.

AGING, HEALTH, SOCIAL, AND MEDICAL TRENDS

It has been almost obligatory for 40 years to begin a gerontological book or article with comments about the rapid aging of society. The social analyst Ann Roberson labeled this phenomenon "apocalyptic demography," in which the escalating increases in the number of older adults will portend social and economic crises. About 20 years ago, we began to see two slight variations of this apocalyptic ritual: Many published works began with comments warning about the *aging of the aged,* and an additional spate of writings were on the coming onslaught of aging baby boomers.

Today, with the vanguard of ***baby boomers*** and the very ***older old*** receiving considerable media attention for different reasons, both ends of the older age spectrum command our full attention. The robust baby boomers crossing the Rubicon of old age make it obvious to all but the most ageist that the vitality of aging persons can remain strong. The stereotype of aging as merely physical and mental deterioration has been convincingly challenged. Also, an increasing number of boomers are tapping into Social Security and Medicare, and this deserves our attention as well.

At the other end of the age spectrum, persons age 85 and older, the growth in the percentage of the very old begins to startle—about a 40% growth per decade. In 1980, there were 2.2 million Americans age 85+; in 1990, about 3 million; in 2000, around 4.3 million; in 2010, about 5.5 million; and in 2020 6.3 million (Caplan, 2023). While the rate of increase slows thereafter, those age 85 and older are expected to reach 14.6 million by 2040 (Administration for Community Living [ACL], 2018). The oldest of the old require considerable medical assistance and long-term services and supports at a significant cost to society.

Along with the increasing breadth of the age span of Americans comes increasing complexity. Fifty-year-olds are eligible for membership in AARP (formerly known as the American Association of Retired Persons but, few members were retired at age 50, hence the use of the acronym only), and they are quite different from 70-year-olds, who in turn are significantly different from 90-year-olds. Moreover, 90-year-olds are different from one another. A few of them are pumping iron and throwing away their canes, whereas others are waiting to die.

Is Health Promotion Cost-Effective?

What aging Americans have in common, be they 50 or 90, robust or frail, is a future with an intensified demand for medical care (euphemistically referred to in America as *health*care) and the ongoing escalation of medical care costs. Driving these demands and costs are the increasing number of aging persons with both chronic and acute medical conditions and an expensive, high-tech, acute care–oriented medical system.

Some argue that the solution to rising healthcare costs is to encourage ***health promotion, disease prevention***, and *chronic disease management*. This may be true, but the evidence is still emerging and not fully encouraging. Health promotion advocates often fail to consider that prevention, promotion, and management entail:

- substantial costs in the attempt to screen and educate people at risk, along with subsidizing subsequent interventions; and additional deferred costs. If health promotion/disease prevention programs work, healthier individuals will live longer on a taxpayer-supported Medicare program, only to die of other costly medical conditions, though some research suggests deaths at older ages are actually less costly. The high cost of dying is due to the high prevalence of medical conditions requiring expensive treatment, not to age per se (Hogan et al., 2001). People dying at later ages are actually less likely to receive aggressive medical care and less likely to survive such care because of diminished physiologic reserve.

Perhaps the skeptics of health promotion's ability to lower healthcare costs support the philosopher Woody Allen's contention: Death is the best way to cut down on expenses.

A Multifaceted Approach

Yes to health promotion! The media has taken a stand, allocating considerable time and space to the merits of promoting good health practices to improve quality of life and realize medical care cost savings. Joining the media are the health professions, which have proclaimed health promotion's importance in the education and training of students; the business community, which has firmly supported a wellness approach for employees; and individual people, who often discuss their attempts at health promotion, both successful and otherwise, with relatives and friends.

If the media, the health professions, the business community, and individual people are willing to hop on the wellness train, the government has been reluctant to subsidize the fuel. Federal and state governments have been concerned more about dealing with rising expenditures than with new disease prevention, health promotion, and disease management initiatives that require additional funding.

Government can share the blame with health professionals who provide mostly lip service to promoting health because they are not reimbursed for it. Health science instructors provide only a modicum of health promotion instruction and training, and experience in applying it is the exception rather than the rule. The business community allocates resources to worksite wellness but has stopped short of focusing on those who need it most—older and more sedentary employees. Rigorous evaluations suggest low returns on worksite wellness programs (Song & Baicker, 2019).

Last but not least, too many people have spent not only more time and money on health promotion, but also more time and money at fast-food restaurants, eating larger portions of food with higher fat, sugar, and sodium content; and on computers, in front of which they sit, unhealthily immobile, for an increasing number of hours. And even though it is true that a smartphone is portable, walking while staring at it is dangerous (particularly when you are walking across the street, which seems to be a pastime with students on university campuses).

POPULATION GROWTH OVER AGE 65

All but the most uninformed know that the average age of the American population has been increasing dramatically. In just 16 years, the U.S. Census Bureau (Federal Interagency Forum on Aging-Related Statistics [FIFARS], 2016) reported that the number of Americans age 65+ increased from 35 million (12.4%) in 2000 to 49.2 million (15.2%) in 2016. The 2020 U.S. Census identifies 55.8 million Americans age 65 and older as 16.8% of the population. The age 65+ population has grown five times as fast as the total U.S. population over the prior 100 years (Caplan, 2023). This growth will continue and reach 20% in 2030 (Figure 1.1).

The percentages in Table 1.3 show why the population "age pyramid"—a few older adults at the top and many children at the bottom—is rapidly becoming an "***age rectangle***."

The Baby Boomers

The *baby boomers* are the 76 million persons who were born in the United States between 1946 and 1964. Most were conceived when the millions of soldiers, sailors, and marines returned home from World War II and created a surge in the number of births that started quickly—there were fewer than 2.8 million births in 1945 but more than 3.4 million in 1946—and lasted 19 years.

FIGURE 1.1 Population age 65+ and age 85+, selected years, 1900 to 2014, and projected years, 2020 to 2060.

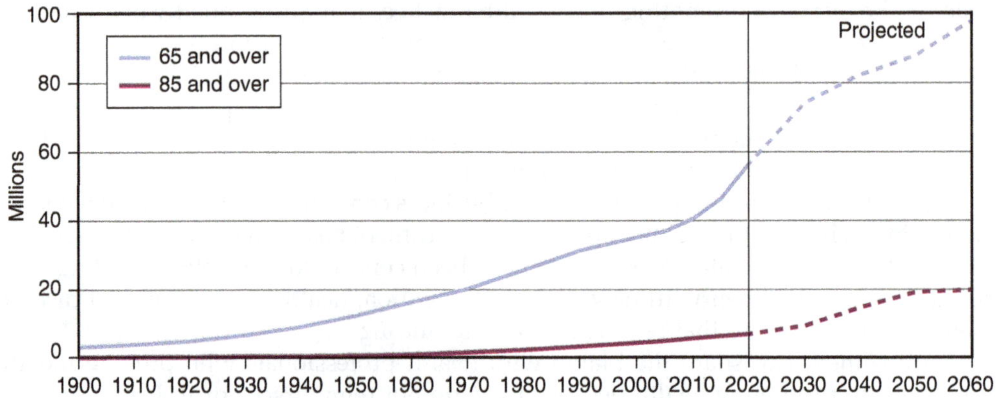

Source: Federal Interagency Forum on Aging-Related Statistics. (2016). *Older Americans 2016: Key indicators of well-being*. U.S. Government Publishing Office. https://agingstats.gov/docs/LatestReport/Older-Americans-2016-Key-Indicators-of-WellBeing.pdf

TABLE 1.3 BECOMING AN AGE RECTANGLE

YEAR	POPULATION UNDER AGE 18 (%)	POPULATION OVER AGE 65 (%)
1900	40	4
1980	28	11
2030	20	20

The boomers challenged U.S. hospital capacity when they were born, the adequacy of the public school system a few years later, society in general when they reached draft age and spurned the politicians who were intent on expanding the Vietnam War, and still later the sufficiency of available housing for raising their families.

The baby boomers' place in history, as they begin to dominate the old age segment of it, is still unclear. Will they be known as the spoiled descendants of the greatest generation or as pioneers in social reform and civil rights? Regardless, their impact on society as older persons will raise a troublesome question, that asks society if it will still need us when we are 64?

If the Beatles had been more knowledgeable about aging, they would have substituted 84 for 64, as it more accurately represents a threshold to frailty. (As far as they were concerned, 64 was the same as 84: too old to differentiate.) Hopefully, we will be able to answer this question in the affirmative by the time the first boomers reach age 84 in 2030.

By 2010, the number of Americans between the ages of 45 and 64 (roughly the boomers at that time) was about twice that of those age 65+: roughly 79 million versus 39 million. And those boomers were bringing into retirement not only their large numbers and a history of advocacy, but also a powerful interest in, and impact on, the integrity of the Social Security and Medicare programs and the adequacy of long-term care alternatives. Their future influence on society is likely to be dramatic and widespread as they become retirees in increasing numbers.

As boomers retire, they will make enormous demands on both the Social Security and Medicare programs, which, at the same time, will be supported by a shrinking taxpaying workforce. By the time the last boomer turns 65 in the year 2029, the retirees drawing Social Security and Medicare benefits will account for one in five Americans.

The profound effect of the baby boomers for population aging in America can be seen in changes in the age–sex pyramid between 2010 and 2020 (Figure 1.2). The boomer cohort has slowly advanced into the upper reach of the pyramid (dark blue, between ages 55 and 75). By 2030, smaller birth cohorts will reach this part of the pyramid and the proportion of those age 65+ will begin to decline. But one implication of this process will be increasing numbers of nonagenarians and centenarians, mostly women but increasingly men as well.

Will boomers be healthier than today's cohort of older adults? Death rates for heart disease and stroke continue to decline, while longevity continues to increase. But diabetes (affecting 20% of boomers and rising), chronic lower respiratory disease, high cholesterol, and hypertension were higher compared to a comparable age cohort two decades earlier. Much of this has to do with the increase in overweight and obesity. Advances in medicine and medical technology may enable boomers to live longer but with substantial morbidity, driven in large part by the greater risk of neurodegenerative disease in later life.

FIGURE 1.2 Population by sex and age: 2010 and 2020.

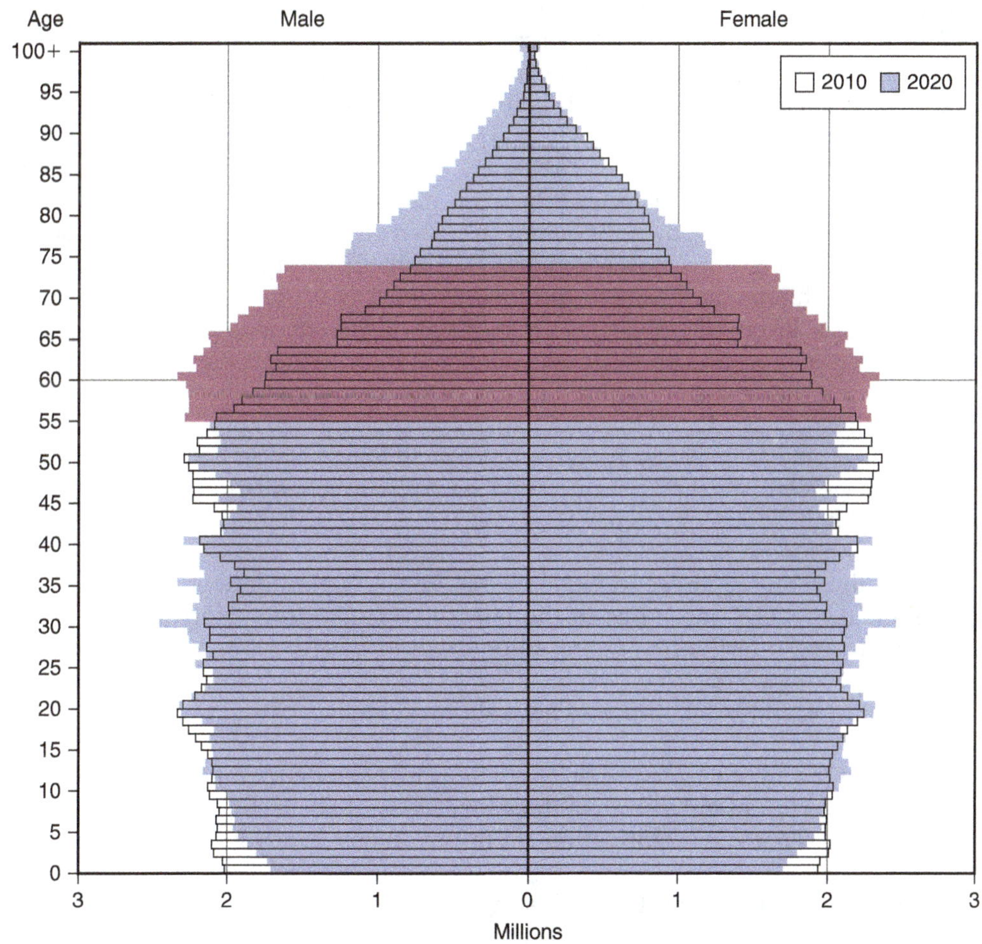

Source: Caplan, Z. (2023). *U.S. older population grew from 2010 to 2020 at fastest rate since 1880 to 1890.* U.S. Census Bureau. Baby boomer cohort shown with magenta color. https://www.census.gov/library/stories/2023/05/2020-census-united-states-older-population-grew.html

The Older Old

The older population itself is getting older. The percentage of persons age 85+ is growing faster than any other age group. As noted earlier, there was a 36% increase among Americans 85+ from 1980 to 1990 (from 2.2 million to 3 million), a 43% increase from 1990 to 2000 (from 3 million to 4.3 million), and a 40% increase from 2000 to 2010 (from 4.3 million to about 6 million). In 2010 to 2020, the 85 to 94 age group saw slower growth (12.6% increase) to 5.7 million; but the population age 95+ grew by 48.6%, from 425,000 in 2010 to 631,000 in 2020 (Caplan, 2023). This growth slows only slightly over the next half-century and is projected to reach 20 million persons over age 85 by 2060 (Figure 1.1).

This demographic trend is significant for two reasons. On the positive side, the rapid growth of this segment of the population has made what was previously an age level rarely attained into an increasingly common stage of the life cycle. Moreover, the percentage of older adults who reach age 75 and beyond and report good, very good, or excellent health is 66%. It is about 85% in the population as a whole.

One analyst reported that 70-year-olds are more like the 60-year-olds of previous generations (Trafford, 2000). Older adults have an even better perception about themselves. The National Council on Aging (NCOA; 2002) together with the Harris National Survey reported that 51% of persons between the ages of 65 and 74 and 33% of persons age 75+ *perceive themselves as middle-aged or younger!* This certainly is evidence that many older adults are redefining old age as beginning later in the life cycle.

On the challenging side, for both families and society, is the significantly greater prevalence of disability among the older old relative to the younger old.

The ***activities of daily living*** (ADL) are a standard measure of personal self-maintenance or adult competencies. These measures of function assess difficulty or need for help with bathing, dressing, eating, transferring, toileting, and indoor mobility. Difficulty ambulating is the most common ADL problem, eating the least. The activities are acquired in hierarchical fashion during childhood (with independence in bathing and dressing the last to be gained), lost in hierarchical fashion with progression of neurologic disease and the end of life (independence in bathing and dressing affected first), and regained in hierarchical fashion through rehabilitation (independence in bathing and dressing the most difficult to secure). ***Instrumental activities of daily living*** (IADL) refer to the ability to perform more complex activities such as home management, money management, meal preparation, making a phone call, medication management, laundry, and light shopping. Figure 1.3 shows that IADL limitations are more common than ADL limitations.

Given the many changes in technologies and accommodations available since development of IADL measures in the late 1960s (including smartphones, the internet, air fryers, and the like), gerontology would benefit from an updated IADL measure.

Studies of ADL and IADL disability have shown that:

- People age 75+ are three times more vulnerable to dependency than the adjoining age category of 65 to 74 (and *more* than three times likely to be institutionalized).
- Age 65 to 74 is not significantly different from younger adult age categories.

Therefore, when it comes to anticipating caregiving challenges to both family and society, and the need for additional resources, age 75—or 80 or 85—is a much more significant cutoff point for analysis than the traditional age 65+ entry into old age.

FIGURE 1.3 Percentage of adults with activity limitations, by age group and type of limitation.

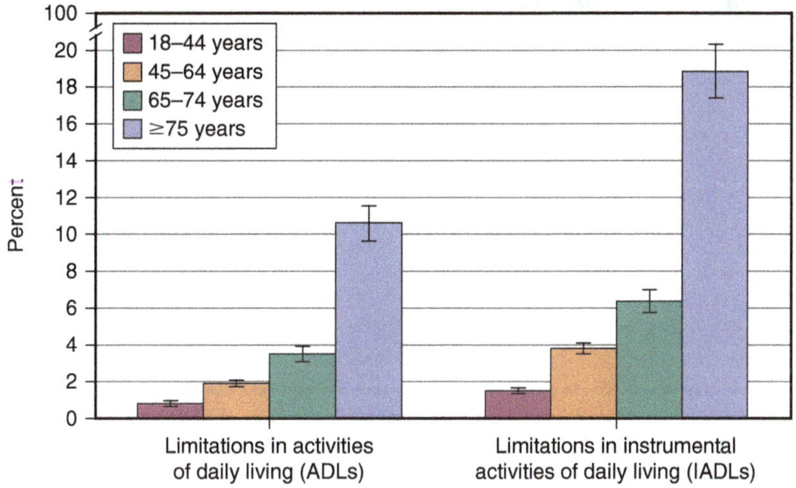

Source: Centers for Disease Control and Prevention. (2016). QuickStats: Percentage of adults with activity limitations, by age group and type of limitation—National Health Interview Survey, United States, 2014. *Morbidity and Mortality Weekly Report*, *65*, 14. https://doi.org/10.15585/mmwr.mm6501a6

Disability and Chronic Conditions

Disability is defined by the U.S. Census Bureau as difficulty with hearing, vision, cognition, ambulation, self-care, or independent living. In 2015, 35% of persons age 65+ had some type of disability, with ambulation difficulty the most likely (23%). In 2019, 10.2 million of 52.8 million people age 65+ living in noninstitutional settings reported "a lot of difficulty" or "cannot do at all" for one or more of these domains of function (National Center for Health Statistics [NCHS], 2023a). Some of the difficulties presented in Table 1.4 may be considered manageable by the older adult, while others require personal assistance and other long-term care services and support.

The leading ***chronic conditions*** among older adults are listed in Figure 1.4. The prevalence of each condition increases in old age, and persons over age 85 often have multiple chronic conditions. The leading chronic conditions are hypertension, arthritis, heart disease, cancer, and diabetes. Women report higher levels of asthma, arthritis, and hypertension; men report higher levels of heart disease, cancer, and diabetes.

The epidemiology of chronic disease in old age was similar in 2020. The most prevalent chronic conditions among adults age 65+ currently include arthritis (47%); cancers (26%); diabetes (21%); coronary heart disease (14%); pulmonary diseases such as emphysema or chronic bronchitis (COPD, 11%); myocardial infarction (9%); and angina (4%) (ACL, 2022). Alzheimer disease and related dementias are missing from this list but should be included as they affect about 10% of people age 65+ (and approximately 30% if we include mild cognitive impairment). Unfortunately, these conditions are not diagnosed or tracked as effectively. The same applies to depression, anxiety, and substance abuse disorders—common mental health conditions similarly affecting 5% to 10% of older adults.

Although chronic conditions and functional limitations increase with age, disability rates for older Americans have been declining. In 1982, the disabled older population in the United States totaled 6.4 million. If the 1982 rate had continued, the number of disabled would have climbed to about 9.3 million in 1999. Instead, it rose to only 7 million—less

TABLE 1.4 PERCENTAGE OF PERSONS AGE 65+ REPORTING DIFFICULTY IN DOMAINS OF FUNCTION, 2021

Self-care	8%
Ambulation	39%
Cognition	28%
Vision	21%
Hearing	29%
Communication	8%
Severe disability	18%

Note: Severe disability is defined as a lot of difficulty/cannot do in one or more domains.
Source: U.S. Census Bureau. (2021). *American Community Survey: Older Americans with a disability*. U.S. Department of Commerce.

FIGURE 1.4 Percentage of people age 65+ who reported having chronic health conditions, by sex, 2013 to 2014.

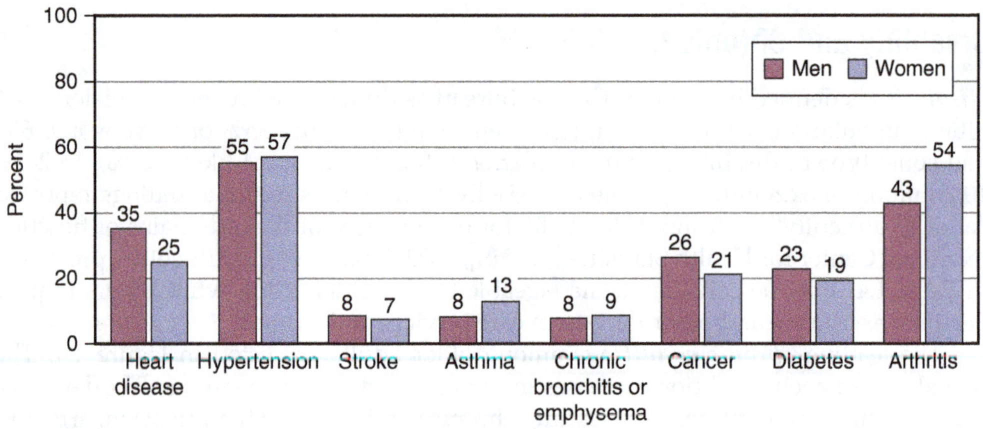

Source: Federal Interagency Forum on Aging-Related Statistics. (2016). *Older Americans 2016: Key indicators of well-being*. U.S. Government Publishing Office. https://agingstats.gov/docs/LatestReport/Older-Americans-2016-Key-Indicators-of-WellBeing.pdf

than a quarter of the increase that might have been expected. More recently, the overall percentage of Americans age 65+ with a disability declined between 2013 and 2015. These trends, however, are hard to interpret. Accommodations that reduce the impact of functional limitation have also become more widely accessible. For example, automatic deposit of Social Security checks reduces the functional significance of cognitive impairment. Walk-in showers, elevators, adapted utensils, ride-share services, speed-dialing smartphones, and home-delivered meals all can reduce disability in the activities of daily living.

Another hopeful research outcome in disability trends is the conclusion that among the very old, disability decline slows significantly. As more people today are living into their 90s and beyond (which is the fastest-growing age segment of society in developed countries), researchers have found that the percentage who are independent changed less than expected between the ages of 92 and 100.

For example, 39% of 92-year-old Danish adults were able to care for themselves, and the same was true of 33% of those who lived to the age of 100 (Christensen et al., 2008). In general, loss of independence among the very old appears to occur close to the end of life and is not significantly more severe or costly for the 100-year-old than for the 90-year-old.

Centenarians

A *USA Today/ABC News* poll reported that only 25% of Americans want to live to be 100 or older. (Do you?) The majority of Americans are concerned that they will become disabled and a burden to their families. And yet many Americans are fascinated by the idea of becoming a ***centenarian*** (or even ***supercentenarian***, age 110+).

In 2019, about 70,000 centenarians in the United States were Social Security beneficiaries. Their number is increasing along with other older age groups: beneficiaries age 65 or older rose from 42.0 million in 2014 to 48.6 million in 2019 (+15.6%), and beneficiaries age 85 or older increased from 5.6 million to 5.8 million over the same time period (+4%) (Social Security Administration [SSA], 2021). Census projections forecast that there will be eight times as many centenarians by the year 2050, when some baby boomers begin reaching age 100.

For every 100 centenarian women, there are only 20.7 centenarian men. Thus, the oldest person alive during any particular year is typically a woman. According to the *Guinness Book of World Records* (www.guinnessworldrecords.com), a French woman, Jeanne-Louise Calment, has lived the longest, reaching 122 years before she died in 1997. She stated: "I just kept getting older and couldn't help it."

(Maybe she did help it. In 2019, skeptics argued that her daughter, Yvonne Calment, took over her identity to avoid estate taxes. If that is the case, Yvonne died at age 99 and the American Sarah Knauss took over as longest-lived, having died at age 119.)

On June 9, 2005, the world's oldest living married couple had an aggregate age of 205 years. Magda Brown, age 100, attributed her 74-year union to Herbert Brown, age 105, to her taking the lead ("I am the strong one") and his following ("He is the easy-going one"). Apparently, Herbert is more than just easy going: He survived the Nazi concentration camp at Dachau.

Supercentenarians

In 2005, the oldest living documented person at that time (able to provide original proof of birth) was a Dutch woman, Hendrikje van Andel-Schipper, who reached 115 years and attributed her longevity to eating a piece of herring every day. In 2015, Jeralean Talley was the longest-lived person and also reached 115 years. She challenged the prior advice and attributed her long life to eating pigs' ears and feet. After Ms. Talley died, a New Yorker, Susannah Mushatt Jones, yet again 115 years old, became the longest-lived person and attributed her longevity in part to bacon.

As of this writing, therefore, bacon seems to be a leading contributor to becoming a *supercentenarian—110 years of age or older*. On the Gerontology Wiki website (http://www.the110club.com) in 2018 there were 257 supercentenarians with validated birth and death dates who ever lived for any length of time in the United States. The website had since been updated to include a list of 332 people who have lived in the United States and reached age 112; 15 were reported to be alive as of 2023 (https://gerontology.fandom.com/wiki/List_of_United_States_supercentenarians_(age_112), accessed December 2023).

Another supercentenarian, Misao Okawa, just left the ranks after being a widow for more than 80 years. Despite (or because of?) her lengthy widowhood, she offered this comment when asked about how she felt about the past 117 years: "It seemed rather short."

Super-Duper-Centenarians

Biogerontology, or geroscience, focuses on the biology, physiology, and genetics of aging. Insights from the biology of aging may lead to new therapies designed to slow the rate of aging. Even with such discoveries people will not live forever; still, the prospect of high function until age 100 is welcome. But even without new "senolytic" therapies designed to reduce senescence, we can expect to see more centenarians. Christensen et al. (2009) suggest that 50% of women born today in the most developed countries will celebrate their 100th birthday. With effective geroscience this upper bound will likely increase.

HEALTH INDICATORS

Life Expectancy

Life expectancy for the U.S. population in 2021 was 76.4 years, a decrease of 0.6 year from 2020 (Xu et al., 2022), reflecting the impact of the SARS-CoV-2 pandemic. Gains in life expectancy have returned beginning in 2023. But life expectancy was already declining in the period before COVID-19 as a result of the increasing impact of the "diseases of despair," such as opioid use disorders, suicide, and firearm violence, The same trend can be seen in the increase in the age-adjusted death rate (a 5.3% increase from 835.4 per 100,000 in 2020 to 879.7 in 2021). Not surprisingly, COVID-19 joined heart disease and cancer as one of the top three leading causes of death in 2020 and 2021. Dips in life expectancy are notable in light of the long run of gains since 1900 resulting from greater affluence and advances in sanitation, medicine, and health behaviors (particularly smoking cessation).

The United States has been trailing other countries in life expectancy for quite some time. Over 30 comparator countries have life expectancies over age 80. Increases in obesity and the related conditions of hypertension and diabetes, the opioid crisis, or other events may foster this trend, while continued advances in medicine in the United States may reverse (WHO 2023a; 2023b).

There is also a gender longevity gap in the United States. The life expectancy of men in 2021 was 73.5 years and for women it was 79.3 years. Life expectancy at age 65 is 19.7 years for women and 17.0 for men. Medical experts speculate that women are working harder, smoking more, and undergoing more stress and that the gender gap may narrow without improvements in men's health. The disparity among Latinx, Black, and White populations persists. In 2021, age-adjusted death rates per 100,000 for men were 915.6 among Latinx, 1,370.2 for Blacks, and 1,055.2 for Whites. Among women, death rates per 100,000 were 599.8 among Latinas, 921.9 among Blacks, and 750.6 among Whites (Xu et al., 2022). The gaps are narrowing but still pronounced. Data for other race–ethnicity groups show similar disparities, with Asians at the lowest mortality risk and American Indian or Alaska Native (AIAN) at the highest.

Heart disease continued to be the leading ***cause of death*** in 2021 (Table 1.5), but during the prior decade, the gap between heart disease and cancer narrowed. Also during this time, respiratory diseases and Alzheimer disease rose in the rankings.

The Centers for Disease Control and Prevention (CDC) notes that the current system of relying on death certificates misses the complexity of dying for many older people and underestimates the impact of Alzheimer disease. The death certificate lists the most

TABLE 1.5 10 LEADING CAUSES OF DEATH AMONG OLDER ADULTS AGE 65+ IN 2021

CAUSES OF DEATH	AGE-ADJUSTED DEATH RATE (PER 100,000)
1. Heart disease	173.8
2. Cancer	146.6
3. COVID-19	104.1
4. Unintentional injury (accidents)	64.7
5. Stroke	41.1
6. Chronic lower respiratory diseases	34.7
7. Alzheimer disease	31.0
8. Diabetes	25.4
9. Chronic liver disease	14.5
10. Kidney disease	13.6

Source: Xu, J. Q., Murphy, S. L., Kochanek, K. D., & Arias, E. (2022). *Mortality in the United States, 2021.* NCHS Data Brief, no 456. National Center for Health Statistics. https://doi.org/10.15620/cdc:122516

immediate cause of death, while Alzheimer disease may have been a major contributor to the person dying from pneumonia (through aspiration of food) or from infections and other problems.

Hospital Stays and Physician Visits

Older adults consume far more medical resources than younger age groups. In 2019, 16.6% of people age 65+ had at least one overnight hospital stay. Among people age 75+, 20% had a hospitalization; and among people age 85+, 26.1% (USDHHS, 2023). In the population as a whole (age 1+), about 7% had a hospitalization.

Although quickening hospital discharges over the past few decades affect all age groups, the growing number of older adults in the United States results in a higher percentage of older patients in the hospital. Older adults accounted for 20% of hospital stays and used one third of the total days of hospital care in 1970; by 2000, they accounted for 40% of hospital stays and almost one half of the days of hospital care (Hall & Owings, 2002), a continuing trend.

For every 100 people, older adults age 65+ made 550 physician office visits in 2018. The rate was half as much across all age groups combined. ED visits were elevated among people age 65+ (45 vs. 40 per 100 overall), and substantially higher among people age 75+ (60 visits per 100 people; USDHHS, 2023). The percentage of time that healthcare practitioners spend with older patients will continue to increase.

Medication Use

Medicare expenditures on medications for noninstitutionalized elders increased at an astounding rate for many years (double-digit increases from 1994 to 2001) but have risen more slowly over the past two decades. These expenditures constitute 15% of overall healthcare spending. A primary reason for the slowing in the rise of medication costs has been an expansion in the availability of low-cost generic drugs, which has increased to 80% of all dispensed prescriptions. This trend toward generic drugs is due to many expensive, brand-name medications coming off patent protection.

This cost saving, however, has been offset by three factors: (a) The escalating costs for brand-name drugs still in use, with costs rising 62% between 2011 and 2015, with the continued demand for these expensive brand-name drugs being fueled by advertising on television. (b) An increase, though slower, in the price of generic drug costs as well. (c) The ability of the pharmaceutical industry to maintain profitability in an era of widespread use of generic drugs through lobbying. As part of the passage of Medicare Part D in 2006, the Medicare program was banned from negotiating future reductions in drug prices. Nearly 20 years later this decision remains contentious.

While overall medication expenditures have risen more slowly lately, medication usage and costs are highly correlated with age. Older adults constitute about 15% of the population but consume 34% of all prescription drugs and 40% of over-the-counter drugs. For instance, a nationally representative sample of community-residing older persons, aged 57 to 85 years revealed that at least one prescription medication was used by 81% of the sample during the prior month, at least one over-the-counter medication by 42%, and at least one dietary supplement by 49%. Also, polypharmacy, use of five or more prescription medications, is common. In an early population-based study, 29% of older adults were taking five or more prescribed medications (Qato et al., 2008). By 2012, the use of five or more prescription drugs increased to 39% of those over 65 years of age (Kantor et al., 2015).

Health Habits

On the brighter side, the health habits of older adults may, on balance, be slightly superior to those of younger adults. People age 65+, for instance, are less likely to smoke, drink alcohol, or report high stress. They eat more sensibly than do younger adults, are as likely to walk for exercise, and are more likely to check their blood pressure regularly. Older adults continue to increase their rate of participation in medical screenings and taking advantage of immunizations. They are more consistent with use of seatbelts.

On the darker side, older adults are more likely to be sedentary or malnourished. And their advantage in being less stressed may be merely the result of less awareness of, or less willingness to report, stress. The lower percentage of smokers may be due in part to the fact that smokers are more likely to die before age 65. Also, when older adults engage in risk behaviors such as excessive alcohol consumption, sedentary behavior, poor nutrition, and failure to use seatbelts, their vulnerability to morbidity and mortality is greater.

To put things in perspective, though, few adults in the United States, young or old, live a comprehensively healthy lifestyle. National data reveal that only 3% of the population engage in all four of the following lifestyle choices: nonsmoking, healthy weight, five fruit and vegetable servings per day, and regular physical activity (Reeves & Rafferty, 2005). Among older adults, one third do not get any leisure-time physical activity, two thirds do not eat five servings of fruit or vegetables a day, and one fifth are 30 pounds or more overweight. The low uptake of these protective behaviors, all with a strong evidence base and increasing access through a robust aging services network, show the challenges of changing health behavior at all ages.

Perceptions of Health

Despite stereotypes to the contrary, most people who are older tend to view their health positively (FIFARS, 2016). Seventy-eight percent of older adults, age 65+, rate their health as being good, very good, or excellent. Among those age 85+, this percentage declines to 68% who report good, very good, or excellent health. (Still a lot higher than you would expect, right?)

Another way to look at perceived health is to note the proportion reporting poor or fair health. In 2019, the proportion of people age 65+ reporting fair or poor health was 25.1%, more than the double the 11.2% across all age groups. The percentage reporting fair or poor health was 29.3% among people age 75+ (NCHS, 2023b).

HEALTH AND OLDER ADULT EXPERIENCE

Volunteering

Many older adults are active and productive, and some choose to engage in volunteer opportunities. In any given year, almost one fifth of older Americans engage in unpaid volunteer work for organizations such as churches, schools, or civic organizations. In addition, an unknown percentage of older adults do other types of volunteer work, such as helping family and friends who are sick or disabled, or assisting with the care of grandchildren.

Surprisingly, those who continue to work after age 65 are not less likely to volunteer than those older adults who retire (Caro & Morris, 2001). Researchers believe that the potential for increasing volunteerism among retired older adults is significant, and that "in the period immediately after retirement there is a heightened receptivity to volunteerism" (Caro & Morris, 2001, p. 349).

Marital Status

Older men are much more likely to be married, 70% versus 46%, and much less likely to be widowed, 11% versus 33%, than older women (Figure 1.5). In absolute numbers, there were more than three times as many widows (8.8 million) as widowers (2.6 million). Divorced or separated older adults represented 15% (steadily increasing since 1980), and single adults 5% of the population (also increasing). All of these categories will increase

FIGURE 1.5 Marital status of persons age 65+, 2017.

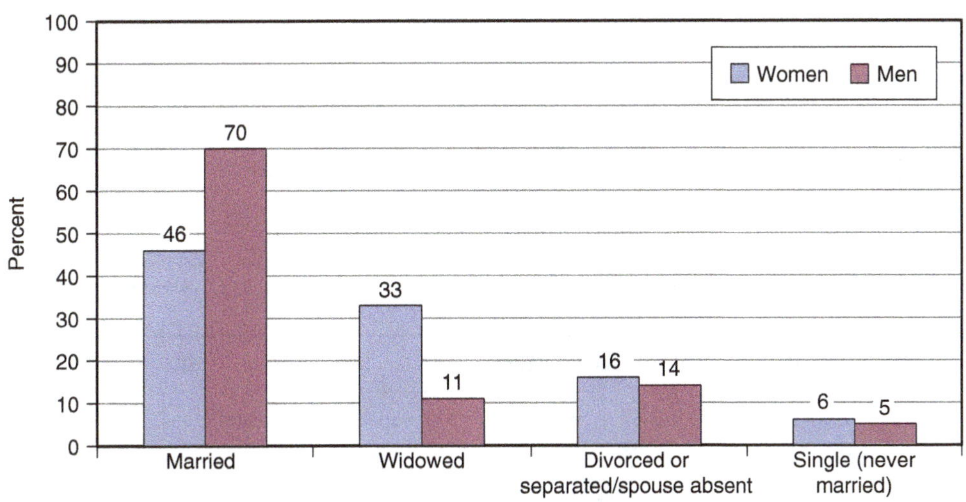

Source: U.S. Census Bureau. (2018, April). *Current population survey: Annual social and economic supplement.* www.acl.gov/sites/default/files/Aging%20and%20Disability%20in%20America/2017OlderAmericansProfile.pdf

in the future with the expansion of the boomers among the old, and their greater acceptance of divorce, separation, and a single lifestyle.

Most women (54%) should expect to spend all or part of their later years without a husband. Are most older women preparing for this, or just dealing with the consequences after it happens?

Not examined in Figure 1.4 is cohabitation, whch increased 75% between 2007 and 2016 (Pew Research Center Report, 2017). Whether cohabitation is taking the place of, or in addition to, marriage has not been determined.

Work

The ***labor force participation rate***, that is, the percentage of a population that is in the labor force, declined from 1960 to 1995 and then began to rise among men age 65+ (Figure 1.6). The 35-year decline may have been due to a combination of factors, such as mandatory retirement policies, fewer work opportunities, age discrimination, declining health, or desire for more leisure time. The rise of labor force participation for older men since 1995 may be due to the opposite of these factors—fewer mandatory retirement policies, more opportunities for older workers, less age discrimination, improved health, or desire for more income or purposeful activities.

The U.S. Bureau of Labor Statistics reported that 60% of older respondents stated financial factors—making money or earning benefits—were a primary influence in choosing to remain in the work force. Thirty-six percent stated they primarily liked their jobs or wanted to stay involved. Older Americans are healthier and living longer and many need extra money and/or seek continued purpose.

Labor force participation rates began to rise 10 years earlier for women than for men, around 1985 (Figure 1.7). While money and continued purpose apply to older women as well, additional factors include an increased opportunity for women to work and the rising expectation that women will work. A disincentive to work is caregiving

FIGURE 1.6 Labor force participation rates (annual averages) of men age 55+, by age group, 1963 to 2015.

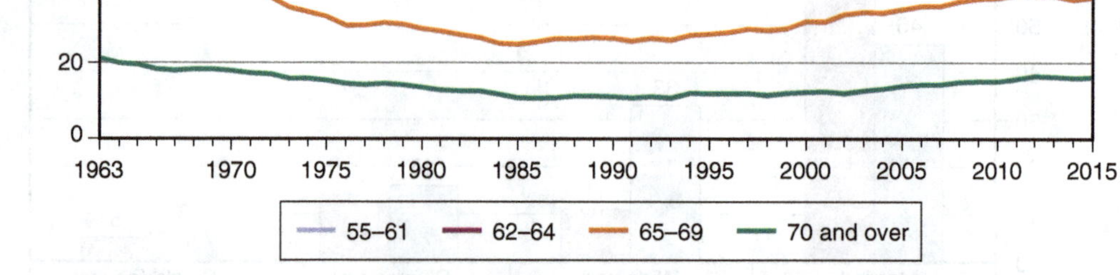

Note: Data for 1994 and later years are not strictly comparable with data for 1993 and earlier years owing to a redesign of survey and methodology of the Current Population Survey. Reference population: These data refer to the civilian noninstitutionalized population.

Source: Data from U.S. Census Bureau. Bureau of Labor Statistics. *Current Population Survey*. https://www.bls.gov/cps/demographics.htm#age

FIGURE 1.7 Labor force participation rates (annual averages) of women age 55+, by age group, 1963 to 2015.

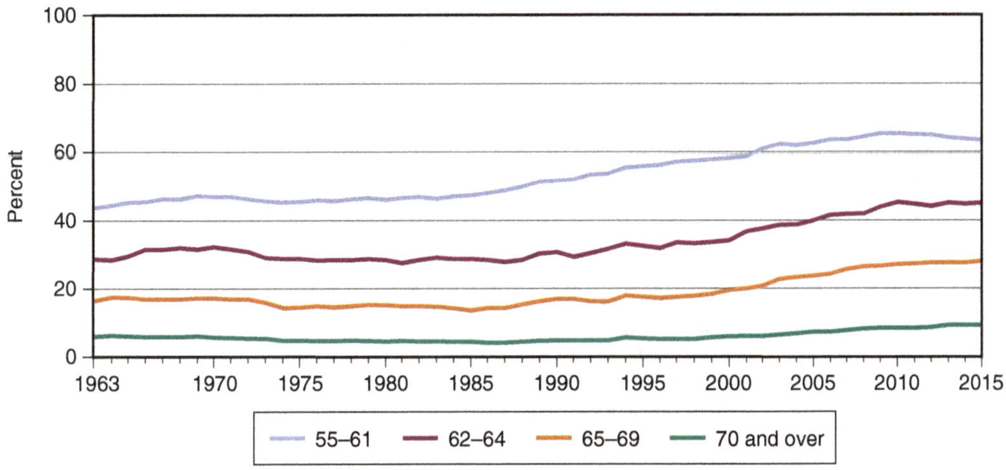

Note: Data for 1994 and later years are not strictly comparable with data for 1993 and earlier years owing to a redesign of survey and methodology of the Current Population Survey. Reference population: These data refer to the civilian noninstitutionalized population.
Source: Data from U.S. Census Bureau. Bureau of Labor Statistics. *Current Population Survey.* https://www.bls.gov/cps/demographics.htm#age

responsibilities, which disproportionately affect women and lead to exit from the workforce and earlier retirement. The difference between the labor force participation of the sexes narrowed for all age groups.

According to a 2012 Gallup survey, 81% of working people reported that they thought they would work part time (63%) or full time (18%) when they reached retirement age. People expecting part-time work were much more likely to state that they would be working because they wanted to, while people expecting to work full time were more likely to work for financial reasons.

Expecting to work during one's retirement years, obviously, will not be perfectly correlated with actually working, given the challenges of finding a job, sustaining good health, and/or dealing with onerous family caregiving responsibilities. In 2015, 19% of Americans age 65+ were in the labor force, including 4.8 million men (23.4%) and 4 million women (15.3%).

With increasing life expectancy, workers can anticipate a longer retirement phase to save for. Complicating matters is that employees are increasingly less able to take advantage of the security and predictability of *defined benefit programs* (i.e., traditional, lifetime pensions provided by employers), and must instead rely on *defined contribution programs* (i.e., do-it-yourself retirement savings plans that are subject to the whims of the stock market).

Labor force participation among older adults in the United States is considerably higher than that in most other countries, including France, Germany, Italy, Sweden, United Kingdom, and Canada, although it is lower than the rate in Japan.

Educational Status

Between 1965 and 2015, the percentage of older persons who had completed high school increased from 24% to 84% (Figure 1.8). In 1965, only 5% had at least a bachelor's degree or more, while in 2015 that figure rose to 27% and 33% in 2021 (ACL, 2022). When the

FIGURE 1.8 Educational attainment of the population age 65+, selected years, 1965 to 2015.

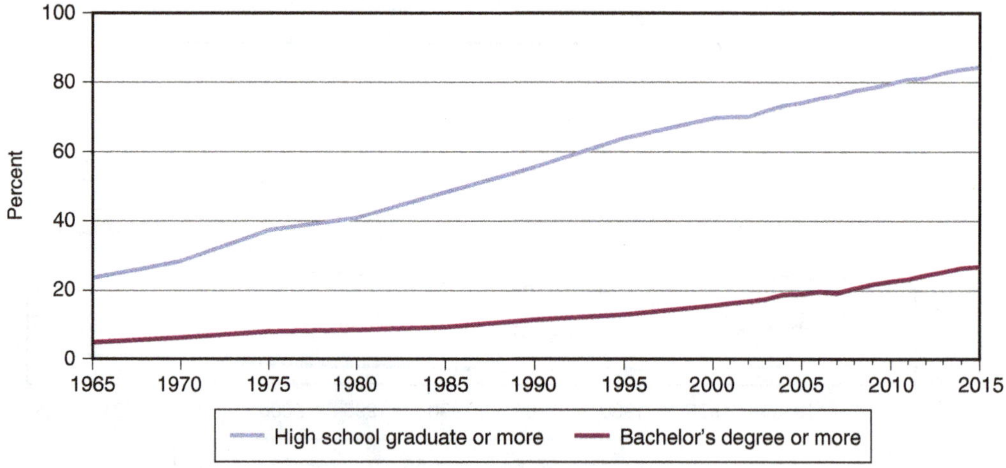

Note: A single question that asks for the highest grade or degree completed is now used to determine educational attainment. Prior to 1995, educational attainment was measured using data on years of school completed. Reference population: These data refer to the civilian noninstitutionalized population.
Source: Data from U.S. Census Bureau. (2016). *Current Population Survey: Annual social and economic supplement.* U.S. Department of Commerce.

last baby boomer reaches age 65 (replacing most of the current cohort of older adults), these percentages will increase to 89% high school graduates and 36%—and counting—college graduates.

Why "and counting?" If Nola Ochs and Phyllis Turner are role models, boomers have *plenty* of time to further increase their college graduation rate. Nola Ochs got her undergraduate degree from Fort Hays State University in Kansas in 2007 at the age of 95. Nola was not the only nonagenarian that year with such an impressive educational achievement. Phyllis Turner, at age 94, received her master's degree in medical science at the University of Adelaide in Australia. Not many boomers are likely to be discouraged from attending college because of their age. They seem to be more serious students too!

In 2010, older men had attained two thirds of the bachelor's degrees, but if current trends hold, this percentage will soon be substantially reversed. Women have constituted about 57% of college matriculation for several years now.

Disparities in higher education among older adults are striking. In 2021, the proportion of older adults completing college was 35% among White, 22% among Black, and 17% among Latinx populations. Because educational attainment is a key predictor of so many factors in American life, including adoption of effective health behaviors, this disparity has important implications for public health and health promotion. Figure 1.9 shows differences in educational attainment by race and ethnicity.

By 2007, there were more than 400 *lifelong learning* programs targeted toward older adults in the United States and Canada, almost all of them linked with colleges and universities and many loosely associated with Road Scholar (formerly Elderhostel, then Exploritas) or the Osher Lifelong Learning Institutes, funded by the Bernard Osher Foundation. There were also a variety of other lifelong learning opportunities, such as the Adventures in Learning programs at Shepherd's Centers, the educational programs at OASIS Centers, and other innovative educational options at community colleges, community centers, art museums, and hospitals.

FIGURE 1.9 Educational attainment of the population age 65+, by race and Hispanic origin, 2021.

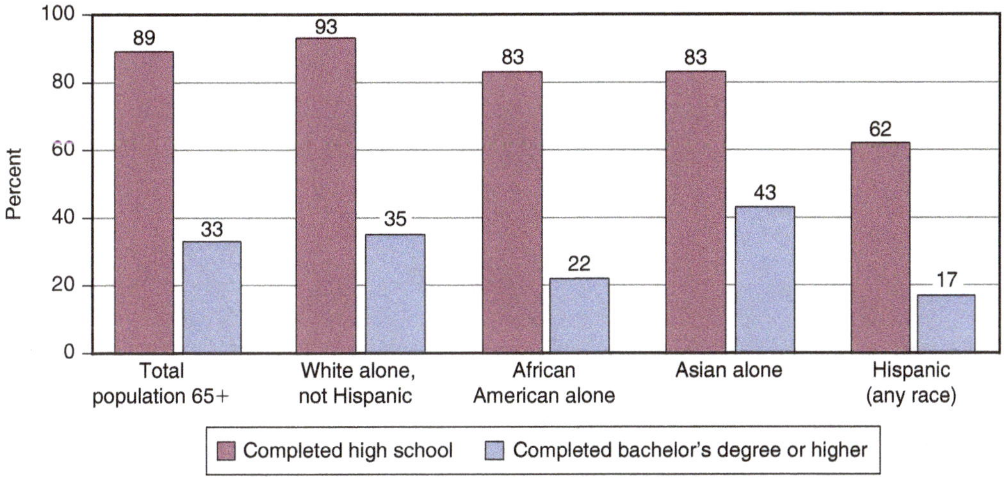

Source: U.S. Census Bureau (2021). *Current Population Survey, Annual Social and Economic Supplement.* U.S. Department of Commerce.

As the educational level of older adults continues to rise, this may well correlate with an increase in their interest in seeking out health information and engaging in health-promoting activities in their communities.

Political Power

The Federal Election Commission reports that older adults are disproportionately likely to vote. In the 2016 presidential election, 71% of those age 65+ voted! This compares to 67% for those age 45 to 64; 59% for those age 30 to 44; and 46% for those age 18 to 29. In 2020, 71.9% of people age 65+ voted compared to 61.3% of the electorate as a whole (O'Neill, 2022). These age discrepancies have been consistent for several decades. When AARP speaks, politicians listen!

There are also significant voting differences among older adults, as they are also influenced by socioeconomic class, ethnicity, gender, and religion (Binstock, 2009). Even when they do throw their weight toward one candidate, they don't always get their way. Older voters in the 2008 presidential election were the only age group that gave a majority of their votes to John McCain—to no avail.

Did older McCain voters become more conservative with age? Or did a specific cohort that was always more conservative remain so? Or did McCain voters just vote for an age peer (McCain was 71 in 2008; Obama was 47)? Unfortunately, only this gerontologist finds these questions interesting. I could not find any research on this topic. What is your opinion, and why?

Internet Access

A 2012 national survey from the Pew Research Center's Internet and American Life Project reported that more than half—a majority for the first time—of adults age 65+ and older had ***internet access***. This is due to the tech-savvy baby boomers moving into the age 65+ ranks. Internet use among those over age 75 was, in contrast, only one third.

FIGURE 1.10 Digital experience among adults, by age, 2012 to 2021.

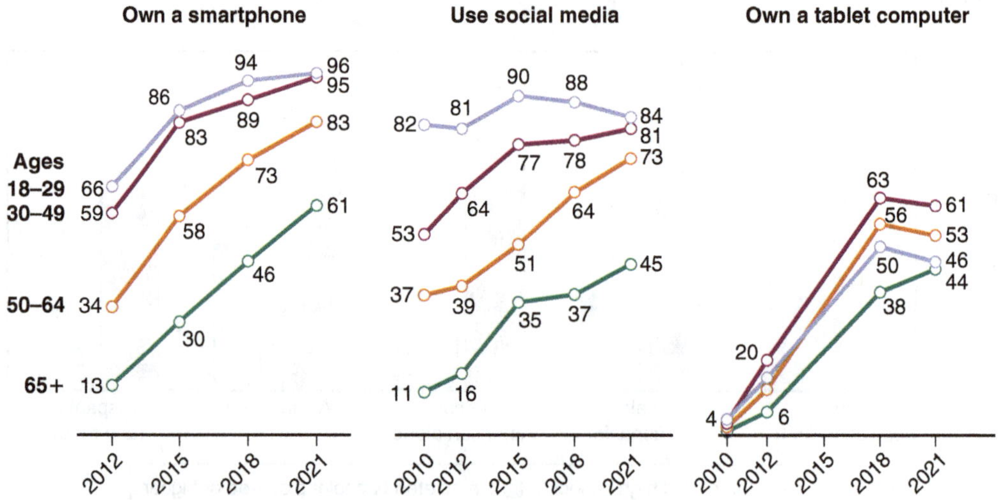

Source: Faverio, M. (2022). *Share of those 65 and older who are tech users has grown in the past decade*. Pew Research Center. https://www.pewresearch.org/short-reads/2022/01/13/share-of-those-65-and-older-who-are-tech-users-has-grown-in-the-past-decade/

In 2021, 75% of people age 65+ reported regular use of the internet. As the latest Pew survey of digital technologies shows, the gap between the oldest and youngest groups of adults in internet use is now half of what it was in 2000. Then it was 56%; now it is 24%. Figure 1.10 shows how older adults have come to resemble younger age cohorts in becoming digital citizens (Faverio, 2022).

Social networking use among internet users ages 65+ quadrupled between 2010 (11%) and 2021 (45%), The Pew study reported that people younger than age 50 used social networking websites primarily to stay in touch with friends, and people older than age 50 reported that they used them primarily to connect with family, particularly those who live far away. They especially want to see photographs of grandchildren. They also use social networking sites to look up old friends and connect with people who share hobbies.

There are no gender differences in overall computer usage, but engagement with social networking sites is greater among older females than older males. Income and education levels still affect differences in the amount and range of computer usage.

Poverty

Poverty kills! According to the Brookings Institution, for a cohort of men born before 1950, life expectancy was 14 years shorter among those in the bottom 10% of earners than among those in the top 10% of earners.

On a more positive note, the poverty rate among older persons had fallen from 35% of those age 65+ in 1969 to 9.5% in 2020. Without Social Security and cost-of-living increases, this rate would have risen to 50% over this time period. Instead, the poverty rate for older adults has, seemingly, fallen below the rate for persons age 18 to 64.

I noted "seemingly" because the declining poverty rate for older adults may be overstated. The U.S. Census Bureau assumes that the costs of food and other necessities are lower for older adults and it does not adequately take into account the rising costs of medical care, transportation, and housing. Also, there are hidden poor among the older

FIGURE 1.11 Poverty among older adults 65+, by race and ethnicity, 2020.

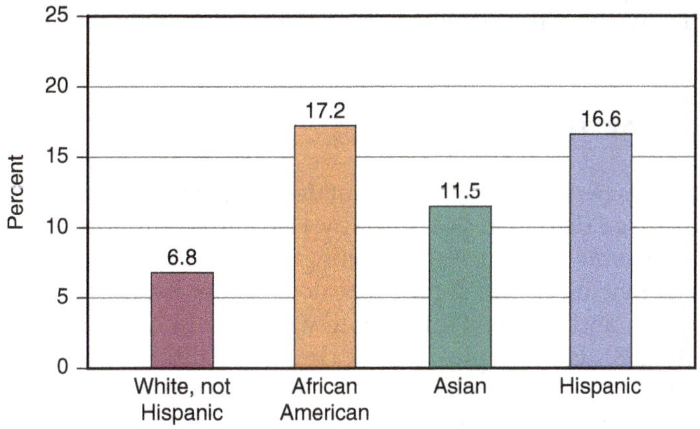

Source: U.S. Census Bureau (2020). *Current Population Survey, Annual Social and Economic Supplement.* U.S. Department of Commerce.

population who reside in nursing homes or who live with relatives and are not counted in the official census statistics (Hooyman & Kiyak, 2011).

The Supplemental Poverty Measure is a U.S. Census research tool that considers previously overlooked costs, like out-of-pocket medical expenses for older adults. It estimated the poverty rate of seniors to have been 14.5% in 2016 instead of the 9.3% noted earlier. The National Academy of Sciences estimated the poverty rate for older Americans even higher at 19%. Perhaps another estimate could be 33%, which is the percentage of older adults who rely on their Social Security check for 90% or more of their total income.

The proportion of older adults living below the federal poverty criterion is more than twice as high for older Hispanics and Blacks (16.6% and 17.2%) than for older Whites (6.8%), as shown in Figure 1.11, and more than 40% higher for older women (10.7%) than for older men (7.6%) (ACL, 2022). Combining gender, ethnicity, and housing, the highest poverty rates were experienced among Hispanic women who lived alone (35.6%).

Racial and Ethnic Composition

The diversity in the ***racial and ethnic composition*** of the older adult population in America is increasing and will continue to increase for the foreseeable future. In 2014, non-Hispanic Whites accounted for 78% of the older adult population in the United States, but this is projected to drop dramatically to 55% in 2060. The fastest-growing minority will be Hispanic elders of any race, almost tripling in percentage between 2010 and 2060 (from 8% to 22%), overtaking Black elders as the dominant minority group. The growth in percentage of Hispanic elders over this half century will be followed by older Asians (4%–7%) and older Blacks (9%–12%).

Although health professionals will need to become more knowledgeable about the ethnic backgrounds of their older clients, there is great diversity within ethnic groups as well. Age, gender, region, religion, English-speaking skills, income, education, lifestyle, physical disability, ***marital status***, place of birth, and length of residence in the United States are examples of important variables to consider within each ethnic group.

There is a continuum of ***acculturation*** that occurs among elders within each ethnic group. *Acculturation* is the degree to which people incorporate the cultural values, beliefs, language, and skills of the mainstream culture. Recognition of the many distinctive ethnic subgroups in the United States, each with a range of acculturation, is a key challenge to effective healthcare delivery and health promotion (Haber, 2005).

DEFINITIONS OF HEALTHY AGING

Health professionals need to be careful about defining good health among older adults. This was the message delivered years ago by Faith Fitzgerald (1994) in an editorial in the *New England Journal of Medicine* cautioning against a narrow or rigid definition of health: "We must beware of developing a zealotry about health, in which we take ourselves too seriously and believe that we know enough to dictate . . . the definition of health" (pp. 197–198). Is it people without chronic health conditions? That would be a highly exclusive club among older adults. Are physical and mental health equally important? Can we rely on the assessment of older adults about their own health? Can we trust the physician's or psychiatrist's judgment? Does the epidemiologist's data provide insight?

QUESTION: What is *your* definition of healthy aging?

What follows is a sampling of definitions of good health.

The Federal Government

A broad and bland definition of *health* is provided by the federal government's USPHS through its Health Objectives for the Nation. It entails three components:

1. *disease prevention,* which comprises strategies to maintain and to improve health through medical care, such as high blood pressure control and immunization;
2. *health protection,* which includes strategies for modifying environmental and social structural health risks, such as toxic agent and radiation control, and accident prevention and injury control; and
3. *health promotion,* which includes strategies for reducing lifestyle risk factors, such as avoiding smoking and the misuse of alcohol and drugs, and adopting good nutritional habits and a proper and adequate exercise regimen.

Extraordinary Accomplishments

One not-so-bland definition of good health in late life is the lauding of ***extraordinary accomplishments*** by older adults who may serve as (unattainable?) role models. You can find these paragons of health everywhere in our multimedia culture. Here are some of my favorites.

Arts

Falstaff, Verdi's last opera, was composed when he was age 80. George Burns won an Oscar, his first, also at age 80. And Anna Mary Robertson, better known as Grandma Moses, had her first showing of her paintings at, you guessed it, age 80, after beginning this artistic pursuit just a couple of years earlier.

Enough with the youngsters. Herman Wouk, Pulitzer Prize–winning author of *The Caine Mutiny,* published his last novel, *The Lawgiver,* in 2012 at the age of 96.

He felt he needed a bit more seasoning before writing his first memoir, which was published in 2015 at age 100 (!) entitled: *Sailor and Fiddler: Reflections of a 100-Year-Old Author.* Mr. Wouk died in 2019, a few days shy of his 104th birthday.

Mieczysław Horszowski, a classical pianist, recorded a new album at age 99. Johannes Heesters, a Dutch-born German singer–dancer–actor, was still appearing on stage at age 101. He announced at that age that he had no plans to take what he called "early retirement" because the stage was his life.

Jumping up to the age of 107, George Abbott collaborated on the revival of the musical *Damn Yankees*. George wasn't the only 107-year-old with an artistic bent. After Sadie and Bessie Delany wrote their bestseller: *The Delany Sisters' First Hundred Years*, Bessie died at age 104. Sadie then went on to author *On My Own at 107: Reflections on Life Without Bessie*. She died 2 years later at age 109.

Politics

In 2006, the average age of a U.S. senator was 62 years, the oldest it had ever been. (It declined slightly since then.) Not surprisingly, the term *senate* derives from the Latin word for "old." Golda Meir became prime minister of Israel at age 71. Former Senator John Glenn completed the rigorous physical preparation necessary to become the oldest space traveler in history at age 77. Former President Jimmy Carter won the Nobel Prize as a global peacemaker at age 78, and in 2018, at the age of 93, authored his 30th book, *Faith*. The former U.S. President died in 2024 at age 100.

Joe Newman, at age 101, ran for a seat in the House of Representatives from Florida's 16th congressional district in 2014. Apparently his long lifetime of experience went unappreciated. Joe got only 220 of the 274,829 votes cast, or 0.1% of the vote. But you have to admire the gumption!

Sports

Kozo Haraguchi ran the 100-meter race in 22.04 seconds, setting a record for the 95 to 99 age group. This 95-year-old Japanese man said he had to run cautiously because the outdoor track was slick with rain. Another runner, Johnny Kelley, won the Boston Marathon twice. Even more remarkable was that he had started this annual race 61 times during his lifetime, completing the entire 26.2 miles 58 times. Mr. Kelley died in 2004 at the age of 97. Another nonagenarian, though, continued to race in 2004. Fauja Singh moved from India to England and decided to take up running at the age of 82. At the age of 92, he set a world record for his age group by running the Toronto Marathon in 5 hours and 40 minutes.

Ken Mink was a basketball player at Roane State, a junior college about 35 miles west of Knoxville, Tennessee. The 6-foot, 190-pound player was listed as a *senior* on the basketball roster. No kidding! Ken Mink was 73 years of age in 2008, more than a half-century older than his teammates. In fact, this septuagenarian was the oldest person ever to play college basketball.

The Seattle Mariners, a 1977 expansion team in major league baseball, set a different kind of record. So I need to add Evelyn Jones to this section of accomplishments. She celebrated her 108th birthday by throwing out the first pitch at a Mariners game, becoming the oldest person to perform this ceremonial pitch. She was an avid fan who watched every game and was given a uniform for this occasion with the number 108 on the back.

Extreme Sports

Japanese mountaineer Tamae Watanabe set a world record in 2012 by becoming the oldest woman to scale Mount Everest, the highest mountain in the world. She did this at the age of 73. In 2013, 80-year-old Yuichiro Miura made it to the summit. Both are relative youngsters compared to Hulda Crooks, who climbed Mount Whitney, the highest mountain in the continental United States, at the age of 91. Centenarians who skydive or scuba dive also make the news (*ABC News*, 2018; KWTX, 2022).

Work

U.S. District Court Judge Wesley E. Brown became the oldest working judge in the nation's history. Near the end of his life, he had to transfer some of his work from his Wichita, Kansas, courtroom to his bedroom at home—because of his health—where he died a few weeks later at the age of 104. Judge Brown, however, was not the oldest worker in the United States. Ray Crist still worked as a research scientist at Messiah College in Pennsylvania at the age of 104. He had earned his doctorate in chemistry from Columbia University at the age of 26 and was still putting it to good use 78 years later.

Religion

In 2009, 10 women ranging in age from 89 to 96 each memorized Hebrew in order to become a bat mitzvah, a Jewish girl who is marking the transition into religious adulthood. Unlike a bar mitzvah for a boy, a bat mitzvah was rare until the 1960s, and these women decided to make up for what they were denied as children. They met weekly with a rabbi for several months to study Hebrew to prepare for their rite of passage at the synagogue of the Menorah Park senior residence in Cleveland, Ohio. Although three of these women used walkers and another carried a small oxygen tank to the podium, all successfully completed their deferred quest.

Marriage

After nearly three decades of dating, George Kirby, age 103, became the world's oldest groom in 2015. His bride, Doreen Luckie, was a mere 91-year-old. George revealed that he didn't get down on one knee because he wouldn't have been able to get up.

Birthing

A California woman named Arceli Keh lied about her age (she said she was 51 but was actually 61) in order to become eligible for a fertility program in which she was implanted with an embryo from an anonymous donor. In 1996, at age 63, she became the oldest woman on record to have a baby. Her record was surpassed in 2006 when Maria del Carmen Bousada, a 66-year-old Spanish woman who had become pregnant after receiving in vitro fertilization treatment, gave birth to twins by cesarean section in a hospital in Barcelona. The wisdom of this accomplishment was called into question in 2009, however, when she died from cancer at age 69, leaving behind boys not yet 3 years old.

Nonetheless, fertility science marches on. In 2013, in the United States, 677 women age 50 or older gave birth, most via in vitro fertilization with donor eggs. The risks are substantial, though, with these older mothers much more likely to become diabetic or hypertensive and babies facing complications from low birth weights.

Bank Robbing

Red Rountree, at the age of 91, became the oldest known bank robber in U.S. history in 2004. Sentenced to a 12-year term in Texas—he died within the first year of his sentence—Red said he robbed banks for fun: "I feel good, awfully good for days after robbing a bank." After two successful heists, the third time apparently was not the charm. The teller at the third bank, responding to his demand for money, asked, "Are you kidding?"

Although I marvel at these examples of unusual achievement by aging adults, I do not personally use them as inspiration for older, or even younger, persons. These models are astonishing, but they do little to enhance the confidence of aging adults who do not believe they can—and perhaps do not want to—come close to achieving similar milestones.

As Friedan (1993) noted in her book *The Fountain of Age*, as an older adult one should not "attempt to hold on to, or judge oneself by, youthful parameters of love, work and power. For this is what blinds us to the new strengths and possibilities emerging in ourselves."

Nonetheless, I had an uproariously good time compiling these accomplishments.

PREVENTION

Prevention is often categorized as primary, secondary, or tertiary (Figure 1.12). *Primary prevention* focuses on the population as a whole, which includes mostly asymptomatic people. Primary prevention of falls, for example, would screen every older person attending a program at a senior center for balance and lower extremity strength, and make referrals for interventions according to performance relative to age-based norms (Albert et al., 2014). Primary preventive measures, such as regular exercise, good nutrition, smoking cessation, or immunizations, are recommended to decrease the probability of the onset of specific diseases or dysfunction. Primary prevention is different from *health promotion* in that it is less broad in scope and tends to be the term used by clinicians in a medical setting.

Secondary prevention is practiced with a preclinical or asymptomatic person in whom actual (rather than potential) risk factors have been identified even though the underlying disease is not yet clinically apparent. A medical screening, as an example of secondary prevention, is cost-effective only when there is hope of lessening the severity or shortening the duration of a pathological process. Blood pressure screenings, cholesterol screenings, and bone densitometries are the most widely implemented forms of secondary prevention.

Tertiary prevention, which takes place after the person with a disease or disability becomes symptomatic, focuses on the rehabilitation or maintenance of function. Health professionals attempt to restore or maintain the maximum level of functioning possible, within the constraints of a medical problem, to prevent further disability and dependency on others.

FIGURE 1.12 Three levels of prevention.

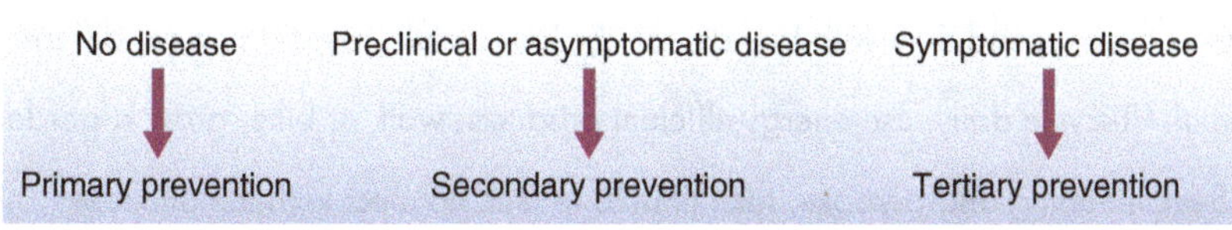

Tertiary prevention corresponds to phase 2 (rehabilitation of outpatients) and phase 3 (long-term maintenance) of the rehabilitation of a cardiac patient (with phase 1 care of a hospitalized cardiac patient). Randomized clinical trials with patients who had myocardial infarctions revealed that programs of tertiary prevention reduced the likelihood of cardiovascular death by 25%.

A focus on prevention may be more appealing to some older adults than an emphasis on health promotion. Older adults are likely to be coping with chronic conditions, and the prevention, delay, or reduction in disability and dependency is a much more salient issue for them than it is for most younger adults.

Moreover, among medical professionals, the relevancy of the term *prevention* is enhanced because the costs of many prevention activities, such as mammograms, are reimbursable through Medicare. Prevention has gotten its foot in the door, so to speak, in the system of healthcare reimbursement, whereas the activities of health promotion have lagged considerably behind.

One advantage of the use of the term *health promotion*, however, is that it encompasses mental, emotional, and spiritual health concerns. In contrast to clients and health professionals fixated on risk factors and the prevention of disease or disability, health promotion or wellness can be viewed as an affirming, even joyful, process. Health professionals who promote health, for instance, can encourage playing with grandchildren or the joy of bird watching to an older client and not concern ourselves with its ability to prevent disease or illness.

Health promotion is also a more proactive approach than primary prevention, which tends to imply a reaction to the prospect of disease. Directing a client's anger or frustration into political advocacy work, for example, is a proactive, health-promoting enterprise that benefits both the client and society.

WELLNESS

Although the term ***wellness*** has had many supporters in the health professions over the years (Jonas, 2000), particularly among persons who conduct health programs at large U.S. corporations (Jacob, 2002), it tends to be embraced less than the terms *health promotion* and *disease prevention*. Nonetheless, wellness conveys an important message that good health is more than physical well-being. In fact, ***seven dimensions*** are usually touted among wellness advocates, as shown in Table 1.6.

Wellness sends a welcome and important reminder about the breadth of health promotion that is not conveyed by most other terms. The only limitation to the term *wellness*

TABLE 1.6 SEVEN DIMENSIONS OF WELLNESS

Physical—Exercise, eat a well-balanced diet, get enough sleep, protect yourself.

Emotional—Express a wide range of feelings, acknowledge stress, channel positive energy.

Intellectual—Embrace lifelong learning, discover new skills and interests.

Vocational—Do something you love, balance work with leisure time.

Social—Laugh often, spend time with friends/family, join a club, respect cultural differences.

Environmental—Recycle daily, use energy-efficient products, walk or bike, grow a garden.

Spiritual—Seek meaning and purpose, take time to reflect, connect with the universe.

is that it tends to be identified with "alternative" activities—acupuncture, homeopathy, spiritual healing, aromatherapy—to the exclusion of more mainstream activities such as exercise and nutrition. Thus, it suggests fringe pursuits or even flakiness to some.

Antiold and Antiaging

Who is healthier, an old person or an older adult? Is this a preposterous question? Maybe not. Do the terms *old person* and *older adult* reflect our prejudices—the frail old person versus the more neutral older adult? One of the leaders in the field of gerontological language, Erdman Palmore, thought so. Palmore suggested that most of the synonyms for old are unhealthy in some way—words like *debilitated, infirm,* and *frail. Older adult,* on the other hand, is a more neutral and relative term—a 40-year-old can be an older adult to a teenager.

Palmore suggested that perhaps the term *elder* connotes the healthiest definition for older persons in society (Palmore, 2000). In Christian churches, for example, an elder is a person who is valued for their wisdom and who holds a position of responsibility and authority. Among the general public, however, the term appears to be viewed no more favorably than other synonyms for old.

Surveys of AARP members have revealed that no synonyms for old are acceptable—not seniors, not elders, not mature adults. As a result, AARP in its magazine entitles its movie review section, "Movies for Grownups." Professional societies and advocates for older people continue to grapple with appropriate language to describe old age. The Gerontological Society of America (GSA) has developed teaching materials and guidance in writing about old age with its "Reframing Aging" initiative (https://www.reframingaging.org). Even gerontologists and aging services professionals can benefit from this careful look at the labels we use and how language often promotes ageist stereotypes.

The challenge is to approach age realistically. Old age, like youth or middle age, has both challenges and virtues. Maggie Kuhn, the founder of the advocacy organization the Gray Panthers, reported on an exchange that she had with President Gerald Ford at a hearing on a pension bill in Washington, D.C. Once she had gotten President Ford's attention, he asked, "And what do you have to say, *young lady*?" Maggie replied, "First of all, I'm not a young lady. I'm an *old woman*." She was making the statement that she was proud of being old, and that she had earned that label.

A related concern is the ***antiaging*** movement and its chief proponent, the American Academy of Anti-Aging Medicine. This professional society is larger than scientific societies seeking to address aging and promotes unrealistic goals for aging. One critic accuses the organization of "pursuing the fountain of youth with their lucrative nostrums and illusory interventions, [while] we geriatricians remain solidly in the trenches caring for our patients, the most aged, complex, frail, and vulnerable—far removed from the fantasies of eternal life, much less the fountain of youth" (Hazzard, 2005, p. 1435).

Not-so-fun fact: There are more physicians in the American Academy of Anti-Aging Medicine (a field not recognized by any legitimate medical certifying body) than there are board-certified geriatricians (who are, in fact, declining in number).

Most proponents of the antiaging movement are focused not on the most aged, but on the middle-aged and the young old, those most concerned with combating the signs of aging. One key weapon in their arsenal is the *cosmeceutical*, a combination of the terms *cosmetic* and *pharmaceutical* that refers to a topical skin treatment formulated to eliminate wrinkles and other signs of aging. If the cosmeceutical intervention proves insufficient, there are Botox injections, microdermabrasion, chemical peels, collagen injections, and plastic surgeries. Antiagers deliver a clear message that aging is a disease that needs to be cured—at least cosmetically and temporarily.

Another segment of the antiaging movement believes in the power of human growth hormone (HGH). Ironically, while the target audience is the middle-aged and the younger-old crowd, Don Ramos of Colorado Springs, age 80, was suspended for 2 years by the U.S. Anti-Doping Agency for testing positive for an anabolic steroid, a growth hormone, at the Pan American Master's Weight Lifting Championships.

A review of 31 randomized, controlled studies, however, concluded that the risks outweigh any potential antiaging benefits of HGH when taken by healthy older adults (Liu et al., 2007). Side effects may include diabetes, hypertension, hardening of the arteries, and abnormal growth of bones or internal organs.

Nonetheless, government officials estimate that 25,000 to 30,000 Americans take injections of HGH for antiaging purposes, paying up to $1,000 a month. Although it is illegal to prescribe HGH for healthy people in the United States, speakers at the annual conference of the American Academy of Anti-Aging Medicine have told physicians in the audience how they can diagnose a mild hormone deficiency so that they can legally prescribe HGH (Wilson, 2007).

We could all benefit from a ***proaging*** movement, one that emphasizes the healthy aspects of aging and the benefits that accrue with age. No longer needing to impress employers, in-laws, or peers, older adults are free to be themselves. The old have the opportunity to be not only freer, but also wiser, more conscious of the present, and more willing to be advocates for a healthy future. Maggie Kuhn certainly practiced a proaging lifestyle.

I am not the first to use the term "proaging." Over the last few years advertisements for Dove beauty products have consistently asked the question "Are you antiage or proage?" Unfortunately, Dove's proage movement consisted entirely of selling moisturizers and other skin products. This is not what I have in mind when I talk about promoting a healthy attitude toward aging. (Not that I have anything against reasonably priced moisturizers.)

Finally, the Me Too movement rose to prominence worldwide at the end of 2017. It took a strong stand against sexual harassment. From a gerontological perspective, though, there is also a lot of work remaining to be done. In Italy, according to Roman prosecutors, older women are exempt from sexual harassment. They dismissed a groping case brought by 53-year-old Elisabetta Cortani. Verdict? She was too old to be distressed by sexual advances!

Compression of Morbidity

By definition, chronic diseases are not curable. The onset of chronic disease, however, may be postponed through the modification of risk factors. As the onset is delayed to later ages and approaches the limit of the human life span, the result is a ***compression of morbidity***. The goal is to live in robust health to a point as close as one can come to the end of the lifespan, so that one can die after only a brief period of illness. In short, spend a longer time living with reasonable health and a shorter time dying.

For most people, though, the prospect of living long past one's 65th birthday is a mixed blessing. With Americans living longer today than ever before, we have come to dread a prolonged period of disability and dependency in late life.

One definition of healthy aging, then, is to be able to live life fully until death. Pessimists argue that the period of morbidity preceding death will lengthen in the future as a result of (a) limited biomedical research funds available to improve the physical and mental capacity of the very old; (b) the fact that some major diseases, such as Alzheimer, have recognized lifestyle risk factors that account for no more than 40% of the risk of the disease (Livingston et al., 2020); and (c) medical advances, such as dialysis and bypass

FIGURE 1.13 Compression of morbidity.

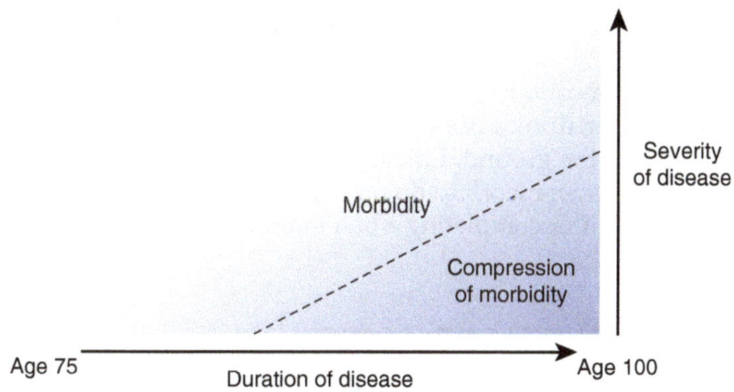

surgery, that will increase the life expectancy of those with disease rather than prevent the occurrence of disease.

Optimists, however, claim that there will be a compression of morbidity (Figure 1.13) in the future due to (a) the likelihood of advances in biomedical research that will prevent or delay the occurrence of disease, and (b) the continued potential for reducing risk factors such as smoking, high blood pressure, poor nutritional habits, and sedentary lifestyles, which will result in better health.

In the original formulation (Fries & Crapo, 1981), improvements in public health, medical care, and health behavior would allow postponement or prevention of serious, disabling disease until very late in a mostly fixed lifespan. Ideally, disease progression would be delayed to the point of never exceeding a clinical threshold of symptoms. A person could live, age, and die at age 80 to 85 with negligible morbidity. A challenge to the theory is the extension of lifespan that accompanies improvements in public health, medical care, and health behavior. We are living longer, which allows more general senescent processes to take their toll, evident in frailty, loss of mobility, and neurodegeneration. Worse yet, if the mortality frontier (evident in population survival curves) moves faster than the morbidity frontier (evident in disability-free survival curves), we may add years of disability to our lives, leading to an expansion, rather than compression, of morbidity.

Research into compression of disability has not reached a consensus. One study, for instance, did not support evidence of a compression of morbidity. Over the prior decade, length of life with disease and deteriorating function of mobility increased (Crimmins & Beltran-Sanchez, 2010). While longevity increased, living with disease increased as well. A later study by one of the same researchers concluded the reverse. Over a 40-year period, 1970 to 2010, disability-free life expectancy in the United States increased for those age 65+ and for those age 85+ (Crimmins et al., 2016).

What seems to be the most credible research outcome is that given the right combination of healthy lifestyle behaviors, compression of morbidity can be accomplished, at least for particular health conditions. One such study supports this conclusion, examining smoking and alcohol habits, physical activity, diet, body mass index (BMI), and social support (Jacob et al., 2016). The FINGER study showed that behavioral changes can delay cognitive decline (Ngandu et al., 2015).

In a given population, the healthier the lifestyles overall, the more likely we will see compression of morbidity. The challenge, of course, is how to encourage healthy lifestyles in a society in which some risk factors are declining (smoking, for instance) while others are increasing (obesity).

Will we be able to foster compression of morbidity? It is not certain at this time. Moreover, will there be improved medical advances and medical access that compress morbidity? Will societal improvements, such as increased education and income, compress morbidity?

My compression of morbidity vision is to live into my 90s, dribble down a basketball court, leap into the air, dunk a basketball, and after I observe the ball falling through the net but before it hits the ground, I die of a heart attack. Now that's compression of morbidity! (I've still got some work to do on the dunking part.) My long-distance runner spouse wants to die after completing a half marathon in her 80s.

HEALTH PERSPECTIVES AND AGING

Health Expectancy Versus Life Expectancy

Almost everyone is familiar with the term ***life expectancy***, a model prediction based on prevailing mortality rates at each age applied to a cohort born at a particular time. Applying death rates to each age group yields the total number of years lived by the cohort and the expected years of life given that someone has reached a certain age. We can consider life expectancy "the average length of time human beings are expected to live" but only given this underlying demographic model. A less familiar term is ***health expectancy***, the amount of time human beings are expected to live in good health and free from functional limitation as applied to this model. Here the person-years used in the calculation are weighted by the proportion without health conditions, yielding disability-free or dementia-free life expectancy, for example. There is, on average, a 5-year gap between life expectancy and health expectancy after the age of 65, according to the CDC's Behavioral Risk Factor Surveillance System.

Place yourself in the shoes of the person who has just reached age 65. Are you primarily interested in remaining alive as long as possible, or are you most interested in how many of your remaining years will find you healthy and functionally independent? Most older adults I have conversed with over the decades indicate the latter is more important to them.

Your *health expectancy* depends to a great extent on your level of physical activity, nutritional intake, social support network, access to good medical care, health education, and utilization of health services. While health expectancy is more important to older adults than life expectancy, unfortunately we have not made adequate progress on this front. As noted in the beginning of this chapter, the goal of *Healthy People 2000* was to increase the number of years of healthy life remaining after age 65 from 11.8 to 14. It increased only to 12.2 years, an advance of 4 months over the decade.

Physical Versus Emotional Aspects of Aging

There is a strong reciprocal relationship between the physical and emotional aspects of health. When our physical health is threatened, so typically is our emotional health. The converse is equally true.

As we age, however, it may be the case that good health becomes less dependent on our physical status than on our emotional status. Studies report shifting perspectives of health over time, with older participants expecting physical health problems because of their age and discounting them somewhat, when they do appear, because of this expectation.

A study of 85-year-olds living in the Netherlands reported that physical function was not the most important component of successful aging. These older adults were able to adapt successfully to physical limitations. The researchers reported social contacts as the most important factor in well-being, and the quality of the contacts was more important than their number (von Faber et al., 2001). Open-ended interviews reveal more than 100 characteristics of health that are important to older adults besides physical health, including the ability to enjoy life and good personal relationships. Many older adults who are frail and sometimes disabled do *not* evaluate their health or life negatively.

Most health professionals subscribe to the notion that health is more than the absence of illness. Were this not the case, they would have to label the vast majority of older adults, 90% of whom are coping with a chronic condition, unhealthy. The chronic diseases that older persons contend with do not necessarily relate to their ability to perform daily activities. Disease, in fact, may not be evident even to the person who has it.

The presence or absence of disease, therefore, may not be a source of great concern to older adults. The ability to perform ADLs, however, *is* of great concern to older adults who desire as much independence as possible. The definition of health, especially among older adults, should not be linked with disease or its absence, as the medical model suggests, but with independence, the ability to accomplish one's goals, and the presence of satisfying relationships.

A health perspective that emphasizes the psychological status of older adults does not view health as a physical continuum ranging from disability and illness at one end to a high level of robustness at the other. Critics of this type of health continuum argue that even a person who is functionally impaired or disabled, and thus residing at one end of the physical continuum, can focus considerable attention on a high level of wellness and psychological growth.

Finally, health professionals walk a fine line with older patients. On the one hand, they have been accused of ignoring some of the medical needs of older adults by discounting the viability of certain medical interventions because of advanced patient age. In fact, most patients in their 80s can benefit as much from surgical interventions as can younger patients (Varghese & Norman, 2004). On the other hand, physician attempts to "de-prescribe," that is, stop a medication when its benefit is no longer evident, are viewed with suspicion and sometimes criticized as therapeutic nihilism.

Without proper guidance, health professionals can unduly focus on the (reimbursable) medical needs of very old clients and neglect the personal values that inform the quality of life of the older adult. Many older adults, if informed, would avoid the prospect of high-risk surgeries that are unlikely to extend quality of life or perhaps even life expectancy. An example is a study of cancer screening in almost 6,000 frail nursing home residents, most of whom were in their 80s and cognitively impaired. The questionable decision to screen for breast cancer led to surgeries that did not extend life and most certainly did not improve their functioning or quality of life (Tang et al., 2018).

Intergenerational Conflict Over Healthcare?

Creating a name for a generation and then generalizing about it is fraught with complexity, and some analysts shy away from it—but many do not. I personally think it is a type of intellectual fun that analysts and the general public find hard to resist. If you are among them, there is an interesting argument to be made that there will be generational conflict over healthcare expenditures in the future. But first, there are three generations to define.

The baby boomers refer to those born between 1946 and 1964. Many argue that people born up to two decades apart are too diverse for one label (Pruchno, 2012). In fact, some differentiate between *leading-edge boomers* (1946–1955) and *trailing-edge boomers* (1956–1964).

Leading-edge boomers are more likely Caucasian, married, college graduates, and more than twice as likely to have served in the military than trailing-edge boomers. The latter difference is due to the fact that the draft ended after all the leading-edge boomers had turned age 18. Is it wise to lump both groups together? Then throw in the technology revolution to complicate matters. Smartphone ownership by leading-edge boomers is only two thirds that of trailing-edge boomers.

The boomers are differentiated from *generation X*, born between 1965 and 1981, and *generation Y*, also referred to as the *millennials*, born between 1982 and 2000. Some argue that these two generations not only differ from each other but are too diverse within each generation for one label per group. Within each of these generations, are there shared values about hard work, trust, respect for authority, teamwork, competition, privacy, independence, optimism, and so forth, as some analysts claim without much supporting data?

Complicating generalizations about the millennials is that they make up one quarter of the U.S. population. In 2015, this huge cohort surpassed the number of boomers.

In one area, though, I can see the utility of differentiating generations and the potential for *intergenerational conflict*, and that is over healthcare. Let's face it. The boomers use a lot more of it, thanks to aging bodies and Medicare, than do generation X and the millennials. There is insufficient national wealth for all Americans to get all the medical care they desire. One can see the boomers wanting to preserve the benefits of Medicare that they currently (or soon will) get, which is costly to all taxpayers, even the ones who will not be able to take advantage of it for several decades—or may eventually take advantage of it with significantly reduced benefits, according to some skeptical millennials.

The younger generations may resent the expensive cost of Medicare and other resources that older adults disproportionately use, versus government support for education, child support, and the other needs that disproportionately affect younger adults. Millennials, though, may have complex feelings about their boomer parents. They may resent the growing debt awaiting them for decades and perhaps for the rest of their lives. But the percentage of young adults between the ages of 18 and 34 who are living with their parents had increased to 32% in 2016 (and for the first time this is a higher percentage than those living with a partner!). It is hard for millennials to resent Medicare and other resources that older adults disproportionately use while at the same time taking advantage of the voluntary generosity of the older generation.

Intergenerational conflict over jobs may be *less* likely than conflict over healthcare. According to Munnell and Wu (2012), there is no evidence that increasing the employment of older persons reduces the job opportunities or wage rates of younger persons.

LEGISLATION

Medicare, Medicaid, and Social Security have had a tremendous impact on health. It is important, therefore, to review these legislative acts, as many people do not even understand the difference between Medicare and Medicaid, so we begin there.

Medicare

Medicare was enacted in 1965 to help persons age 65+ pay for medical care. In 2016, Medicare covered 48 million older adults and 9 million younger persons with disabilities. It is a major player in the U.S. healthcare system, costing $702 billion in 2017, an increase in costs of 40% from a decade earlier and currently 15% of the entire federal budget.

Ironically, despite the generous reimbursements that beneficiaries received through the Medicare program in 2014 ($11,000 per beneficiary), older Americans spent more money out of pocket (about $5,000 per beneficiary after controlling for inflation) than they did prior to the inauguration of Medicare. These costs include Medicare premiums, deductibles, and coinsurance; eyeglasses and hearing aids along with vision and hearing tests; dental care; over-the-counter drugs; and long-term care. Out-of-pocket medical care costs consume more than one third of the average Social Security check.

Medicare Part A is referred to as hospital insurance, and most people do not have to pay a monthly premium for this insurance because they are eligible through the taxes they paid while working. Part A includes hospital care ($1,632 deductible in 2024), inpatient psychiatric care (190-day lifetime maximum), skilled nursing facility care (100 days), rehabilitation or home care following a hospitalization, and hospice care for the terminally ill. There are restrictions on what kinds of conditions are covered and the length of coverage. Copayments apply as well.

Medicare Part B is referred to as medical insurance and covers physician services, outpatient hospital care, and other medical services such as physical and occupational therapy and some home healthcare. Part B requires a monthly premium ranging from $244.60 to $594.00, depending on income. (In 2024, an individual with gross annual income of $103,000 and a married couple with $206,000 or less pay the minimum monthly premium of $240.) Part B includes most medical screenings and clinical laboratory tests but does not cover dental services, hearing aids, eyeglasses, and most long-term care services. Chronic conditions are, for the most part, not covered by Medicare Part B, and prevention coverage is limited primarily to medical screenings and immunizations.

Beginning in 2007, Medicare shifted, for the first time, to *means-based testing* for Part B premiums. At that time, only persons earning less than $85,000 a year ($170,000 for married couples) pay the base premium; those who exceed this income level have their premiums increased based on how much additional income they earned. Use of this type of *income indexing* will continue to increase in the coming years, and some project that beneficiaries with high incomes will soon pay at least three times the basic premium amount.

Medicare Part C refers to private health insurance plans that provide Medicare benefits; that is, *Medicare Advantage* plans. A subsidy at taxpayers' expense granted to private insurers has led to substantial increases in enrollment in these plans. In 2023, Medicare Advantage enrollees numbered 30.8 million, 51% of all eligible beneficiaries (Ochieng et al., 2023). The number of Part C private health insurance beneficiaries will continue to increase because these HMO-like plans provide additional preventive services and simplified billing. However, they restrict medical services to preferred provider networks as a way of controlling costs and thus narrow patient options for medical care, which may become important with cancer care or other severe medical challenges. Another factor that is likely to increase enrollment in Medicare Advantage plans is coverage for nonskilled in-home services for selected beneficiaries, beginning in 2019.

Medicare Part D refers to the Medicare prescription drug plan, which went into effect on January 1, 2006. This part is also administered by private health insurance companies. Thanks to powerful lobbyists during the Bush administration, Medicare Part D does not allow the government to negotiate with drug companies to lower prescription drug costs for beneficiaries, despite the fact that Medicaid and Veterans Affairs are able to do this to control costs. We can expect changes to this policy in coming years as expenses for new therapies continue to grow.

About one fourth of federal health expenditures for older adults is for Medicare, and these expenditures have been rising (and will continue to rise) rapidly. It is not surprising, therefore, that even though the single largest component of out-of-pocket costs for older adults is for much needed long-term care, it will not be enacted by Medicare anytime soon. Except for the rare initiative, the federal government has resisted overtures to include substantial long-term care coverage under Medicare. One attempt, the CLASS Act (Community Living Assistance Services and Supports Act—one of many ridiculous acronyms you will see throughout this book), was proposed under the Affordable Care Act (ACA). However, this revolutionary proposal was quickly dropped because it was designed as a voluntary program—politically desirable but financially unfeasible.

An interesting line of research has shown that Medicare spending across the country varies greatly, but health outcomes tend to be the same regardless of how much money is spent in a particular region. Some argue, therefore, that Medicare costs could be reduced significantly if the entire nation could bring its costs down to match the lower spending regions.

Landrum et al. (2008) agree with this premise, with one caveat. Although increased area-level spending does not correlate with improved patient outcomes overall, in certain cases increased spending is beneficial. The problem is that high-spending areas also spend too much money on healthcare problems where little or no benefit results. The authors concluded that Medicare could save money not by capping costs, but by implementing evidence-based results from *comparative effectiveness studies*; that is, determining which treatments work best for which patients, and whether the benefits are commensurate with the costs.

The Centers for Medicare & Medicaid Services (CMS) oversees all financial and regulatory aspects of the Medicare and Medicaid systems. For additional information, call 800-MEDICARE (800-633-4227) or go to the Medicare website (https://www.medicare.gov).

Medicaid

Medicaid is different from Medicare in that it is:

- not focused primarily on older adults;
- state-run, not federally managed;
- funded jointly by the states and the federal government; and
- the largest source of public funding for medical and health-related services for people with limited income.

Because it is state run, Medicaid policies for eligibility, services, and payment vary considerably by state. A Supreme Court decision on June 28, 2012 allowed states to opt out of the Medicaid component of the ACA, making this variation even more extreme, though by 2023 only 10 states had not expanded Medicaid coverage (Glied & Weiss, 2023). One aspect of Medicaid that has not varied much across states is that costs have increased steadily throughout the years and now constitute, on average, a quarter or more of each state's budget. Medicaid spending totaled $824 billion in 2022 (Kaiser Family Foundation [KFF], 2023).

On a gerontological note, one third of Medicaid's budget goes to fund long-term care for the frail elderly and the disabled, most of it to nursing homes. It pays for about 60% of nursing home care, and an increasing amount of home- and community-based long-term care. Medicaid is based on the premise that people pay out of pocket until they become impoverished and eligible for coverage. Moreover, an older person cannot shelter money by giving it away to a relative within a 5-year period of qualifying for Medicaid-subsidized long-term care.

Medicaid, unlike Medicare, has no influential constituency advocating on its behalf. It is recognized by the general public as a program for low-income people and many do not feel generous with their tax dollars to support it. With federal deficits looming as far as the eye can see, and with Medicaid the largest cost item in most states' budgets, the pressure to reduce Medicaid expenditures is and will continue to be enormous. This is likely to have a strong and negative impact on the quality of long-term care for low-income older adults and disabled persons.

Social Security

Few would argue that inadequate income is irrelevant to health. It is important, therefore, in a book focused on health and aging to examine Social Security. ***Social Security*** is a federal program designed to protect people and their families from loss of earnings due to retirement, disability, or death. (When signed into law in 1935, it covered only retired workers.) It was believed by historians that President Franklin Roosevelt was interested not only in the economic security of older adults, but in reducing the politically sensitive high unemployment rate at the time.

Social Security is a progressive benefit, replacing a higher proportion of preretirement earnings of low lifetime earners than higher lifetime earners. Additional protection was provided in 1975 when the Social Security benefit was to be adjusted annually to reflect increases in prices (i.e., the Cost of Living Adjustment, or COLA).

It is an entitlement in that to receive retirement benefits, a person must contribute through payroll tax contributions for 10 or more years. Workers and employers are both responsible for paying half of the payroll tax—6.2% each, with the self-employed paying the full 12.4%, up to a taxable maximum of $168,600 (in 2024) of earnings.

In 2023, 67 million Americans (i.e., retired workers; spouses, children, and survivors; and the disabled) received Social Security benefits, about 90% of those age 65 and older. The average monthly benefit for retired workers in 2023 was $1,837 and for disabled workers $1,486. In 2023, "among Social Security beneficiaries age 65 and older, 12% of men and 15% of women [relied] on Social Security for 90% or more of their income" (SSA, 2023). Without access to Social Security, 58% of women and 48% of men above the age of 75 would be living below the poverty line.

Another problem is a societal one; that is, meeting the financial obligation. In 1935, only 6% of the population was age 65 or over; in 2016, that percentage had increased to 15%. Contrary to this increase in older adults, there were approximately four workers per beneficiary in the 1960s. In 2023, there were an estimated 2.7 covered workers for each Social Security beneficiary. By 2035 this number will decline to 2.3. The widening gap between those paying into Social Security and those receiving Social Security means that full benefits will likely be reduced in 2034 to about 81% of scheduled payments if changes are not made.

HEALTHCARE, MEDICAL CARE, QUALITY CARE

In a democratic society there is stiff competition for societal resources that are taxpayer subsidized. However, healthcare (most of our ***healthcare*** expenses are actually for ***medical care***) has consistently maintained its status in this country as a very high priority for these limited resources.

The growth in national expenditures for healthcare has been nothing short of phenomenal (Figure 1.14). U.S. healthcare spending grew 4.1% in 2022, reaching $4.5 trillion or $13,493 per person. This is 17.3% of the U.S. gross domestic product or GDP (CMS, 2022). In fact, the winds may be shifting. The proportion of GDP dedicated to

QUESTION: Why do we call medical care "healthcare"?

FIGURE 1.14 Total national health expenditures as a percentage of gross domestic product, 1970 to 2017.

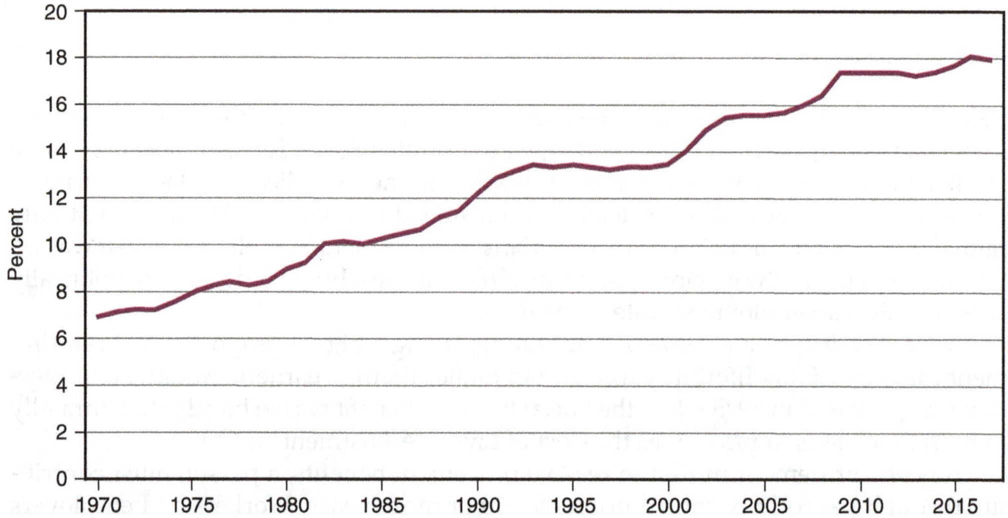

Source: Kamal, R., & Cox, C. (2018, December 10). *How has United States' spending on healthcare changed over time?* https://www.healthsystemtracker.org/chart-collection/u-s-spending-healthcare-changed-time

healthcare declined in 2022. It reached its maximum in 2020 at 19.5%. Reasons for the decline are unclear.

While the United States is spending about 17% of its GDP on healthcare, other developed countries spend between 9% and 11% with most having single-payer systems. In this latter category falls Denmark, which spends 10% of overall expenditures on healthcare, yet this country ranks the highest among developed countries for patient satisfaction with their healthcare system—90% satisfied or very satisfied (Pederson et al., 2012).

Much of this discrepancy in U.S. healthcare costs compared with other countries began in 1980 with the rise of private healthcare insurers in the United States (and their profit-making motivation) and the greater use of sophisticated, and expensive, medical technology in this country. In the past three decades, health expenditures doubled in other countries, but more than tripled here.

Although we spend more on healthcare than any other country, this does not necessarily mean we have the best healthcare. "Best" can be defined in a number of ways, such as the already mentioned patient satisfaction, but also as access to medical care by the greatest number of citizens, or as a system that prioritizes disease prevention and health promotion, or as in contemporary America, a system that prioritizes costly specialized medical procedures.

The World Health Organization (WHO) and others have measured population health and quality of healthcare and, by almost any measure, we do not do well. Relative to other countries, the United States is 40th in life expectancy, with a life expectancy at birth (men and women) of 78.5 (WHO, 2023a). The United States ranks last overall of 11 comparable high-income countries in quality of healthcare, despite spending far in excess of other countries. Top performers were Norway, the Netherlands, and Australia. The low U.S. ranking reflects poor performance on access to care, administrative efficiency, equity, and healthcare outcomes (Schneider et al., 2021). In short, we just do not get enough "bang for our buck." Regarding number of *healthy* years we have to live—a more important measure of quality of life than mere life expectancy—we spend more than double in healthcare expenditures per capita than Japan, but have 8 fewer healthy years (74.1 vs. 66.1); that is, years free of disease or injury (WHO, 2023b).

One international study compared the United States, Australia, Canada, France, Germany, the Netherlands, New Zealand, and Britain, and suggested that the supremacy of American healthcare may be limited to a handful of preeminent medical centers (Schoen et al., 2009). Although the United States does well in such important aspects of healthcare as providing prompt access to some of the best specialists in the world, 43% of *insured* (!) Americans skipped care at some point during the year because they could not afford the high out-of-pocket costs (Schoen et al., 2009).

Healthcare Versus Medical Care

It is estimated that 60% of early deaths in the United States are due to behavioral, social, and environmental circumstances, versus 10% that result from shortfalls in medical care (with genetic predisposition responsible for the remainder; McGinnis et al., 2002). Paradoxically, however, the behavioral, social, and environmental components of healthcare have not constituted a high priority for the healthcare dollar. In fact, only about 3% of the nation's healthcare expenditures are targeted toward health-promoting and disease-preventing activities.

Most of that 3% goes either to the physician's office or to other clinical settings for preventive measures, such as medical screenings and vaccinations (about one third), or toward health protection in the physical environment, such as toxic agent and radiation control (also about one third). And only a portion of the remainder is spent on changing unhealthy behaviors.

Although there has been undeniable financial stinginess at the federal level in addressing unhealthy lifestyles among the American people, public attention has at least been engaged by this problem behavior ever since the publication of the initial *Healthy People* report in 1979. This report provided considerable credence to the idea that major gains in health and independence in the future can come from personal lifestyle changes.

Dr. John Rowe, director of the MacArthur Foundation's Consortium on Successful Aging, supported this report's message by concluding that our vigor and health in old age are mostly a matter of managing how we live. A classic article in the *Journal of the American Medical Association* (McGinnis & Foege, 1993) suggested that we no longer should view death as being due to heart disease, cancer, stroke, and chronic obstructive pulmonary disease; rather, we should see it as the result of tobacco use, inactivity, poor diet, alcohol abuse, microbial and toxic agents, risky sexual behavior, motor vehicle injuries, and illicit or inappropriate use of drugs.

A 2000 update confirmed this approach to the "actual causes of death." The major cause of death included tobacco (435,000 or 18.1% of total U.S. deaths), poor diet and physical inactivity (400,000 or 16.6% of deaths), and alcohol consumption (85,000 or 3.5% of deaths). These were followed by microbial agents, toxins, motor vehicle crashes, firearm violence, sexual behaviors, and illicit use of drugs (Mokdad et al., 2004). In 2020, tobacco-related deaths (400,000) still dwarfed deaths from COVID-19 (300,000; Kamerow, 2020).

We undoubtedly will continue to devote most of our money to medical care, but we need to focus more of our attention and resources on healthcare.

QUESTION: In your opinion, what are two of the most important changes we need to make to convert our medical care system into a healthcare system? How can we make these changes?

SUMMARY

The field of health promotion has come a long way since it was initially defined as exercise, nutrition, and smoking cessation. Moreover, older adults were typically excluded from early writings on health promotion and disease prevention. They were old after all, perhaps resistant to change, and without much of a future.

Health promotion and aging now cover dozens of topics. Here is just a sampling: the improved health habits of older adults regarding exercise, diet, nonsmoking, and the search for reliable health information; the impact of increasing education and empowerment with age on health status; the reduction in poverty and its impact on the health of older adults due to the success of Medicare and Social Security; the burgeoning and exciting healthy aging program initiatives at the national, state, and community levels; the influence of older adults on politics and public policy on health and income due to their greater involvement in leadership positions and the high percentage of older voters; the participation of older adults in environmental advocacy and the health of our planet; the encouraging research into the association of age with wisdom, emotional resilience, spirituality, volunteerism, and social connectedness; the extraordinary accomplishments in many fields of endeavor by older adults; the confrontation with and reduction in ageism; the increase in not only life expectancy, but health expectancy; the potential for compression of morbidity in old age; and so much more. Anyone who is interested in life is interested in health promotion and aging.

Which brings us to aging. While many health science students have preferred to focus on children and young adults because of the potential to influence persons over a lifetime, others increasingly believe the real action is with older adults. Why? First reason: There are so many older adults. For the first time in American history. older adults will outnumber children under the age of 18 in 2034. Keeping older adults as independent as possible saves countless dollars and resources (disproportionately spent on older patients) that can improve the health and prosperity of society in general. Second reason: There is an immediacy to disease prevention and health promotion in late life that leads to an openness to learn and change. Older adults realize that there is no longer a seemingly endless amount of time left and are enthusiastic learners and doers.

SPRINGER PUBLISHING CONNECT™ | **A robust set of instructor resources designed to supplement this text is located at http://connect.springerpub.com/content/book/978-0-8261-8386-6. Qualifying instructors may request access by emailing textbook@springerpub.com.**

REFERENCES

Only key references appear in the print edition. The full reference list can be accessed by visiting www.springerpub.com/courseconnect. See inside front cover and tear-out card for CourseConnect details.

Albert, S. M., King, J., Boudreau, R., Prasad, T., Lin, C. J., & Newman, A. B. (2014). Primary prevention of falls: Effectiveness of a Statewide Program. *American Journal of Public Health, 104*(5), e77–e84. https://doi.org/10.2105/AJPH.2013.301829

Hogan, C., Lunney, J., Gabel, J., & Lynn, J. (2001). Medicare beneficiaries' costs of care in the last year of life. *Health Affairs, 20*(4), 188–195. https://doi.org/10.1377/hlthaff.20.4.188

Livingston, G., Huntley, J., Sommerlad, A., Ames, D., Ballard, C., Banerjee, S., Brayne, C., Burns, A., Cohen-Mansfield, J., Cooper, C., Costafreda, S. G., Dias, A., Fox, N., Gitlin, L. N., Howard, R., Kales, H. C., Kivimäki, M., Larson, E. B., Ogunniyi, A., ... Mukadam, N. (2020).

Dementia prevention, intervention, and care: 2020 report of the Lancet Commission. *The Lancet*, *396*(10248), 413–446. https://doi.org/10.1016/S0140-6736(20)30367-6

Ngandu, T., Lehtisalo, J., Solomon, A., Levälahti, E., Ahtiluoto, S., Antikainen, R., Bäckman, L., Hänninen, T., Jula, A., Laatikainen, T., Lindström, J., Mangialasche, F., Paajanen, T., Pajala, S., Peltonen, M., Rauramaa, R., Stigsdotter-Neely, A., Strandberg, T., Tuomilehto, J., … Kivipelto, M. (2015). A 2 year multidomain intervention of diet, exercise, cognitive training, and vascular risk monitoring versus control to prevent cognitive decline in at-risk elderly people (FINGER): A randomised controlled trial. *The Lancet*, *385*(9984), 2255–2263. https://doi.org/10.1016/S0140-6736(15)60461-5

Qato, D. M., Alexander, G. C., Conti, R. M., Johnson, M., Schumm, P., & Lindau, S. T. (2008). Use of prescription and over-the-counter medications and dietary supplements among older adults in the United States. *Journal of the American Medical Association*, *300*, 2867–2878. https://doi.org/10.1001/jama.2008.892

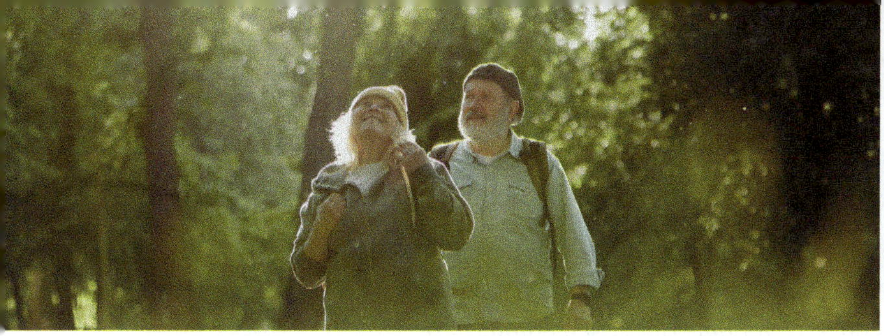

2

CLINICAL PREVENTIVE SERVICES AND AGING

KEY TERMS

accuracy, reliability, and effectiveness
annual physical
aspirin prophylaxis
breast cancer and mammography
cervical cancer, Pap test, and human papillomavirus (HPV)
cholesterol, low-density lipoproteins, high-density lipoproteins, and statins
colorectal cancer and colonoscopy
diabetes and prediabetes
hearing loss
hepatitis C
hypertension and prehypertension
lung cancer
medical screenings
Medicare prevention
menopause, hormone replacement therapy, and the Women's Health Initiative
oral healthcare
osteoporosis, osteopenia, and densitometry
Polypill and Polymeal
prophylaxis
prostate cancer and prostate-specific antigen (PSA) screening
skin cancer
thyroid cancer
vaccinations: influenza, pneumococcal, tetanus, and shingles
visual acuity

LEARNING OBJECTIVES

- Describe the benefits and risks of the *annual physical* examination.
- Define *accuracy, reliability, and effectiveness* of screening tests.
- Examine the decision to cover *lung cancer* screening.
- Contrast breast self-examination, clinical examination, and mammography.
- Critically evaluate routine screenings for prostate cancer.
- Contrast fecal occult blood/DNA test, sigmoidoscopy, and colonoscopy.
- Analyze colonoscopy compliance.
- Review *cervical cancer, Pap smears, and human papillomavirus.*
- Review screening for *skin cancer*.
- Analyze the risk of routine *thyroid cancer* screening.
- Critically evaluate the effectiveness of mammography.
- Explain the Women's Health Initiative, and review the research into hormone replacement therapy.
- Explain the high systolic blood pressure threshold controversies.
- Differentiate osteoporosis and osteopenia, and define densitometry.
- Review the effectiveness of bisphosphonates.
- Examine the cholesterol guidelines and their consequences.
- Analyze the potential of, and concerns regarding, statins.
- Define prediabetes and the utility of this concept.
- Examine *hearing and vision* problems.
- Review *oral healthcare.*
- Review immunization guidelines.
- Examine *hepatitis* C and the baby boomers.
- Define shingles and analyze the use of Zostavax versus Shingrix.
- Review ***aspirin prophylaxis.***
- Examine the *Polypill and Polymeal.*
- Critically evaluate *Medicare prevention* coverage.

Medicine is a science of uncertainty and an art of probability.

—*William Osler*

MEDICAL SCREENINGS AND PROPHYLAXIS: CONSIDERABLE CONTROVERSY

Medical screenings (tests with the potential for the early diagnosis of medical problems) and ***prophylaxis*** (medical prevention) have received justifiable acclaim as well as concern over the years. Many of these interventions remain controversial. It is important that health providers, health educators, and older adults become informed, and that older patients take some responsibility in the decision-making process. Clinicians are not equally well informed about the latest research findings, and even if they are, decisions are often still not clear cut.

Medical screenings and prophylaxis have benefits, but they also have risks—medical, psychological, and financial. Only 20% of respondents in one large survey agreed with the (correct) assertion that the harms of screening tests sometimes outweigh the benefits (Roberts et al., 2018). While some older adults, at their peril, avoid all screenings and prophylaxis, others falsely believe in always opting for screening interventions because it is "better to be safe than sorry."

To weigh benefits versus risks, one can seek out information from the many professional associations such as the American Cancer Society (ACS), the American Heart Association (AHA), the American Thyroid Association (ATA), or the American Urological Association (AUA). But what if a professional association disagrees with a recommendation from a more evidence-based organization, like the U.S. Preventive Services Task Force (USPSTF), a not uncommon occurrence? And what if your physician recommends a medical screening or prophylaxis at odds with the latest research?

The likelihood is that the typical patient will never know about these disagreements and will rely on the recommendation of the physician, more likely than not made during an ***annual physical.***

Annual Physical

Many physicians and patients value an ***annual physical*** because they can address health issues before they become a problem, such as gradual weight gain. Or the physical can provide an opportunity for a yearly conversation about staying well. Also, many adults, particularly older adults, have a chronic medical problem or a lifetime medication that warrants yearly monitoring.

Not only do physicians endorse this annual practice for promoting health, safety, and prevention (Prochazka et al., 2005), but the general public does as well (Oboler et al., 2002). Regarding patients, 92% of Americans say it is important to get an annual physical examination, according to a Kaiser Family Foundation poll. In that same poll, 62% said they went to the doctor every year for their physical examination.

The problem with the annual physical, however, is that it can lead to medical screening tests being recommended too frequently and sometimes inappropriately. Regarding excessive medical testing, consider a study of 1,266 primary care physicians. They were asked if they agreed with a hypothetical scenario of an 80-year-old patient with advanced lung cancer receiving a colorectal cancer screening. Despite the fact that the older patient would not benefit from this screening, 25% of the physicians agreed with this recommendation (Haggstrom et al., 2013).

Consider the 78-year-old mother with advanced lung cancer. Upon visiting her in the hospital, her son found her in recovery following a colonoscopy. She was exhausted, in significant discomfort, and said that the physician was unable to conduct the exam successfully. Here is an example of inappropriate screening. It is inappropriate because the expected years of life gained from screening (and treatment) are unlikely to be realized, given her condition. In fact, she died 40 days later with more appropriate palliative care.

To combat excessive medical screenings, annual physicals that included screening recommendations were replaced by periodic reviews, based on the unique health risk factors, age, and sex of individual clients. This began with the first comprehensive effort to assess the effectiveness and timing of a wide array of medical interventions by the Canadian Task Force on the Periodic Health Examination in 1976. This task force developed explicit criteria for assessing the quality of evidence in published clinical research, and then established decision rules to guide clinicians.

A follow-up effort was begun in 1984 by the USPSTF, which also created a manual, *Guide to Clinical Preventive Services* (USPSTF, 1989). Recommendations in this manual were based on a rating system that gave the most weight to research based on randomized controlled trials, followed by well-designed trials without randomization. The least weight was given to the opinions of respected authorities or expert committees (much to the chagrin of disease-specific professional associations), descriptive studies, and case reports.

Because changes in recommendations are not uncommon, the *Guide to Clinical Preventive Services* is no longer in print. Instead, these recommendations can be accessed online: https://www.uspreventiveservicestaskforce.org/uspstf/

Examining USPSFT screening recommendations with the highest level of evidence ("A" rating) for the "senior" age group yields just four recommendations: screening for syphilis, colorectal cancer, hypertension, and cervical cancer. Even these guidelines are unclear in the case of the very old and mostly left to the discretion of healthcare professionals and patients. "A" ratings indicate "high certainty that the net benefit is substantial" and require that Medicare cover such screenings as part of reimbursed services.

Relaxing ratings to include "B" level evidence yields another 15 recommendations. These cover screening for anxiety and depression, latent tuberculosis, chlamydia and gonorrhea, prediabetes and diabetes, lung cancer, hepatitis B and C, substance use, abdominal aortic aneurysm, asymptomatic bacteriuria, *BRCA* genetic testing (for breast and ovarian cancer), alcohol use, intimate partner violence, osteoporosis, and breast cancer. "B" ratings indicate "high certainty that the net benefit is moderate or there is moderate certainty that the net benefit is moderate to substantial" (https://www.uspreventiveservicestaskforce.org/uspstf/about-uspstf/methods-and-processes/grade-definitions). Both "A" and "B" ratings mean the service is recommended by the task force for universal or primary prevention. "C" ratings indicate that the screening is appropriate only for select subpopulations, and "D" and "I" indicate potential harm or insufficient evidence, respectively.

Note that these screenings are part of a physical exam, not part of the Medicare annual wellness visit (https://www.medicare.gov/coverage/yearly-wellness-visits). The wellness visit focuses on health risk assessment (biometry, medical history, prescriptions, advance care planning, and brief cognitive assessment). Based on the wellness visit, a physician may refer patients for screening.

Should recommended screenings be part of the annual physical exam? Following the "A"-rated recommendations, tempered by expected years of life over which benefits can accrue, seems reasonable. The value of lower-rated recommendations is less clear.

In any case, uptake of preventive health services is a problem. *Healthy People 2030* notes that the proportion of adults who get recommended evidence-based preventive healthcare is currently quite low. The *Healthy People* indicator (drawn from self-reported measures used in the Medical Expenditures Panel Survey [MEPS]) includes physician counseling for preventive behaviors (weight management, alcohol and tobacco use, depression, blood pressure, cholesterol); preventive medical screenings (mammogram, colorectal screenings, prostate-specific antigen screening [PSA], Pap); and immunizations. Only 8.5% of adults aged 35 years and over received all of the recommended high-priority clinical preventive services in 2015 (https://health.gov/healthypeople/objectives-and-data/browse-objectives/health-care-access-and-quality/increase-proportion-adults-who-get-recommended-evidence-based-preventive-health-care-ahs-08). For older adults age 65+, only 5.1% (95% Confidence Interval [CI] 3.9%–6.2%) in 2020 met the criterion. The 2030 target for this age group is 11.5%.

Accuracy, Reliability, and Effectiveness of Medical Screenings

To evaluate medical screenings, a few definitions are necessary:

Accuracy refers to the sensitivity and specificity of screening tests.

Sensitivity of a screening test is defined as the percentage of persons who actually had the disease and tested positive when screened. A test with poor sensitivity will miss persons with the condition and produce a large proportion of *false-negative* results. Persons who receive false-negative results will experience delays in treatment.

Specificity refers to the percentage of persons without the condition who correctly test negative when screened. A test with poor specificity will result in healthy persons being told that they have the disease and will produce a large proportion of *false-positive* results. Persons who receive false-positive results may experience expensive follow-up tests or unnecessary treatment that might not be completely safe.

Even if the test is accurate, that is, sensitive and specific, it must also be reliable and effective.

Reliability refers to the ability of a test to obtain the same result when repeated. The reliability of some screenings, such as mammograms and Pap smears, has increased owing to the initiation of federal certification and annual state inspections of facilities.

Effectiveness refers to whether the test is worth the cost, time, and bother; that is, whether there is a subsequent clinical intervention for a positive finding that can prevent or delay the disease. So, even if a test has good sensitivity, specificity, and reliability, it does *not* necessarily mean the screening will be effective.

These terms come up repeatedly within the following review of medical screenings and prophylaxis measures.

CANCER DEATHS

According to the ACS's *Cancer Facts & Figures 2023*, the three leading cancer killers for women and men are age-related; the older you get, the more likely you will be vulnerable to them. In the United States in 2023, cancers with the greatest annual mortality included cancers of the lung and bronchus (59,910 deaths), breast (43,170), and colon and rectum (24,080) for women, and lung and cancers of the bronchus (67,160), prostate (34,700), and colon and rectum (28,470) for men (*Cancer Facts & Figures 2023*). The good news is that the majority of cancer *survivors* are also over age 65, with older cancer survivors expected to double in number from 2016 to 2040, and to reach 19 million older adults (Bluethmann et al., 2016). More good news: Some of these cancer deaths can be avoided by making modifications in lifestyle (Song & Giovannucci, 2016).

We first examine the four different cancers listed in Table 2.1 and their related screenings, and then consider additional diseases and prophylaxis measures. The numbers indicate improvement, considering increasing numbers of older adults over the half decade.

TABLE 2.1 LEADING CANCER DEATHS, 2017 AND 2023

	WOMEN			MEN	
	2017	2023		2017	2023
Lung and bronchus	66,020	59,910	Lung and bronchus	76,650	67,160
Breast	41,760	43,170	Prostate	31,620	34,700
Colon and rectum	23,380	24,080	Colon and rectum	27,640	28,470

Source: Nutrition Action Healthletter, April, 2019, p. 5 and *Cancer Facts & Figures 2023*, Table 1. https://www.cancer.org/content/dam/cancer-org/research/cancer-facts-and-statistics/annual-cancer-facts-and-figures/2023/mr3-sex-cases-and-deaths-2023-cff.pdf

LUNG CANCER

Lung cancer is a malignant lung tumor that is characterized by an uncontrolled, abnormal growth of cells that invade and destroy healthy pulmonary tissue. Smoking causes most, but not all, lung cancers. Treatments include surgery, chemotherapy, radiation, and other options.

In 2015, Medicare began to cover annual lung cancer screenings for older Americans with a long history of heavy smoking, which includes about 4 million older adults. A "long history" is defined as at least a pack a day for 30 years or the equivalent (e.g., two packs a day for 15 years). The USPSTF recommends that for those with this type of history, an annual screening is recommended between the ages of 55 and 80.

The scans are free and apply to beneficiaries through age 77 (there is an age limit because the risk of death during lung cancer surgery increases with age). Typically, Medicare initiates reimbursement of charges, followed by private insurers. In this instance, though, the Affordable Care Act mandated reimbursement of lung cancer screening for private insurers, and Medicare followed suit a few years later.

Because lung cancer is by far the number-one cancer killer, affecting over 120,070 Americans a year in 2023 (*Cancer Facts & Figures* 2023), why the delay? In part, it was to wait for evidence that CT scans can detect much smaller tumors than the traditional chest x-ray, which seldom caught lung cancer early enough for surgery to be effective.

The delay also brought about the government requirement that lung cancer scans are to be conducted by accredited centers, with up-to-date equipment and thoroughly trained personnel. The concern with previously conducted CT scans was that they detected abnormalities that looked like cancer, which led to invasive biopsies or unnecessary surgery. Accreditation reduces, but does not eliminate, this concern. Between 23% and 50% of lung nodules identified by CT scans are false positives (Huo et al., 2019). This leads to biopsies, bronchoscopies, and thoracic surgeries. The high false-positive rates discourage some from being screened.

Another factor in whether to screen for lung cancer, however, was that in 2018 treatment options became more effective. Lung cancer was not an automatic death sentence. Immune checkpoint blockers (a type of immunotherapy) combined with chemotherapy or radiation resulted in more successful outcomes than chemotherapy or radiation alone.

The USPSTF lists three factors for *foregoing* lung cancer screening: (a) if you stopped smoking more than 15 years ago, (b) if you have limited life expectancy, or (c) if you are unwilling to proceed with lung cancer surgery even if the screening produces positive results.

According to the American Lung Association, cancer screening is recommended for more than 14 million U.S. adults, but only 5.8% of this eligible group were screened in 2021 (https://www.uspreventiveservicestaskforce.org/uspstf/recommendation/lung-cancer-screening). Moreover, screened patients are counseled to return for annual follow-up screening, but falloff is substantial. In one study, only 22.3% of patients returned for screening the following year and under 10% of patients returned within 2 years (Silvestri et al., 2022).

BREAST CANCER

Breast cancer is the second leading cause of death from cancer among women (after lung cancer), accounting for an estimated 43,700 deaths in 2023. An estimated 297,790 new cases of breast cancer were diagnosed in women in 2023 (less than 1% of breast cancers are diagnosed in men). The median age at the time of breast cancer diagnosis is 61 years, with 57% of deaths from breast cancer occurring at age 65+.

The three screening tests for breast cancer are breast self-examination, clinical examination, and x-ray mammography. *Breast self-examinations* have never been demonstrated to reduce breast cancer deaths, but the ACS—along with many physicians—encourages self-examinations on a regular basis. The encouragement is based on the belief that the procedure may be effective, and it is simple, safe, and free.

In one study, however, 266,000 women in Shanghai factories were randomly assigned to either breast self-examination or no intervention. (This experiment could not be conducted in the United States, but because mammography was not widely available in China in the old days, self-examination was the best option available for most women at that time.) The breast self-examinations were supervised and were done correctly and regularly. After 5 years, there was no difference in mortality between the two groups (Thomas et al., 2002). A Cochrane Review summarized this study and other evidence related to self-examination (Kösters & Gøtzsche, 2003) and found no benefit and perhaps harm. In a Russian study, more cancers were found in the breast self-examination group but also almost twice as many biopsies with benign results. Although larger tumors are more likely to be discovered through self-examination, they are unlikely to be found in a timely manner. Also, the accuracy of self-examination is quite low.

An annual *clinical breast examination* for women older than 40 is recommended by the USPSTF. It is unclear, though, whether breast examinations performed by clinicians provide added benefit when conducted in conjunction with mammography.

Consensus on the utility of ***mammography***, low-dose x-ray imaging of breasts, has grown tremendously beginning in 1987. In that year, only 23% of women age 65+ had a mammogram within the preceding 2 years. By 2017, that percentage more than tripled to 72%. The percentage in 2019 was 78% for women age 65 to 74 and 54% for women age 75+ (ACS, 2022, p. 32).

Back in 1987, there was great disparity among White, Black, and Hispanic women, with the latter two groups having a little more than half the percentage of mammograms as the former. But by 2011 that race-ethnic difference had disappeared when controlled for socioeconomic status. Socioeconomic status, though, has remained a problem. Among middle-income women, 75% reported having had a mammogram versus 51% for low-income women (Federal Interagency Forum on Aging-Related Statistics, 2012). More recent data suggest narrowing of this gap by income. Among women age 50 to 74 years, 79% with incomes greater than 200% of the federal poverty level reported having a mammogram. For women below the federal poverty income level, 68% reported mammography.

What accounts for the growth in mammography usage in the past three decades? It was the onset of Medicare coverage and the improvements in the quality of mammograms. In 1992, Medicare began offering partial reimbursement for routine mammograms conducted every 2 years (which increased to annually in 1998). In 1994, Congress approved the Mammography Quality Standards Act, which regulated equipment and personnel, including technologists and physicians, and required federal certification and annual state inspections of facilities.

Despite the annual coverage and quality improvements with the procedure, the specificity of mammograms still left much to be desired. Fifty percent of women who have had 10 mammograms over the past decade or two will have had one false-positive result that required further testing and unnecessary stress and expense. As many as 20% of these false alarms have led to a breast biopsy in which tissue is removed from the suspected tumor.

Ductal Carcinoma In Situ

The effectiveness of early detection is a concern as well, particularly with ductal carcinoma in situ (DCIS), a cluster of cancer cells limited to the milk duct. Although these clusters may eventually spread, the chance of this happening and subsequent death from DCIS is only 3.3% at 20 years. Yet, with advanced digital detection, almost 25% of the clusters are being found in about 60,000 women annually and most recently 51,400 in 2022 (Giaquinto et al., 2022). Most are routinely treated with surgery, radiation, and chemotherapy.

Despite the removal of thousands of DCIS lesions each year, there has not been a reduction in the incidence of invasive breast cancer. Researchers have now differentiated high-grade from low-grade DCIS, with the former being of abnormal shape and more likely to progress to invasive carcinoma. But the latter tends to be treated aggressively as well.

A group of physicians at the Society of Surgical Oncology's 66th Annual Cancer Symposium in 2013 argued not to treat DCIS until invasive cancer appears, as it is almost always treatable at that stage. Dr. E. Shelly Hwang from Duke University reported that it is best to avoid the side effects of premature breast cancer treatment if possible. One way to cut down on premature treatment is for physicians to be careful with the terms they use with patients. If DCIS is labeled noninvasive cancer or Stage 0 breast cancer, about half of the patients studied chose surgery, but if it is called a lesion, or abnormal cells, only one-third opted for surgery. Similar to other "pre" conditions that we examine later (e.g., prediabetes, prehypertension, predementia), Dr. Hwang notes that immediate medical intervention is not necessarily the preferred strategy.

Mammography Controversies

The controversies surrounding mammography began in the mid-1980s and continue today. At issue is whether mammograms should be prescribed starting at age 40 or 50, and whether they should be annual or biennial.

On one side of the debate is the National Cancer Institute and the American Cancer Society (ACS), which recommended (at first) that annual mammograms begin at age 40 and continue indefinitely. On the other side is the USPSTF, which recommended starting at age 50 and conducting them every 2 years until age 75 when individual consultation is recommended.

In 2015, the ACS belatedly moved halfway toward the research-based USPSTF recommendation: annual screenings to begin at age 45 and biennial screenings at age 55 and older.

The age at which mammography screenings should be terminated also generated controversy. The USPSTF recommends the discontinuation of *routine* mammogram screenings after age 74 in consultation with a physician in asymptomatic women whose results had consistently been normal on previous examinations. Yet studies reported that routine mammography was not uncommon in women after age 80, and that a substantial percentage of screened women were unlikely to benefit (Badgwell et al., 2008; Schonberg et al., 2004).

Beginning in 2001, the focus became the effectiveness of mammography *at any age*. Two Danish researchers' revised report (Olsen & Gotzsche, 2001) challenged the long-prevailing orthodoxy that seven large studies conducted in the mid-1980s and involving 500,000 women demonstrated the effectiveness of this screening tool. The Danish researchers reported that five of the seven studies were too flawed to be credible, and the remaining two studies showed that mammography did not save, or even prolong, lives. Their conclusions were endorsed by *The Lancet* journal and by an expert panel sponsored by the National Cancer Institute.

The surrounding publicity following Olsen and Gotzsche's report was nothing short of astonishing. Major professional organizations and experts expressed uncertainty, or they argued either for or against mammograms. In February 2002, Tommy Thompson, Secretary of Health and Human Services, declared by fiat that if you are a woman age 40 or older, you need to get screened for breast cancer with mammography every year. A not irrelevant fact was that Secretary Thompson's wife was a breast cancer survivor whose tumor was detected by mammography.

Peter Gotzsche, the original Danish researcher who started the mammography controversy, concluded that breast cancer mortality rate is reduced by 15% through mammography, but for every woman who has her life prolonged there are 200 healthy women who experience the distress of false-positive findings, and 10 healthy women who have been treated unnecessarily—sometimes with negative consequences (Gotzsche & Nielsen, 2009).

He also reinforced the idea that there are cancers that do not need to be found because they will do no harm if left alone but can create harm by being unnecessarily treated through biopsies and other procedures. Conversely, lethal breast cancers tend to grow quickly and even an annual mammogram (and its cumulative radiation) will do no good.

Doubters of mammography suggested that perhaps the decline in breast cancer death rates was *not* due mostly to early detection, but to the increasing effectiveness of treatments like the drug tamoxifen.

So what is a woman to do?

Mammography Update

The ACS, which has long been a staunch defender of cancer screenings, unexpectedly announced in October 2009 that American medicine had overpromised when it came to mammograms. This announcement followed the USPSTF's latest evidence-based recommendations (though their recommendations were not, and still are not, endorsed by the ACS). Here are the USPSTF's recommendations (USPSTF, 2009):

1. Women without risk factors should undergo screening beginning at age 50 instead of age 40. The risks of mammograms before age 50 exceed the benefits of early detection (Grade C recommendation).
2. Women age 50 to 74 without symptoms or risk factors (e.g., family history) should undergo mammography every other year rather than annually. For every breast cancer death averted in this age group, 838 women must undergo screening for 6 years, generating thousands of screens, hundreds of biopsies, and many cancers treated as if they were life-threatening when they are not. Age is critical in this appraisal of risk and benefit. For every 10,000 women screened by repeat screening, the number of breast cancer deaths that would be avoided over 10 years would be 8 in women age 50 to 59, and 21 in women age 70 to 74 (*Cancer Facts & Figures, 2023*).
3. There is insufficient evidence either for or against a screening recommendation for women age 75+. Women should consult with their physicians at that age.
4. Physicians should stop teaching patients to perform breast self-examinations because there is no evidence they are effective and may produce a false sense of confidence.

Task force members concluded that widespread screening has increased the detection and treatment of small, slow-growing tumors that may never cause harm—and in some cases may even disappear—while failing to detect aggressive tumors because they arise between screenings and grow quickly. There is also a small risk posed by decades of repeated radiation exposure.

QUESTION: What would you say to a client who is asking you for advice on whether to get a mammogram and, if so, when and how often? Why would you answer that way?

A 25-year follow-up study of almost 90,000 women who were randomly assigned either to annual mammograms or no mammograms found that the cumulative mortality rate from breast cancer was almost identical between the two groups. Moreover, the Canadian researchers concluded that the excess of breast cancer identified in the mammography group represented an overdiagnosis of tumors not destined to cause future problems (Miller et al., 2014).

A European meta-analysis of 12 million women in 26 screening programs in 18 countries supported the conclusions of the USPSTF. The chances of saving a woman's life and minimizing the negative effects of overscreening and false-positive results are best with screenings every 2 years between the ages of 50 and 69, with follow-up to age 79 (Paci, 2012).

Dr. Otis Brawley, former chief medical officer at the ACS, reported that "the overwhelming majority of folks over age 75 should not be getting cancer screenings." Nonetheless, in 2011, among women 75 to 79 years old, 62% received a mammogram in the past 2 years, as had 50% of women age 80 and older (Bellizzi et al., 2011). In 2019, among women 75+, 54% received a mammogram in the past 2 years (ACS, 2022).

Over the first two decades of this millennium, we have witnessed an increasing number of women getting routine annual screenings in their 40s (a majority of physicians still recommend it) and over age 75. After the 2009 USPSTF recommendations, it is unclear whether screening decisions have changed (Dehkordy et al., 2015; Wharam et al., 2015). Screening guidelines continue to evolve without clear consensus (Mack & Lapane, 2019).

What is clear is that mammographic techniques have become more expensive because of replacing film with digital mammography and the use of computer-aided detection. Thus, Medicare spending on mammography increased 47% between 2000 and 2010 without an improvement in outcomes (Elmer & Gross, 2014). False-positive mammography screenings and subsequent testing carry a cost of $852 per result. False positives and overdiagnoses in breast cancer screening total perhaps $4 billion per year (Mack & Lapane, 2019).

PROSTATE CANCER

As far as controversy goes, prostate cancer screening does not take a back seat to breast cancer screening. This will become clear by the end of this (apologetically long) section.

More than half of all men over age 60 are bothered by *benign prostatic hyperplasia*, a gradual enlargement of the prostate—a walnut-size gland between the bladder and the penis—that occurs with age. A much more serious diagnosis, though, is ***prostate cancer***, a disease that is second only to lung cancer in cancer deaths in men. About 288,300 men in the United States were diagnosed with prostate cancer in 2023, and about 34,700 men died from it (*Cancer Facts & Figures, 2023*).

Prostate-specific antigen (PSA) screening is a blood test discovered in the 1980s that measures elevated protein levels made by the prostate that might (or might not) be an indicator of cancer. Although the test is recommended for routine use by the ACS, the American College of Radiology (ACR), and the AUA, it is not routinely recommended by the more evidence-based (and less financially influenced) USPSTF. In fact, in 2012, the USPSTF went from no recommendation to recommending *against routine screening*. For men 70+ years, USPSTF still recommends against PSA with a Grade D recommendation; for men age 55 to 69 years the recommendation is Grade C (https://www.uspreventiveservicestaskforce.org/uspstf/recommendation/prostate-cancer-screening).

The USPSTF found that one man in every 1,000 given the PSA test may avoid death as a result of the screening. However, one man for every 3,000 tested will die prematurely because of complications from treatment *and* up to 43 men per 1,000 will be seriously harmed. These 43 men may undergo prostate biopsies that can cause pain, infection, and emotional distress, or a cancer diagnosis that typically leads to surgery or radiation treatment. This, in turn, can render a man impotent and/or incontinent, but not necessarily extend longevity as most men have an indolent form of the disease.

A meta-analysis of five randomized controlled trials (n = 722,000 men!) concluded that routine PSA tests had no effect on all-cause mortality, and only a small effect on prostate-specific mortality—one less death per 1,000 men screened over 10 years versus 29 men who would experience either erectile dysfunction, urinary incontinence, or hospitalization for sepsis (Ilic et al., 2018).

One study reported that the decline of routine prostate cancer screening led to biopsies of prostate tissue with a higher rate of advanced cancers being detected via *Gleason scores*, which measure the percentage of abnormal versus normal cells (Ahlering et al., 2019). The European Randomised study of Screening for Prostate Cancer (ERSPC), however, found a reduction in prostate cancer mortality attributable to PSA testing, which increased between 9 and 13 years postscreening. Still, screening averted just one prostate cancer death per 781 men invited for screening, or only one per 27 additional prostate cancer detected, leading the authors to stress the need for assessment of harms before introducing PSA for universal prevention (Schröder et al., 2014).

Although autopsy studies indicate that prostate cancer is present in about 70% of men at age 80, only 3% of men die from it. A large proportion of prostate cancers are indolent; that is, unlikely to produce clinical symptoms or affect survival. Moreover, many men may live with slow-growing prostate cancers that never cause any problems; but removing them, or radiating them, can cause urinary or bowel incontinence, impotence, painful defecation, or chronic diarrhea without providing any benefit. Nonetheless, studies show that many men in the general population are willing to accept considerable risk for harm to achieve a small reduction in risk of death from prostate cancer (Vernooij et al., 2018).

Routine prostate cancer screening is still promoted by many physicians in the United States despite the unsupportive research findings, as well are conducted at state fairs, workplaces, and shopping malls. It is also promoted by famous people like the comedic actor Ben Stiller, who publicly pronounced (in 2016 at age 49) that the PSA test had saved his life and encouraged all men (even older men) to get routinely screened. In other developed countries, however, it is not recommended to be done on a routine basis by celebrities, or for that matter physicians or researchers.

Why is the United States an outlier? First, in the United States, the media portrays PSA testing as unequivocally beneficial. Behind this media support is the endorsement of routine prostate cancer screenings by both the AUA and the ACS. This led 80% of patients in one sample to agree with the statement that "doctors are sure that PSA tests are useful" (Chan et al., 2003). Second, aggressive medical care is practiced more in the United States than in any other country. Thus, 90% of men in the United States with early-stage prostate cancer will undergo immediate treatment with surgery or radiation.

Did the negative recommendation toward routine PSA screenings by the USPSTF in 2012 have an effect on reducing such screenings? Studies have reported a modest decline in screenings (Li et al., 2015), though this is more likely to have been the case among better-trained, board-certified primary care physicians than with nonboard-certified primary care physicians (Goodwin et al., 2014). Among those who are screened, the rate of watchful waiting versus opting immediately for surgery or radiation has increased from 14% in 2010 to 42% in 2015 (Mahal et al., 2019).

There are other aspects of PSA testing that are challenging. Not only is it questionable whether high PSA scores are predictive of prostate cancer mortality, but people with low PSA scores—about 15% of patients who score below the standard 4.0 ng/mL threshold—may nonetheless have prostate cancer (Thompson et al., 2004). Another uncertain issue is the rapidity with which PSA levels rise. Some researchers have reported this may be a promising line of investigation (D'Amico et al., 2004), while others reported that PSA velocity does not improve the prediction of cancer outcomes (Vickers, 2011).

Let me summarize the discussion of routine PSA screening with a comment from Richard Ablin, the *research professor who discovered PSA in 1970!* Dr. Ablin says that PSA use for routine screening has been a "hugely expensive public health disaster," and he wrote a book titled: *The Great Prostate Hoax: How Big Medicine Hijacked the PSA Test and Caused a Public Health Disaster* (Ablin & Piana, 2014).

Treatment Options

Treatment options for benign and malignant prostate problems vary, and include drug therapy, surgery, radiation, heat, freezing, herbs, and vaccines. The increasing use of saw palmetto, a plant-based remedy for *benign* prostate problems, was deemed promising, providing mild to moderate improvement in earlier studies. A subsequent study, however, reported that there was no significant difference between saw palmetto recipients and placebo recipients (Bent et al., 2006).

A vaccine called Provenge was approved by the Food and Drug Administration (FDA) in 2010 after the vaccine produced promising results with prostate cancer during a clinical trial. This vaccine does not prevent disease, but it may accelerate the body's own immune system to fight cancer after it has developed. The results, however, were controversial, since one would expect the vaccine to extend life by being effective in those under age 65 who were more immunocompetent, but in fact it was more beneficial to those over age 65. Also, the vaccine is expensive—$93,000!

Another expensive option, proton beam radiation, at a cost of up to $100,000 per patient, does not produce any better results than less expensive options (Sheets et al., 2012). In fact, these proton-treated men had more stomach-related side effects. Nonetheless, its appealing high-tech dazzle has led to hundreds of millions of dollars of extra Medicare expenses.

COLORECTAL CANCER

In 2023, there were estimated to be about 153,020 new cases of ***colorectal cancer (CRC)*** and 52,550 CRC deaths, making it the third leading cause of cancer-related death in both women and men (*Cancer Facts & Figures, 2023*). Risk for CRC increases with age, with most new cancers affecting persons age 75 and older. The USPSTF has given an A Grade for CRC screening for adults age 50 to 75 years and a B Grade for adults age 45 to 49 years (https://www.uspreventiveservicestaskforce.org/uspstf/recommendation/colorectal-cancer-screening). Some practitioners feel that the recommendation should have been limited to colonoscopy, and not include other CRC screening modalities. The likely rationale is that the inferior screening alternatives are better than no screening at all, and that those results might subsequently lead to a colonoscopy.

The USPSTF has recommended stool-based tests as well. These include the high-sensitivity guaiac fecal occult blood test (gFOBT), fecal immunochemical test (FIT), and stool DNA test (https://www.uspreventiveservicestaskforce.org/uspstf/recommendation/colorectal-cancer-screening). These tests can have high false positives, and inadequate sensitivity, especially when it comes to their inability to detect nonbleeding polyps. Currently, the only stool DNA test approved by the FDA is a multitarget stool DNA test that also includes a FIT component.

Digital (finger) *rectal examinations* are of limited value because few colorectal cancers (about 10%) can be detected by this procedure.

Sigmoidoscopy, insertion of a flexible tube connected to a fiberoptic camera, is recommended every 5 years for average-risk patients aged 45 to 75. A sigmoidoscopy, however, examines only about 40% of the colon (about 2 feet), and research supports the need for a *colonoscopy,* which examines the entire length of the colon (about 5 feet).

Colonoscopy is the gold standard of colorectal screening, beginning at age 50. The USPSTF recommends colonoscopy screening every 10 years for all adults age 45 to 75 years. Since 1975, the incidence of CRC after age 50 declined 40% and mortality rates declined by 50%. In the absence of evidence, several theories are being offered for this good news, with the three most popular (though not necessarily accurate) being earlier detection of polyps, better diets, and the increased use of aspirin for primary prevention. By contrast, the incidence of CRC has increased among adults under age 50, which has been linked to obesity, sedentary behavior, and diets increasingly characterized by highly processed foods (https://www.cancer.gov/news-events/cancer-currents-blog/2020/colorectal-cancer-rising-younger-adults).

Colonoscopies are most effective when done by high volume gastroenterologists (who perform multiple examinations each day) who are skilled at recognizing flat and indented polyps or serrated lesions in the right side of the colon. In patients tracked for as long as 20 years, the death rate from CRC was reduced by 53% in those who had the test and whose doctors removed precancerous growths, known as adenomatous polyps (Zauber et al., 2012).

While preparation for the test is uncomfortable and, for some, embarrassing, colonoscopies have been increasing among older adults—from 54% in 2008 to 67% in 2016 and 69.7% in 2020, based on estimates from the Centers for Disease Control and Prevention (CDC) Behavioral Risk Factors Surveillance System (BRFSS; https://www.cdc.gov/cancer/colorectal/statistics/use-screening-tests-BRFSS.htm). However, those in the target gerontological group, age 65 to 75, did not have a much higher percentage of screenings than those age 75 and over—the age group with the least chance of benefiting because of limited life expectancy (Schonberg et al., 2015). In the United States in 2019, 25.2% of adults age 65 to 75, 17.2% age 76 to 84, and 8.0% age 85 years and older in the United States reported CRC screening in the prior 12 months (Hornschuch et al., 2022).

One possible way to increase colonoscopies among younger older adults is to have an age peer undergo one on television. There was a 20% increase in CRC screenings over a 9-month period after Katie Couric, then host of the morning

TV show *Today*, whose husband had previously died of colorectal cancer, had the procedure done live on television in March 2000 (Cram et al., 2003). This increase in screenings, however—referred to as the *Couric effect*—was a temporary one.

Medicare covers a fecal occult test annually, a flexible sigmoidoscopy every 4 years, and a colonoscopy every 10 years (more frequently if medically indicated). There is no upper age limit to sigmoidoscopy or colonoscopy when it comes to Medicare coverage, though researchers suggest that this test can be discontinued at age 80 with minimal loss in life expectancy (Lin et al., 2006; Rich & Black, 2000). Beginning at age 75, limited life expectancy and the increased risk of perforating the intestinal lining outweigh the benefits.

Innovative Colorectal Cancer Screenings

The discomfort of preparing for a colonoscopy discourages some from participation and has inspired less intrusive alternatives—none of which are ready for prime time yet. A "virtual" colonoscopy utilizes a scanner that takes hundreds of x-rays at different angles from the outside, and then uses sophisticated software to combine the data to produce a three-dimensional image of the colon. At the current level of technology, however, this type of scan misses growths identified by a traditional colonoscopy, and abnormal results will still require a follow-up with a traditional colonoscopy.

Another approach to colorectal screening involves the swallowing of a small camera to scan from the inside (Hara et al., 2004). Patients do not have to worry about returning the camera; the capsule in which the camera is placed will do what food does.

Another test looks for abnormal DNA in stool samples, and researchers at the Mayo Clinic in Minnesota believe a simple stool test may detect not only colon cancer, but eventually stomach, pancreatic, bile duct, and esophageal cancer as well. USPSTF has endorsed stool DNA screening. One such DNA screening test, Cologuard, was approved by the FDA in 2014, and is quite sensitive in detecting advanced lesions. However, it cannot detect nonbleeding precancerous polyps, is expensive ($600), and a follow-up colonoscopy is recommended.

Funded research is also underway to develop a blood test (e.g., Epi proColon) to determine colon cancer risk. These innovative strategies are in the experimental stage, and a higher rate of compliance for colon cancer screening is likely to be dependent on the success of one of them or on an as yet untested alternative.

OTHER CANCERS

Skin Cancer

Skin cancer is the most common form of cancer in the United States. More than half of skin cancer–related deaths occur in people over age 65. Many years of sun exposure, exacerbated during an earlier time by ignorance of the danger of sunburn and the absence of sunscreen protection, makes the older adult a prime candidate. The American Academy of Dermatology (AAD) estimates that one in five Americans will develop skin cancer in their lifetime (Stern, 2010).

There has been a cultural trend for decades in which people associate being tan with being fit and even successful. This inspired the popularization of tanning beds beginning in the 1980s. Subsequently, in a four-decade study that included this time period, there was an eightfold increase in skin cancer among 40- to 60-year-olds (Lowe et al., 2014).

Basal cell cancer (65%–85% of cases) and *squamous* (15%–30% of cases) cell cancer are the most common malignant skin tumors, increasing in incidence with age, but highly treatable. *Melanoma* (about 3% of cases) is the most lethal type of skin cancer, and it too increases in incidence with age. It can be cured if detected early, but if it persists to metastatic melanoma, it is usually fatal within a year. There is new hope, however, in this type of cancer.

In 2023, the ACS estimated 97,610 new melanoma cases in the United States, with about 7,990 deaths. When melanoma spreads to the brain, the survival rate had been less than 20% at 1 year with traditional care. However, a study testing a new immunotherapy technique, combined with radiation, produced a survival rate of 72% for patients with melanoma and asymptomatic brain metastases (Tawbi et al., 2021). Former President Jimmy Carter (who was not in the study) had melanoma that metastasized to his brain and liver in 2015 that would likely have killed him within a year with traditional treatment. Four years later, after immunotherapy and radiation, a scan revealed no sign of cancer. This type of immunotherapy, referred to as "checkpoint inhibitors," costs $100,000 with significant side effects for slightly over half the sample. (Jimmy Carter lived to be 100 years old.)

The key for all malignant skin tumors is not to ignore a suspicious mole, wart-like growth, area that bleeds easily, persistent sore that won't heal, or a rough and scaly red spot. Any of these signs warrants a trip to the dermatologist. Prevention consists of applying and reapplying sunscreen, wearing a protective hat and clothing, and avoidance of sun during midday hours.

The AAD recommends melanoma screening for all persons age 50 and older, and suggests that it is cost-effective and comparable to other cancer screening recommendations. The USPSTF, however, found insufficient evidence for or against this recommendation. The type of prospective randomized controlled trial that provides the highest level of evidence, and has brought many other screening methods into widespread use, has not been conducted for skin cancer. A population-based mass screening effort in Germany, initially promising, turned out to be inconclusive with longer follow-up and more careful ascertainment of skin cancer mortality (Stang et al., 2016).

The USPSTF also concluded that (a) primary care counseling had only a minor impact on increasing sun-protective behaviors and the modest results may not be clinically meaningful, and (b) sunscreen use had no clear protective effect on melanoma risk (Lin et al., 2011). According to the USPSTF, current evidence is insufficient to assess the value of visual skin examination by a clinician (https://www.uspreventiveservicestaskforce.org/uspstf/recommendation/skin-cancer-screening).

Cervical Cancer

Until the 1940s, more American women died of ***cervical cancer*** than from any other type of malignancy. However, the ***Pap test***, named for its creator, George Papanicolaou, reduced the death rate from cervical cancer by 70%. Consequently, cervical cancer deaths are much less prevalent in the United States than in countries that perform far fewer screenings. Yet, in 2023, there were still 13,960 new cases of cervical cancer in the United States, and 4,310 cervical cancer deaths.

Although cervical cancer rarely develops after middle age, more than 20% of cases of cervical cancer are found in women over 65, though these cancers infrequently occur in women who have been getting regular screening tests for cervical cancer (https://www.cancer.org/cancer/types/cervical-cancer/about/key-statistics.html). Cervical cancers diagnosed after age 65 are largely due to lack of regular Pap smears or ***human***

papillomavirus (HPV) tests earlier in life. Many older women have not had regular screenings and no longer visit gynecologists, the physicians most likely to recommend the test.

The cervix is the narrow organ at the bottom of the uterus that connects to the vagina. If cancer occurs in the cervix, it rarely presents symptoms in its early stage. Therefore, regular Pap smears and HPV tests are important. Medicare covers Pap screening and pelvic examination for older women every 2 years. A *Pap smear*—the collection of cells from the cervix—is recommended for women by the USPSTF beginning at age 30, and it should be repeated every 3 years. Pap smears may be discontinued at age 65 if there have been two consecutive annual Pap smears that are normal (neither cancer cells nor precancerous lesions). The USPSTF concludes that the harms of continued routine screening after age 65, such as false-positive tests and invasive procedures, outweigh the benefits of continued screening.

A *DNA screening test for HPV*—the primary cause (more than 90%) of cervical cancer—has been recommended since 2012 by the USPSTF, in combination with Pap testing, for women ages 30 to 65 on a routine basis every 5 years. An 8-year study in India with 132,000 healthy women demonstrated that a single screening with the HPV DNA test significantly outperformed the Pap smear (Sankaranarayanan et al., 2009). In the United States, HPV detects cervical cancer significantly earlier and more accurately than Pap smears (Ogilvie et al., 2018). Nonetheless, Pap smears are conducted much more frequently than HPV tests because of resistance to change, higher costs, and insufficient research studies comparing the two interventions in the long term.

In 2006, an HPV vaccine named *Gardasil* was approved by the FDA. The vaccine is effective in blocking viruses that cause 90% of cervical cancer cases. The vaccine works best when given to girls before they begin having sex, and preferably between the ages of 11 and 26 (the earlier the better). The vaccine is administered in three shots—two doses if under age 15—over 6 months.

A report from the CDC concluded that the safety profile of Gardasil has been similar to that of other vaccines (Haug, 2009), and there is no evidence that it is unsafe despite the claims by those who are skeptical of the scientific evidence for vaccinations of any type. The negative publicity, however, has had an impact on compliance. In 2014, only 40% of girls had completed the series, and the rate for boys was 22%. (The CDC recommended Gardasil for boys in 2012, 6 years after the recommendation for girls.) In a national telephone survey conducted by the CDC from 2015 through 2020, researchers found increases in HPV vaccination and a decrease in the gender gap. In 2020, 73.7% of males had received at least one dose compared to 76.8% of females (Lu et al., 2022).

The $300 cost for this vaccine was initially a barrier until most health insurance companies began to cover it with no copay. The cost is still a problem with states that do not cooperate with the expanded Medicaid program implemented through the Affordable Care Act. It is an even bigger financial barrier in the developing world, where the incidence of cervical cancer is much higher than in the United States.

Some conservative Christians negatively view the cervical cancer vaccine as a tacit license for the young to engage in sexual activity. One study reported that HPV vaccinations did not lead to increased sexual activity among adolescent and young women (Liddon et al., 2012).

Thyroid Cancer

The thyroid is an endocrine gland located above the collar bone, which controls metabolism and produces more hormones when the body needs more energy. In addition to age as a risk factor in ***thyroid cancer,*** older adults are far more susceptible to thyroid dysfunction, such as *hypothyroidism*, or underactivity, and *hyperthyroidism*, or overactivity, than younger adults; the USPSTF does not recommend routine screening in asymptomatic adults (https://www.uspreventiveservicestaskforce.org/uspstf/recommendation/thyroid-cancer-screening). The task force reports that subclinical thyroid disease is not uncommon in the United States (it is estimated that 15% have subclinical hypothyroidism and 1%–2% have hyperthyroidism) and could lead to unnecessary detection and harmful treatment (Bekkering et al., 2019).

Nonetheless, the ATA recommends routine screening beginning at age 35 and every 5 years thereafter. Because the American Thyroid Association's (ATA) recommendation has *not* been widely implemented in the United States, we do not know what the consequences would be if enacted. However, we do know the consequences of widespread screening for thyroid cancer in South Korea. In 1999, the South Korean government initiated a national health screening program that included thyroid cancer screening (Ahn et al., 2014). Over the subsequent decade-plus, what was once a rare cancer became the most common cancer in South Korea. Paradoxically, this dramatic increase in discovery of thyroid cancer did not alter the number of deaths from thyroid cancer. It did, however, lead to an onslaught of expensive lifelong thyroid replacement therapy, involving the determination of the right dose, with uncomfortable fluctuations in energy and weight along the way to obtaining it.

Thus, routine ultrasound screening for thyroid cancer in South Korea begat an epidemic of costly, uncomfortable, and unnecessary treatment. In the United States, researchers have realized that there is a major difference between noticing symptoms like a lump on the neck or hoarseness and obtaining a thyroid screening, versus establishing a formal and widespread routine screening program to find problems. It is estimated that over one third of adults will have thyroid cancer detected when autopsies are conducted, but we also know that, like prostate cancer, people tend to die with it and not of it.

Another issue is that the prescription, Synthroid (for an underactive thyroid), was the most widely dispensed prescription drug in the United States in 2015, with about 15% of older adults taking it. Typically, an older patient reports fatigue to their physician, which is a common geriatric symptom with a wide variety of causes. The physician orders a TSH (thyroid-stimulating hormone) blood test. The results come back slightly positive, and Synthroid is prescribed. The result? Research suggests that there is no difference in improvement between the drug and a placebo (Stott et al., 2017).

One should conclude that getting a screening is not always the wise choice just because it is "better to be safe than sorry." We should also recognize that not all clinicians base their recommendations on the most current research findings and recommendations.

For screening, as in consumer purchases, caveat emptor (Latin for "Let the buyer beware!").

MENOPAUSE

Menopause is the permanent cessation of menses—the monthly flow of blood from the female genital tract—and begins on average at age 51 (there is also perimenopause, in which the onset of symptoms begins on average at age 45). In the United States, more than 1 million women a year experience menopause (https://www.nia.nih.gov/health/menopause).

There is no definitive medical screening for menopause and its existence is primarily documented by the onset and eventual termination of a variety of symptoms. These symptoms typically include irregular menstrual cycles, hot flashes, changes in mood and cognition, insomnia, night sweats, headache, fatigue, vaginal dryness, dry skin, and weight gain.

Some women do not view menopause as "symptoms" or a medical problem and do not seek a consultation with a physician. At the other end of the spectrum, menopause may be viewed as an estrogen-deficiency disease. Similarly, there is considerable cultural variation in attitudes toward menopause. For instance, a symptom such as vaginal dryness is 20% less likely to be reported as a complaint in Italy than in Canada (Minkin et al., 2015).

Hormone Replacement Therapy

The debate over the use of ***hormone replacement therapy (HRT)*** to relieve the symptoms of menopause and prevent disease was intense and even surpassed the controversies over mammography. It began with serious questions about the validity of the research that had been conducted over the past couple of decades.

The early reports that provided optimism about HRT were based on observational studies in which large groups of women were tracked for years. In these studies, the patients themselves decided whether to take HRT. We later found out that the sample populations for these studies were more affluent, better educated, younger, thinner, and more likely to exercise, and they had greater access to healthcare than women in general. In other words, the sample populations were healthier and had better health habits than other women, and the outcomes were due to sampling bias rather than to the intervention of HRT.

Under the leadership of Bernadine Healy, the first woman to head the National Institutes of Health (NIH), the ***Women's Health Initiative*** was launched in the 1990s and it included the Heart and Estrogen/Progestin Replacement Study (HERS) and its follow-up (HERS II). Using a more rigorous methodology, HERS and HERS II produced different results by correcting the previous sampling bias. Dr. Healy provided the resources to conduct a placebo-controlled clinical trial with random assignment, the gold standard in medical research.

To the surprise of many people, the randomized clinical trials did not agree with several decades of producing consistently positive results from observational studies. Even more surprising, the HERS studies reported that there were negative results, an *increase* in heart attacks, strokes, breast cancer, and blood clots in the legs and lungs among healthy women taking HRT, compared with those on the placebo.

In 2001, the AHA reversed its support of HRT, and for women with cardiovascular illness a recommendation was made to avoid the therapy. In 2002, the NIH became sufficiently convinced about the problems associated with HRT that it sent letters to the 16,000 women participating in the HERS II study, recommending that the therapy be terminated. This announcement had broader implications. On June 21, 2002, there were 379,581 prescriptions filled for Prempro, a popular HRT; on September 20, 2002, only 211,249 prescriptions were filled (Elliott, 2002), a decline of 44% in 3 months.

Physicians now became more cautious with HRT, using lower doses, focusing on menopausal symptoms, and reassessing its effectiveness and continuation more quickly. For disease prevention, there are better options than HRT for heart disease (e.g., statins, aspirin) and osteoporosis (e.g., bisphosphonates).

HRT Update

Between 2002 and 2012, the percentage of postmenopausal women in the United States who reported having ever used HRT dropped from 40% to 20%. However, as later revisions to the Women's Health Initiative appeared (this study continued for more than

15 years and involved more than 160,000 women), the HRT decline stopped because of its low-risk probability for medical events and the strong need some women have to treat menopausal symptoms such as hot flashes, night sweats, and vaginal dryness.

The main criticism of the Women's Health Initiative has been that most of the study participants were women already in their 60s and 70s, a decade or more past menopause. A better target group would have been women within a few years of menopause who were not at a high risk for breast cancer (i.e., family history), blood clots, or heart disease. Short-term hormone treatment, up to 5 years, to control life-disrupting menopausal symptoms would have outweighed the small risks involved with HRT.

Given updated studies, many argue that HRT is a better option for the disruptive effects of menopause than the use of alternative treatments that have turned out to be comparable to placebos. Although over-the-counter herbal supplements like black cohosh are increasingly popular for alleviating symptoms, there is no supporting research on their effectiveness beyond the placebo effect. Black cohosh and a variety of soy products (i.e., weak plant-based estrogens) result in the alleviation of symptoms in up to 40% of menopausal women, but this is about the same percentage of improvement that placebos elicit!

An analysis by a federal task force updated recommendations about HRT use (Nelson et al., 2012), which were similar to the 2012 North American Menopause Society guidelines. They can be summarized as follows:

- HRT is an acceptable choice for women age 50 to 59, or within 10 years of menopause, and who are healthy and bothered by moderate to severe menopausal symptoms.
- The decision to use HRT at any age should be made on a case-by-case basis.
- Low-dose estrogen alone is recommended for women without a uterus and with only vaginal dryness or discomfort during intercourse.
- The North American Menopause Society (2022) advises against hormone therapy for women more than 10 years from menopause onset or who are aged older than 60 years because of the greater absolute risks of coronary heart disease, stroke, venous thromboembolism, and dementia.
- Progesterone and estrogen are recommended for women who still have a uterus, to prevent uterine cancer.
- HRT increases the risk for blood clots in the legs and lungs; this risk is low in women 50 to 59 years old.
- Breast cancer risk increases when HRT is taken continuously for more than 5 years—and possibly earlier. The risk declines when HRT is stopped.

QUESTION: What would you say to a client who is asking you for advice on whether to start HRT? Why did you answer that way?

HIGH BLOOD PRESSURE

The proportion of adults aged 18 and over with hypertension (i.e., measured high blood pressure and/or taking antihypertensive medication) stands at 48.1% (2017–2020; https://www.cdc.gov/nchs/fastats/hypertension.htm). Close to 120 million U.S. adults—one in three—were diagnosed with high blood pressure, and only about one quarter were able to reduce their blood pressure to a safe level (CDC Hypertension Cascade, 2023).

High blood pressure, or ***hypertension***, is defined as the excess force needed to move blood through the vessels. In 2017, the American College of Cardiology (ACC) and the AHA published new guidelines for hypertension management and defined high hypertension as a blood pressure at or above 130/80 mmHg. Stage 2 hypertension is defined as a blood pressure at or above 140/90 mmHg (Whelton et al., 2017). *Systolic blood pressure* refers to the contraction of the left ventricle, and is typically written as the upper or first number. A rise in systolic blood pressure among older adults is age related, but the diastolic blood pressure, or the relaxation of the ventricle and the lower or the second number, is not. Systolic blood pressure, therefore, is the focus of geriatric interest.

The AHA and ACC threshold of 130 mmHg for high blood pressure emerged from data showing that people in the 130 to 139 mmHg systolic range are at double the risk of heart attack or stroke compared with those under 130 mmHg systolic. With this decision, the number of adults with high blood pressure rises to nearly 50%, and among older adults to nearly 80% (https://millionhearts.hhs.gov/data-reports/hypertension-prevalence.html). Some leaders in the blood pressure field, like H. Gilbert Welch, professor of medicine at Dartmouth Institute for Health Policy and Clinical Practice, believe this decision will lead to overmedication of many older adults.

There are typically no symptoms with high blood pressure, and it is therefore referred to as the "silent killer." The lack of symptoms and daily dosing schedule reduces motivation to adhere to a blood pressure medication regimen. The consequences of nonadherence, though, are severe, as there is an increased chance of heart attack, stroke, peripheral vascular disease, chronic kidney disease, retinal damage, cognitive decline, and death.

Interventions to promote medication adherence address a host of patient-specific barriers, typical of many management challenges. These include depression and other comorbidities, low health literacy, medication complexity, cost, recourse to alternative therapies, lack of trust in medical providers, discrimination, poor communication or provider–patient relationships, medication side effects, cognitive impairment, inadequate social support, caregiving responsibilities, and self-neglect (Peacock & Krousel-Wood, 2017).

The risk factors for high blood pressure include age, high sodium intake, ethnicity (Blacks, Latinx), obesity, excess alcohol usage, smoking, inactivity, and stress, but age is the most powerful risk factor. Researchers associated with the Framingham Heart Study of the National Heart, Lung, and Blood Institute reported that Americans aged 55 and over face a 90% chance—let me repeat that, a 90% chance—of developing hypertension over the remainder of their lives (Vasan et al., 2002).

The good news about blood pressure is that it has widespread awareness, especially among older adults. It is estimated that three out of four adults, but 90% of older adults, have had their blood pressure measured within the preceding year (Figure 2.1), though more recent survey data show that less than half (47.9%) of those with hypertension or blood pressure–related health conditions (BPHCs) regularly monitored their blood pressure (Springer et al., 2022). Other good news is that nearly all the drugs used to treat high blood pressure are now generic and low cost. The bad news is that among those with high blood pressure, many are not being treated successfully. Some are unaware of their hypertension, some choose to do nothing, and some are being treated and still do not achieve adequate blood pressure control.

Blood Pressure Thresholds

The USPSTF, as of this writing, has remained with the 140 mmHg threshold for high systolic blood pressure, based on a panel of experts from the NIH, which issued

FIGURE 2.1 Nursing student teaching older adult to take a blood pressure reading.

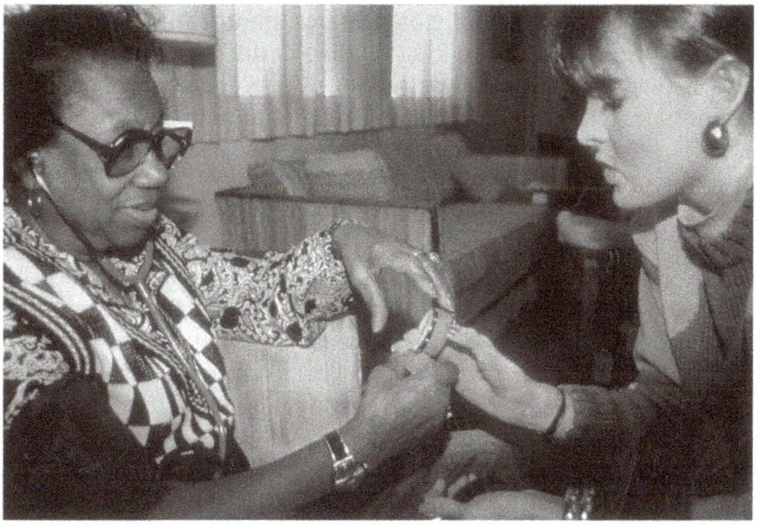

federal guidelines stating that there should *also be a prehypertensive* range. Readings of 121 to 139 mmHg systolic should be considered a transition phase due to likely damage to blood vessels. Although hypertension quadruples the risk of heart disease or stroke, ***prehypertension*** doubles the risk. A designated prehypertension range, however, did not seem like adequate warning according to the AHA and ACC—too vague, perhaps; hence they revised the systolic threshold to 130 mmHg.

So which threshold should clinicians strive for with their patients? The answer is more complicated than 140 versus 130. In fact, there are proponents for 150 and 120 as well!

Regarding the former threshold, the 2014 blood pressure guidelines proposed by expert panel members on the Eighth Joint National Committee on Blood Pressure recommended *less* restrictive blood pressure targets for adults aged 60 and older. These experts stated that the evidence for achieving 150 mmHg systolic blood pressure or lower was as persuasive as the previously recommended 140 mmHg or lower (Weber et al., 2014).

Regarding the latter threshold, though, the SPRINT (Systolic Blood Pressure Intervention Trial) study sponsored by the NIH reported the opposite: The systolic threshold should be lowered to 120 mmHg because the risk of heart attack, heart failure, and strokes declined by one third and the risk of death by nearly one quarter (Supiano & Williamson, 2017). A follow-up SPRINT study reported that intensive systolic blood pressure control may also reduce the risk of cognitive impairment (The SPRINT MIND Investigators for SPRINT Research Group, 2019). A SPRINT reanalysis estimated improvements in survival by 6 months to 3 years, depending on the age at which this more aggressive blood pressure control begins (Vaduganathan et al., 2020).

It took, on average, three medications in the SPRINT study to achieve the lower systolic blood pressure level among persons over age 50 with at least one risk factor for heart disease, but the NIH-sponsored researchers claimed there was no evidence of increased medication interaction effects among drugs, or an increase in the side effects of dizziness and falls.

Proponents and opponents of the SPRINT study findings agree that the research was rigorously conducted. But the critics remain skeptical for a few reasons. The results measured relative decline among older participants rather than absolute decline (8% lowered to 6%, for instance, is a 25% relative deduction, which sounds clinically significant, but is only a 2% absolute deduction). Also, rigorously controlled randomized trials do not always produce the same results in actual clinical practice. Additionally, the incidence of acute kidney injury was twice as high in the group that was aggressively treated to reach the 120 mmHg systolic level. And, finally, the research sample criteria could only be generalized to 35% of those age 75+ in the United States (Wu et al., 2018).

The greatest controversy is over what to do with those age 80 and older. Several studies report that aggressive lowering of blood pressure below 140 mmHg leads to a higher mortality rate (Delgado et al., 2017; Finestone, 2009; Rastas et al., 2006). Many physicians are considering a stepwise approach recommended by Aram Chobanian, MD, at the 2016 American Geriatrics Society Annual Meeting: Set modest target levels for reduction and, if tolerated, reduce the level gradually.

Mary Tinetti, former chief of geriatrics at the Yale School of Medicine and the foremost expert on fall prevention among older adults, reported that older adults who were moderate users of antihypertensives were 40% more likely to have a serious fall than those who did not take antihypertensives. What about the SPRINT study that averaged *three* medications to achieve the 120 mmHg systolic threshold without undue harm? This study needs replication with a sample of adults age 75+. The jury is still out on the risks of inadequate blood circulation and weakness, dizziness, falls, and kidney disease among those over a certain age who aggressively attempt to reach the 120 mmHg systolic threshold.

Treatment

In one study, more than 4,000 hypertensive patients were randomly assigned to take a blood pressure medication or a placebo. Consistent adherence to the blood pressure medicine for more than 4 years added about 1 day each month of extra life, or almost 2 years of extra life for someone who started treatment at age 40 (Kostis et al., 2011).

Nonpharmacological therapies such as exercise, sodium restriction, weight reduction, decreased alcohol intake, smoking cessation, and stress management are promising in lowering mildly elevated blood pressure (Elmer et al., 2006), but these lifestyle changes can be complicated by biological factors (e.g., hypertensive patients who are not salt sensitive) and behavioral factors (e.g., a person's ability to maintain weight loss or sustain an exercise program). Implementation makes a difference: Delivering therapies with behavioral counseling and gradual titration improves adherence (Peacock & Krousel-Wood, 2017).

Finally, there is counseling in the outpatient clinic. Medicare does not provide specific coverage for blood pressure screening (though it is considered part of the overall care covered by Medicare), despite the fact that uncontrolled high blood pressure among older adults is widespread with costly consequences. If Medicare coverage of periodic blood pressure screenings *with counseling* was instituted, it would draw more attention to the problem, encourage more reliable screenings (taking into consideration *white-coat hypertension*; i.e., increased anxiety in the medical office), and encourage follow-up action in a timely manner (Haber, 2001, 2005).

OSTEOPOROSIS

Osteoporosis is a disease in which the bones become progressively more thin, brittle, and susceptible to fracture. Half of all women over age 50 will have an osteoporosis-related fracture in their lifetime. Men lose bone more gradually than women, though they are still at risk. The International Osteoporosis Foundation estimates one in three women and one in five men over age 50 will experience osteoporosis fractures in their remaining lifetimes (https://www.osteoporosis.foundation/health-professionals/fragility-fractures/epidemiology).

Without intervention, about 5% to 10% of trabecular bone, the inner, soft, spongy part of the bone, is lost during the first 2 years after menopause—up to 20% in the 5 to 7 years following menopause—followed by a more gradual loss thereafter. The outer, harder cortical bone thins as well.

Osteoporosis is technically defined as a bone density that is 2.5 or more standard deviations below the young-adult peak bone density, which occurs about age 30. ***Osteopenia*** is a weakening of the bones and can be considered a warning on the way to osteoporosis. It is technically defined as 1 to 2.4 standard deviations below the young-adult peak bone density. It is most accurately assessed through ***densitometry*** (the measurement of bone density), typically through dual-energy x-ray absorptiometry. This screening test is accurate and emits very little radiation.

Osteoporosis and low bone mass are common. In 2010, 10.2 million older adults (2 million men) had a diagnosis of osteoporosis, but overall low bone mass (osteopenia) was 43.9%, leading to an estimate of 43.4 million older adults with low bone mass (Wright et al., 2014). Osteoporosis causes 1.5 million fractures in the United States each year (Office of the Surgeon General 2004). Slightly more fractures are vertebral, followed closely by hip and wrist fractures. Multiple vertebral fractures lead to *kyphosis* or dowager's hump, a painful spine condition that affects height, posture, and the rib cage. This disease can compress the heart and lungs, diminish respiratory and cardiac function, and restrict vision because the head is tilted downward.

A study of more than 200,000 mostly healthy women age 50 and older found osteoporosis in 7% of the women and osteopenia in another 40% (Siris et al., 2001). The fracture rate of women with osteoporosis in the following year was four times higher than for the women with normal bones, and two times higher in women with osteopenia. These study results were surprising not only in detecting the widespread prevalence of osteopenia, but also in the researchers' ability to detect, within a year, a significant increase in fracture rate.

The USPSTF recommends routine densitometry screening beginning at age 65 for all women, though not for men. (Because 20% of older men will experience an osteoporotic fracture in their lifetime, some evidence-based endocrinologists recommend that men over age 74 be screened.) It is not clear how often women should undergo screenings. Medicare pays for a bone density test every 2 years even though researchers suggest that this is too frequent (Gourlay et al., 2012). There was even less consensus at what age—or even if—screenings should be discontinued.

For women ages 50 to 64.5, assessment is often based on risk factors, such as a combination of some of the following: age, sex, Caucasian or Asian race, slender build, bilateral oophorectomy prior to natural menopause, early onset menstruation, smoking, alcohol abuse, physical inactivity, the use of steroid hormones to treat a variety of medical conditions, insufficient calcium intake, and excess caffeine, protein, or salt in the diet (https://www.uspreventiveservicestaskforce.org/uspstf/recommendation/osteoporosis-screening).

For ages 50 to 64.5, risk fracture risk can be estimated with the *FRAX instrument* (Fracture Risk Assessment Tool). Based on a combination of the prior risk factors noted, if the 10-year overall risk of fracture is 9.3% or greater, follow-up dual-energy x-ray absorptiometry screening is recommended.

Treatment

Surprisingly, studies that identify osteoporosis in women report that detection does not necessarily lead to follow-up intervention. In three independent samples, only one fourth (Andrade et al., 2003), one third (Gehlbach et al., 2002), and less than half (Feldstein et al., 2003) of those who had suffered an osteoporosis-related fracture received drug treatment or another intervention for osteoporosis within about one year following the fracture. We identify low bone mineral density well, but use of calcium, vitamin D, and bisphosphoate therapy is underutilized (Elliot-Gibson et al., 2004).

Several years later, interventions have become even less frequent. Only 20% of patients discharged from a hospital with a broken hip had been prescribed bone-strengthening medications—*bisphosphonates® such as Fosamax®, Actonel®, Boniva®, and Reclast®* (Kolata, 2016), despite the high risk of recurrence and even though the medications are off patent and inexpensive. The consequences are severe as only 36% of patients return to independence after a hip fracture after age 65, with the remainder experiencing a significant decline in their ability to perform activities of daily living or death within a year (Tang et al., 2017).

There may be several reasons for this negligence: (a) Advertising of bone-strengthening medications plunged after they went off patent (brand names bring in significant profits; generics do not). (b) After 2007, bone scan reimbursements for physicians were severely reduced resulting in fewer diagnoses (Hardy, 2013). (c) The risks of osteonecrosis (fracture of the jaw) or fracture of the upper femur, which affect one in 1,000 patients, was given disproportionate publicity compared to the 50% risk women have of suffering an osteoporotic fracture in their lifetimes. (d) The side effects of osteoporosis drugs (but not infusions), particularly heartburn, discourage some women.

Among those who have not yet suffered an osteoporosis-related fracture, the disease often goes undetected. Women who are most in need of detection through densitometry—women age 75+—are the least likely to get it. In the 3 years after Medicare reimbursement for osteoporosis screening began, 27% of women age 65 to 70 were tested, but fewer than 10% of women age 75+ (Neuner et al., 2006). This percentage has increased to about 40% a decade later among those aged 75+ (Amarnath et al., 2015), but this is still a dismally low percentage.

This negligence with both screening and treating weakened bones has led to an increase in osteoporotic bone fractures in the United States after 2012, following a plateau with minor fluctuations over the prior 16 years. The overall age- and sex-adjusted fracture rate decreased from 14.67/1,000 person-years (py) in 2007 to 11.79/1,000 py in 2013, followed by a plateau for the next 3 years and then an increase to 12.50/1,000 py in mid-2017 (Lewiecki et al., 2020).

Fosamax (alendronate sodium), the first medication approved by the FDA in 1995, reverses osteoporotic bone loss. It increased bone density by 3% to 9% in one sample of postmenopausal women, whereas a placebo group lost bone (Liberman et al., 1995). This study also reported that women with osteoporosis who took Fosamax were only half as likely to break a hip as women who did not take it.

In 2006, the first generic—that is, no longer patented, and therefore low-cost—version of Fosamax was approved. Boniva, Reclast, and Actonel became generic afterward. All substantially reduce the incidence of new vertebral fractures. For women who do not tolerate oral dosing well, IV injections are available. Having a variety of medications to choose from is fortunate because it increases the likelihood of avoiding side effects that can include muscle pain, leg cramps, joint pain, heartburn, throat irritation, hot flashes, and blood clots.

The FDA has cautioned against the long-term use of bisphosphonates (Black et al., 2012). The agency's analysis found reduced benefit and possible harm from the drugs after 3 to 5 years of use for two thirds of women—the primary exceptions being women who have a history of spinal fracture or an existing fracture. After a 3- to 5-year interval, it is recommended that a patient take a 1- or 2-year break from the drug, with monitoring to determine whether it should be resumed or terminated.

Two interventions for preventing cumulative bone loss are an increase in dietary calcium, or calcium and vitamin D supplementation. However, excess calcium supplementation of about 1400 mg or more a day, or vitamin D intake more than 2000 mg or IU a day, can lead to a risk of kidney stones or even kidney damage. The lifestyle intervention of weight-bearing exercise (walking, not swimming) can be effective if implemented sufficiently prior to a diagnosis of osteoporosis.

CHOLESTEROL

Cholesterol is a lipid—a waxy, white fatty substance that is manufactured by the liver and supplemented through the diet. Excess cholesterol can cling to the interior walls of the arteries and restrict the flow of blood; over time, it can narrow the arterial passages enough to cause a heart attack or stroke.

Cholesterol can be measured by a blood test that monitors two types of lipoproteins. ***Low-density lipoproteins*** (LDLs) carry cholesterol toward the body cells, leading to plaque buildup; hence the name the bad cholesterol. ***High-density lipoproteins*** (HDLs) carry cholesterol away from the cells to the liver, to be further processed and excreted. HDL is referred to as the good cholesterol.

At one time, the cholesterol guideline was a rather simple affair: A total cholesterol level of 240 mg/dL or higher was considered abnormal because it had a substantial association with coronary heart disease. Over time, though, the guidelines have become complex and thresholds have been lowered.

Low-Density Lipoprotein

The National Cholesterol Education Program (NCEP) guidelines got increasingly complex over the years (Expert Panel on Detection, Evaluation, and Treatment of High Blood Cholesterol in Adults, 2001). Determining risk involved more than the simple calculation of a total blood cholesterol level; it involved the calculation of several risk factors, such as LDL, HDL, total cholesterol level, systolic blood pressure, one's 5-year age category, smoking status, abdominal obesity, diabetes, and a family history of heart disease.

In the 2004 update to the NCEP guidelines (Grundy et al., 2004), there was a more aggressive focus on keeping those with a specific type or quantity of risk factors below specific LDL levels. In Table 2.2, *low-risk* people have zero or one of the risk factors noted previously; *moderate-risk* patients have two or more risk factors; and *high-risk* patients have coronary heart disease or its risk equivalent, such as diabetes. Some researchers have added a *very high-risk* category for those with a prior heart attack or stroke and ongoing risk factors.

TABLE 2.2 LOW-DENSITY LIPOPROTEIN (LDL) CHOLESTEROL TARGETS

<70 mg/dL	Optimal for *very high-risk* patients
<100 mg/dL	Optimal for *high-risk* patients
100 – 129 mg/dL	Optimal for *moderate-risk* patients
130 – 159 mg/dL	Optimal for *low-risk* patients

This more aggressive approach increased the number of people who were recommended to take a statin, from 13 million under the 1993 guidelines, to 36 million under the 2001 guidelines, to 43 million under the 2004 update (to 56 million under the 2013 guidelines, discussed in the next section).

Paralleling the aggressive new NCEP guidelines were broader age ranges for assessment purposes. The USPSTF eliminated its upper age limit of 65 for routine cholesterol screening and endorsed Medicare coverage of cholesterol screening every 5 years with no upper age limit.

At the other end of the age spectrum, the USPSTF recommended testing every 5 years or more frequently, depending on cholesterol level, for all men age 35+, women age 45+, and both men and women age 20+ with risk factors for heart disease.

High-Density Lipoprotein

Not all cholesterol guidelines consider HDLs in their formula. Several years ago, researchers suggested that the higher the HDL level, the better. Subsequent research has not borne this out. Instead, HDL levels below 30 mg/dL and above 70 mg/dL are considered risk factors. HDL levels between 40 and 60 mg/dL may act like an arterial cleanser, removing cholesterol from blood vessels and preparing for it to be removed from the body. This level of HDL cholesterol in the blood serum has been linked to lower rates of heart attack and stroke, at least in the short term.

Researchers who have extensively studied the link between cholesterol levels and cardiovascular disease report that it is difficult to assess the long-term benefits of HDLs in terms of protective effects on the heart. As a consequence of the uncertainty in the field, guidelines for desirable and undesirable ranges of cholesterol levels tend to be focused more on the LDLs (Khambhati et al., 2018).

2013 and 2018 Cholesterol Guidelines

The guidelines released at the end of 2013 by the AHA and ACC ignore *regular* monitoring of LDL—once on a *cholesterol-lowering statin drug*, you stay on it. The rationale? The continued fixation on reaching a specific LDL level led to the use of multiple drugs and repeated adjustments of doses. These adjustments did not always correspond with the goal of reducing heart attacks and strokes.

Under the 2013 guidelines, statins were recommended for even more adults, substantially raising the number of Americans advised to take statins. (Some leaders in the field support guidelines that would recommend a statin for 87% of men age 60+ and 54% of women age 60+ [Brody, 2018].) The number of individuals in the general population who reported taking any statin climbed from 31 million (12%) in 2008 to 2009, to 92 million (35%) in 2018 to 2019, nearly a doubling (Matyori et al., 2023).

The 2013 guidelines for statin recommendations include:

- patients with clinically evident atherosclerotic cardiovascular disease,
- patients with primary LDL levels of 190 mg/dL or higher,
- patients with type 1 or 2 diabetes and an LDL of 70 mg/dL or higher in patients age 40 to 75, and
- patients with a 10-year risk of cardiovascular disease of 7.5% or higher using the Atherosclerotic Cardiovascular Disease Risk Calculator (ACDRC), and an LDL of 70 mg/dL or higher, in patients age. 40 to 75 years.

It is the fourth subgroup that increased the number of American adults recommended for statins—those with risk factors but *without evidence of cardiovascular disease.* This was the first time this category of patients has been included in cholesterol guidelines. Some experts question the use of the ACDRC and point out that nearly half of the panel members who came up with these recommendations had financial conflicts of interest.

While recommendations were not made for those over age 75, many older adults in this age category without cardiovascular disease are also on statins. For instance, a study of people over the age of 79 with no history of coronary heart disease, stroke, or vascular disease reported that one third were on a statin (Johansen et al., 2015). This percentage had steadily risen from 9% in 1999 to 34% in 2012.

The 2018 cholesterol guidelines basically supported the recommendations of the 2013 guidelines with a few modifications. For instance, nonfasting assessments of cholesterol would be considered not just more convenient but equally effective at assessing cholesterol levels. More important, there would be less reliance on the ACDRC that computes the 10-year risk of cardiovascular disease for persons age 40 to 75 to be 7.5% or greater (USPSTF recommends 10% or greater), which then triggers a statin recommendation (see the next section on statins). In short, there would be more flexibility with, and individualizing of, statin recommendations from a physician rather than relying on the computed ACDRC score.

Finally, there would be greater emphasis on lowering the LDL cholesterol level for high-risk secondary prevention patients, that is, those with prior heart attack or stroke and ongoing risk factors. This new guideline recommends the maximally tolerated statin therapy for this high-risk group, and the use of one of the expensive PCSK9 inhibitors, Praluent or Repatha, which were unavailable when the 2013 guidelines were formulated, to get the LDL level as low as possible.

Statins

Statins are cholesterol-lowering drugs that most people believe are primarily responsible for reducing the prevalence of cardiovascular disease and lowering the risk for a cardiovascular event. The drugs work primarily by lowering blood levels of LDL cholesterol or stabilizing existing plaque that might break off and trigger a heart attack or stroke. The two most widely used statins are generic equivalents to the well-known brand-name drugs, Lipitor and Zocor. The generic drugs have significantly lowered the costs of these medications.

Given the lower costs and the huge increase in the number of people who are now recommended to take a statin, the percentage of adults on a statin between the ages of 40 and 75 has risen to about one third. What is surprising is that despite the lack of research findings for older adults age 75+, and the absence of a recommendation from any medical, professional, or research organization, the percentage of adults older than 75 taking a statin, according to the CDC, slightly exceeds one third!

While the benefits of statins for secondary prevention—those with cardiovascular disease or prior heart attack or stroke—have been well documented, many controversies remain. The concerns relate to (a) side effects, especially with high-dose statins; (b) taking statins for primary prevention; and (c) taking statins among those age 80+.

Many statin users complain of side effects, although the incidence of side effects due directly to statins is in some dispute. About 25% of older patients complain of muscle and joint pain—some refer to this as *statin-related myalgia*—according to observational studies and clinical experience (Curfman, 2018). This compares to only 5% of older patients complaining of myalgia in clinical trials. Some researchers believe this discrepancy is due either to the anticipation of well-known side effects or to other factors such as arthritis, which are better controlled for (i.e., eliminated as factors) through more rigorous clinical trials.

Another side effect is the increase in blood sugar levels in patients who take statins. Two longitudinal studies (of 10- and 15-years duration) reported a 38% and a 33% increased risk of new-onset diabetes in statin users, respectively (Ahmadizar et al., 2019; Jones et al., 2017). Blood sugar levels and new-onset diabetes increased even more with the higher-dose statins.

About 10% of statin users discontinue usage because of the adverse effects of symptoms (Newman et al., 2018). The side effects of myalgia and increased blood sugar were legitimate enough to have prompted the FDA in 2012 to issue a change in the safety information mandated on the labels of statins, warning of the side effects. The FDA also rejected efforts to sell statin drugs over the counter, in part because of the potential for side effects.

The use of statins for primary prevention at age 75 or older is common but controversial. One study reported no benefit for primary prevention with statin users age 75+, and there was even a nonsignificant direction toward an *increase* in all-cause mortality (Han et al., 2017). The use of statins for primary prevention for those age 75+ without diabetes did not lower risk of cardiovascular disease or all-cause mortality; with diabetes, the effectiveness of statins was less potent after age 85 and disappeared among nonagenarians (Ramos et al., 2018).

A National Institute on Aging expert panel concluded that there was insufficient research to recommend statins for primary prevention for adults age 75+ (Singh et al., 2018), while others suggest more caution regarding the harms of taking a statin for primary prevention (Richman & Ross, 2018).

The use of statins for secondary prevention has been questioned as well when it comes to patients age 80+. One study of statin use by octogenarians who had been hospitalized with coronary artery disease reported no significant effect on long-term survival rates compared with those who did not take a statin (Rothschild et al., 2016).

QUESTION: **There has been a trend toward lowering the threshold for intervention from medical screenings for blood pressure, blood glucose, and cholesterol. This can allow people to take action before the problem gets too serious. It can also lead to more people being on medications and the greater medicalization of healthcare. What do *you* think?**

None of these studies question the benefit of statins if properly targeted and dosed. But they do question whether statins are overprescribed for those at low risk, for primary prevention for those age 75+, and for downplaying the side effects of statins, particularly high-dose statins that become more problematic with advanced age.

There are other concerns as well. Statins interact with a wide range of drugs taken by older adults, including proton pump inhibitors, blood pressure and heart medications, and many antibiotics. Another concern is with daily adherence at the prescribed dose. Data on almost 30,000 Medicare patients age 66 to 75 who had been hospitalized for a heart attack and had been prescribed Lipitor or Crestor revealed 59% adherence at 6 months after discharge and 42% after 2 years (Colantonio et al., 2017).

Americans love the ease and effectiveness of pills, particularly when the alternative, at least early in the disease process or as a preventive measure, is the much more difficult lifestyle commitment to regular exercise and good nutrition. While many physicians support lifestyle changes, they are pessimistic that patients can sustain healthy behavior changes.

Also, at what age or level of frailty does a dietary recommendation for lowering fat or cholesterol levels just foster malnutrition in highly compliant older clients (Figure 2.2)? Malnutrition is not an uncommon issue when it comes to older adults, and avoidance of cholesterol or fat in the diet that triggers malnutrition is a legitimate concern.

Finally, for those who are statin intolerant, or who need to reach a very low LDL level (typically below 70 mg/dL for very high-risk patients), two injectable drugs were approved by the FDA in 2015: Praluent, which when first available was $14,600 a year,

FIGURE 2.2 The late Elizabeth "Grandma" Layton took her first art class at age 68 (in 1977), and drew a picture of her husband, Glenn, on a bathroom scale when he was concerned about weight loss and malnutrition. By drawing pictures of herself and her husband, Elizabeth cured a 30-year depression and had a show at the Smithsonian when she was 82 (elizabethlayton.com).

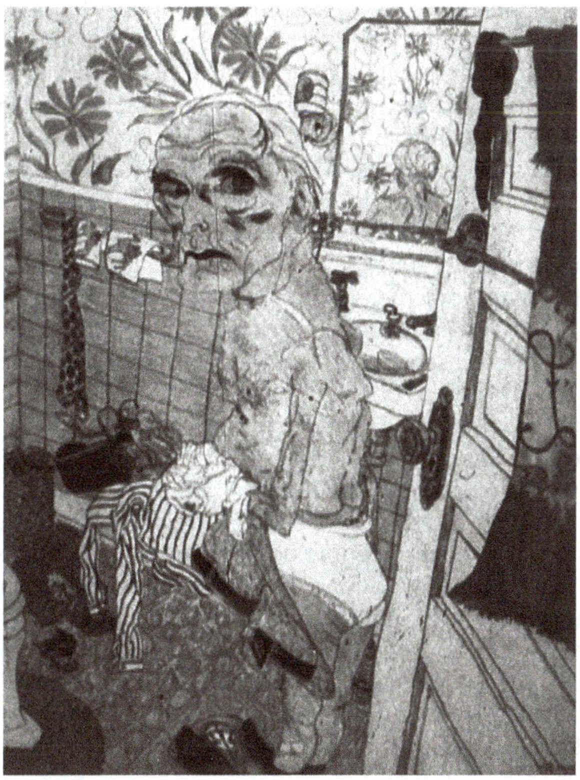

and Repatha, $14,100 a year, were lowered to $5,850 in 2019, but that is still quite high! These two drugs reduce LDLs to levels not obtained previously, but were not being utilized by many patients in 2018 for two probable reasons:

1. It was not until the 2018 guidelines came out that the AHA and ACC declared that these two drugs were effective for lowering the risk of heart attacks, heart failure, and strokes for high-risk patients (in conjunction with statins or in place of statins).
2. Even if their effectiveness becomes more widely known, many patients who would be responsible for a hefty copayment will not be able to bear this cost. Moreover, how will insurance companies bear the cost of Praluent and Repatha, which are *lifetime* drugs, and if broadly used would be the most costly class of medications ever?

DIABETES

Type 2 diabetes (previously called adult-onset diabetes until it started showing up in the teenage years) is the form of the disease related to obesity and inactivity. It refers to a person's increased resistance to insulin, the hormone that is produced by the pancreas and used for metabolizing and utilizing glucose (blood sugar). This resistance leads to *hyperglycemia*, or increased blood sugar, which if uncontrolled leads to the potential for a wide range of diseases, dysfunctions, or death. Lifestyle changes or drugs become necessary. *Hypoglycemia*, or low blood sugar, can be a side effect of antidiabetes medications.

Diabetes is defined as 126 mg or above of glucose per deciliter (mg/dL) of blood. The prevalence of Americans age 65+ with this level of blood sugar is 27% and rising. Alternatively, a hemoglobin A1c level ≥6.5% (≥48 mmol/mol) is recognized by the American Diabetes Association (ADA) and the World Health Organization (WHO) as diagnostic for diabetes. The incidence of diabetes is increasing due to rising obesity and increases in the number of older minorities (Asians, Latinx, and African Americans) with higher incidence rates. Approximately 20% (21.4%) of adults age 65+ years are aware of a diabetes diagnosis, but another 16% is unaware. From 1997 to 2010, the prevalence of diabetes in older adults increased by 62% (Laiteerapong & Huang, 2018). Consequences of untreated disease can be severe. The higher the blood sugar, for example, the greater the vulnerability to physical deterioration as well as the greater decline in mental function (Yaffe et al., 2001).

The ADA, with the endorsement of the NIH, recommended that Americans over age 45 have their blood sugar screened every 3 years. In 2014, the USPSTF was more conservative, recommending screening for all adults age 45 and over, but only for those with diabetes risk factors such as obesity, family history, ethnicity, high blood pressure, or dyslipidemia (high cholesterol). In 2021, the USPSTF expanded diabetes screening to include people age 35 to 70 with overweight or obesity.

Medicare prevention policy is consistent with the USPSTF's recommendation. While it does not routinely cover diabetes screening, in practice Medicare reimburses most older adults for an annual screening because most older adults have one or more of the previously mentioned risk factors. Older adults with diabetes can also receive outpatient self-management training that includes nutrition and exercise education.

For those with prediabetes, Medicare screening can be reimbursed every 6 months. ***Prediabetes*** refers to blood sugar level ranging between 100 and 125 mg/dL (or A1c between 5.7 and 6.4). This continues a trend over the years, when the blood sugar screening threshold for diabetes was lowered from 140 to 126 mg/dL and now, for prediabetes, reduced even lower.

With an estimated 41 million Americans falling within this 100 and 125 mg/dL range, many more cases can be identified in which diet and exercise can prevent or delay the disease. Through diet and exercise, prediabetics can reduce by 60% their chances of eventually developing diabetes. This finding was reported in 2000 at the termination of a behavioral intervention demonstration project called the *Diabetes Prevention Program*. It then took 18 years, beginning on January 1, 2018, before there was Medicare coverage under Part B for participation in this program, with the impetus coming from the Affordable Care Act.

The National Diabetes Prevention Program is available for those with prediabetes, and the content covers stress reduction, dietary coaching, and moderate physical activity. Eligible Medicare beneficiaries attend sixteen 1-hour weekly sessions, followed by monthly sessions thereafter (https://www.cdc.gov/diabetes-prevention/index.html).

One study compared diet, exercise, and weight loss with the use of the drug metformin for preventing the onset of diabetes. Changing lifestyle habits, such as exercise and diet, was nearly twice as effective as using the medication, particularly in people age 60+ who were helped little by the drug (Knowler et al., 2002). Once diabetes is diagnosed, high-intensity resistance training in addition to physical activity or aerobics can improve glycemic control in older persons (Dunstan et al., 2002).

What does the future hold? The CDC (Cheng et al., 2013) reported that diabetes grew by 45% over the past two decades, with the greatest increase among older adults age 65+. Older adults are also living longer with diabetes (Geiss et al., 2014), which may be a mixed blessing. The longer life comes with rising healthcare costs and the quality-of-life burden of living with this chronic disease, which may include impaired kidney function, eye disease, and neuropathy.

HEARING

It is important to deal with ***hearing loss*** because studies consistently report that those with hearing loss are more susceptible to depression, anxiety, isolation, balance problems, falls, and even dementia—less cognitive input, less brain function (Deal et al., 2018). Memory and other cognitive functions may be strained by the extra processing required from hearing-impaired people attempting to comprehend words (McCoy et al., 2005).

Over 50% of adults in their 70s, rising to over 80% of adults in their 80s, have at least mild to moderate hearing loss, according to the National Health and Nutrition Examination Survey. Yet only 15% of older adults who need hearing devices actually have them. In one nationally representative sample of 2,803 older adults, 65.3% (representing 21.5 million individuals) of those age 71+ had hearing loss, as did 96.2% of adults age 90+. However, only 29.2% of those with hearing loss used hearing aids (Reed et al., 2023).

A major barrier is cost—it is not covered by Medicare (with the exception of partial reimbursement through some Medicare Advantage plans), and the typical range is from $2,400 to $5,600 for both ears. Other barriers include vanity, denial of a problem, dissatisfaction with past devices, and fear of technology, which has become quite sophisticated for hearing devices.

It would seem likely that baby boomers will have worse hearing problems, thanks to the popularity of loud rock concerts and headphones for music at too high a volume or too long an exposure. Yet, when researchers conducted the first study to examine generational differences in hearing loss, they tentatively concluded that boomers retain good hearing longer than previous generations (Zhan et al., 2010). The researchers suggested that offsetting the negative influences are fewer noisy jobs, a decline in smoking, and better medical care.

Presbycusis is an age-related hearing loss that results in the inability to register higher frequency sounds. Consonants with higher frequency sounds blend together, and a hearing aid that merely amplifies will not be effective. Interventions for hearing loss, though, have improved markedly over the last decade. Digital hearing aids have a precision enabling them to selectively enhance frequencies that older analog models cannot, and they are able to create a signal that is more finely tuned to the hearing loss of older adults.

Good digital hearing aids, for instance, have directional microphones that prioritize sound from where the person is looking. Sound is amplified in front and is dampened from behind and to the sides, which helps in a room with a lot of low-density, easier-to-hear background noise, like what you find in restaurants. A 2011 survey by AARP and the American Speech–Language–Hearing Association found that 82% of Americans older than age 50 were satisfied with their hearing aids, a large increase from a decade ago. Hearing aids are now connected to smartphones through Bluetooth technology, handy for telephone conversations and podcasts.

Hearing tests are inexpensive and effective, with no known drawbacks except the financial one for obtaining them. Yet, in 2012, the USPSTF did not advise for or against screenings for hearing loss (https://www.uspreventiveservicestaskforce.org/uspstf/recommendation/hearing-loss-in-older-adults-screening). The task force noted that there was only a single randomized clinical trial on the effects of screening for hearing loss. This study reported that adults who tested positive for hearing loss were only slightly more likely to use a hearing aid 1 year later (Yueh et al., 2010). And this study was flawed in that most participants already knew they had a hearing problem before they were screened.

Before buying a hearing aid, clients should consider having an evaluation by an otolaryngologist (ear, nose, and throat specialist) to rule out impacted ear wax and other correctable medical conditions. This should be followed by a thorough audiological examination in a soundproof room, and finally, a visit to a hearing aid practitioner who will work with the client if repeated adjustments are needed. Unfortunately, some practitioners who dispense hearing aids receive a commission from a hearing aid maker, affecting their objectivity in choosing the most appropriate aid for a client (Age, Hearing Loss and Hearing Aids, 2000).

Primarily because of the barrier of cost, legislation was passed in 2017, titled the *Over-the-Counter Hearing Aid Act*, which gave the FDA 3 years to create a regulatory category for such devices and to establish standards for safety, effectiveness, and labeling. Hearing aids and personal sound amplification products (PSAPs) received FDA regulatory oversight in 2022 and are available over-the-counter (https://www.fda.gov/regulatory-information/search-fda-guidance-documents/regulatory-requirements-hearing-aid-devices-and-personal-sound-amplification-products). Because Medicare and most health insurers do not pay for hearing aids, it may be helpful to contact *Hear Now* (800-648-HEAR), which can provide hearing aids to persons whose income level qualifies them for assistance.

VISION

Although less common than hearing impairment, blindness is one of the most-feared disabilities. Although impaired ***visual acuity*** can eventually lead to blindness, effective treatments are available for certain conditions. Nonetheless, the USPSTF does not recommend routine visual screening for older adults because there is no direct evidence yet that screening in primary care settings is associated with improved outcomes (Chou et al., 2009; https://uspreventiveservicestaskforce.org/uspstf/recommendation/impaired-visual-acuity-screening-older-adults).

Presbyopia, a universal age-related change in the ability to focus on nearby objects, begins in most persons in their 40s. Despite this age-related change, visual acuity in the absence of a disease should be correctable to 20/20 even in very old persons.

A *cataract* is a clouding of the lens that reduces visual acuity. In patients over age 75, slightly more than half have visually significant cataracts, which increases to 68.3% for people age 80+ (https://www.nei.nih.gov/learn-about-eye-health/eye-health-data-and-statistics/cataract-data-and-statistics/cataract-tables). Most cataracts can be successfully managed through changes in corrective lenses, and more advanced cataracts can be successfully removed through surgery by replacing the eye lens with an artificial lens. Surgery should be performed when desired activities cannot be performed, rather than on the basis of which stage of the cataract. The surgery can be performed under local or topical anesthesia, has very low morbidity rate and almost no mortality, and 92% report improved visual function after surgery (Lee & Beaver, 2003).

More than 3 million Americans have cataract surgery each year. At a cost of about $3,600 per eye (Medicare copay is 20%), total Medicare costs are about $22 billion. While this is a significant cost, it means greater independence for millions of people. In 2019, 2,361,653 cataract surgeries were performed by 9,171 surgeons in 1,103 U.S. counties (Bhatnagar et al., 2023).

Glaucoma is a condition that occurs when fluid in the eye does not drain and the increased pressure damages the optic nerve. Although it cannot be cured, eye drops can prevent further deterioration. Unfortunately, half of the 3 million Americans afflicted by glaucoma do not know they have it because they do not have their eyes tested often enough. In 2023, about 3.5 million Americans have open-angle glaucoma (https://www.nei.nih.gov/learn-about-eye-health/eye-conditions-and-diseases/glaucoma).

Glaucoma tests should preferably be done every year or two. Medicare covers an annual dilated eye examination for persons at high risk of glaucoma. High risk is defined as having diabetes, having a family history of glaucoma, or being African American. Glaucoma is five times more likely to occur in African Americans.

Macular degeneration, the loss of central vision (see https://www.macular.org), is the leading cause of blindness among older adults and can be self-detected by looking at a dot in the middle of a cross-hatched grid (the Amsler grid) and seeing wavy lines. Approximately 25% of persons age 65+ and 33% of those over 80+ have signs of macular degeneration. Though damage from macular degeneration cannot be reversed, early detection may help slow the progression of the disease. It can be confused with other retinal conditions, however.

The National Eye Institute's Age-Related Eye Disease Study reported that antioxidant vitamins with zinc may slow the progress of macular degeneration in certain subsets of people with the disease. A vitamin E supplement by itself, however, does not appear to slow the progress of macular degeneration (Taylor et al., 2002).

In 2012, University of California–Irvine ophthalmologists implanted tiny telescopes into the eyes of two patients (ages 85 and 94) suffering from age-related, end-stage macular degeneration, and the devices restored limited vision by projecting an image onto the undamaged section of the retina. The patients were able to recognize faces, read, and perform daily activities.

A wide variety of low-vision aids are available, such as large-type books, talking clocks, high-intensity lamps, magnifiers, and computer adapters. These devices are not covered by insurance. Those who are age 65+ may qualify to have a volunteer ophthalmologist perform a comprehensive medical eye examination and provide up to 1 year of care at no out-of-pocket cost. Visit EyeCareAmerica.org. The Seniors Program connects eligible seniors 65+ with local volunteer ophthalmologists who provide a medical eye exam, often at no out-of-pocket cost, as well as up to 1 year of follow-up care for any condition diagnosed during the initial exam (https://www.aao.org/eyecare-america).

ORAL HEALTH

The Surgeon General has reported that Americans' mouths have shown steady improvement from decades ago. For instance, there has been a steady decline in the level of *edentulism* (loss of all teeth) among successive cohorts of older adults. Nonetheless, about 20% of U.S. adults over the age of 65 were edentulous in 2015, increasing to 33% among those age 85+. In 2023, 17% of older adults had lost all of their teeth, a drop of 10% compared to 1999 to 2004 (https://www.cdc.gov/oral-health/index.html).

Income level is the major divider, according to the report, *Older Americans 2016: Key Indicators of Well-Being* (Federal Interagency Forum on Agency-Related Statistics, 2012). Among those living below the poverty level, edentulism is almost twice as high as among those living above the poverty line; those above age 85 have about one-third greater levels of edentulism as those between the ages of 65 and 84. Smoking is another major risk factor. Among older adults who are current smokers, 43% are edentulous, three times the prevalence of those who never smoked.

As the American population ages, visits to physicians increase, but visits to dentists decrease. Only 60% of older Americans reported a dental visit in 2014. The lack of reimbursement by traditional Medicare for dental care is no small factor in this neglect. As older adults retire, many lose employer-based dental insurance and, at the same time, deal with a reduction in income.

The one-third of Medicare beneficiaries who opted for Medicare Advantage plans in 2018 were significantly more likely to have dental coverage than those on traditional Medicare plans. However, these Plan C dental insurance programs are saddled with premiums, copays, and overall caps on what they pay out. Not surprisingly, about 20% of those age 65+ have untreated cavities (this percentage more than doubles for low-income older adults) and an increasing number are choosing to travel to Mexico each year for dental work at much lower prices.

Older adults are also significantly more likely to have to deal with oral cancer or periodontal disease. The latter is a particularly significant problem for older adults, affecting about 70% (with the possibility of bacteria circulating elsewhere and contributing to other health problems such as pneumonia, heart disease, or stroke).

Professional ***oral healthcare*** may be particularly important in nursing homes. A study of older residents in two nursing homes reported that professional oral healthcare given by dental hygienists was associated with a reduction in the prevalence of fever and fatal pneumonia due to aspirated bacteria (Adachi et al., 2002). Other researchers suggest that aggressive oral care might reduce nursing home pneumonias by as much as 40% (Terpenning, 2005).

One public policy initiative that could benefit older adults is the promotion of water fluoridation in the 33% of communities that, as of 2014, still do not treat their public water supplies. A study of more than 3,000 women age 65+ concluded that fluoridation not only enhanced the prevention of dental caries but also appeared to increase bone density in the hip and spine and to slightly reduce the risk of fractures at these sites (Phipps et al., 2000).

Of interest, dental x-ray studies can show the beginnings of low skeletal bone mineral density (Taguchi et al., 2006). A woman may be more likely to be alerted to osteopenia or osteoporosis from a trip to the dentist's office than to get checked for osteoporosis by her physician.

Resources are available to makes it easier for older adults and their caregivers to find low-cost dental care nationwide by identifying community dental clinics, providing dental referrals, locating transportation resources, and identifying other community resources (https://www.hhs.gov/answers/health-insurance-reform/where-can-i-find-low-cost-dental-care/index.html). Your local school of dentistry may offer discounted services by supervised dental students.

HEPATITIS C

According to the CDC, one in 30 baby boomers has been infected with hepatitis C, and about half do not know it. ***Hepatitis C*** is a blood-borne virus that is spread through shared needles, blood transfusions that took place before routine screening began in 1992, and other exposures to infected blood. The virus can also be spread through sexual contact. Hepatitis C causes serious liver disease, such as liver cancer and cirrhosis, and contributed to 34,000 deaths in 2016. It is also the primary cause of liver transplants in the United States. Hepatitis C-associated deaths during 2020 increased 4% (3.45 deaths per 100,000 people), compared to 2019 (3.33 deaths per 100,000 people; https://www.cdc.gov/hepatitis/statistics/2020surveillance/hepatitis-c.htm).

In 2012, the CDC, followed by the USPSTF in 2013, recommended hepatitis C testing for every person born between 1945 and 1965 (roughly comparable to baby boomers, who were born between 1946 and 1964). Routine blood tests can address the largely preventable consequences of the disease, especially in light of newly available and highly effective antiviral therapies that can cure around 90% of infections and have fewer harmful side effects. Unfortunately, the plea for screening has gone largely unheeded, with only 14% of boomers complying by 2016.

Chronic infections from this disease may cause no symptoms for 30 or 40 years, but then people may see symptoms from liver disease thereafter. And once symptoms of liver disease appear, such as jaundice, there is already significant damage to the liver.

If hepatitis C is a virus most often transmitted via blood and body fluids, why does the CDC recommend screening all boomers rather than just those who had a blood transfusion before 1992 or engaged in risky drug or sex behavior in the 1960s? Because people in their 60s may not have perfect memory of what happened in their youth, and it is estimated that about half of those who have hepatitis C do not know they have it. Even more persuasive is that baby boomers account for 2.8 million of the 3.5 million Americans who are infected with this blood-borne disease. The CDC estimates that if all boomers were screened, an estimated 800,000 cases of hepatitis C would be found and 120,000 deaths would be prevented.

While the drug Sovaldi was a wonderful breakthrough in 2014, its cost implications were staggering. Medicare spent more than $3 billion in the first year alone on this one drug, which costs $84,000 for a 12-week treatment. The cost was largely borne by U.S. taxpayers who pay for most of Medicare's underfunded Part D prescription drug program. The good news is that both costs and length of treatment have gone down since the launching of Sovaldi in 2014, followed by Harvoni in 2015 and Mavyret in 2017—from 24 to 8 weeks and from $84,000 to $26,000. Still, the costs remain daunting for clients (20% copayment) and Medicare alike.

Globally, about 150 million people have hepatitis C, and Gilead Science, the drug manufacturer of Sovaldi, offered a generic version to some undeveloped countries at a considerable cost savings. Egypt, once the country with the highest rate of hepatitis C in the world, may become the first to eliminate it. The price of treatment in Egypt is just $80 per person, and the country has already cured 1.6 million cases. Manufactured at just dollars per course of treatment, even the low rate of $80 is profitable for Gilead—not to mention that they already brought in more than $55 billion in revenue between 2014 and March 2018 (Alcorn, 2018).

Other countries, but not the U.S. government (as of this writing), are advocating for lower medication costs, so they can cover more people. Pharmaceutical companies in the United States have lobbied successfully to make sure that Medicare cannot negotiate lower rates. However, in 2023 the United States announced Medicare will negotiate prices for 10 prescription drugs directly with manufacturers, a promising start (https://www.whitehouse.gov/briefing-room/statements-releases/2023/12/07/fact-sheet-biden-harris-administration-announces-new-actions-to-lower-health-care-and-prescription-drug-costs-by-promoting-competition/).

The denial rate for individual hepatitis C coverage is 52% for private insurance companies, 35% for Medicaid programs, and 15% for the Medicare program. In 2015, U.S. prisons were treating less than 1% of inmates known to be infected (Alcorn, 2018).

ARE SCREENINGS GOING TO THE DOGS (AND CATS)?

In 1989, two London dermatologists described the case of a woman asking for a mole to be cut out of her leg because her dog would constantly sniff it. One day the dog tried to bite it off. It turned out that she had a malignant melanoma that was caught early enough to save her life. Similar cases have been reported by a variety of other physicians in regard to dogs detecting skin cancer.

The dog's hypersensitive nose appears to detect changes in blood sugar levels as well. When blood sugar levels fall to dangerously low levels and the person is about to have a hypoglycemic attack, dogs react by whining, barking, licking, or performing some other agitated display (O'Connor et al., 2008). One study reported an 81% predictive value when glucose levels were out of the target range (Rooney et al., 2019). Four of the intervention dogs achieved 100% accuracy.

Dogs are currently being trained in Britain to warn diabetic owners that their blood sugar level has fallen to a dangerously low level. Trained animals are certified as Diabetic Hypo-Alert dogs and are dressed in a red jacket in order to identify them as working assistance animals. One study reported a sensitivity of 83% among trained dogs for detecting a hypoglycaemic episode (Rooney et al., 2019).

An experiment was set up to determine whether dogs could correctly select urine from patients with bladder cancer. The dogs were briefly trained and were able to identify the cancer 41% of the time, compared with 14% expected by chance alone (Willis et al., 2004). In another experiment using breath samples, dogs were accurate in identifying lung cancers 99% of the time and breast cancers 88% of the time (McCullough et al., 2006). Cancer tumors exude tiny amounts of alkanes and benzene derivatives not found in healthy tissue, and it is believed that a dog's sense of smell is between 1,000 and 10,000 times more acute than that of a human being.

Dogs have also been trained through operant conditioning methods over a 24-month period to sniff urine for early detection of prostate cancer. When half of a sample had prostate cancer and the other half did not, the sensitivity and specificity rates were both 91% with 66 patients (Cornu et al., 2011).

Nonetheless, if your dog starts sniffing you repeatedly in a specific area, it is probably not a good idea to begin chemotherapy right away. I would suggest taking a bath first, and if that does not work, head for an open-minded physician and see whether a biopsy is recommended.

We end this chapter with *Oscar the Cat*, a feline who was able to screen for impending death. When Oscar was alive, he had an uncanny ability to predict death at the nursing center where he resided. He presided over the deaths of 25 residents on the third-floor dementia unit at the Steere House Nursing and Rehabilitation Center in Providence, Rhode Island. His presence at the bedside or on the bed of a particular patient was viewed by physicians and nursing home staff as an indicator of impending death. It usually meant that the patient had less than 4 hours to live.

Every day Oscar would make his own rounds, just like the doctors and nurses. When Oscar would sniff the air and decide to curl up on the bed of a resident, the first attending staff person who noticed this would grab the medical chart and quickly make phone calls to notify family members. The priest would also be called to deliver last rites. If there were no family, Oscar provided companionship for those who otherwise would have died alone. After the death of a resident, Oscar would quickly depart.

A geriatrician at this facility, David Dosa, wrote about this phenomenon in *The New England Journal of Medicine* (Dosa, 2007). On the wall of the rehabilitation center where Oscar did his work is a commendation from the local hospice agency, with this inscription on a plaque: "For his compassionate hospice care, this plaque is awarded to Oscar the Cat."

IMMUNIZATIONS

Influenza

Everyone is familiar with the flu, as it affects tens of millions of people in the United States each year. Influenza is a viral infection that affects the entire body but is most evident in the throat and lungs. The CDC estimates that the flu resulted in 9.4 to 41 million influenza-like illnesses, 100,000 to 710,000 hospitalizations, and 4,900 to 52,000 deaths annually between 2010 and 2022 (https://www.cdc.gov/flu/vaccines/index.html).

What is less known about this virus is that 90% of influenza deaths occur in persons age 65+—about 23,000 annually on average (Pilkinton & Talbot, 2015). In the flu season 2017 to 2018, the CDC reported that flu deaths had reached 52,000 and hospitalizations 710,000, both record-breaking numbers for the past century (https://www.cdc.gov/flu/about/season.html). The devastating 1918 flu pandemic is in a class by itself and led to an astounding 675,000 deaths in the United States alone, within a much smaller overall population than today. The 2017 to 2018 vaccine was less effective due to the not uncommon phenomenon of a mutating flu virus that can occur after the vaccine is developed and before it reaches the public.

Because it is contagious, older adults in congregate settings are particularly vulnerable during peak season of late fall and winter. Therefore, it is important not only for older adults to get their annual ***influenza vaccination*** but also for the healthcare workers serving them. Compliance for both older adults and their healthcare workers could stand improvement. Regarding older adults, compliance varies slightly year to year. On average, only two thirds of older adults get vaccinated, with older Whites at a significantly higher rate than older Blacks and Latinx. Belief in the myth that a "flu shot causes the flu" is not uncommon among older adults. During the 2021 to 2022 season, influenza vaccination coverage was lower among Latinx (37.9%), American Indian and

Alaska Native (40.9%), Black (42.0%), and other/multiple race (42.6%) adults compared with White (53.9%) and non-Latinx Asian (54.2%) adults (Black et al., 2022).

Although there are reactions to flu shots, they are rare. An individual allergic to egg products can still be administered a flu shot if the reaction is only hives. If a serious reaction is possible, a consultation with an allergist is necessary.

There is a *high-dose influenza vaccination*, called Fluzone, which delivers up to four times the amount of hemagglutinin in a normal dose. It is recommended for persons age 65 and over. In one study, older adults who took a high-dose flu vaccine during the 2012 to 2013 influenza season were 36% less likely to die in the 30 days following a hospitalization or emergency department visit that included an influenza diagnosis than those who received the standard-dose flu vaccine (Shay et al., 2017). Similarly, nursing home residents who received a high-dose flu vaccine showed a 13% relative reduction in the incidence of hospitalization for respiratory disease, compared with those who received a standard-dose flu vaccine (Gravenstein et al., 2017). Significant benefits were also obtained with older adults at the Veterans Health Administration (Young-Xu et al., 2018).

And yet, hundreds of older adults reported that from 2017 to 2019 only the standard-dose flu vaccines were offered—unless specifically requested by the patient. One researcher noted that the high-dose flu vaccinations cost more and perhaps this and ignorance (i.e., providers were unaware of the cost-effectiveness and public health benefits of the high-dose vaccine) are factors (Raviotta et al., 2016).

Regarding staff vaccination rates, according to the Association for Professionals in Infection Control and Epidemiology, more than 7,000 nursing home residents die of the flu each year, yet only about half of nursing home staff got the flu vaccine during the 2010 to 2012 seasons. Nearly 40% of the staff incorrectly thought that the vaccine could cause the flu. Others did not believe the vaccine was effective, did not find the time, or were unmotivated.

Some states, such as New York and Rhode Island, now require healthcare workers who serve older adults to get a flu shot or wear a mask when near older patients. Because unvaccinated and unmasked workers are more likely to infect, and possibly kill, vulnerable older adults, this legislation makes sense, except perhaps to my libertarian readers who are against all legislation that makes specific health behaviors mandatory (Centers for Medicare & Medicaid Services, U.S. Department of Health and Human Services, 2005). Medicare and Medicaid programs; condition of participation: immunization standard for long term care facilities. Final rule. Federal Register, 70(194), 58833–58852).

It should be noted, though, that while the *Healthy People* objectives call for the mandatory immunization of 90% of healthcare personnel, one study reported that once the vaccination rate of healthcare workers in a specific facility reaches about 50%, there is no further reduction to be obtained in the rate of patients with facility-acquired influenza (Dionne, 2015).

The flu vaccine is far from 100% effective, but over a 6-year period, an analysis from the CDC estimates that about 13.6 million illnesses, 5.8 million medical visits, and 112,900 hospitalizations were prevented by using the vaccine (Reed et al., 2014).

And let us end this section on a happy note—literally! British researchers followed up 138 people age 65 to 85 who got the 2014 to 2015 flu vaccine. A positive mood on the day the influenza vaccination was received predicted vaccine effectiveness. The more positive one's mood, the lower the cortisol (stress hormone) level, the higher the blood levels of antibodies released by the shot, and the better the immune response (Ayling et al., 2018). Next time you get a flu shot, consider watching your favorite stress-reducing movie (for this author, *Groundhog Day*).

Pneumonia

Pneumonia is the inflammation of the alveoli, or small air sacs of the lungs, and surrounding tissues. There are many potential causes, including influenza and other viruses, bacteria, chemical irritants, aspiration of food or liquid, inactivity, and—like influenza—living in close quarters. About 1 million adults are hospitalized for pneumonia and influenza in the United States each year (statisticians find it difficult to estimate separate hospitalizations due to comorbidity), with roughly 50,000 annual deaths from pneumonia. Older adults are significantly more vulnerable than younger adults for both hospitalization and death by pneumonia.

The *pneumococcal vaccine* should be administered to persons 65 and older at least once during their lifetime, with possible revaccination for older persons with severe comorbidity after 5 years (https://www.cdc.gov/vaccines/vpd/pneumo/hcp/who-when-to-vaccinate.html). Vaccinations increased dramatically in the 1990s largely because of Medicare reimbursement. For example, only 10% of older adults in the community had received the ***pneumococcal*** vaccination in 1989; by 1997, 46% of Medicare beneficiaries had received the vaccine. The one-time vaccination rate had increased to 67% in 2016, but still fell well short of the *Healthy People 2020* goal of 90%. As with the flu shot, there is considerable racial disparity with the pneumococcal vaccination, with less than 50% compliance among older Blacks and Latinx.

As of 2014, the PCV-13 (also called Prevnar 13) was recommended as a supplemental vaccination to the previously recommended PPSV-23 (also called Pneumovax 23) at the age of 65. The two vaccines work in different ways and together offer broader protection.

> **QUESTION:** What do you believe accounts for the racial disparity in immunization rates, and what can be done about it?

For those who already had the PPSV-23, the PCV-13 should be added after a year's wait. Those who have not received their first vaccination should receive the PCV-13 first, followed by the PPSV-23 6 to 12 months later. If given at the same time, they can produce a counteracting immune response. Compliance rates for older adults who have received both shots are not yet available.

Tetanus

The ***tetanus*** disease is sometimes called lockjaw, because the first symptom is often a contraction, or stiffening, of the muscles around the mouth. It is caused by a bacterial toxin that affects the nervous system, which enters through a cut or wound that becomes contaminated with the tetanus bacteria.

Most children receive three doses of the vaccine tetanus, diphtheria, and pertussis (Tdap), with a booster for adolescents and adults. If an older adult has not received a Tdap booster, then it is recommended as soon as possible. A one-time Tdap booster, followed by a routine tetanus and diphtheria (Td) vaccine every 10 years, is recommended. Rates of tetanus have declined by 95% since the introduction of the vaccine.

Medicare does not cover tetanus immunization under Part B, but it is covered under Part D (https://www.medicare.gov/coverage/tdap-shots). Less than 50 tetanus cases are reported each year in the United States, with about 70% of the cases leading to death and occur in persons over age 65. Only 58% of older adults have had a tetanus shot in the past 10 years. Even fewer (14%) received the recommended dose of the Tdap vaccine against tetanus, diphtheria, and whooping cough.

Shingles

Shingles, caused by the varicella-zoster virus, is a painful skin rash and blistering on the trunk, but can also affect the face and other areas of the body. The rash begins as irritated red spots that soon develop into vesicles or fluid-filled sacs. This can be accompanied by fever, chills, muscle pain, headache, itching, or numbness. One in six individuals with shingles will develop a chronic condition called postherpetic neuralgia (PHN). Its frequency and severity increase with age, with 20% of people age 60 to 65 years and more than 30% of people age 80+ years progressing from acute shingles to PHN (Fashner & Bell, 2011).

The virus that causes chickenpox in a child latently resides in the nerve roots and manifests as shingles with an increasing incidence with age (Pilkinton & Talbot, 2015). It can reactivate as people's immune systems wane due to age, stress, or an immune-weakening disease such as cancer. Among adults who previously had chickenpox (about 95% of adult Americans), roughly 30% become afflicted with shingles. About a million cases of shingles are reported annually in the United States, with the risk for shingles increasing with age.

A vaccine called Zostavax, roughly equivalent to 14 doses of the pediatric chickenpox vaccine, was approved by the FDA in 2006 to reduce the risk of shingles in people age 60+. In 2018, a new vaccine called Shingrix was recommended for people age 50 and older, even if they have had the prior Zostavax vaccine (which achieved only 31% compliance by 2017). Shingles vaccination among adults age 60+ increased from 6.7% in 2008 to 34.5% in 2018 (https://www.cdc.gov/nchs/products/databriefs/db370.htm). Zostavax is no longer available for use in the United States, as of November 18, 2020 (https://www.cdc.gov/shingles/vaccines/index.html). Why? Shingrix is 97% effective in persons in their 60s, and only declines to 91% in their 70s and 80s. Zostavax, however, is only 64% effective in persons in their 60s and declines to 38% in their 70s and to 18% in their 80s.

There are other differences. Whereas both vaccines are reimbursed under Part D, Zostavax is one shot (about $240, or $48 copay) and Shingrix is two shots, 2 to 6 months apart (about $280, or $56 copay). Older adults report a stronger reaction to the Shingrix shot, with most people experiencing soreness at the injection site for about 2 days, and 10% reporting more significant myalgia, headache, fatigue, and/or fever.

Finally, Shingrix, unlike Zostavax, may protect people with compromised immune systems due to chemotherapy, transplants, HIV, steroids, and so forth. Whereas Zostavax was made with a weakened live virus, Shingrix is made from a synthetic, purified protein which is safer for immune-compromised older adults.

CARDIOVASCULAR DISEASE AND ASPIRIN PROPHYLAXIS

The USPSTF in 2022 recommended against low-dose aspirin for the primary prevention of cardiovascular disease in adults 60 years or older (Grade D; https://www.uspreventiveservicestaskforce.org/uspstf/recommendation/aspirin-to-prevent-cardiovascular-disease-preventive-medication). This position is consistent with the most recent (2019) guidelines from the ACC and AHA and the European Society of Cardiology in 2021 (Cofer et al., 2022). The likelihood that aspirin will prevent a first heart attack may not be greater than the chance that it will cause harmful side effects, including increasing the prospect of stomach bleeding by about two thirds, and a possible increase in the rare event of a hemorrhagic stroke. Among adults without established cardiovascular disease, aspirin was not associated with a reduction in the incidence of all-cause mortality;

moreover, it was associated with an increase in the incidence of major bleeding. The routine use of aspirin for primary prevention for adults, therefore, was questioned (Mahmoud et al., 2019).

Professional associations and experts agree, however, that once having had a heart attack or stroke, a daily baby aspirin is recommended. Daily aspirin can prevent clots from forming in arteries that can cause another stroke or heart attack, and it has anti inflammatory properties that can prevent these plaques from becoming unstable and leading to a blockage. For a person who has had a heart attack or stroke caused by a blocked artery, daily aspirin reduces the risk of a second event by 25% to 30%. In a meta-analysis of secondary prevention trials, 6.7% of people receiving aspirin experienced a serious vascular event compared to 8.2% in controls. Aspirin was also associated with reductions of about a fifth in total stroke (2.08% vs. 2.54% per year) and coronary events (4.3% vs. 5.3% per year), with only a nonsignificant increase in hemorrhagic stroke (Antithrombotic Trialists' [ATT] Collaboration, 2009).

Aspirin, though, is a blood thinner that can cause bleeding events even with the use of a daily baby aspirin (a low dose of 81 mg), the recommended dose for prevention. One third of aspirin users, however, use dosages stronger than that of baby aspirin, which increases the chance of internal bleeding (Williams et al., 2015).

The use of daily aspirin for *prevention* of cardiovascular disease (CVD) has been adopted by 52% of the population between the age of 45 and 75, and the percentage has been rising steadily. There was a 57% increase in usage between 2005 and 2010 among those who have never had a heart attack or stroke. Older adults over the age of 65 were slightly more likely to be on aspirin for primary prevention than those between the age of 45 and 64, despite the increased risk for bleeding past age 60 and especially past the age of 75. Recent trends, however, suggest a downturn. Among adults age 40+ years without CVD, 23.4% (approximately 29 million persons) reported taking daily aspirin for prevention of CVD. Of these, 22.8% (6.6 million persons) did so without a physician's recommendation. Nearly half of adults aged 70 years or older without CVD reported daily aspirin use (O'Brien et al., 2019).

Researchers found in two studies that after 3 years of daily aspirin use, the risk of developing colorectal cancer was reduced by almost 25% when compared with a control group; after 5 years, the risk of dying of cancer was reduced by 37%; and daily aspirin use reduced the risk of cancer progressing to metastatic disease (Algra & Rothwell, 2012; Rothwell et al., 2012). A rigorous randomized clinical trial (n = 16,000) of adults with diabetes taking an aspirin for primary prevention of colorectal cancer, however, did not produce significant differences between those getting an aspirin versus those receiving a placebo (Bowman et al., 2018). The USPSTF recognized the benefit of low-dose aspirin for major cardiovascular disease events but also small absolute increases in major bleeding and less robust results for colorectal cancer (Guirguis-Blake et al., 2022).

Bottom line? If you're an older adult who has had a heart attack or stroke, aspirin is still recommended, but if you are taking it for primary prevention, the balance of risk and benefit is not favorable and the ratio becomes more unfavorable the older you get. The jury is still out on the use of aspirin prevention for colorectal cancer.

THE POLYPILL VERSUS THE POLYMEAL

Much controversy was created by a proposal from Wald and Law (2003) for a single daily pill to be recommended for all persons age 50 and over. This would contain a statin, three half-dose antihypertensives, aspirin, and folic acid. The authors suggested that such a pill if universally implemented for older adults, even those without a history of cardiovascular disease, could reduce the risk of both cardiovascular disease and stroke with minimal adverse side effects. Their formulation was based on the results of meta-analyses of randomized trials and cohort studies. They concluded that the ***Polypill*** would be acceptably safe and "with widespread use would have a greater impact on the prevention of disease in the Western world than any other single intervention." As one colleague put it, "If you are a male over age 50, you should be taking an antihypertensive, a statin, and a baby aspirin daily until proven otherwise!"

After several years of hypothesizing, the researchers had a chance to implement a study and evaluate it. The health implications were impressive. In a placebo-controlled, crossover trial (each person took the Polypill for 3 months and a placebo for 3 months, in random sequence), an estimated 28% of the participants would have avoided or delayed a heart attack or stroke during their lifetime, according to the researchers (Wald & Wald, 2012).

The researchers also estimated that even if only 50% of the population of the United Kingdom (where the research took place) took the Polypill, about 94,000 heart attacks and strokes would be prevented each year. Although single studies can be promising, they are far from conclusive.

In 2019, almost two decades after Wald and Law first proposed their Polypill, progress for its implementation has been slow going. One issue has been a regulatory hurdle: How do you regulate a single pill that combines multiple classes of medications? A second hurdle: Who will subsidize this experiment on a mass scale? Research findings continue to produce positive results but not of a sufficient magnitude or rigor to overcome this hurdle. One review notes, "There are still gaps in its efficacy in primary prevention and reducing total mortality" (Lopez-Lopez et al., 2023).

An argument could be made that lifestyle interventions would be even more powerful than a pill and have no side effects. Interventions to increase physical activity and to improve dietary habits, along with public policies regarding poor-quality food (e.g., banning junk food and vending machines in public schools) and reducing sedentary behaviors (e.g., urban planning to encourage sidewalks and attractive places to walk to) could provide a nonmedical alternative for the prevention of disease and the promotion of health.

A team of researchers from the Netherlands suggested that a ***Polymeal*** would be even better than a Polypill (Franco et al., 2004). The long title of their article provided a good summary of it: "The Polymeal: A More Natural, Safer, and Probably Tastier (Than the Polypill) Strategy to Reduce Cardiovascular Disease by More Than 75%." The Polymeal consists of wine, fish, dark chocolate, fruits, vegetables, garlic, and almonds.

Proponents of nonmedical approaches believe that government policies and research funding for the promotion of health have been inadequate to date. Opponents argue that nonmedical approaches have been tried and proved to be inadequate at best (Green, 2005). This same argument—medical versus lifestyle perspective—plays out in the policy arena of Medicare prevention.

MEDICARE PREVENTION

If you review the USPSTF recommendations inserted into the specific screening summaries in this chapter, you will undoubtedly conclude that the USPSTF recommendations and ***Medicare prevention*** are often out of sync. Much of the content of Medicare prevention interventions (Box 2.1) appears to have been influenced much more by medical

BOX 2.1 Medicare Prevention

One-Time "Welcome to Medicare" Physical

Within 12 months of initial enrollment

Physician takes history of modifiable risk factors (coverage makes special mention of depression, functional ability, cognitive impairment, home safety, falls risk, hearing, vision), height and weight, blood pressure, ECG, advance directives

Annual Wellness Visit

Personalized prevention plan services, similar to Welcome to Medicare, except on an annual basis

Cardiovascular Screening

Every 5 years

Ratio between total cholesterol and HDL, triglycerides

Cervical Cancer

Covered every 2 years, if inadequately screened prior to age 65

Pap smear and pelvic examination

Lung Cancer

Covered annually through age 77 and averaged 1 pack per day for 30 years, or the equivalent (2 packs for 15 years, etc.)

Colorectal Cancer

Covered annually for fecal occult test

Covered every 4 years for sigmoidoscopy or barium enema

Covered every 10 years for colonoscopy

Densitometry

Covered every 2 years

Diabetes Screening

Annually, those with prediabetes every 6 months

Not covered routinely, but includes most people age 65+ (if overweight, family history, fasting glucose of 100–125 mg/dL [prediabetes], hypertension, dyslipidemia)

Mammogram

Covered annually

Prostate Cancer

Covered annually

Digital rectal examination and PSA test

Smoking Cessation

Two quit attempts annually, each consisting of up to four counseling sessions

Clinicians are encouraged to become credentialed in smoking cessation

(*continued*)

BOX 2.1 Medicare Prevention (*continued*)

Immunization

Influenza vaccination covered annually; two pneumococcal vaccinations covered one time each, revaccination after 5 years dependent on risk

Other Coverage

Diabetes outpatient self-management training (blood glucose monitors, test strips, lancets; nutrition and exercise education; self-management skills: 9 hours of group training, plus 1 hour of individual training; up to 2 hours of follow-up training annually [co-pay and deductible apply])

Medical nutrition therapy for persons with diabetes or a renal disease: 3 hours of individual training first year, 2 hours subsequent years

Glaucoma screening annually for those with diabetes, family history, or African American descent

Hepatitis C screening if born between 1945 and 1965, have received a blood transfusion prior to 1992, or used federally prohibited injectable substance

Persons with cardiovascular disease may be eligible for comprehensive prevention programs developed by Drs. Dean Ornish and Herbert Benson: coverage for 36 sessions within 18 weeks, possible extension to 72 sessions within 36 weeks; only in states where offered

Abdominal aortic aneurysm, one-time screening by ultrasound for men aged 65 to 75 years who have ever smoked

Obesity screening and intensive behavioral therapy; face-to-face counseling weekly for a month by a medical provider in a primary care setting, then five more monthly sessions, and then six additional monthly sessions if progress is being made

Depression screening annually, if in a primary care setting that can provide follow-up treatment and referrals

Alcohol misuse counseling annually; if screened positive in a primary care setting by a qualified provider, up to four brief face-to-face counseling sessions annually

Frequency and Duration

The following are *estimates* of what researchers recommend, relying most heavily on the USPSTF recommendations, but not exclusively on them:

Blood pressure: Begin early adulthood, annually, ending around age 85

Cholesterol: Begin age 35 for men, age 45 for women, every 5 years, no consensus after age 75

Colorectal cancer: Begin age 50 (age 45 for African Americans), every 10 years for a colonoscopy, ending around age 80

Mammogram: Begin age 50, every other year, no consensus after age 74

Osteoporosis: Begin early adulthood for women, no frequency recommended

Pap test: Begin at age 21, two normal consecutive annual screenings, followed by every 3 years; two normal consecutive annual screenings around age 65, then discontinue

Prostate cancer: Do not do routinely, except if there is a family history or African American heritage, or in consultation with a physician

(*continued*)

BOX 2.1 Medicare Prevention (*continued*)

Definitions

Hypercholesterolemia: LDL above 160/130/100 mg/dL (low/moderate/high risk), HDL below 40 mg/dL, ratio (total/HDL) 4.2 or above

Diabetes: Fasting glucose 126 mg/dL and above; prediabetes, 100–125 mg/dL

High blood pressure: Over 140 mmHg systolic; between 121 and 139 mmHg systolic, prehypertensive

Osteopenia: 1 to 2.4 standard deviations below young-adult peak bone density

Osteoporosis: 2.5 standard deviations or more below young-adult peak bone density

Note: No deductibles or copayments, unless noted.

ECG, electrocardiogram; HDL, high-density lipoprotein; LDL, low-density lipoprotein; PSA, prostate-specific antigen; USPSTF, U.S. Preventive Services Task Force.

lobbyists advocating for specific segments of the medical industry (e.g., oncology, urology, orthopedics) than by policy derived from evidence-based medicine (Haber, 2001, 2005). You will notice that Medicare coverage errs on the side of starting medical screenings earlier, ending later (if at all), and more frequently in between.

Nonetheless, the expansion of Medicare prevention has been consistent over the years, with major improvements in 1998 and 2005, and then in 2010 when the Affordable Care Act was enacted. The Affordable Care Act eliminated all cost sharing for prevention services, that is, deductibles and co-payments, to maximize access.

Although the expansion of Medicare prevention undoubtedly benefits older Americans, the bottom-line question remains: What is the most effective and cost-effective way to promote health and prevent disease through the Medicare program? How do you get the most bang for your buck? The present system, although consistently improving, still falls far short of ideal.

Mammogram screening is an example of a benefit unduly influenced by medical lobbyists. This benefit was increased to annual screening for all Medicare-eligible women age *40* and older. The USPSTF noted, however, that the earlier, more frequent mammogram screenings, without an upper age limit, is expensive, will not result in reduced mortality rate, and will increase risk of unnecessary additional intervention. The task force raised the prospects of more false-positive results and additional biopsies as a consequence.

Bone mass screening procedures covered by Medicare every 2 years are also unnecessarily frequent and expensive. In women whose bones test normal at age 65, many can safely wait at least 5 years due to potential bone loss developing slowly in most women.

Little criticism can be leveled at the Medicare benefits for colonoscopy for all Medicare-eligible individuals age 50 and over, but continued coverage at age 80+ is not based on the evidence. One could also argue that the sigmoidoscopy, barium enema, and fecal occult test are not worth the expense. However, the most relevant issue—how to increase the unacceptably low compliance rate for colorectal cancer screening—is not being addressed by Medicare policymakers.

Another example of the effects of lobbying is the routine coverage for an annual prostate cancer screening for Medicare-eligible men over age 55. This coverage is made

BOX 2.2 Medicare Prevention and Sex Differences

Medicare was developed by men and began with a sex bias. Older women are more likely to be afflicted with debilitating arthritis, osteoporosis, and other conditions that lend themselves to chronic care. Women are also likely to live longer than men with these debilitating conditions. Older men are more likely to encounter life-threatening acute conditions that require hospitalization. Thus, Medicare reimbursement, with its emphasis on hospital coverage and neglect of tertiary prevention and chronic care support services in the home, favors older men.

Medicare prevention messages may be more effective if tailored by sex. For example, given that only a minority of men have osteoporosis, messaging to encourage densitometry screening may be targeted to women. When it comes to smoking cessation counseling, women have different concerns than men. Research reveals that they have greater anxiety about gaining weight if they should stop smoking.

Finally, America is made up of many cultures, and in some cultures there are differences in the way healthcare providers should communicate with female and male patients, as well as the way the body may be examined.

available despite the lack of evidence that routine screening among older men improves survival. Prostate screening also carries a strong risk of screening results leading to expensive and invasive interventions, whereas the original condition may have posed no harm during the man's life expectancy. The USPSTF does not recommend routine screening—yet Medicare prevention not only reimburses for it but will do so annually.

For information regarding Medicare prevention differences between men and women, see Box 2.2.

Another example of medical lobbying influence is the coverage of an initial electrocardiogram (EKG), despite a USPSTF recommendation against it because it would be inconclusive in terms of how it would change the course of treatment. Moreover, false-positive results will lead to unnecessary invasive procedures, and overtreatment will outweigh any benefit of the test.

The expansion of Medicare benefits for the management of diabetes is not controversial, including the introduction of risk-reduction counseling for prediabetics that began in 2018. Health-promotion advocates, though, are hoping that this would pave the way for routine nutrition and exercise counseling for all Medicare recipients.

In general, there are two criticisms about the cost-effectiveness and effectiveness of Medicare prevention: (a) reimbursement for too-frequent medical screenings is unnecessarily costly and can lead to unintended consequences; and (b) there needs to be a better balance between overly generous medical screenings versus inadequate counseling for risk reduction.

The authors have noted that it would be more effective—and cost-effective—to focus on counseling in the areas of sedentary behavior, inadequate nutrition, smoking and tobacco use, and alcohol abuse (Albert et al., 2018; Haber 2001, 2005). Since that time, several positive steps have been implemented, many of them a product of the Affordable Care Act:

- an initial physical examination that includes prevention counseling;
- annual wellness visits;
- smoking cessation—no longer limited to those who have an illness caused by or complicated by tobacco use;

- comprehensive health promotion programs developed by Dean Ornish and Herbert Benson for beneficiaries with heart problems, in certain states;
- obesity screening and behavioral therapy;
- depression screening in a primary care setting that can provide follow-up and referral;
- alcohol misuse assessment and counseling sessions;
- elimination of deductibles and copayments for prevention services to enhance access;
- screening for social needs in primary care; and
- efforts to deprescribe; that is, stop prescription medications that are inappropriate or unnecessary.

The next steps are (a) to consider judicious expansion of prevention counseling to include both exercise and nutrition, and (b) to publicize all prevention programs. An annual wellness visit through Medicare, for instance, is a good idea, but would be an even better idea if we could increase the proportion of eligible older adults who took advantage of this option. One analysis found an increase among Medicare beneficiaries in yearly appointments for preventive medical care following introduction of the Medicare annual wellness visit in 2011, from 19% to 38% (Chung et al., 2018).

A FINAL WORD

Medical screenings and immunizations are undeniably important tools for disease prevention, but the data collected by the USPSTF years ago resulted in a surprising—at the time—conclusion: The most effective interventions available to clinicians for reducing the incidence and severity of the leading causes of disease and disability in the United States are not clinical activities such as diagnostic testing, but rather those that address the personal health practices of patients. Counseling and patient education need to occupy a central role of the clinician.

To be fair to clinicians, a study reported that the average patient in a family practice waiting room needs 25 preventive services (Yarnall et al., 2003). Using a base panel of 2,500 patients (considered average by the American Board of Family Physicians), the researchers conservatively estimate that 7.4 hours a day, apart from treating emergent illness, would be needed to provide the recommended preventive care in a typical practice. The authors recommended a system for prioritizing prevention services based on the patients' characteristics and behaviors, and a team approach toward prevention, involving health educators and other practitioners in the clinic. Collaboration with health-promoting practitioners in the community is essential as well.

SUMMARY

We live in a world where direct-to-consumer advertisers target consumers with prescription medication advertisements in order to encourage them to influence their physicians. While I am against this idea—I personally want to get drug information from more reputable sources—there is a kernel of appropriate patient advocacy in this practice. The topic of clinical preventive services and aging is best not left solely to clinicians for decision-making. First, older consumers need to express their values and preferences and make these values and preferences a part of medical care decision-making. Second, not all clinicians are up to date on the latest, ever-changing research recommendations.

And third, even when they are, the decisions to be made are often not clear cut and can benefit from patient collaboration.

The realm of chronic care requires that patients participate in their medical care in partnership with clinicians. The word *chronic* tells us right away that we have to be alert to day-to-day changes in our condition, to the effects that medications are having on us, and to collaborate with our health provider on how to make their recommendations easier to follow.

One such category of recommendation, immunizations, is supported by rigorous research; yet one third (pneumonia and flu) to two thirds (shingles) of older adults do not adhere to these recommendations. And among those who receive immunizations, there are decisions to be made—determining which month to get the flu shot and whether it should be a high-dose shot are just examples. Regarding medical screenings, professional medical associations are consistently more aggressive in their recommendations than the USPSTF. Which recommendations does your physician support, and will they explain why?

About half of older adults take a statin and/or baby aspirin. To which half do you belong and why? These decisions become particularly problematic *after the age of 75*, as most research has excluded this age group, and side effects are increasingly common with age. Even though these preventive measures can sometimes reduce heart attacks and strokes, and save lives, they can also cause serious internal bleeding, myalgia, and high blood sugar.

Why do the majority of older women not get a bone scan, and when they do, increasingly decide not to take one of the bisphosphonates? Fractures are not only increasingly likely to happen with age, but their consequences can impact hugely on quality of life, as well as life itself.

Thresholds keep lowering for blood pressure, hyperlipidemia, and glucose levels. Which threshold the clinician recommends or the patient follows has significant repercussions. Regarding prostate cancer, can men resist getting *routine* PSA screenings or, if a high PSA score is obtained, show restraint when watchful waiting may be a sensible alternative? Do Medicare beneficiaries know which free preventive services it provides? Why do so few take advantage of these services?

There are two recommendations: (a) The concept of "better be safe than sorry" when it comes to aggressive medical care in the United States makes little sense. (b) Leaving decisions completely up to the medical provider is not in one's self-interest. At the least, constant self-monitoring and sharing of health goals with providers are basic requirements in the era of chronic care.

REFERENCES

Only key references appear in the print edition. The full reference list can be accessed by visiting www.springerpub.com/courseconnect. See inside front cover and tear-out card for CourseConnect details.

Guirguis-Blake, J. M., Evans, C. V., Perdue, L. A., Bean, S. I., & Senger, C. A. (2022). Aspirin use to prevent cardiovascular disease and colorectal cancer: Updated evidence report and systematic review for the US Preventive Services Task Force. *Journal of the American Medical Association, 327*(16), 1585–1597. https://doi.org/10.1001/jama.2022.3337

Han, B., Sutin, D., Williamson, J., Davis, B. R., Piller, L. B., Pervin, H., Pressel, S. L., Blaum, C. S., & ALLHAT Collaborative Research Group. (2017). Effect of statin treatment versus usual care on primary cardiovascular prevention among older adults: The ALLHAT-LLT randomized clinical trial. *Journal of the American Medical Association Internal Medicine, 177*(7), 955–965. https://doi.org/10.1001/jamainternmed.2017.1442

Lewiecki, E. M., Chastek, B., Sundquist, K., Williams, S. A., Weiss, R. J., Wang, Y., Fitzpatrick, L. A., & Curtis, J. R. (2020). Osteoporotic fracture trends in a population of US managed care enrollees from 2007 to 2017. *Osteoporosis, 31*(7), 1299–1304. https://doi.org/10.1007/s00198-020-05334-y

Lopez-Lopez, J. P., Gonzalez, A. M., Lanza, P., & Lopez-Jaramillo, P. (2023). Benefits of the polypill on medication adherence in the primary and secondary prevention of cardiovascular disease: A systematic review. *Vascular Health and Risk Management, 19*, 605–615. https://doi.org/10.2147/VHRM.S421024

North American Menopause Society. The 2022 Hormone Therapy Position Statement of the North American Menopause Society (2022). *Menopause, 29*(7), 767–794. https://doi.org/10.1097/GME.0000000000002028

Raviotta, J., Smith, K., DePasse, J., Brown, S. T., Nowalk, M. P., & Zimmerman, R. K. (2016). Cost-effectiveness and public health effect on influenza vaccination strategies for U.S. elderly adults. *Journal of the American Geriatrics Society, 64*, 2126–2131. https://doi.org/10.1111/jgs.14323

Reed, N. S., Garcia-Morales, E. E., Myers, C., Huang, A. R., Ehrlich, J. R., Killeen, O. J., Hoover-Fong, J. E., Lin, F. R., Arnold, M. L., Oh, E. S., Schrack, J. A., & Deal, J. A. (2023). Prevalence of hearing loss and hearing aid use among U.S. Medicare Beneficiaries aged 71 years and older. *Journal of the American Medical Association Network Open, 6*(7), e2326320. https://doi.org/10.1001/jamanetworkopen.2023.26320

Stang, A., Garbe, C., Autier, P., Jöckel, K. H. (2016). The many unanswered questions related to the German skin cancer screening programme. *European Journal of Cancer, 64*, 83–88. https://doi.org/10.1016/j.ejca.2016.05.029

Vaduganathan, M., Claggett, B. L., Juraschek, S. P., & Solomon, S. D. (2020). Assessment of long-term benefit of intensive blood pressure control on residual life span: Secondary analysis of the Systolic Blood Pressure Intervention Trial (SPRINT). *Journal of the American Medical Association Cardiology, 5*(5), 576–581.

[illegible]

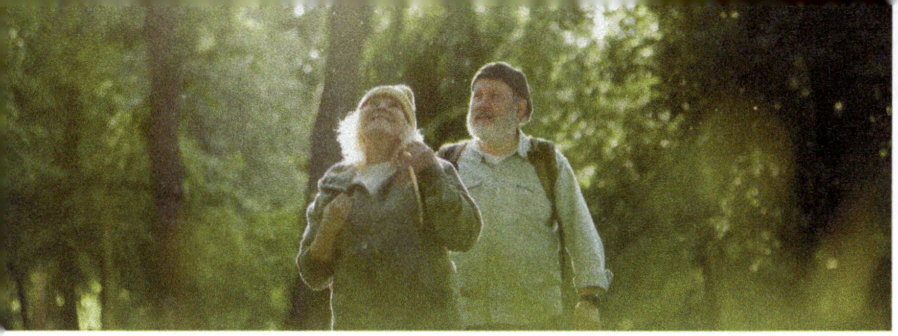

3

EMPOWERING OLDER ADULTS

KEY TERMS

- andragogy
- behavioral and cognitive management
- chronic disease self-management programs
- client versus patients
- communication barriers
- efficacy versus effectiveness
- empowerment
- environmental support
- food behavior diary
- health contract and health calendar
- health risk appraisals
- healthy pleasures and self-monitoring
- informational processing
- interpersonal effectiveness
- jargon and elderspeak
- measurable and modest goals
- motivation
- positive thoughts
- PRECEDE-PROCEED
- problem-solving
- program
- reinforcement
- self-efficacy
- social and behavioral support
- social cognitive theory
- social support
- stages of change
- stress management
- theories versus concepts

LEARNING OBJECTIVES

- Examine ways to encourage *empowerment*.
- Review U.S. Preventive Services Task Force recommendations for health education.
- Identify barriers to effective community health referrals.
- Examine ways to encourage empowerment.
- Explore ways to make a profession more health promoting.
- Review likely sources of health promotion in the community.
- Define and give examples of *andragogy*.
- Examine communication skills associated with ***interpersonal effectiveness***, ***informational processing***, and *social and behavioral support*.
- Assess the credibility of health information on the internet.
- Describe internet deception.
- Review health-promoting resources on the internet.
- Identify *communication barriers* between health professionals and older clients.
- Examine the five spheres of influence on early deaths.
- Evaluate *health risk appraisals* and reflective health assessments.
- Describe *stages of change*, and explore precontemplation in particular.
- Describe the health contract technique.
- Implement a health contract with an older adult.
- Describe the *PRECEDE* model.
- Describe and apply the 10 tips for changing a health behavior.
- Differentiate among behavior management, cognitive management, healthy pleasure, social cognitive theory, self-efficacy, health locus of control, and health belief model.
- Analyze the impact of a *food behavior diary*.
- Distinguish between efficacious and effective *chronic disease self-management programs*.
- Contrast *theories versus concepts*.

EMPOWERING OLDER ADULTS AS EFFECTIVE PATIENTS AND PARTNERS IN SECURING HEALTH

Empowerment for an older person means having the opportunity to learn, discuss, decide, and act on decisions. From the perspective of the health professional or health educator, empowerment of older patients in the clinic setting or clients at a community site means not only to provide service, but also to collaborate with them and encourage their participation.

We begin with the health educator and the older client. The health educator empowers a client to overcome passivity, negativity, ignorance, and other barriers. This is a challenging goal because of both the limited time available in a professional/client encounter and the complexity of the challenges. Consider the following:

- An older client with unhealthy lifestyle habits expresses the desire to eat less and get more exercise, but is discouraged because of repeated and unsuccessful past attempts. Moreover, their latest diet, which they enthusiastically embrace, is not based on sound nutritional principles.
- A chronically impaired older client, or a member of their family, is disgruntled by the lack of some long-term care service, such as home care or respite, that could enhance the client's independence or the family caregiver's mental health. However, this service is not covered by Medicare or a Medigap insurance policy, and the family cannot afford it as an out-of-pocket expense.
- An older client is recovering from cancer surgery and appears to be isolated and discouraged. Because of shyness and privacy reasons, they resist joining a support group with people who are coping with similar challenges.
- An older client who takes multiple medications on an ongoing basis is having trouble complying with their medication regimen despite repeated educational efforts of clinicians. Moreover, the client believes in some questionable over-the-counter drugs.

Passive, negative, or uninformed clients or family members have little hope of rectifying any of these situations on their own. Despite the challenges, health educators have an opportunity to assist and empower. They can motivate, educate, refer, and follow up.

QUESTION: The term *empowerment* can easily be viewed as a buzzword (thrown around a lot, signifying much but meaning little). Do you feel that way? Can you give an example of how you or someone you know became a more empowered student, teacher, practitioner, patient, or client?

The U.S. Preventive Services Task Force (USPSTF) lists recommendations for health educators that are useful for empowering clients. These recommendations are liberally paraphrased as follows:

- Consider yourself a consultant and help your client remain in control of their own health choices.
- Recognize and be informed about the differences you will encounter with your client, who will differ from you in some important ways, such as age, educational level, gender, religion, or culture.
- Make sure your client understands the relationship between behavior and health. Knowledge is necessary, but not sufficient, to change a behavior.
- Assess your client's barriers to change, including possible lack of skill, motivation, education, resources, and social support.
- Encourage your client to commit to change, involving them in the selection of risk factors to eliminate and methods to achieve this.
- Use a combination of strategies, including behavioral and cognitive techniques, the identification and encouragement of social support, and appropriate referrals.
- Monitor progress through follow-up e-mails, texts, telephone calls, and appointments.
- Be a role model.

Community Health Promotion Programs

Referral to an appropriate and effective community health ***program*** is an essential skill for a health educator. Why is it a skill? Because of the challenges of identifying *appropriate* and *effective* services. The past decades have witnessed a proliferation of low-cost or free educational opportunities for older adults within the community (with the exception of many rural areas). Thus, there are a considerable number of health-promoting opportunities to choose from.

These opportunities may include programs sponsored by the local senior center, area agency on aging, YMCA/YWCA, hospital, religious institution, AARP organization, health professional association, health advocacy group, support group, university- or community college–affiliated program such as Road Scholar or Osher Lifelong Learning, mall-walker program, corporate preretiree or retiree program—to name just a few possibilities.

QUESTION: How familiar are you with the health-promoting resources in your community? Find one that you are unfamiliar with but that you believe may be important for older persons.

Summarize it sufficiently to answer most questions that older adults might have about it.

After identifying relevant community health organizations or resources, additional considerations come into play. Cost, transportation access, and instructor competency with older persons are obviously important factors. It is also important to be knowledgeable about which community health services and programs may be best suited for a particular client. To effectively refer a client, it is important to gather feedback from prior older clients (this should be done in an ongoing and systematic way) and other health practitioners about the effectiveness of community health programs.

Community health programs are likely to be more successful with older clients if they are based on andragogical principles. ***Andragogy*** is the art and science of teaching adults, versus *pedagogy*, which is the education of children. Andragogy is based on a different set of assumptions about learning than are found in traditional pedagogy. These assumptions, which have received limited empirical examination, are threefold:

1. *Active involvement*. Active involvement on the part of older persons is preferable to the more traditional passive role. Older adults learn best (as do other age groups) when actively participating in an experience, such as helping to set goals, individualizing instruction to meet their needs, and helping to assess their own progress.
2. *Peer interaction*. Learning is fostered when age peers provide support, information, and assistance to one another. Community health programs that allow for peer interaction and support may be more effective than those that rely on authoritarian leadership.
3. *Short-term, doable goals*. Older adults do best with a ***modest goal*** over a limited period of time, perhaps along the way to a loftier goal.

Empowering Older Patients

The art of medicine consists of amusing the patient while nature cures the disease.

—*Voltaire, French physician and author*

Most health educators use the term ***client*** in the community, while health professionals in the medical setting are dealing with ***patients***. (Aging service providers prefer "consumer.") The term *patient* is derived from a Latin word meaning "to suffer," and suffering is an appropriate adjective for some patients. Patients are also associated with another adjective—*passive*. Passivity is not a good option when it comes to acute care, but it is worse when it comes to ongoing, long-term challenges, such as managing chronic conditions, promoting health, and preventing disease, activities that require initiative and repeated decision-making.

Voltaire's quotation appears to endorse passivity, as he knew that many medical conditions can be self-limiting, and that benignly amusing the patient is often all that is needed while a naturally occurring remission takes place. (He was also appropriately skeptical of 18th century medicine.) Benign amusement, however, is not the way to go even in the clinical setting, when unexpected questions arise:

Should I supplement chemotherapy with visualization techniques? Am I likely to be more adherent with one medication regimen versus another? Should I seek a second opinion and if it is different, which one should I choose? Decision-making can produce anxiety, but it is also healthy. In a classic study, residents in a long-term care setting who made decisions became more sociable, showed improvement in mental health, and even lived longer than residents who adopted a passive lifestyle (Rodin & Langer, 1977).

When the patient is passive, it may not be the primary care physician who makes the choice, but the specialty area to which the patient is referred. For example, the selection of the best treatment for prostate cancer—surgery, radiation, or some other option—is difficult to make. The choice may depend, however, on whether a patient is referred to a urological surgeon, a radiation oncologist, or another provider. Depending on the referral, you may not even find out that active surveillance, or watchful waiting, could be your best choice.

The role of the passive patient evolved from the belief that the healthcare arena is too complex to be understood by a layperson and that the doctor knows best. Through a number of surveys, the American Board of Family Practice has noted that the endorsement of this attitude among older adults is changing, particularly among the baby boomers. They are educated and interested in collaboration.

But there are exceptions that prove the general rule. Patients may not always want to be empowered or collaborate. They may want to give up responsibility to the healthcare provider under certain circumstances. A focus group study of coronary artery disease patients, for instance, reported that older patients were likely to prefer that doctors make decisions for them when the decision-making process is complex and uncertain (Kennelly, 2001).

Regarding metastatic colon cancer that has been diagnosed in older patients, only 44% in one study wanted complete information about their condition (Elkin et al., 2007). They were also willing—older women in particular—to leave treatment decisions to their physician. Interviewed separately, though, physicians predicted with only modest success their older patients' preferences in life-and-death matters.

Unfortunately, some physicians expect less from their older patients. One study of patients at primary care clinics reported that physicians were less willing to provide education and collaborate on decisions with their older patients versus their younger patients (Callahan et al., 2000). Patients older than age 60 with high blood pressure were less likely than younger patients to receive advice from their physicians about lifestyle modifications that could help lower their blood pressure (Viera et al., 2007). This bias cannot be explained by less interest in health information among older patients. One study has shown that older and younger people did not differ in preferences for health information and participation in decision-making about standard treatments (Xie et al., 2014). Communicating with older adults in clinical settings may need to take into account challenges of cognitive impairment, family caregiver involvement, hearing loss, and related factors (Backman et al., 2020).

Meta-analyses suggest that shared decision-making (SDM) is not always easy for patients and providers and is more likely to be effective when certain conditions are met. Patient barriers include cognitive and physical impairments, and involvement of families can hinder SDM if they differ in treatment choices or appraisal of the patient's competence. Provider barriers include poor interpersonal skills and inadequate time to spend with patients. However, "SDM could be facilitated when patients share information about personal values, priorities and preferences, as well as information about

BOX 3.1 Health-Promoting Occupations

It is not much of a leap in imagination to construct a health-promoting role for a nurse or physician, even if the person's current position makes such additional activity difficult. But what about a profession that is not known for being health promoting, or is known for having a narrow perspective on health promotion?

Take the profession of a minister, for example. Clearly, the health-promoting focus is on the specific dimension of spiritual health. How could the minister take a broader approach and include other dimensions of health promotion? The minister could provide free space in their church for an Alcoholics Anonymous (AA) or drug-free support group. The religious institution might be a more trusting and supportive environment for this type of behavior change than an alternative site. The minister could encourage a church-based exercise class or nutrition program, perhaps run by a qualified congregation member. Or the minister could launch a parish nurse program. Or the minister could arrange for periodic sermons on Bible-related topics such as "the body as God's temple" or any topic on physical, emotional, or social healthcare that relates to the spiritual dimension.

Select a profession of interest to you that traditionally does not include health promotion and that has older adults among its clients (a car salesperson, for instance). What could you do in that role to promote health? (Hint: For car salesperson, think safety.)

quality of life and functional status" (Pel-Littel et al., 2021, p. 10). A systematic review found that interest in self-management and desire to foster partnerships with healthcare professionals promote SDM (Holm et al., 2016).

Does greater SDM lead to better outcomes for patients? One review suggests strong benefit for "affective-cognitive patient outcomes" but less clear results for effective management (Shay & Lafata, 2015). The challenges of choosing the right outcome for this assessment are clear, as SDM is likely to be most important for patients with multiple chronic conditions at high risk of health declines.

Philosophical orientations among health practitioners—and nonhealth practitioners—vary (Box 3.1). Some health practitioners want a *professional-centered relationship* with patients. They want to be in control of the interaction and prefer brief responses to their questions. This approach is guided by highly structured questions to patients. Others are more *empowering*. They ask open-ended questions, value information on the psychosocial aspects of the health problem, restrict their use of jargon, elicit the patient's perception of the health problem, and encourage the patient to participate in the decision-making process.

COMMUNICATION

Open-ended inquiries and empathic listening skills are important communication aids to the health educator. Taking the time to explore the values and beliefs of clients can help the professional overcome ***communication barriers*** erected by differences in educational attainment, cultural beliefs, socioeconomic status, ethnicity, religion, language, immigration status, gender, and age.

While the health educator in the community generally has more time than the clinician in the medical setting, both can get impatient when time is limited and may want the older adult to focus and get to the point. Yet good communication skills cannot be rushed. A good source of ideas for communicating effectively with older adults is provided by a paper by the Gerontological Society of America, titled *Communicating With Older Adults* (https://gsaenrich.geron.org/communicating-with-older-adults) or the National Institute on Aging titled *Talking With Your Older Patients* (https://www.nia.nih.gov/health/health-care-professionals-information/talking-your-older-patients).

Personality Characteristics of an Effective Health Educator

Certain personality characteristics, such as patience, tolerance, and a positive attitude, enhance the health educator's chances for collaborating successfully on a health goal.

Encouraging health change requires *patience*; client progress tends to be slow, incremental, and characterized by lapses or reversals. Health educators are unrealistic if they expect to achieve health goals with their clients in the same time period required for the reversal of some acute care problems.

Tolerant health educators are nonjudgmental about the health habits of clients. These habits should no more be viewed as character weaknesses than a physical illness would be. If a client senses self-righteous judgment on the part of a health educator, even though it may not be verbally expressed, any mutual health endeavor is doomed to fail.

Health educators with a *positive attitude* should begin any health endeavor by identifying the personal assets of clients that will facilitate a change in health behavior. If, for instance, a client has a receptive attitude toward health, the educator should acknowledge it. It is also important to acknowledge past successes in a health area; positive personality traits, such as persistence or a sense of humor; the support of a spouse or friend; or the educational and financial resources that will help the client access community health resources or education programs.

How Effectively Do You Communicate?

The following questions are designed to help assess the effectiveness of one's communication skills. Some of these questions were stimulated by a presentation made by Kate Lorig, a health educator at Stanford University; others borrowed from other health educators; and the rest based on personal experience.

Interpersonal Effectiveness

1. Do you make eye contact?
2. Do you have a caring but not condescending tone of voice?
3. Are you and your client comfortable with touching? If so, will this enhance rapport?
4. Do you engage in reciprocity of information by self-disclosing when useful?
5. Do you let your client talk enough, or provide someone who will listen, or refer the client to a support group that will listen?
6. Are you well informed about your client's religious or cultural restrictions regarding privacy, touching, speaking to a woman alone, or engagement in other types of intimate interactions?
7. Do you try to be sensitive to your client's unique "cultural interpretation?" Cross-cultural issues are not just racial, religious, or ethnic in nature. We all interpret our health and diseases uniquely (i.e., we try to make sense of things within our belief system).

8. Are you able to resist the urge to counter your client's beliefs that are not harmful and instead just add to them? "Yes, the sin you stated you committed may be contributing to your pain, but pain is also caused by other factors." Do you give your client power by adding to their data bank, rather than contradicting it?
9. Is it possible to gain insight into a client's lifestyle by making a home visit or getting feedback from someone who has?

Informational Processing

1. Do you know if your client understands what you said—can they paraphrase it back to you?
2. Do you know what your client means—can you paraphrase it back to them?
3. Do you supplement your verbal instructions with clear written instructions?
4. Do you ask your client to write down any questions between visits and bring the questions on the next visit?
5. Do you encourage your client to bring along a helpful family member or friend to help with communication? Do you talk directly to your client and not primarily to their support person?
6. If appropriate, have you screened for cognitive impairment?
7. Are you aware of the impact that medication side effects may have on your client? Do these side effects interfere with their ability to communicate?
8. Does your client have an interest in the science (e.g., the anatomy and physiology) of the medical problem, or are they just interested in practical skills and knowledge?
9. Do you provide data in a manner that is preferred and easily understood?

Social and Behavioral Support

1. Do you motivate through positive incentives, rather than rely exclusively on fear tactics such as warning your client about morbidity or mortality risks?
2. Do you rely exclusively on talk to change your client's behavior, or do you combine talk with other strategies, such as behavioral management techniques?
3. Do you involve your client's social support system, such as family and friends, in the plan to change or maintain a health behavior?
4. Do you have an adequate reminder system to provide timely follow-up support for a client attempting to make a health behavior change?
5. Do you make appropriate referrals to community health programs or services when necessary and, equally important, do you seek feedback from a client for the benefit of other clients and to help determine future referrals?
6. When making referrals, do you consider programs and resources that are offered at culturally relevant and supportive sites, such as neighborhood religious institutions?
7. Do you ascertain your client's goal, see the underlying importance of this goal even if it is seemingly grandiose or trivial, and help your client redefine it to make it more achievable?
8. If you refer a client to a support group with lay leaders, do you know if they are receiving appropriate information from this group? Does the group invite professional expertise, and are you interested in contributing health education to this group?

CRUISING THE INTERNET

Face-to-face communication with health professionals has become increasingly limited in our healthcare system. Consumers, therefore, rely on other sources of health information. For decades, Americans relied on television as their primary source of health information, followed in priority by physicians, magazines, and journals.

It is not surprising that television had been the primary source of health information. A survey of 122 local news stations in the top 50 markets reported that 40% of television broadcasts contained at least one segment on health (Pribble et al., 2006). The researchers also noted, however, that an alarming number of stories included factually incorrect information and sometimes dangerous advice. Time limitations may have been responsible for some of the distortions aired on television—a problem also shared by newspaper coverage with its limited space.

However, the source of health information that now dominates among baby boomers, as well as the young, is the internet. Regarding the boomers, a survey in the *AARP Bulletin* (December 2008, p. 4) revealed that boomers age 50 to 64 were twice as likely as persons age 65+ to use the internet to research health information. Nearly two decades later, these boomers are now in their 70s and 80s, replacing some of the noncomputer-literate older adults who have died. The differences in where health information is being sought are quickly vanishing: The internet rules!

People living with chronic conditions, which are mostly older people, are more likely than others to fact check what they find online with a medical professional (https://www.pewresearch.org/internet/2013/11/26/part-two-sources-of-health-information/), though the quality of internet health searches is variable (Zhao & Zhang, 2017). Sharing information obtained from web searches with healthcare professionals is increasingly common (Huo et al., 2019). Use of large language models, such as ChatGPT, will become more prominent among older adults searching for health information (Coşkun et al., 2024). Disparities persist in access and recourse to web-based information (Wang & Cohen, 2023).

Merely accessing online consumer health information is insufficient; consumers need to be savvy about the validity of such information. Internet health information is often not the result of peer reviewed, high quality research; therefore, finding information that is accurate, timely, relevant, and unbiased is a challenge to web surfers. In one study, about half the websites on Lyme disease contained inaccurate information (J. Cooper & Feder, 2004).

Credentials matter. A comparison of websites offering nutrition services managed by registered dietitians revealed differences from sites managed by nondietitian nutrition consultants. Websites controlled by the registered dietitians ranked higher in accuracy (Hires et al., 2005). Another issue is whether the website contributor has a financial stake in the products or information presented—which brings us to Dr. Koop.

Case Study in Web Deception: DrKoop.com

During his 8 years as U.S. surgeon general (1981–1989), Dr. C. Everett Koop (who died in 2013 at the age of 96) became one of the most trusted and recognizable public figures in the area of public health. He was best known for leading campaigns to deter cigarette smoking and to raise AIDS awareness. In June 1999, a decade after leaving office, Dr. Koop cashed in on his fame and reputation and launched an online health information website. The initial public offering of drkoop.com sold 9 million shares and earned close to $90 million. A bull market for e-health stocks at the time resulted in a start-up value of more than $500 million for this website. By August 1999, it was the most visited health website, with about 3.5 million users.

It was downhill from there, unfortunately, owing to a series of ethical lapses. Millions of dollars were made by Dr. Koop and his investment partners when they sold shares of their stock soon after the initial public offering, in direct violation of securities law (Biesada, 2000). Nor did visitors to the site know that 14 hospitals described on the site as "the most innovative and advanced healthcare institutions in the country" had each paid a $40,000 fee to be included on this list (Noble, 1999). Repeated examples of the inability to distinguish between advertising and health education on the site continued to surface.

By May 2002, questionable dietary supplement formulas were being peddled by "the doctor you KNOW you can trust," and free psychic readings were being promoted. A few months later, drkoop.com filed for bankruptcy (Dr. Koop to Cease Operation, 2002), and in July 2002 its assets were sold for a paltry $186,000 (at one time it had been valued at $1 billion) to a company that sold discount vitamins.

According to one investigative reporter, WebMD, which regained its dominance in web-based medical information, earned revenues of $504 million in 2010, primarily by becoming a front for the Big Pharmacy industry (Heffernan, 2011). Heffernan found that WebMD drove consumer traffic to pharmaceutical companies. For instance, she plugged "headache" and "Mayo Clinic" into Google, and was directed to information on fostering healthy habits, finding effective nondrug treatments and, later on, using medications appropriately. She then plugged "headache" and "WebMD" into Google and was quickly referred to medications to prevent or stop headaches.

Websites

Potential problems aside, more and more health consumers are finding the internet to be an incredibly useful tool. Following are a few websites that are mostly .gov or .org, which are much more credible than most .com sites.

Before you begin reviewing them, two cautions are in order: (a) *cyberaddiction*—finding yourself lost in cyberspace for hours; and (b) *cyberchondria*—a malady among people who increase their anxiety about their health by reading health information online. "Doom scrolling" captures these cautions well.

Government

- https://healthfinder.gov (considered by many to be the premiere site for health information, including publications, clearinghouses, databases, websites, self-help or support groups, etc.)
- https://nih.gov (National Institutes of Health, with links to more than 100 government databases and a list of consumer health publications)
- https://medlineplus.gov (a database with references to 4,000 medical journals, a medical encyclopedia and dictionary, a drug reference guide, and hundreds of links to reputable health organizations)
- https://fda.org (U.S. Food and Drug Administration provides the latest information on new drugs and recently identified risks)
- https://health.gov (Office of Disease Prevention and Health Promotion provides fact sheets and links to publications)
- https://ahrq.gov (Agency for Healthcare Research and Quality provides information on the best treatments for specific health problems)

- https://clinicaltrials.gov (details on 5,200 clinical trials, most of them government funded). ClinicalTrials.gov provides information about research studies, and registration on the site is increasingly a requirement for research funding and publication. Note that no government agency reviews or approves the safety or scientific value of studies.

Wellness

- https://drweil.com (Dr. Weil is director of integrative medicine at the University of Arizona; this site is broad in scope but focuses on dietary supplements)
- https://welcoa.org (Wellness Councils of America focuses on worksite wellness programs and products)
- https://nationalwellness.org (the National Wellness Institute offers conferences, programs, and wellness assessment tools)
- https://nccam.nih.gov (National Center for Complementary and Alternative Medicine)
- https://quackwatch.org (identifying dubious alternative healthcare claims)

Professional Organizations

- https://n4a.org (National Association of Area Agencies on Aging), now USAging. "USAging is the national association representing and supporting the network of [U.S.] Area Agencies on Aging and advocating for the Title VI Native American Aging Programs" (https://www.usaging.org/about)
- https://cancer.org (American Cancer Society)
- https://www.heart.org/ (American Heart Association)
- https://diabetes.org (American Diabetes Association)
- https://lung.org (American Lung Association)
- https://www.bonehealthandosteoporosis.org/ (National Osteoporosis Foundation)
- https://geron.org (Gerontological Society of America focuses on research), "the oldest and largest interdisciplinary organization devoted to research, education, and practice in the field of aging."
- https://aghe.org (Academy for Gerontology in Higher Education focuses on education)
- https://ncoa.org, https://asaging.org (National Council on Aging and the American Society on Aging sponsor many community service and educational programs, including a joint conference)
- https://nhpco.org (National Hospice and Palliative Care Organization will help you find a hospice near you and draft a living will)
- https://aarp.org/research (AARP policy and research information for professionals in aging)
- https://agingstats.gov (Federal Interagency Forum on Aging-Related Statistics is a collaborative effort among 12 federal agencies that produce or use statistics on aging)
- https://hrs.isr.umich.edu/ (Health and Retirement Study surveys more than 22,000 Americans age 50+ every 2 years on physical and mental health and related topics; data available at no cost)
- https://afar.org (American Federation for Aging Research focuses on disease, biology, and healthy aging)
- https://civicengagement.org (National Academy on an Aging Society provides data profiles and issue briefs about older Americans, with emphasis on public policy research on population aging)

Specific Health Content Areas

- https://caregiveraction.org (National Family Caregivers Association provides education, support, and advocacy for caregivers)
- https://acefitness.org (American Council on Exercise provides certification for training and fitness continuing education)
- https://active.com (event locator for individual and team sports, and park and community activities)
- https://eatright.org (Academy of Nutrition and Dietetics offers daily nutrition tips and reliable answers to nutrition questions, including where to find a dietitian)
- https://wheatfoods.org (Wheat Foods Council provides everything you want to know about grains)
- https://cspinet.org (Center for Science in the Public Interest, and publisher of Nutrition Action Healthletter)
- https://nutritionletter.tufts.edu (Tufts University Health & Nutrition Letter)
- https://niaaa.nih.gov (National Institute on Alcohol Abuse and Alcoholism)
- https://nida.nih.gov (National Institute on Drug Abuse)
- https://nia.nih.gov (National Institute on Aging)
- https://samhsa.gov (Substance Abuse and Mental Health Services Administration)
- https://www.adec.org (Association for Death Education & Counseling)
- https://alz.org (Alzheimer's Association)
- https://diabetes.org (American Diabetes Association)

Older Consumer

- https://aarp.org (AARP provides health news, information on a wide range of activities, and links to other sites)
- https://seniornet.org (teaches adults age 50+ to use computers, with links to 600 discussion groups)
- https://thirdage.com (tips on a wide variety of topics, from retirement savings to clothing colors that flatter gray hair)
- https://assistedlivingstore.com (lists devices for assisted living)
- https://webmd.com (wide range of health and medical topics)
- https://roadscholar.org (lists nearly 8,000 educational tours sponsored throughout the United States and in 90 other countries)
- https://mayohealth.org (Mayo Clinic covers a wide range of health topics)

Electronic Resources

Positive Aging

Psychologists Ken and Mary Gergen edit this electronic newsletter devoted to positive approaches to aging. This newsletter not only offers a uniquely positive perspective, but summarizes a variety of research that is useful to practitioners. For a free subscription go to https://taosinstitute.net/positive-aging-newsletter-sign-up. Currently, only archived materials are available.

Antiageism

A clearinghouse for educating about ageism and dismantling it. Established in 2018. Contact: OldSchool.info

Public Policy and Aging

Quarterly newsletter that highlights key developments in the field of aging policy: https://agingsociety.org/agingsociety/publications/public_policy/index.html

Today's Research on Aging

Published by the Population Reference Bureau with the goal of increasing awareness of research results and their application to public and private decision-making, https://www.prb.org/collections/todays-research-on-aging/

SELECTED COMMUNICATION BARRIERS

Race and Gender

Familiarity helps with communication. Health professionals who are similar to their clients or patients are viewed as better communicators and more participatory. One study, for example, reported that African American patients who visited physicians of the same race rated their medical visits as more satisfying and participatory (L. A. Cooper et al., 2003).

The benefits of racial familiarity, though, are not limited to visit satisfaction. When Black patients were assigned to a Black doctor, 63% agreed to a recommended diabetes screening versus 43% when assigned to a White or Asian doctor. Also, when Black patients were assigned to a Black physician, 62% agreed to a recommended cholesterol test versus 36% when assigned to a physician who was not Black (Alsan et al., 2018).

Why might this be? The researchers speculated that perhaps more nonverbal cues to communicate empathy were given to patients of the same race. Another observation was that the communication was more personal, with more laughter evident in the doctor–patient relationship. One Black physician who was interviewed reported that he understood minority barriers to compliance and took extra steps to overcome them. Several Black patients interviewed reported that they felt more comfortable and relaxed with a physician of the same race. These encounters promote trust in recommendations and reassurance that providers have the patient's best interest in mind.

A study of 580,000 heart attack patients admitted to Florida emergency departments between 1991 and 2010 reported that there was a higher mortality rate among female patients when treated by a male physician. With female physicians there were no discrepancies between male and female patient results (Greenwood et al., 2018).

A review of studies comparing male versus female physicians reported the following: (a) Medicare patients treated by a female physician were less likely to die or be readmitted to the hospital over a 30-day period than those who were cared for by a male doctor. (b) Women doctors spent on average 2 extra minutes with patients compared with male doctors. (c) Female primary physicians waited an average of 3 minutes before interrupting a patient whereas male doctors waited an average of 47 seconds (Parker-Pope, 2018). To end on an encouraging note, the more female patients a male physician treated, the more these discrepancies between male and female doctors were reduced (Greenwood et al., 2018). However, a study involving simulated patients did not find strong bias in patient encounters varying in patient and physician race (Solnick et al., 2020).

Cross-Cultural Communication

Cross-cultural communication, however, is not simply an issue of race or gender. Many cultural differences that emerge between health professionals and clients are also based on differences in age, religion, ethnicity, socioeconomic class, and education. Every health professional must deal with these types of cross-cultural issues.

Open-ended questions can help the health professional understand the patient's point of view: How would you describe your health problem? Why do you think this problem occurred? Do you have sources of relief that I don't know about? Apart from me, who do you think can help you get better? Has anyone made recommendations to you? Did you try any of them? (For more cross-cultural questions, organized by content area, see Haber, 2005.)

Some managed-care organizations are recognizing the importance of helping health professionals communicate more effectively with minority patients. In Southern California, for instance, Kaiser Permanente has a medical anthropologist on staff to help health professionals work more successfully with minority patients and to develop special programs for minority members.

For those interested in the topic of racial and cultural biases in the healthcare setting, and improvement in communication skills between health professionals and clients, the American Academy of Family Physicians provides a CD (#724) or a video (#723) entitled *Quality Care for Diverse Populations* (call 800-274-2237). The U.S. Agency for Healthcare Research and Quality (AHRQ) has also developed guidance on cultural competence (Butler et al., 2016). Recognizing the importance of these biases, more recently the U.S. Department of Health and Human Services has begun to promote "culturally and linguistically appropriate services" (CLAS; https://thinkculturalhealth.hhs.gov/clas/what-is-clas): "By tailoring services to an individual's culture and language preferences, health professionals can help bring about positive health outcomes for diverse populations." The principal aim of the national CLAS standards is to "provide effective, equitable, understandable, and respectful quality care and services that are responsive to diverse cultural health beliefs and practices, preferred languages, health literacy, and other communication needs."

Communication With Older Patients

The satisfaction of older patients is positively associated with the length of their visits with physicians, and with physicians' support of topics initiated by the patient. Using audiotapes and other tools, however, researchers have found that doctors seem reluctant to discuss psychosocial and prevention issues with older clients and are less receptive to these issues when raised by older patients than when raised by younger ones (Callahan et al., 2000; Gaspar et al., 2016; Kennelly, 2001).

QUESTION: Describe an example of ageism that you experienced, witnessed, or heard about in a health professional–patient, health educator–client, or teacher–student encounter. What made it ageist?

Physicians give older patients considerably less cardiac risk-reduction advice regarding diet, exercise, weight control, smoking, and stress management, than they give younger clients. Thus, older patients are systematically denied the opportunity to lessen their risk of future heart problems by adopting the behavioral advice of the physician.

How well do nurses communicate with older patients? A meta-analysis of 34 studies reported that more patients were satisfied with care from a nurse practitioner than they were with care from a physician. Some of the studies reported that the nurse practitioner gave more time, information, and advice on self-care and management of disease (Horrocks et al., 2002; Htay & Whitehead, 2021). However, this key difference between nurse practitioners and physicians may be diminished in the future as nurse practitioners find themselves with less time to spend with patients.

A survey of 552 pharmacists in Indiana reported that 88% were willing to participate in continuing education courses to learn more about health education and promotion involving patients, including older adults. Despite this willingness to learn, though, the pharmacists reported persistent barriers to health education in the pharmacy setting, such as lack of time, reimbursement, privacy, training, and management support (Kotecki et al., 2000).

In primary care practices, about one third of older patients bring a companion to the doctor's office, and 16% have the companion come into the examination room (Schilling et al., 2002; Wolff & Greenberg, 2012). A majority of physicians, and an even higher percentage of patients, find this arrangement to be helpful. The two major drawbacks are with patient confidentiality and patients' possible reluctance to reveal necessary information when someone close to them is in the room.

Older men are less likely than women to bring a companion when visiting a doctor, but if they do bring a companion to the clinic, they are more likely to bring that companion into the examining room to help them communicate with the doctor. Older women tend to bring companions primarily for transportation or companionship, visiting with the doctor alone (Mitchell et al., 2020).

A patient's companion can provide a vital service to both the health professional and the patient, serving as an independent monitor of a person's condition and providing helpful feedback on patient collaboration with treatment regimens. A companion can make sure that questions are asked and answers are understood. In contrast, health professionals can be seduced into communicating with younger and more articulate companions and ignoring their older patients.

Jargon

Jargon is language—often technical or obscure used by people who work in a particular profession or area of interest. The lower the educational level of a patient, including the older patient, the fewer terms they will understand.

The reasons health providers use incomprehensible language, which continues despite many efforts to make medical language more accessible (Miller et al., 2022) include:

- habit,
- the belief that comprehension of a medical problem might increase the older adult's stress level,
- the fact that hard-to-understand terms may be conversation stoppers, making more time for other patients or clients, and
- the belief that the use of jargon elevates one's authority.

Transcripts of 86 conversations between medical residents and standardized patients reveal that a large number of jargon words were still being used by medical residents and that they impeded patient understanding of cancer screening tests (Deuster et al., 2008).

Jargon affects the older adults' ability to understand and to feel warmth and concern from the health professional. When communication is effective, the older adult remembers more, has greater trust, and litigates less.

Jargon complicates *health literacy*, a person's ability to understand basic health information needed to make appropriate health decisions and avoid harm (Gotlieb et al., 2022). Whereas 53% of American adults have an intermediate level of health literacy, the percentage falls to 38% among those age 65 and older (Span, 2018). Factors for this age discrepancy include lower formal educational levels, reduced cognitive acuity, hearing and visual decline, and coping with more complicated medical issues such as comorbidity, polypharmacy, and multiple specialists.

Elderspeak

Elderspeak, the gerontology counterpart to baby talk, is a term used to describe the sometimes sweet, but always infantilizing, way of communicating to older adults. Elderspeak can be addressing an older adult with such endearments as "Sweetie" or "Honey." Or it can be addressing an unfamiliar older adult by their first name without asking permission first. Or it can be using only simple words, spoken slowly or loudly.

Even demented older adults can detect elderspeak, often by the tone rather than the content. One study reported that elderspeak inspired resistance to care by older adults with dementia in nursing homes, or stimulated more aggressive behaviors, whereas those who were addressed normally were more cooperative (Williams et al., 2009).

Communication training has been shown to reduce the use of elderspeak among nursing staff and other care providers (Williams et al., 2023). Many providers believe that it conveys affection or caring and is easier to understand, without realizing that elderspeak conveys the message that older adults are incompetent and baby-like. This may be particularly upsetting to early-stage dementia patients who are losing cognitive abilities and trying to maintain their personhood. Older adults without cognitive problems may also feel that they are being addressed in an infantile manner and find it upsetting.

HEALTH BEHAVIOR CHANGE

In their article "The Case for More Active Policy Attention to Health Promotion," McGinnis et al. (2002) examined the impact of five spheres of influence on early deaths in the United States. Using the best available data, their estimates are as follows, in ascending order:

- environmental exposures (5%),
- shortfalls in medical care (10%),
- social circumstances (education, poverty; 15%),
- genetic dispositions (30%), and
- behavioral patterns (40%).

McGinnis and colleagues observe that behavioral patterns—contributing to 40% of early deaths—are important contributors to quality of life as well. They noted that "what we choose to eat and how we design activity into (or out of) our lives have a great bearing on our health prospects" (McGinnis et al., 2002, p. 82). This updates an earlier analysis from 1993 suggesting that 40% of deaths involve behaviors that in principle could be changed with the proper mix of education, incentives, and supports (McGinnis & Foege 1993).

As mentioned in Chapter 1, it is instructive to compare the distribution of causes of death identified in death certificates with what have been called "actual causes of death." In the United States in 2022, major killers (with number of deaths in parentheses) included heart disease (702,880), cancer (608,371), unintentional injuries (227,039), COVID-19 (186,552), stroke (165,393), chronic lower respiratory diseases (147,382), Alzheimer disease (120,122), diabetes (101,209), kidney disease (57,937), and liver disease (54,803; (https://www.cdc.gov/nchs/fastats/leading-causes-of-death.htm). But many of the conditions involve health behaviors, thus the "actual causes of death," by contrast, involve tobacco, poor diet, sedentary lifestyle, alcohol consumption, illicit drug use, sexually transmitted disease, and accidents and injuries (including firearm deaths). No update for the attributable fraction of deaths due to these behavioral factors is currently available, but an analysis dated 2000 suggested that approximately 40% to 45% of deaths could be attributed to behavioral risk factors (Mokdad et al., 2004).

Despite the prominence of behavioral factors in prevention of premature deaths, more than 95% of the money we spend on healthcare in America goes toward medical care; less than 5% to prevention; and only a small amount of that is allocated to improve health behavior patterns. Research funding shows the same mismatch: In 2023, less than $12 billion of $317 billion was awarded to primarily behavioral science studies (https://report.nih.gov/funding/categorical-spending#/). This budgetary allocation may seem out of balance to the health-conscious reader, but it is undeniably good for certain businesses and practitioners, such as medical institutions, medical professionals, pharmaceutical companies, tobacco growers, alcohol producers, food manufacturers, and advertising companies.

The health education profession, in contrast, is a modest industry with practitioners who toil away in relative obscurity. There are few millionaires and fewer lobbyists who seek concessions from congressional leaders. As a consequence, the healthcare industry in America is primarily a medical care industry dominated by medical organizations and practitioners. In the remaining section of this chapter, however, I will focus on health behavior assessments, interventions, and concepts—the tools of health educators.

ASSESSMENTS AND INTERVENTIONS

Health Risk Appraisals

Unlike the specific medical screenings detailed in the last chapter, and which tend to be conducted in a clinical setting, ***health risk appraisals*** (HRAs) and other health behavior assessments are typically comprehensive in scope and are implemented in nonmedical settings. Health promotion advocates in the community believe that a comprehensive health behavior assessment gives clients a broad, holistic perspective and a sense of the priority areas that they may want to work on.

This big picture, though, may also discourage persons who discover an array of lifestyle risk factors that need attention. A good health assessment may be broad in scope, but it also has to guide the client, who must be able and willing to start with one achievable health behavior change.

HRA instruments in the context of worksite wellness were launched in the 1970s. By 2014, according to a study for the Labor Department by RAND reseach insititute, about half of employers with at least 50 workers offered some type of HRA or wellness program and this increased to 90% in companies with more than 50,000 employees. Among large firms, in 2023 54% offered health risk assessments, 42% biometric screening, and 80% access to wellness programs. Firms continue to provide incentives for participation in prevention programs (https://www.kff.org/report-section/ehbs-2023-section-12-health-screening-and-health-promotion-and-wellness-programs-and-disease-management/), and the number of HRA instruments continues to grow, with some even offering estimates of biological age.

One study of 3,000 Canadians reported that showing coronary risk profiles to subjects, to help them narrow their gap between their actual age and a reduced "cardiovascular age," led some to achieve modest success with lipid control (Grover et al., 2007). The greater the gap, the greater the motivation and success.

An interesting study of 1,000 people over a 20-year period, from ages 18 to 38, revealed that *even by midlife* there emerged tremendous variability in "biological ages." Those who were aging faster biologically already showed by age 38 evidence of cognitive decline through lower IQ scores, and physical decline through difficulty with basic tasks such as climbing stairs and carrying groceries (Belsky et al., 2015). At the same chronological age of 38, the biological age of these persons ranged from age 30 to age 60.

The methodological issues with HRAs for older adults, though, remain unresolved (Shekelle et al., 2003). Risk calculations have been based on younger and middle-aged adults and are not as accurate for older adults. Moreover, HRAs tend to focus on premature mortality, which is less relevant to older adults than health expectancy, the number of years remaining with good health. The process of evaluating the suitability of HRA instruments for older populations is a work in progress.

In a review of 20 HRAs, including ones from such well-known organizations as the National Wellness Institute and Johnson & Johnson Health Management, all claimed versions of their instruments that were appropriate for, or adaptable to, specific age groups, ranging from high school to older adults. The goal of these assessments is "to activate multidimensional, multicultural, whole-person wellness where individuals live, work, learn, play, and reflect" (https://nationalwellness.org/resources/).

Among the instruments we note the following:

1. They are computerized and available for commercial use. Most offered individual and aggregate reporting, immediate individual feedback, and data security.
2. At minimum, they include medical questions involving such measures as blood pressure and cholesterol level, and health habits such as smoking, exercise, and nutrition.
3. There was no consensus on length. Some instruments were deliberately short, about 15 questions; others included upward of 150 questions.
4. They were quantifiable, comparing actual age with an earned age. The apparent assumption is that learning whether your days are running out faster or slower than expected is motivating to clients.
5. They used outdated or debatable scientific evidence. This was not surprising, because research results are changing more rapidly than patented HRA instruments.
6. They had a health education component to motivate clients to change undesirable health behaviors in order to reduce specific risk factors. In most instances, this health education component relied on tailored written resource materials, although some provided follow up by a health educator, or linked specific risk factors identified by the HRA to appropriate health programs in the work or community setting.

The Centers for Disease Control and Prevention (CDC) also offers guidance on HRA design and use (https://stacks.cdc.gov/view/cdc/23365), and Medicare has developed guidance for health risk assessment in its Medicare Wellness Visit (https://www.cdc.gov/policy/paeo/hra/hraawvguidancereportfinal.pdf#page=23.99).

The RAND research institute reviewed 267 studies of HRAs, eventually paring them down to 27 controlled studies, 13 of which were randomized controlled trials. They concluded that about 44% of HRA interventions reported positive health outcomes. Among these studies, the more limited the feedback and support to participants, the more limited the beneficial results. Feedback and support ranged from general written materials to personalized written materials, to incentives, to counseling, and to the opportunity to participate in a health program. Few interventions involved vulnerable or minority populations, and most HRA methodologies designed for older adults were not tested for effectiveness on that population (Shekelle et al., 2003).

A Reflective Health Assessment

In contrast to specific responses to a series of focused risk-reduction questions posed by HRAs, the Andrew Weil Center for Integrative Medicine offers patients a unique health assessment tool that encourages patient reflection and initiative (Weil, Finding Mastering [podcast]). Dr. Weil begins with the following questions: *What does good health mean to you? How do you attain it? Additional questions include: Does your life have meaning to you? Are you happy?*

Dr. Weil also asks clients unique questions about specific content areas: *What is your relationship with food? What is your relationship with exercise? Do you have satisfying personal relationships? How do you deal with your stress?*

When you complete these questions, it is time for you to reflect on your answers. You may never have examined your health in this way. You will explore your attitudes toward your health, identify your health goals, recognize the obstacles to achieving your goals, and discover the personal resources you can assemble to accomplish them.

Reflecting on your answers may give you a better understanding of what is contributing to your health problems. You may be more aware of what kind of support you would like from your family, friends, and healthcare providers. Also, defining terms for yourself, assessing your own priorities, and designing self-tailored strategies to achieve your health goals may help you feel more empowered.

Another type of reflective health assessment is delivered by health coaches in a business setting. *Health coaches* encourage employees to improve their health behaviors by helping them reflect on their risk factors and ways to change them. The goal of health coaching for the employer is to reduce absenteeism and medical care costs and improve productivity (Dolan, 2007). Some health coaching is offered at reduced rates in the employer setting, but rarely is it coordinated with the employee's primary care physician.

Huffman (2007) believes health coaching is based on three principles: (a) asking open-ended questions, (b) affirming the client's strengths and building their confidence, and (c) listening carefully and demonstrating that you have listened. She also encourages health coaching to be used in the home healthcare setting with older clients. A number of studies have reported benefit for health coaching interventions (Kivelä et al., 2014), but few health coach efforts involve a fully whole-person approach, and separate coach encounters (e.g., one for diabetes management and another for mental health) can be counterproductive.

Stages of Change

Another type of health assessment, one that is typically not comprehensive in scope, is the stages-of-change instrument, also referred to academically as the transtheoretical model (Hilliard et al., 2018). This popular assessment tool was developed and subsequently refined and expanded by Prochaska et al. (2009) to help health professionals assess a client's readiness to change a specific health habit. The ***stages of change*** are as follows:

1. precontemplation—no intention to change behavior in the foreseeable future;
2. contemplation—awareness that a problem exists but no commitment to action;
3. preparation—intention to take action in the next month, typically preceded by unsuccessful action taken in the past year;

4. action—modification of behavior, experiences, or environment for a time period ranging from 1 day to 6 months in order to overcome a problem; and
5. maintenance—an indeterminate period, perhaps a lifetime, in which to actively prevent termination or relapse.

The authors report that relapsing and recycling through the stages of change is the rule rather than the exception, and this process could be viewed as a spiral rather than a linear model. If clients become more aware of the relapsing phenomenon, they might feel less guilt, embarrassment, and discouragement after an unsuccessful attempt. If health professionals become more aware of the relapsing process, they might be more patient with their clients' attempts at change.

Persons who are in the precontemplation stage are, by definition, not ready for action-oriented programs. A study of 20,000 people found that only 20% of the population is ready to make a specific behavior change (Noar, Chabot, & Zimmerman, 2008). So what happens to those who are *not* ready? According to Prochaska et al. (1993), they can be helped through the stages by giving them stage-matched messages and support.

Precontemplators, for instance, are denied immediate support (justified on the basis of limited personnel resources) and are offered literature in the hope that someday they may be more ready to make a behavior change. Contemplators, however, receive both information about the pros and cons involved with changing a behavior, and the support to increase confidence and to explore ways to overcome barriers. The last three stages of change—preparation, action, and maintenance—are behavior-change oriented.

Despite the enormous popularity of the stages-of-change framework in the psychology literature, not everyone is a true believer. One analyst reported that the vast majority of studies testing this model are cross-sectional rather than longitudinal. As a consequence, there have been serious flaws, such as the assignment of arbitrary time periods to particular stages. Also, there is an overlap in the definition of the different stages. Finally, there is the overpromotion of meager and inconsistent research results (Sutton, 2001).

One behavioral scientist questioned the ethics of too quickly ignoring reputed precontemplators, or postponing interventions with them, when they constitute the section of the population with the greatest need. She suggested that this model may lead to discrimination against those who are poor, less educated, and frail (Whitehead, 1997; see Box 3.2).

BOX 3.2 Perhaps There Are No Precontemplators?

My first reservation with the stages-of-change framework occurred when I was interviewing several older people in an African American church. They reported to me that they were not interested in exercise and also not interested in joining my soon-to-be-launched, church-based exercise program (Looney & Haber, 2001). Had I allowed this initial report of disinterest to result in my labeling them "precontemplators," I would have offered them literature and moved on to seek other people who may have been ready to join my exercise program.

Instead, a few days later, along with several of my health science students, we recruited these congregation members and others, and gave them a 20-minute demonstration of an exercise program that would not only be good for their health, but fun. Accompanied by church music, easy banter, humor, and scripture that we read ("to take care of God's temple [the body]" and "above all else, guard your heart for it provides health to a man's whole body"), many people signed up for, and then successfully completed, the 10-week program—including the several alleged precontemplators!

An interesting variation on the stages-of-change framework is to focus on specific aspects of a particular behavior change. A team of researchers examined the topic of weight loss, for instance, and instead of asking people whether they were ready to make changes leading to weight loss, the researchers asked which changes they were most interested in making. Six aspects of weight loss were targeted: decreasing dietary fat, improving portion control, increasing vegetable intake, increasing fruit intake, increasing physical activity, and implementing an exercise regimen. The researchers found that respondents may have been precontemplators in some aspects of weight loss, but they were ready to make a change in at least one other area (Logue et al., 2000).

A similar strategy with a much broader focus is to present older persons with different categories of potential behavior-change goals to choose from. Presented with sufficiently diverse options, older adults may be more motivated to choose one behavior change that is of high priority to them (Haber, 1996). Here is a partial list of diverse health promotion categories that were presented to older adults, accompanied by a brief and individualized health assessment in each of the categories (Haber, 2001):

1. Complete one of several (listed) medical screenings or immunizations.
2. Increase physical activity level: Begin a brisk walking program; join an aerobics, yoga, or Tai chi class; start a strength-building program; or begin a flexibility routine.
3. Decrease dietary fat, implement portion control, increase vegetable or fruit intake, or increase fluid consumption.
4. Initiate a stress management routine.
5. Establish a sleep hygiene routine.
6. Implement a fall prevention or home safety plan.
7. Join a smoking cessation program.
8. Enroll in a memory improvement course.
9. Join one of the disease-specific peer support groups in the area.
10. Implement an alcohol-in-moderation plan.

Among 48 older adults who were presented an array of health promotion options, 44 were able and willing to select a health goal. Using the technique of a health contract, 75% achieved substantial success with their goal (Haber & Looney, 2000).

An interesting new wrinkle on stages of change is to target those who have had a recent and serious medical diagnosis, such as heart disease or diabetes. When these patients are contacted at this propitious time, they are more likely to quit smoking or, to a lesser extent, lose weight (Keenan, 2009). It may prove advantageous if businesses or healthcare systems could target, in a timely fashion, those who may be particularly ready to make a health behavior change.

Health Contracts

A health assessment and intervention tool used with older adults is a ***health contract*** (Figure 3.1) and ***health calendar*** (Figure 3.2). It is based on a self-management application of *social cognitive theory* (Bandura, 1977), which will be examined in more detail in the theory section.

Self-management refers to clients who, with the help of a health educator, can choose an appropriate behavior-change goal and create and implement a plan to accomplish that goal. The statement of the goal and the plan of action can be written into a health contract format. A health contract is alleged to have several advantages over verbal

FIGURE 3.1 Health contract.

Health contract

My **health** goal is: ______________________________

My **motivations** for my health goal are:

1. ____________
2. ____________
3. ____________

My plan of action

For social or emotional **support,** I will . . .

To **remind** of new behaviors I will . . .

Problems that may interfere with reaching my health goal and **solutions:**

____

My **signature**/date

Support person's **signature**/date

FIGURE 3.2 Health calendar.

Health calender

Month: ____________ ____________

Backup plan:

Weekly success
#days completed/
#days contracted

Sunday	Monday	Tuesday	Wednesday	Thursday	Friday	Saturday	
							___/___
							___/___
							___/___
							___/___
							___/___

communication alone, especially when the communication tends to be limited in direction; that is, mostly from health professional to client. The alleged advantages of a health contract are that it:

- is a formal commitment that enhances motivation;
- clarifies goals and behaviors and makes them explicit;

- requires the active participation of the client;
- enhances the therapeutic relationship between provider and client (though a health contract can be completed without assistance);
- provides a structured means for involving significant others (e.g., family, friends) in a supportive role;
- provides a structured means of ***problem-solving*** around barriers that previously interfered with the achievement of a goal; and
- can include (this is optional) incentives to reinforce behaviors.

The health contract incorporates a set of instructions that help older adults state a health goal (Box 3.3), identify benefits that provide motivation, establish a plan of action that helps the older adult remember to perform new behaviors and to elicit social support, and identify potential problems to achieving the health goal and encourage solutions to overcome these barriers.

BOX 3.3 Health Contract Directions for Exercise

Exercise Motivation

Review a list of potential motivations (see the 10 Tips section), and help the client choose among "improved function" and "disease prevention" motives. Record up to three motivations on the health contract.

Encourage the client to write down one motivation and keep it in their wallet or purse, smartphone, calendar, or in a conspicuous place. The client may want to state the motivation aloud on a daily basis.

Exercise Modality

Review the list of exercise modalities; help the client choose one before working on a health goal (e.g., community exercise program, aerobic options in the home, walking alternatives, increasing physical activity, strength building, flexibility/balance).

Exercise Baseline

If the client is sedentary, set a minimum goal; if the client is not sedentary, assess the client's baseline and progress from there. Review the last week for exercise/physical activity frequency, duration, and intensity. If last week was not typical, substitute a typical week. Establish a goal of slightly above baseline for the first week, gradually increase it over the remaining weeks, and set a modest goal for the last week of the month.

Frequency and duration should be assessed by number of days per week and total minutes each day. Moderate intensity level should be assessed by asking the client to notice increases in body warmth and breathing rate during exercise or physical activity. If no change is observed, increase the intensity level.

Health Goal

Write a specific statement about what the client will do by the end of the first month, and include the following information: how often (days/week), how much (duration/day), and how intense (light/medium).

(*continued*)

BOX 3.3 Health Contract Directions for Exercise (*continued*)

The goal should be *modest* and *measurable*—no more than 5 days a week, one half-hour a day, one unit over baseline for the first week, with week-by-week gradations until the health goal is reached during the last week of the first month. A client may choose to exceed these parameters, but not as part of the stated health goal.

Reassess the health goal at the end of the first week, and change if necessary. Set a day and time to meet at the end of the first month to assess progress and possible change for the next month; record the meeting on the health calendar.

Plan of Action

Social Support. Review the list of social support possibilities. The client should select one (or more) socially supportive person, state the ways support is to be expected, and the frequency of support desired. Client may opt for no social support.

Reminders. Attach the health contract to the refrigerator. Have a friend or family member call to remind the client of goals. Associate new behaviors with an established habit, such as engaging in brisk walking just before a meal. Keep exercise-related reading materials visible around the house. Keep workout shoes by the door. Exercise at the same time each day. Hang a picture on the wall that shows the client or others exercising.

Problems/Solutions

Consider problems that arose when similar goals were set in the past, or anticipate new problems that might arise in the coming month.

Positive Thoughts. A solution for the negative thinker is to deliberately verbalize ***positive thoughts*** about achieving the health goal on a daily basis. The positive thought can also be written on paper and read—something like "I am confident of success, though not perfection."

Reinforcement. Encourage ***reinforcement***. The client should seek praise: Swallow modesty and tell people about successes and solicit additional praise from them. Seek internal motivation: Pay attention to the signs of feeling better. Seek external motivation: Buy theater tickets or enjoy another (nonedible) treat if success is achieved at the end of a week or month.

Environmental Support. Alter immediate surroundings. Place walking sneakers by the front door, distribute exercise-related literature around the house, place exercise band on the coffee table, keep pictures on the wall of healthy people exercising.

Stress Management. Stress can sidetrack a person from the goal. To manage stress, consider: deep breathing, muscle relaxation, meditation, prayer, listening to music, playing with a pet, taking a walk. Schedule these activities on a regular basis.

Problem Solve. Brainstorm about problems that arose from past attempts at behavior change. Brainstorm about problems that might arise in the future. Find solutions. Be especially attentive to issues of pain and fatigue. Record under Problems/Solutions.

Signatures

The client signs the contract, along with someone who will be offering support and is willing to sign the contract. If no one comes to mind, the health educator can sign it.

Health Calendar

Follow directions for recording activities on the health calendar. Place checkmarks on successful days. Calculate percent success. Aim for 75% or higher success rate.

The health contract is signed by the older adult and a support person. Progress is typically assessed after 1 week, and the success of the contract is reviewed at the end of a month (Haber, 2007; Haber & Looney, 2000; Haber & Rhodes, 2004). Health contracts have been applied with varying degrees of success to a wide variety of behaviors, such as drug use, smoking, alcohol abuse, nutrition, and exercise.

Health contracts can be uniquely designed by a practitioner. For instance, a weight loss contract developed by Joseph Chemplavil, a cardiac endocrinologist in Hampton, Virginia, consists of the following: "I (patient's name), hereby promise to myself and to Dr. Chemplavil, that I will make every effort to lose my (agreed-upon) weight, and I will pay $1 to Dr. Chemplavil's Dollar for Pound Fund, for every pound of weight that I gain, on each visit to the office, by cash. I also understand that I will receive $1 from the same fund for each pound of weight that I lose." Dr. Chemplavil paid out $1,044 to 118 patients and received $166 from 30 patients, with two patients breaking even (Kazel, 2004).

Research into health contracts has been limited (and often marred) by small sample sizes, lack of random assignment to treatment and control groups, and lack of replication. In addition, there are several uncertainties about the effectiveness of health contracts in terms of ability to identify which components work best (e.g., health education, social support, the professional–client relationship, memory enhancement, motivation building, contingency rewards), whether contracts work better with one type of client than another, and determining the content and amount of training required for health educators or clinicians to administer health contracts effectively.

Even without a definitive body of research, health contracts are widely used. They are simple to administer, time efficient, and cost-effective. The health contract can also be successfully implemented with students in the classroom (Haber, 2007).

PRECEDE-PROCEED

The ***PRECEDE*** framework (Green & Kreuter, 1999) offers a broad conceptual guideline that can also be used for assessing the readiness of adults to change or maintain a health behavior. PRECEDE is an (awkwardly constructed) acronym for *p*redisposing, *r*einforcing, and *e*nabling *c*onstructs in *e*ducational/*e*cological *d*iagnosis and *e*valuation. ***PROCEED*** refers to *p*olicy, *r*egulatory, and *o*rganizational *c*onstructs in *e*ducational and *e*nvironmental *d*evelopment (https://ctb.ku.edu/en/table-contents/overview/other-models-promoting-community-health-and-development/preceder-proceder/main).

Predisposing factors are the knowledge, attitudes, and beliefs a person holds about a health behavior. For instance, if an older person believes exercise will aggravate arthritis or cause unnecessary fatigue, exhortation to exercise will be ineffective. It is necessary that health professionals ascertain these types of predisposing barriers before attempting to change a health behavior.

Often it is better not to attempt to change a belief, but to add a new one. If older persons believe, for example, that God will take care of their health, the health professional can agree with this assertion and then simply add Sophocles's declaration, "Heaven never helps the man who will not act" (Lorig, 1992).

Predisposing factors can be determined by finding out what clients know about the health area of concern, whether they believe they have a problem, whether they have cultural habits that must be taken into consideration, and whether they believe behavior changes will help. Older adults, for instance, may believe that because of their age it is too late to change or to do themselves any good. It may be helpful to respond with data on how rapidly health improvements can take place after the age of 65. A significant number of older adults may believe they get all the exercise they need when in fact, according to indicators of exercise frequency, intensity, and duration, they do not.

Enabling factors are those resources necessary for engaging in health-related activities—specifically, access and skill level. Before making recommendations to clients, health professionals need to determine whether there are appropriate programs with experienced leaders who are trained to work with older adults, whether these programs are accessible to those with limited transportation and financial means, whether clients have the necessary skills for modifying their behavior, whether recommended materials needed by older adults are affordable and available, and whether older adults perceive their environment to be safe enough to implement a program.

Practitioners need to be resourceful; it may be necessary to help older adults find accessible programs or gain necessary skills. It is also important that health professionals facilitate ways in which older persons can help themselves rather than solve problems for clients and thereby foster dependency.

Reinforcing factors refer to the peers, significant others, and health professionals who can support the continuation of new health behaviors. Older adults may be widowed, uninvolved in former occupational groups, and relatively isolated from other persons who are interested in maintaining health. Practitioners ought to consider whether their clients have sufficient family, peer, or professional support to reinforce health behavior changes.

PROCEED involves evaluation of the intervention: implementation, process evaluation (was the intervention delivered in the required "dose" to the expected audience?), and impact and outcome evaluation (did it have the desired effect?).

10 Tips for Changing Health Behaviors

After years of working with health science students to help older adults change health behaviors, it would be wonderful if I could offer the reader a simple formula for increasing the probability of success. Unfortunately, I fall victim to the "kitchen sink" syndrome that I think also afflicts the PRECEDE model just described. Many factors can influence the success or failure of a person's attempt to change a health behavior, and research has not helped us much in understanding which factors are more important for which types of people.

Over the years, therefore, I developed my own framework for helping older adults make a desired health behavior change. "Model" is too sophisticated a word to describe this framework, so I refer to it as the "10 Tips." With each older client willing to attempt a behavior change, a review of the 10 Tips is likely to produce strategies that will help the person succeed. From personal experience and research projects, I believe this approach will be helpful. If you examine the health contract/calendar technique previously summarized, along with the directions for completing it, you will notice that the 10 Tips are incorporated into this technique.

In order to make these ideas more practical, I focus on the specific goal of increasing exercise or physical activity. This also happens to be the health goal most likely to be chosen by older adults when given a choice among many options (Elder et al., 1995; Haber & Looney, 2000).

1. Motivation
2. Modest
3. Measurable
4. Memory
5. Positive thoughts

6. Reinforcement
7. Environmental support
8. Stress management
9. Social support
10. Problem-solve

Motivation

It is obvious that a person must be motivated to change a health behavior. I have found, however, that the first ***motivation*** identified by an older adult is not necessarily the one that lights up their eyes with authenticity. Those contemplating a reason for overcoming their sedentary ways may first come up with a politically correct motivation that elicits the approval of others, including the health educator they are working with, rather than one that is heartfelt.

For instance, avoiding heart disease may truly be the most motivating reason for someone to take on the challenge of a new exercise routine. Or it may not be. With a little probing on the part of the health educator, it may come to light that the person is more passionate about achieving better sleeping habits, or regularity in bowel habits, or additional energy in order to play longer with the grandchildren. It is best to spend a sufficient amount of time discussing what motivates the client and to examine the client's facial expressions for clues to what is of importance.

To assist the client, the practitioner may provide a list of possible motivations to choose from. This list includes disease categories that the client may want to avoid or alleviate, such as arthritis, stroke, obesity, hypertension, heart disease, peripheral vascular disease, diabetes, osteoporosis, colon cancer, and depression; and areas of potential functional improvement, such as constipation, forgetfulness, low energy, sleeplessness, stress, weakness, stiffness, and falls. Once the primary motivation has been identified, write it down (on the health contract if that is the technique of choice), and encourage clients to remind themselves about their motivation on a regular basis.

Also, if the goal is exercise, the client should identify which type: brisk walking, joining an aerobics class, increasing physical activity over the course of the day, or something else the client is likely to stick with? Motivation is enhanced by choosing an intervention a person enjoys, or at least by avoiding the more burdensome options.

Modest

No one is ever disappointed if they meet or exceed the goal established. Yet, it is an uncommon event when an older adult initially declares a goal that is modest enough to elicit the health educator's confidence that it can be achieved or exceeded. It is more common for someone to state an overly ambitious goal, like exercising *every* day. It is important to make one's goal modest. If a client sets a goal to exercise four times a week and meets or exceeds that goal, motivation will be sustained. But if the goal is to exercise every day, 4 days is a failure, and motivation may be compromised.

If the person establishes 60 minutes of daily walking as the goal, reduce it by half and give "extra credit" (perhaps in the form of more praise) for exceeding that goal. Encourage the sedentary client to build up to the 30-minute goal by establishing a target of 10 minutes of walking for the first week, 20 minutes for the second week, and 30 minutes for the third and fourth weeks. Allow clients to walk a *cumulative* 30 minutes a day if they choose, rather than limit them to 30 consecutive minutes.

The opposite problem can also reduce motivation: the client setting a goal that is too easy and then losing interest in it. This is an unusual occurrence, especially if the person has identified the appropriate motivation. Once you understand what motivates a client, help that person modify their goal during the first month so that it is neither grandiose nor undemanding.

A goal using a 1-month time period is often successful—hence the monthly contract/calendar. One month does not extend too far into the future, and with the use of the 1-month calendar, the end is in sight. It is also a long enough period of time to allow for adjustment of the goal, or the behaviors to achieve the goal, in the first week in order to increase the likelihood of success. Even if the goal turns out to be less motivating than was initially thought, the client may still have a good chance of successfully completing it in 1 month and carrying over that confidence to another, more motivating health goal the following month.

Measurable

Measurability has several components. With exercise, how much will the older adult be doing—how many minutes of exercise and on how many days of the week? How intensely will the person be doing it—will they establish a brisk walking pace that is twice the pace of normal walking? Will they monitor their breathing and body heat, making sure that they achieve sufficient intensity to produce deeper breathing or body heat (up to or including sweating), but not so much intensity that talking while walking becomes difficult? Will they monitor intensity level, building up in the beginning and slowing down near the end?

Measurability also implies recordkeeping, which is another reason the contract/calendar technique is appealing. People are used to recording on their calendars the activities that they need to be reminded of. I encourage clients to measure and compare the number of days they actually complete the contracted behavior each week with the number of days they had contracted for. Monitoring weekly success can lead to greater confidence, or to the periodic need to revise the health goal.

Memory

Habits take up a large part of the day. We give little thought to many of the activities that constitute our daily routines, and at the same time we rarely forget them. How do we switch to a new behavior, one that is a bit challenging to adopt, and make it a new habit? The answer is by enhancing our memory in as many ways as possible.

What cues can be established to help remind us? For example, we can place our walking shoes by the front door; place the health contract on the refrigerator door; ask a family member or a friend to remind us or check on us; associate the new behavior with an established one, like walking before dinner every night (perhaps adding a well-placed cue—a note near the dinner table that reads, "Did you walk yet?").

Positive Thoughts

Substitute positive and hopeful thoughts for negative, self-defeating ones. For each negative thought like "I've never been able to maintain exercise routines before," substitute a positive argument like "It may be difficult, but this time I will persist and accomplish my goal." It may be helpful to record affirmations and place them in conspicuous locations. Other avenues of positive support are to find books, magazines, or podcasts that inspire clients, encourage them to associate with persons who model what they are attempting to accomplish, and have them seek friends or acquaintances who are willing to be supportive of their goal.

For those who like irony and want to use negative reinforcement to promote positive thinking, keep a rubber band unobtrusively around your wrist, and when a negative thought about the health goal occurs, snap the band and replace the negative thought with a positive one.

Reinforcement

Most psychologists rely on positive rather than negative reinforcement. If success is achieved at the end of the first week, for instance, encourage clients to treat themselves to a movie or purchase a book. If success is observed at the end of the month, perhaps the spouse will take over one of your errands. Reinforcements tend to be more effective when they fall in close proximity to achievement.

External reinforcement does not necessarily involve spending money. Praise can be an important reinforcement. Encourage clients to speak highly of themselves when they are doing well with their goal, and ask them to be a bit immodest in their solicitation of praise from others. External incentives are helpful to some people but not to others. If the motivation to achieve a goal is strong, the successful efforts themselves may be sufficiently rewarding. External incentives may, in fact, distract from internal rewards.

Though most psychologists prefer positive reinforcement to negative reinforcement, I heard of a diabolically clever form of punishment that I will pass along. Identify an issue about which a person feels strongly (e.g., death penalty) and then have the client make out several small checks to an organization that promotes a belief *contrary* to their own belief. Let the person know that when punishments are to be administered, the checks will be mailed to the offending organization by someone other than the client.

Environmental Support

Another term for ***environmental support*** is *stimulus control.* The best example of this applies to weight management. If you want to contribute to weight maintenance or loss, make sure that the client does not keep junk food in the house.

Exercisers also have options in this regard. Placing sneakers by the front door is an example of environmental support. Locate the stair-stepper in front of the television set. Keep the elastic exercise band on the coffee table as a visible reminder.

Stress Management

It is the rare person who does not feel stress these days. Not only do we live in a fast-paced society, but we are also likely to contend with the automobile driver who is releasing road rage, cope with a frustrating physical disability, struggle with a personal loss, or encounter countless hassles and annoyances. Stress is a common barrier to achieving a health goal. If possible, build into the plan of action a few ***stress management*** techniques that can be practiced on a regular basis, preferably daily. A useful and easy stress management technique is deep breathing, which can be combined with an everyday activity.

Social Support

I suggest that some thought be given to ***social support*** for every client. For many, but not all, older adults, social support is desirable, perhaps essential. It may be a good idea to build social support into the statement of the health goal itself.

Ideally, a person has multiple sources of social support: perhaps a health educator, a spouse, a friend, a physician or nurse, a pastor, or a neighbor. Suggest to your client that they announce the health goal to others in general, even acquaintances, to increase the chances that additional people will offer support and approval.

Clients who unexpectedly find social support lacking or inconvenient ("My spouse doesn't always want to walk when I want to"), unreliable ("My friend doesn't always show up"), or overly critical will need to seek other sources of social support. A physician who does not muster enthusiasm for their client's health goal may cause the client to consider finding another, more health-oriented healthcare professional. Clients needing more social support than is currently available to them may need to explore the option of joining a class in the community.

A community class that has a leader of the same age and gender as the client may provide a better role model. Fellow classmates who are also peers in age, gender, disability, or other relevant variables may provide extra social and emotional support for behavior change and maintenance.

Problem-Solve

Finally, chances are good that the client has tried to achieve this exercise goal or a similar one before. It typically takes multiple efforts to achieve a goal. Explore what might have gone wrong in the past, or what might go wrong in the immediate future. Spend a little time identifying likely barriers and ways to overcome them.

An example of a problem to be solved is an older adult who lives in Oregon who likes to walk briskly outdoors. Either learn to love the rain or find a backup plan, like walking in a shopping mall; turning on music and dancing alone in the living room; or dragging out the vacuum cleaner to do some energetic sweeping.

Another problem—quite common among older adults attempting to increase their exercise level—involves working around aches, pains, and fatigue. The solution may be to modify an exercise, change the exercise modality, or alter the time that the exercise is to be performed. The challenge is to identify problems from the past, imagine possible problems in the future, brainstorm solutions, and increase the chance of success.

HEALTH BEHAVIOR THEORIES

Theories can help us understand what influences health behaviors, and thus help us plan effective interventions. Theories may focus on different levels (e.g., psychological, social, institutional, community) and are subject to change based on new evidence. They may also be applied singly or in combination in order to address behavior-change challenges.

The preceding section, "Assessments and Interventions," overlaps with this one. I describe some of the theories upon which those strategies were based in a bit more detail, and succinctly describe a few more. First, three brief overlapping definitions: A ***theory*** of behavior change attempts to explain the processes underlying learning. A *model* draws on a number of theories to help people understand a problem. A ***concept*** is the primary element of a theory or model.

Behavioral and Cognitive Management

Operant conditioning, Skinner's (1953) model of behavior control, is based on the premise that behavior is determined by its consequences, that is, the kinds of rewards and punishments that follow behavior. Behaviors followed by rewards will increase in frequency, whereas behaviors followed by punishments will decline.

Operant conditioning has spawned a number of principles. *Immediate rewards and punishments*, for instance, are more effective than delayed ones. *Intermittent reinforcement* is more resistant to extinction than constant reinforcement. Careful observation of conditions that promote or discourage behavior can help shape future success.

Cognitive conditioning—unlike operant conditioning, which focuses on external behaviors—deals with internal changes in thoughts and feelings. Cognitive-conditioning advocates assert that behavior and feelings are influenced not by their consequences, but by antecedent thoughts.

The first step toward cognitive restructuring, therefore, is the identification of undesirable and unrealistic thoughts. The next step is the substitution and regular repetition of positive thoughts in order to shape future behavior. Once we have positively restructured our thoughts, we engage in fewer cognitive distortions, experience less emotional distress, and perform fewer maladaptive behaviors (Burns, 1980).

Because operant and cognitive conditioning are practiced universally, they do not appear to constitute a formal learning model. All of us use praise and punishment to influence the behavior of others as well as ourselves, and we often substitute positive thoughts for negative ones. Unlike informal methods for influencing others or ourselves, however, formal ***behavioral** and **cognitive management*** techniques are applied systematically and typically include these three steps:

1. *Clearly define the problem.* A need to exercise is vague. The ability to climb the steps in one's home without having to stop to rest is clear.
2. *Implement a systematic and measurable response to the problem.* To exercise as often as possible is vague. To exercise three times a week, 30 minutes at a time, and periodically assess one's perceived exertion level at moderate intensity is both systematic and measurable.
3. *Implement scheduled evaluations.* To feel one is making progress is vague. To assess the effectiveness of a health plan on a monthly basis and alter the plan of action or the health goal as necessary is explicit.

Healthy Pleasures

In contrast to the behavioral and cognitive management theories, which are based on structure and self-discipline, is the theory of ***healthy pleasures***. Advocates of this theory propose that healthy behaviors will be sustained when these behaviors are based on joy, intuition, and self-trust. Advocates suggest that a growing reliance on one's ability to listen to the body's internal cues for feeling good can replace behavior-change decisions based on scientific guidelines. For additional ideas on this topic, read *Healthy Pleasures* (Ornstein & Sobel, 1989).

My own bias is that healthy pleasures and management techniques are not an "either/or" proposition. Joyful and intuitive activities may be consistently practiced, even if not always in their spontaneous form, and a disciplined routine may be temporarily relieved by spontaneous and joyful forms of exercise. Whatever sustains motivation for a healthy lifestyle is the way to go.

Self-monitoring can be viewed as a strategy that borrows from both the healthy pleasures and management strategies. It consists of systematically recording one's own pattern of behavior for a specific period of time (management technique), but only for the purpose of awareness and without an effort to conform to a pattern of behavior (healthy-pleasures technique).

One example of self-monitoring is to keep a written record, or *food behavior diary*, of everything you eat and drink (see Exhibit 3.1). During a 3-day period (including a weekend day if your weekend eating pattern differs from that of weekdays), record what you eat, how much you eat, the quality of what you eat (which corresponds to the rings of the nutrition bull's-eye to be described in Chapter 5, "Nutrition and Weight Management"), where you eat, with whom you eat, what you are doing while you eat, and how you feel when you are eating. Make no effort to control this pattern of behavior, and make no effort to not control it. Just be aware of what you are doing and how you are feeling, and record it.

EXHIBIT 3.1 FOOD BEHAVIOR DIARY

What is a food behavior diary?

The diary is for recording and monitoring the foods and drinks that you consume each day, so that you can understand what, how, and why you consume what you do.

What information do I put in my food behavior diary?

- ✓ **What** foods or drinks did you consume?
- ✓ **How much** did you eat? (not enough, okay amount, too much)
- ✓ **Quality** of food you ate? (refers to the three rings of the Nutrition Bull's-Eye in Chapter 5: 1—bull's-eye; 2—middle ring; 3—outer ring)
- ✓ **Where** did you eat? (home, office, restaurant, school, car, etc.)
- ✓ **Who with?** (family member, friend, business colleague, alone, etc.)
- ✓ What were you **doing?** (activity)
- ✓ What was your **emotional state?** (happy, sad, anxious, angry, etc.)

FOOD/DRINK	AMOUNT	QUALITY	WHERE	WHO	ACTIVITY	MOOD
Oatmeal	Okay	1	Living room	Son	Watching TV	Energetic
Skim milk	Okay	1				
Grilled cheese	Too much	3	Kitchen table	Son	Reading newspaper	Anxious
Water	Not enough	1				
Chips	Too much	3	Living room	Alone	On the phone	Tired
Pepper steak	Too much	2	Restaurant	Family	Dinnertime/ talk	Excited, happy
Brown rice	Okay	1				
Skim milk	Not enough	1				

When you carefully monitor your eating behaviors, you not only increase your awareness of what triggers unhealthy eating patterns but you also often begin to modify them as part of the self-awareness process. One study reported that people who kept daily food diaries lost twice as much weight as those who kept no records (Hollis et al., 2008).

By monitoring food intake you might realize, for instance, that you eat automatically and in greater quantity, in front of the television set and when you socialize in certain settings, even when you are not hungry. You may choose to eliminate the former because it provides no extra pleasure, but maintain the latter—allowing yourself to indulge at parties that serve food because they happen infrequently and are more enjoyable.

QUESTION: Complete a food behavior diary for 3 days. What did you learn about your eating and drinking habits? Did the monitoring process lead to changes in your eating pattern? If so, did these changes occur easily and naturally, or through discipline?

Social Cognitive Theory

One broad learning perspective, referred to as ***social cognitive theory***, has a lengthy history (Bandura, 1977, 1997; Rodin, 1986; Rotter, 1954). It addresses both the psychosocial dynamics underlying health behavior and the methods of promoting behavior change. This perspective actually encompasses a wide range of learning concepts that include role modeling, guided mastery of tasks, verbal persuasion, physiological state, and self-efficacy. The last one is the most applied component, perhaps a theory unto itself.

Role modeling is an important component of social cognitive theory. It is most effective when the role model shares many characteristics with the participant, such as age, race, physical impairment, gender, and socioeconomic status. Professional leaders of health education classes who are not role models in this sense should consider sharing teaching responsibilities and problem-solving strategies with class members who are. McAuley and Courneya (1993) suggest that role modeling with older program participants "may be particularly salient. In such cases it is common to look to other people, especially those that bear similar physical characteristics to ourselves, for motivation and information regarding our own prospects of success" (p. 73).

Guided mastery involves learning and practicing appropriate behaviors through the assignment of small, graded (i.e., increasingly challenging) tasks that are to be accomplished in a specific period of time. Achieving mastery over a difficult or previously feared task through guided personal experience may be the most potent source of self-efficacy (this is discussed in more detail in the next section).

Persuasion is another social cognitive strategy, one that is probably more popular than effective. Persuasion is most effective when health providers and educators ensure that it is accompanied by realistic goals and includes supervision of tasks on a step-by-step basis. It is also important that messages be positive and direct ("You can do it," not "Try and do it") and delivered by a respected source. Persuasion focuses on identifying the risk along with the intervention that can reduce the risk, and convincing clients that they can successfully engage in the intervention and have a positive outcome.

Physiological state can provide information that affects performance. High physiological arousal, for instance, can impair performance. People are more likely to expect failure when they are tense or agitated prior to starting something new. Someone experiencing fatigue, aches, or pains just before starting an exercise session is likely to question the effort needed to perform. Easing of physiological arousal may enhance the ability to perform.

Self-Efficacy

Self-efficacy may be the most widely utilized and tested concept in social cognitive theory. It is a belief in one's capabilities to implement a course of action. Self-efficacy is synonymous with having *confidence* about behavior change or maintenance within a specific behavioral domain (Bandura, 1997).

Self-efficacy can be manipulated experimentally with success. In one classic study, psychological tests were administered to a group of volunteers in a smoking cessation program. Half the subjects were then randomly assigned to a treatment group and told that in their tests they had demonstrated great potential to quit smoking. The other half were told the truth, which was that they had been *randomly* assigned to a control group. Fourteen months after treatment, smoking frequency had been reduced by 67% within the efficacy-enhanced group and by 35% within the control group (Blittner et al., 1978).

After reviewing the literature, McAuley and Courneya (1993) concluded, "If practitioners and clinicians fail to organize, present, and develop their programs in such a way as to cultivate efficacy beliefs, participants are likely to perceive the activity negatively, become disenchanted, discouraged, and discontinue. On the other hand, adequately organizing [programs] in a manner such that a strong sense of personal efficacy is promoted will result in the individual displaying more positive affect, evaluating their self-worth more positively, embracing more challenging activities, putting forth more effort, and persisting longer. In short, they will be in a position to successfully self-regulate their behavior" (p. 72).

The relationship between self-efficacy and behaviors is interactive, not unidirectional. Just as enhancing self-efficacy beliefs may increase the likelihood of sustaining a new health behavior, ongoing adherence to a new health behavior may continue to increase self-efficacy. Extreme optimism regarding one's self-efficacy, however, may relate *inversely* to successful performance (Rakowski et al., 1991).

Other cautions apply as well. Self-efficacy is limited to a person's belief in a specific, not a general, ability. People may, for example, perceive themselves to possess the self-efficacy to implement a walking program but not to follow through on a diet. Self-efficacy in one area of behavior does not necessarily carry over to another. Also, the perceived ability to change a health habit or adopt a new health behavior does not guarantee that a person has the necessary skill level, role model, peer or professional support, or access that might be required. Self-efficacy may be a necessary, though not a sufficient, condition for clients attempting to improve a health behavior.

Self-efficacy was an important part of the *Arthritis Self-Help (ASH) course* (Lorig et al., 1989) developed at Stanford University in 1978 by Kate Lorig, a nurse and health educator, and physicians Halsted Holman and James Fries. More than 100,000 persons with arthritis completed the ASH course, usually in groups of 15 or fewer and typically led by trained nonprofessionals with arthritis. During the 12-hour program, students were taught about arthritis and how to (a) design an exercise program around their limitations, (b) manage pain through relaxation techniques, (c) improve nutrition, (d) fight depression and fatigue, and (e) communicate more effectively with physicians. Participants who completed the program reported a 15% to 20% reduction in pain, were more active, and visited a physician less frequently. Among those who were depressed when starting the program, fewer depressive symptoms were reported by the end of the program.

The researchers were surprised to find that although changes in behavior, such as exercise and stress management, occurred as a consequence of the program, the factor most closely linked to outcomes (improvements in pain control, depression management, and activity level) was an increase in self-efficacy. In one group of successful patients, self-efficacy was still 17% higher 4 years after they completed the course (Lorig et al., 1989).

The ASH program and the follow-up *Chronic Disease Self-Management Program* (CDSMP; see Chapter 9, "Community Health") were developed and evaluated by Kate

Lorig and colleagues at the Stanford University Patient Education Research Center. These programs have demonstrated effective management of chronic disease through reductions in fatigue, emotional stress, and—most important to insurers—visits to physicians and emergency departments (see www.ahrq.gov/research). A national evaluation of CDSMP demonstrated strong improvements in self-rated measures and healthcare utilization but did not include a control arm (Ory et al., 2013). Worksite and health plan implementation, as well as longer follow-up and extension to varied clinical populations, have all confirmed benefit. Similar chronic disease management programs, however, have generated controversy (Box 3.4).

BOX 3.4 Chronic Disease Self-Management Programs

In medicine, ***efficacy*** measures how well an intervention works in clinical trials or laboratory studies when researchers exert a considerable amount of control over the experiment. ***Effectiveness***, however, relates to how well a treatment works in the real world on a large-scale basis.

Chronic disease self-management programs have raised questions about whether these types of programs are effective, or just efficacious when researchers utilize small samples and exert a good deal of control over the intervention (and, some argue, the evaluation). A number of researchers report that the results of chronic disease management programs in general have been equivocal or negative (Buszewicz et al., 2006; Chodosh et al., 2005; Newbould et al., 2006).

As an example, Medicare funded a chronic disease management pilot program that had nurses periodically check on whether patients were managing their drugs and seeing the right doctors, as well as monitoring their laboratory results (Abelson, 2008). Not only were there no savings to Medicare, but the program was hard pressed to even be budget neutral. A meta-analysis reported that 13 of 15 Medicare demonstration programs designed to improve chronic care, communication, and patient adherence through nurse monitoring and patient education did not yield net Medicare savings (Peikes et al., 2009).

Conversely, though, a nurse-led disease management program with early-stage heart failure patients cost about $2,200 per patient, but this was offset by savings of about $2,400 per patient in lower hospitalization rates (Hebert et al., 2008). A randomized controlled trial examining a chronic care model, called Guided Care, in which nurses focus on the sickest and most complex older patients, cost health insurers 11% less than the control group (Leff et al., 2009). Guided Care patients had 24% fewer hospital days, 37% fewer skilled nursing facility days, 15% fewer emergency visits, and 29% fewer home healthcare episodes. The program realized annual net savings of $75,000 per nurse.

The challenges with evaluating chronic disease self-management programs are the variation in program content and evaluation techniques. Some chronic disease management programs use clinicians, whereas others use lay persons; some take place over the telephone, others in medical settings or in community settings; some report low attrition rates and others high rates; some link the efforts of medical and community staff, whereas others do not; some focus on patients with complex diseases and comorbidity and others do not; and few use the same measurement tools, with some tools well validated and reliable, while others are not.

An excellent program producing consistent benefits may be quite efficacious, but when taken out into the real world with a large and diverse patient and provider populations and different health goals or cost objectives, it may not be effective. This type of research takes plenty of time and money before convincing results can be obtained.

Health Locus of Control

Health locus of control refers to the idea that health can be controlled through the person's ability to control their own behavior (internal locus), or through powerful others or luck (external locus). One's health-locus-of-control orientation, similar to perceived self-efficacy, is of limited utility when persons do not place much value on seeking better health.

Also, medical practices and outcomes, unlike health practices, may not be within one's sphere of influence. Therefore, it is important that health professionals who encourage their clients to take personal responsibility for their health practices discourage them from overestimating their personal control over medical events. It may be necessary to help clients differentiate between the realistic goals they may be able to control—increasing energy, reducing stress, enhancing feelings of well-being, increasing knowledge and decision-making ability—and the less realistic goal of curing a medical condition.

One's health locus of control may become more external with age. For instance, older patients are more likely than younger ones to prefer that health professionals make health-related decisions for them (Woodward & Wallston, 1987). This increased externality among older adults, however, may be due to *cohort factors* such as (a) the cultural orientation of specific older cohorts who believe in an authoritarian health professional role (not the case with most baby boomers), or (b) the lower education level of the oldest cohort, which leads to reluctance to engage with health professionals in a dialogue they might not understand.

Increasing externality with age, though, may also be due to maturational factors. For example, the increased physical vulnerability that occurs with age may, over time, diminish a person's sense of personal control. This feeling of loss of personal control may not be associated with a negative attitude. A belief in powerful others, such as physicians, who can influence the course of an illness may lead older patients to become more hopeful about the future.

Information seeking does not always lead to better adjustment. Information about an illness can both raise and lower anxiety. When combined with the adoption of a relaxation technique, however, information seeking may be less prone to being anxiety producing.

One classic study matched subjects by their health-locus-of-control profiles. Those with internal control matches in self-directed programs and external control matches in peer support groups were more satisfied and lost more weight than nonmatched subjects (Wallston et al., 1976). However, another possible (and perhaps more powerful) explanation was not examined—that combining both internal *and* external sources of support may lead to better perceptions and results.

The success of *Alcoholics Anonymous* (AA), for example, may be attributable to its reliance on both internal and external sources of control. On the one hand, AA members must take responsibility for their problem; on the other hand, they are required to acknowledge their inability to control alcoholism without the help of a higher power and the other members of AA.

Related to the study of locus of control are two landmark studies focused on personal control. Both reveal that seemingly insignificant opportunities to control events can affect both physical and mental health. In one study, the residents of two floors of a nursing home were given responsibility for such activities as taking care of a plant, deciding on when to see a movie, and rearranging furniture. The residents of the other two floors were also beneficiaries of a plant, weekly movie, and furniture, but were given no control over these activities; the staff took care of the plants, decided when the movie would be shown, and rearranged the furniture.

Despite the fact that the residents were similar in physical health, mental health, and prior socioeconomic status, the residents with personal control were physically and mentally healthier, and 18 months later only 15% of those with enhanced control had died, versus 30% of those without (Langer & Rodin, 1976; Rodin & Langer, 1977).

The second study was Schulz's (1976) experiment with residents of a retirement home. It revealed that student visits to residents led to more active, happier lives among the residents. However, unlike the nursing home experiments in which personal control opportunities for residents were on a continuing basis, the removal of the students from the retirement home precipitated a significant decline in health.

The rationale underlying the desirability of internal health locus of control is that decisions and actions will more likely produce advantageous outcomes. Studies show that perceived internal control is associated with reduced stress, increased motivation, improved health, and enhanced performance. Perceived internal control, however, can have negative effects under certain conditions; for example, when perceived internal control or confidence exists without sufficient information or skill to support a positive outcome; when excessive demands are made on a person's time, effort, and resources; and when clients accept responsibility for complex medical problems or blame for medical outcomes outside their control.

Health Belief Model

One model of health behavior change focuses on perceived threats, benefits, and barriers. The health belief model was developed during the early 1950s by a group of social psychologists at the U.S. Public Health Service to explain why people did not participate in screening tests for the early detection of asymptomatic disease (Rosenstock, 1990). The researcher reported that people chose to take or not take preventive action depending on their perception of threats, benefits, and barriers.

Perceived threats refer to the person's perception of their *susceptibility* to a particular condition and the degree of *severity* of the condition that they fear. Persons who perceive no threat lack a reason to act. Perceived susceptibility to and severity of a condition together produce fear. For instance, when heart patients see a scan showing plaque accumulation in their own arteries, their adherence to a lipid-lowering drug regimen increases significantly. Moreover, the more severe the plaque accumulation, the more likely the patient is to stay on the medicine (Kalia et al., 2006).

Fear is an effective motivator, yet the optimal level of fear for motivating client behavior is unknown. Too little fear may not motivate, but too much can lead to denial and inaction. An important consideration in fear-inducing interventions is that fearful people, regardless of their motivation, may lack the necessary skills or confidence to change their health behaviors.

Perceived benefits refers to the belief that specific actions on the part of a person will reduce the threat of negative outcomes or increase the chance of positive outcomes. Perceived benefits must outweigh perceived barriers before a person will initiate an action. *Perceived barriers* may include financial considerations, inconvenience, lack of transportation, lack of knowledge, or potential pain or discomfort.

Evaluations of the health belief model conducted exclusively with older persons have been limited. One such study, though, assessed health beliefs related to osteoporosis—specifically, the likelihood that the older adults in the study would adopt exercise behaviors and increase their calcium intake (Kim et al., 1991). The authors concluded that it is particularly important to focus on overcoming the perceived barriers of older adults, such as their difficulty with changing old habits and the difficulty of incorporating new habits into a daily routine.

Where do people get their ideas about severity and susceptibility, benefits or barriers? Recent efforts, spurred on by computational modeling, yield a dynamic picture of social influence and awareness of disease trends as key factors driving health behavior change. Figure 3.3 shows a schematic using the health belief model to assess the dynamics of health behavior change, following a model proposed by Durham and Casman (2012).

In this approach, people observe illnesses in their social networks and in the world at large through media messages; this perception gives rise to an appraisal of personal susceptibility (SUSC). They observe the prevalence of protective or risk behaviors among friends and family, or when using public transportation, and so on. This gives rise to appraisals of barriers to adopting a behavior (BEN/BAR). They learn of disease trends, hospitalization, and mortality from media, public service announcements, CDC recommendations, internet misinformation, and so forth. This gives rise to appraisals of severity (SEV). Individuals ("agents") use this information external to the agent to compute a single score, which if greater than some threshold, leads them to adopt a protective behavior. They can then influence others at a subsequent time point to change or maintain a health behavior. This simple computational model can generate testable predictions about the likelihood of health behavior change under specified conditions (Albert, 2023). Even if overly simple, this approach may be valuable for assessing the dynamics of health behavior change. However, additional factors may need to be considered, including physiological dependency, economic limitations, environmental influences, skill development, and self-efficacy.

FIGURE 3.3 Computational schema for the health belief model.

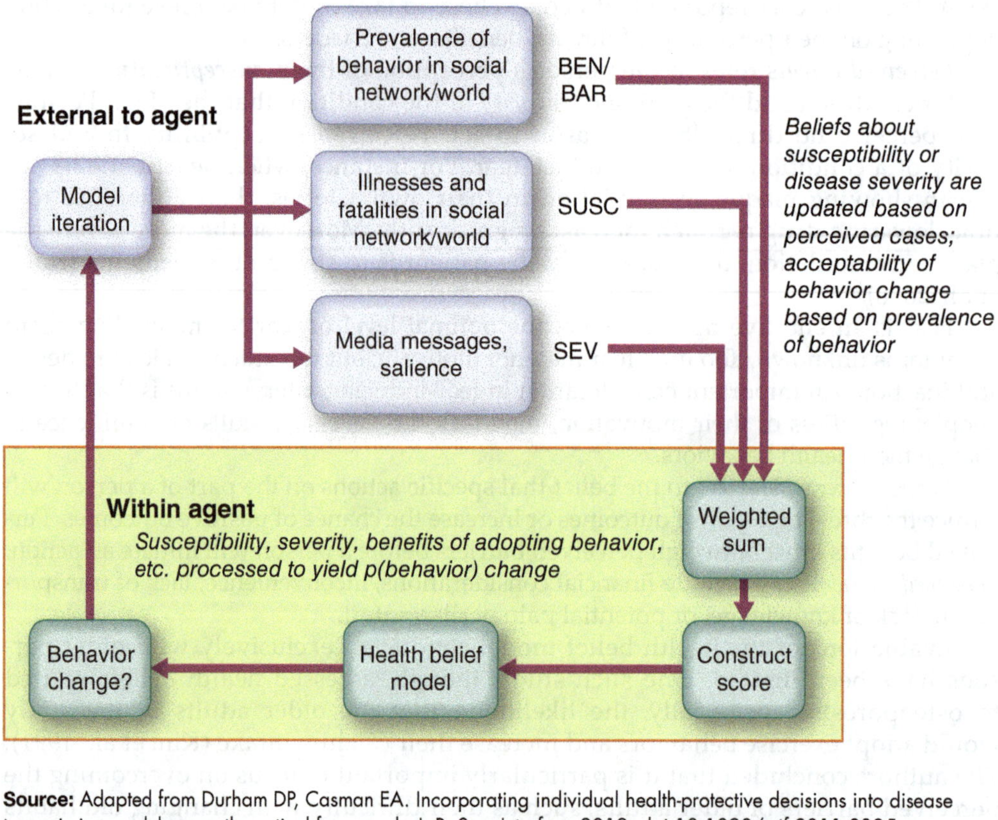

Source: Adapted from Durham DP, Casman EA. Incorporating individual health-protective decisions into disease transmission models: a mathematical framework. J. R. Soc. Interface 2012; doi:10.1098/rsif.2011.0325

Other Theories

The *theory of reasoned action* focuses on attitudes that precede potential behaviors (Fishbein & Ajzen, 1975). One aspect of this theory is its focus on taking into account what a person's relevant others think that person should do. An older person may finally relent and join a smoking cessation program based on the perception of their physician's or spouse's wishes.

The *theory of planned behaviors*, an extension of the theory of reasoned action, has an additional focus on the perceived ease or difficulty of performing a behavior (Ajzen, 1988). The older smoker may intend to quit but does not believe there is access to a program that will provide the skills to quit.

There are theories that focus on *individual empowerment*, which most practitioners endorse, but the outcomes of empowering people may not lead to what practitioners think will be the best course of action. Harvath (2008), for example, recounts her nursing experiences and reports that empowered older adults may choose to remain in their homes despite repeated falls and injuries, rather than transfer to a safer nursing home environment. Also, empowered older adults with dysphagia may choose textured foods despite the risk of aspiration, because these foods play such an important role in their lives.

There are also *community empowerment* theories that emphasize collective education and social action to promote the participation of people, organizations, and communities in gaining control over their lives (Wallerstein & Bernstein, 1988). Community empowerment initiatives to address health problems usually must surmount challenging cultural, social, and historical barriers.

Community-oriented primary care (COPC) is another community-level theory that encourages clinicians to view their patient populations, not just individual patients, and to involve other community organizations and community leaders to help with population-based behavior change (Nutting, 1987). Examples of applying COPC in the community are provided in Chapter 9, "Community Health."

A surprising article, at least to sociologists like myself, reports that, in general, well-funded large-scale programs designed to change the larger community in which people live to get people to improve their health behaviors have not turned out to be successful (Syme, 2003).

THEORIES VERSUS CONCEPTS

You might wonder why health behavior theories are placed near the end of this chapter given that they are the foundation for empowering older adults. Perhaps because the behavior-change theories are not sufficiently powerful to stimulate the shaping of a health intervention; however, several concepts embedded in the theories may be useful once a health intervention has progressed to the development phase. Furthermore, a theory attempts to relate a set of concepts systematically to explain and predict events and activities. Concepts, however, are the primary elements of theory, and each theory has a concept or two that is particularly well developed and helpful in guiding a community intervention and evaluation.

QUESTION: **If you were writing a grant proposal to help older adults exercise more in the community, which two health behavior concepts described in this chapter would you find most helpful for guiding your intervention? Explain your answer.**

So, a question was raised from community experience rather than theory. Was a health promotion directory being utilized by older adults (Haber & Looney, 2003)? How effective was a health contract/calendar for behavior change (Haber, 2007; Haber & Looney, 2000; Haber & Rhodes, 2004)? Were African American churches good sites for exercise programs (Looney & Haber, 2001)? How effective were health science students as exercise leaders (Haber et al., 2000)? How effective was a health promotion intervention with older adults (Haber, 1986; Haber & Lacy, 1993)? If we provide personalized information on risk of falls, with referrals for remediation, can we reduce the incidence of falls (Albert, 2014)? Will a lifestyle intervention involving diet and activity improve healthy eating, promote weight loss, and improve gait speed (Albert et al., 2021)?

SUMMARY

In the olden days, the doctor prescribed a pill, usually described by its color, to an older patient, with no questions asked. Other medical decisions came from "on high" (the physician-god) as well. Times are changing with older adults. They are much better educated than before, they have the internet to surf, and they have a different attitude toward healthcare. With the exception, perhaps, of some complex medical circumstances, older patients want to participate in medical care decision-making.

Although there are undeniable benefits for older adults to be empowered, there are risks as well. The quality of internet content is inconsistent. Some medical decisions are so complex that taking even partial responsibility can be stressful. And knowing how important a healthy lifestyle is does not necessarily make it easier to follow through. Behavior change is enormously difficult.

Several health-promoting strategies may help. For those who are behavior management-oriented and like recordkeeping, the health contract might be helpful. These clients may also benefit from keeping a food diary over several days. For those who want group support, joining a chronic disease self-management group is an option. An older worker might take advantage of an HRA or other worksite wellness initiatives. There are support groups to help with chronic diseases, caregiving, coping with loss, and alcohol or other addiction problems. Fitness facilities and religious institutions are taking an interest in both the physical health and mental health of their older participants.

A behavioral cognitive intervention will be more effective than a sleeping pill in dealing with sleep problems over the long term. Bringing notes and questions to a physician visit can help focus on issues, or even remember them in a stressful environment. Health providers need to know that *all* patients are cross-cultural, because this term can refer not only to different ethnicities, but also to other gaps in understanding due to provider–patient differences in age, education, income, gender, religion, and so forth. A truly progressive and caring health provider might organize among patients the sharing of similar challenges among age peers with arthritis, cancer, heart disease, chronic obstructive pulmonary disease (COPD), stroke, or diabetes.

Empowerment, with its rewards and risks, is fast becoming a requirement in the era of chronic healthcare conditions that must be managed, sometimes for decades.

REFERENCES

Only key references appear in the print edition. The full reference list can be accessed by visiting www.springerpub.com/courseconnect. See inside front cover and tear-out card for CourseConnect details.

Albert, S. M., Venditti, E., Boudreau, R., Kieffer, L., Rager, J., Zgibor, J., Bilt, J., Danielson, M., Burke, L., Glynn, N., Jakicic, J., Smith, K., Semler, L., & Newman, A. (2021). Weight loss through lifestyle intervention improves mobility in older adults. *The Gerontologist*, *62*(6), 931–941. https://doi.org/10.1093/geront/gnab048

Belsky, W., Caspi, A., Houts, R., Cohen, H. J., Corcoran, D. L., Danese, A., Harrington, H., Israel, S., Levine, M. E., Schaefer, J. D., Sugden, K., Williams, B., Yashin, A. I., Poulton, R., & Moffitt, T. E. (2015). Quantification of biological aging in young adults. *Proceedings of the National Academy of Sciences*, *112*(30), E4104–E4110. https://doi.org/10.1073/pnas.1506264112

Butler, M., McCreedy, E., Schwer, N., Burgess, D., Call, K., Przedworski, J., Rosser, S., Larson, S., Allen, M., Fu, S., & Kane, R. L. (2016). *Improving cultural competence to reduce health disparities.* Report No. 16-EHC006-EF. Agency for Healthcare Research and Quality (US).

Hilliard, M. E., Riekert, K. A., Ockene, J. K., & Pbert, L. (2018). *The handbook of health behavior change* (5th ed.). Springer Publishing Company.

Huo, J., Desai, R., Hong, Y. R., Turner, K., Mainous, III, A. G., & Bian, J. (2019). Use of social media in health communication: Findings from the health information national trends survey 2013, 2014, and 2017. *Cancer Control*, *26*(1), 1073274819841442. https://doi.org/10.1177/1073274819841442

Langer, E., & Rodin, J. (1976). The effects of choice and enhanced personal responsibility for the aged: A field experiment in an institutional setting. *Journal of Personality and Social Psychology*, *34*, 191–198. https://doi.org/10.1037/0022-3514.34.2.191

Lorig, K. (1992). *Patient education: A practical approach*. Mosby-Year Book.

McGinnis, J. M., Williams-Russo, P., & Knickman, J. R. (2002). The case for more active policy attention to health promotion. *Health Affairs*, *21*, 78–93. https://doi.org/10.1377/hlthaff.21.2.78

Mokdad, A. H., Marks, J. S., Stroup, D. F., & Gerberding, J. L. (2004). Actual causes of death in the United States, 2000. *Journal of the American Medical Association*, *291*(10), 1238–1245. https://doi.org/10.1001/jama.291.10.1238

Ory, M. G., Ahn, S., Jiang, L., Lorig, K., Ritter, P., Laurent, D. D., Whitelaw, N., & Smith, M. L. (2013). National study of chronic disease self-management: Six-month outcome findings. *Journal of Aging and Health*, *25*(7), 1258–1278. https://doi.org/10.1177/0898264313502531

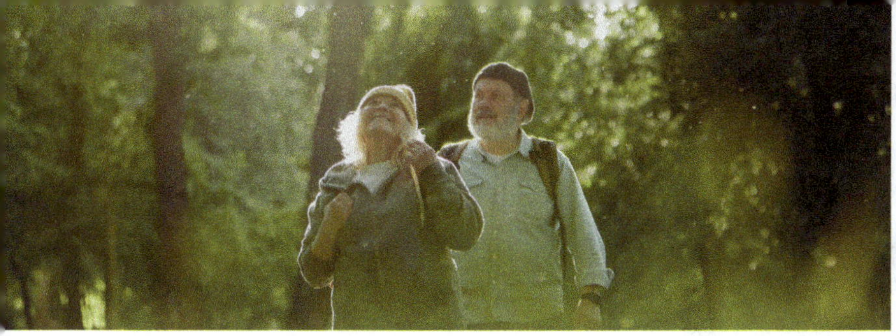

4

EXERCISE AND AGING

KEY TERMS

activity pyramid
aerobics
arthritis and other barriers to exercise
barriers and cautions
brisk walking
disease prevention/functional improvement through exercise
elastic bands, free weights, machine weights, and isometrics
excuses versus benefits of exercise
exercise as a weight management strategy
exercise most days of the week
exercise settings
flexibility and balance
healthy neighborhoods
intensity, fractionated exercise versus continuous exercise
model community exercise program
osteoarthritis
pedometer and fitness trackers
personal trainer
prolonged sitting
sarcopenia
strength building
Surgeon General's Report on Physical Activity and Health
target heart rate versus Borg perceived exertion
target heart rate zone
Valsalva maneuver
Wii-hab
yoga, tai chi, swimming, dance, and other exercise options

LEARNING OBJECTIVES

- Explain the four basic principles endorsed by the *Surgeon General's Report on Physical Activity and Health.*
- Review the benefits of *brisk walking.*
- Examine the dangers of prolonged sitting.
- Recognize the importance of *walking neighborhoods.*
- Review research into the beneficial effects of exercise on disease and functional impairment.
- Examine the importance of *exercise for weight management.*
- Examine the basic components of a ***model community exercise program.***
- Differentiate between aerobic and anaerobic exercise.
- Contrast *target heart rate* with the Borg technique.
- Recognize the importance of music for exercise.
- Define *sarcopenia* and identify the exercise needed to alleviate it.
- Contrast *elastic bands, free weights, machine weights,* and *isometrics.*
- Define the *Valsalva maneuver*, and explain the need to avoid it.
- Contrast *yoga* with flexibility movements.
- Explore *tai chi, swimming,* and *other exercise options.*
- Identify balance exercise options.
- Recognize different benefits for different exercises.
- Describe the *activity pyramid.*
- List exercise precautions and safety measures.
- Respond to exercise *excuses* and *barriers.*
- Contrast health club, home, and religious ***exercise settings.***
- Evaluate *personal trainers* and online exercise options.
- Examine *Wii-hab* as an exercise technique.
- Recognize the importance of a health educator in the medical clinic.

Those who have no time for exercise will sooner or later have to find time for illness.

—*Edward Stanley*

SURGEON GENERAL'S REPORT ON PHYSICAL ACTIVITY AND HEALTH

In her exercise video "Shopping for Fitness," the late comedienne Joan Rivers espoused walking the malls for aerobic conditioning, lifting shopping bags for weight training, and trying on jeans that are one size too small to motivate oneself for weight reduction. According to Rivers, "Everybody's got a tape out, Buns of Steel, Breasts of Iron and Bunions of Teflon. They just don't get it, that it should be fun." Although many of her comments on the video are satirical, the ***Surgeon General's Report on Physical Activity and***

Health supports what she espouses. The Surgeon General's report, *Vision for a Healthy and Fit Nation,* covers physical activity at schools and workplaces and across communities (U.S. Office of the Surgeon General, 2010).

The initial Surgeon General's Report (Blair et al., 1996) represented a collaborative effort between the Centers for Disease Control and Prevention (CDC) and the President's Council on Physical Fitness and Sports. It was the most comprehensive review of the research up to that time on the effects of physical activity on people's health. According to the Surgeon General's Report, regular ***exercise*** and physical activity improved health in a variety of ways, including a reduction in heart disease, diabetes, high blood pressure, colon cancer, depression, anxiety, excess weight, falling, bone thinning, muscle wasting, and joint pain.

However, at the time of the initial report in 1996, 60% of adults did not achieve the recommended amount of physical activity, and 25% of adults were not physically active at all. Inactivity increased with age; by age 75, 36% engaged in no physical activity. Inactivity was more common among women and people with lower income and less education. Little has changed. The proportion of adults reporting no participation in the past month in "any physical activities or exercises such as running, calisthenics, golf, gardening, or walking for exercise" was 24.4% in 2016, 24.5% in 2018, and 23.8% in 2020 (Van Dyke et al., 2023).

Figure 4.1 shows that adults age 65+ are more likely to report no leisure-time physical activity. Women, minority groups, rural residents, and people with lower incomes and education are all similarly more likely to report no physical activity. Gradients across levels of education and income are particularly impressive. For example, less than 15% of college graduates report no physical activity compared to over 40% of people who did not graduate from high school. These disparities by sociodemographic status are typical of many health behaviors and suggest an important role for social determinants, or structural factors beyond individual behavior, in the uptake of protective health behaviors.

Surgeon General reports often go unnoticed, but some have had a major impact. For example, an early report of the Surgeon General on the health hazards of tobacco, published in 1964, had a major influence on public awareness, the policies of government and business, and the percentage of Americans who smoked. The report on physical activity and health, three decades later, also had a major influence on society, but in a different way. While the number of people who participated in a regular exercise routine increased modestly at best, there was a major rethinking in how we exercise. I highlight the four principles embodied in the report.

1. The report agreed with Ms. Rivers that most sedentary Americans are not going to rigorously pursue buns of steel, and of those who do, all will fall short of the goal. Instead, it is important to make the first step for most Americans achievable; and to do so requires a large degree of modesty in setting goals and expectations for persistence and enjoyment. Hence the emphasis on being more active and having fun with it, perhaps by shopping—as Joan suggested—while walking briskly, rather than exclusively focusing on a narrow adherence to a rigid exercise regimen.
2. Another basic premise of the Surgeon General's Report was that Americans should get at least 30 minutes of physical activity, ***most days of the week.*** This statement provided a major perspective shift from previous recommendations by government and exercise leaders. Instead of raising the exercise ***intensity*** level to a ***target heart rate*** for a specific period of time, three times a week, the report recommended that Americans become more concerned about expending calories through physical activity and exercise on a near-daily basis (every day is perfect, but humans are not).

FIGURE 4.1 Prevalence of no leisure-time physical activity, 2018–2020, by sociodemographic status.

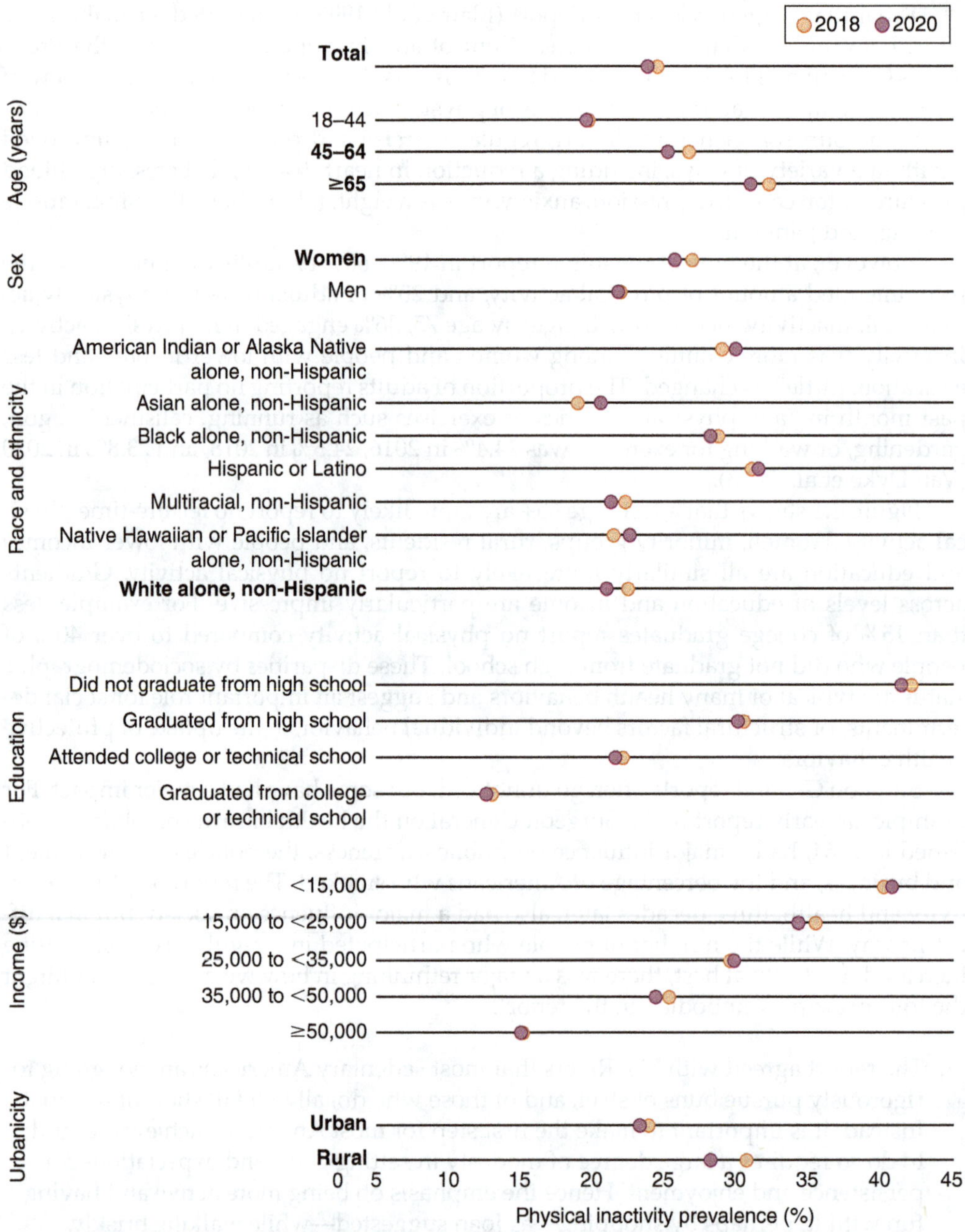

Source: Centers for Disease Control and Prevention. Behavioral Risk Factor Surveillance System. Van Dyke, M. E., Chen, T. J., Nakayama, J. Y., Moore, L. V., & Whitfield, G. P. (2023). Changes in physical inactivity among U.S. adults overall and by sociodemographic characteristics, behavioral risk factor surveillance system, 2020 versus 2018. *Preventing Chronic Disease*, *20*, 230012. https://doi.org/10.5888/pcd20.230012.

3. Also, instead of fixating on measuring target heart rate to assess intensity level, just raising one's respiratory and heart rate each day is sufficient—and this can be done by assessing one's own intensity level through two physiological changes that are apparent to the participant: quicker breathing rate and greater body warmth.
4. The report also suggested not being rigid about the length of a physical activity or exercise session. It was no longer deemed essential to obtain 30 consecutive minutes of exercise. For Americans, the large majority of whom are not too active, accumulating shorter activity spurts throughout the day may be more accessible. Got a spare few minutes? Then briskly walk the shopping malls like Joan did, or climb a few stairs.

Regarding the fourth principle, a review of the research literature concludes that accumulating several 5- or 10-minute bouts of physical activity over the course of the day provides beneficial health and fitness effects comparable to a single prolonged session of an equivalent length (Berrigan et al., 2018). Why should being less sedentary on and off throughout the day in small bouts be as good as or better than a regular 30-minute daily workout? Research suggests that people completing such workouts may reward themselves with sedentary behavior afterward, when not exercising. These dynamics suggest the many challenges involved in altering health behaviors.

One study reported that ***"fractionized" exercise*** may be more effective than ***continuous exercise*** (Angadi et al., 2012). Three bouts of 10 minutes of walking led to lower average 24-hour blood pressure readings than one 30-minute session. Another study reported similar benefits with exercise "snacks," or "bite-size portions of exercise"; they were more effective with controlling blood sugar throughout the day than a comparable longer session (Francois et al., 2014).

QUESTION: The principles of the Surgeon General's Report on Physical Activity and Health were widely accepted, though the percentage of Americans who engaged in regular physical activity and exercise lagged behind. Can you suggest an effective dissemination plan to policymakers, health providers, and consumers that would lead to more Americans practicing what this Surgeon General's Report preached?

Also, many older Americans will find a 10-minute session less daunting to initiate than a longer exercise period. Even more good news is that only one or two of these 10-minute sessions per day may produce significant results. A study of 416,000 Taiwanese over 12 years reported that as little as 15 minutes a day of physical activity reduced the all-cause mortality rate compared to those who were inactive (Wen et al., 2012).

Regarding exercise itself, it is difficult for adults to go from inactivity to an exercise routine. Thinking about how to accumulate short bouts of activity, therefore, is a useful way to get started on better health and fitness. For example, wash your car or your kitchen floor more briskly than you normally do (even if it means doing it in shorter segments throughout the day), or put more energy into raking leaves, mowing the lawn, gardening with enthusiasm, or dancing by yourself to music on the radio. Rather than focus on the length of time you exercise or engage in physical activity, emphasize increasing your breathing rate and elevating your body warmth. A growing industry of activity monitors and related wearable devices makes it easier to track exercise and provides important personalized feedback (Channa et al., 2021), even when unwanted!

Given that the sedentary population in the United States has remained stable—about 25% between 1996 and 2020—it is important to not fixate on a daunting 30 minutes or more of exercise each day, but rather to promote any small increase in movement. Minor increments will have a major impact on all-cause mortality levels (Sparling et al., 2015).

To repeat one of the Surgeon General's conclusions, Americans need to be active most days of the week. Therefore, aim for the habit of everyday exercise, but do not allow the occasional lapse to discourage you. Making exercise a near-daily routine is more likely to become an enduring habit than the previously recommended three times per week or seeking the perfection of 7 days per week.

This topic is more than just a health issue; it is a financial one as well. One study of more than 20,000 people over two decades, beginning with an average age of 51 and ending with an average age of 72, reported that participants who exercised routinely had 38% lower medical costs measured by Medicare and other insurance claims than those who failed to exercise regularly. The authors suggested that perhaps people who are able to document regular exercise should be able to share in the financial benefit gleaned by their insurers (Bachmann, 2012). An updated systematic review confirms this reduction in healthcare expenses but reminds us that better health means greater longevity and ultimately greater healthcare costs over the lifetime (Duijvestijn et al., 2023).

THE MOST POPULAR ACTIVITY: WALKING

Older adults need not become triathletes or engage in other high-intensity activities to reap the ***benefits of exercise*** (Bai et al., 2022). For most older adults, a ***brisk walking*** program will provide sufficient intensity for a good ***aerobics*** program. A landmark 8-year study of more than 13,000 people indicated that walking briskly for 30 to 60 minutes every day was almost as beneficial in reducing the death rate as jogging up to 40 miles a week (Blair et al., 1989). The authors of a study of 1,645 older adults reported that simply walking 4 hours per week decreased the risk of future hospitalization for cardiovascular disease (LaCroix et al., 1996). Taking more daily steps is associated with a decreased risk of cardiovascular disease (CVD). Tracking steps can also be useful for clinician–patient communication for CVD risk (Paluch et al., 2023).

The Nurses' Health Study was a long-term research project, spanning three decades and involving 122,000 nurses. A prospective study of 72,000 of these nurses over an 8-year period revealed that brisk walking 3 hours a week offered as much health benefit as engaging in vigorous exercise. Among the brisk walkers, the incidence of coronary events (nonfatal myocardial infarction or death from coronary disease) was reduced between 30% and 40% (Manson et al., 1999). A subset of this sample containing 5,100 diabetic walkers produced a similar reduction in heart disease risk (Hu et al., 2001).

A study on brisk walking defined it as 100 steps per minute (or count how many steps you take in 6 seconds and multiply by 10 (Han & Aguiar, 2018). Vigorous walking requires about 130 steps per minute, while jogging generally starts at about 140 steps per minute.

The National Center for Health Statistics reported that walking has much greater appeal for older adults than high-intensity exercise. Only 37% of older adults meet the aerobic recommendation (150 minutes per week of vigorous-to-moderate physical activity) proposed in the U.S. Physical Activity Guidelines, and only 19% meet the muscle-strengthening recommendation (2 days per week of exercises involving weights; U.S. Department of Health and Human Services, 2023). While participation in sports declines linearly with age, walking for exercise remains constant across the lifespan and its frequency declines only after age 55. People in their 80s continue to walk and average about 70% as much walking as 55 year olds (McPhee et al., 2016).

Brisk walking is the most popular aerobic activity for older adults. As the Acting Surgeon General Rear Admiral Denise Hinton emphasized in her report, most Americans can benefit from activities like brisk walking and not concern themselves about target heart rate. Many older adults are concerned about unfavorable weather, though, and may abandon their walking routine as a consequence. Prolonged hot or cold spells may sabotage a good walking program. Rather than discontinue this activity because of the weather, adults may choose to walk indoors at their local shopping malls. Many shopping malls—about 2,500 nationwide—open their doors early, usually between 5:30 and 10:00 a.m., for community residents, whether they shop or not. Malls have accommodated indoor walking well, with some providing places to leave coats, extra benches, and the like (King et al., 2016).

Walking in the Neighborhood

There is a relationship between neighborhood and health (Office of the Surgeon General, 2015). Residents who are dependent on a car to get to most places and have few sidewalks for safe walking are likely to be more obese and have chronic medical conditions that affect health-related quality of life (Booth et al., 2005; Sturm & Cohen, 2004). For every extra 30 minutes commuters drive each day, they have a 3% greater chance of being obese; in contrast, people who live within walking distance of shops are 7% less likely to be obese (Frank et al., 2004). Older persons who believe their neighborhoods are accessible by walking are considerably more physically active (Cerin et al., 2017; King et al., 2003; Li et al., 2005a).

Living in an urban area where commercial spaces are near residential areas leads to more frequent and lengthier durations of walking among all age groups, including older residents (Gauvin et al., 2012). Another group of researchers surveyed 2,285 adults age 45 to 84 and found that one third of them lived in ***healthy neighborhoods***, defined as neighborhoods with easy access to nearby walking, visibility of other residents walking in the neighborhood, availability of exercise facilities, and access to fresh produce (Auchincloss et al., 2009). Over a 5-year follow-up, those living in ***healthy neighborhoods*** were 38% less likely to develop diabetes than those who did not.

Another option for older adults is to join a noncompetitive walking or hiking club, or participate in a nearby walking or hiking event. Two such possibilities are the American Walking Club (Volkssport Association) at www.ava.org and a local Sierra Club chapter (contact the national headquarters at 415-977-5500 or at www.sierraclub.org).

Traveling to another city can also be an excuse not to exercise, or it can be an opportunity to gather information from the local newspaper or chamber of commerce about the city's walking tours. These can be an enjoyable way to get exercise and a unique way to learn about offbeat aspects of a neighborhood's history. Most, if not all, big cities have walking tours, and some sound particularly intriguing—like Oak Park, Illinois's walking tours of Frank Lloyd Wright homes (708-848-1976, www.gowright.org); Big Onion walking tours of New York City's ethnic communities and restaurants (212-439-1090, www.bigonion.com); city walks in European capitals (https://www.city-walks.info/index-en.html); or walks organized specifically for people with health limitations, such as tours organized by the Arthritis Foundation.

Walking is so popular that it has spawned many magazines, newsletters, and books. It may appear that there is not much of a need to read about walking—we have been doing it, after all, since we were toddlers—but proper technique improves benefits and reduces injuries. A good walking technique involves proper posture (head erect, chin in, shoulders relaxed, and back straight), a bent-arm swing, and a full natural stride. Good walking shoes should have flexible soles, good arch supports, and roomy toe boxes. Shoe inserts, called orthotics, may be helpful for cushioning impact or to prevent the feet from turning in or out. Trekking poles offer many benefits (Saller et al., 2023).

Pedometers

A sedentary person is estimated to walk about 3,500 steps a day, and the average American about 5,130 steps. Fitness advocates believe Americans should aim for 10,000 steps a day, or about 5 miles. One study reported that up to 7,500 steps a day is correlated with a decrease in mortality–with walking intensity not relevant, just the number of steps (Lee et al., 2019). Workplace physical activity, particularly among blue-collar occupations, helps some people reach a 7,500 daily-step target, leaving retired older adults and sedentary workers most likely to be at risk (McCormack et al., 2006). Men age 65 to 69 years take the most steps per day (more than 9,126) and women age 85+ the least (less than 276 steps per day; Tudor-Locke et al., 2013).

A ***pedometer*** is a small device used to count steps. Pedometers first appeared in Japan in 1965 under the name manpo-meter (*manpo* in Japanese means 10,000 steps). Their introduction into America took another few decades, but they have been increasing in popularity—even McDonald's distributed them several years ago as part of an adult Happy Meal called Go Active (salad, bottled water, and a pedometer for $4.99 in 2004: https://money.cnn.com/2004/05/11/news/fortune500/mcdonalds_happymeal/).

In general, studies have been supportive of the benefits of using a pedometer to motivate walkers and increase physical activity. A meta-analysis of 26 studies (eight randomized controlled trials and 18 observational studies) with 2,767 participants (mean age 49 years) reported significant increases in physical activity and significant decreases in body mass index and blood pressure (Bravata et al., 2007) when steps or distances were tracked. Having a step goal (such as 10,000 steps per day) was a significant influence on individual outcomes. Two 12-week pedometer-based walking interventions in primary care (PACE-UP and PACE-Lift) found that increases in physical activity were maintained at 3 and 4 years (Harris et al., 2018). For more tech-oriented baby boomers, and even some who are quite a bit older, there are ***fitness trackers***. Rupert Murdoch, the international media mogul in his mid-90s, told an Australian audience that he wore one. "I have a bracelet that keeps track of how I sleep, move, and eat—transmitting that information to the cloud."

Current fitness gadgets measure not only the number of steps, but energy expenditure, intensity and duration of activity, and sleep patterns, and provide a 24/7 heart rate monitor. While you get more information than you would from a pedometer, be prepared to spend more on a sophisticated device. Many of these extended functions are standard now in smartwatches, smart rings, and phone apps, and provide feedback on changes in physiologic measures (such as heart rate) or patterns of activity (stairs climbed, steps walked). These are increasingly linked to recognition of activity, such as a fall, with automatic alerts to emergency services and social contacts.

THE MOST POPULAR INACTIVITY: SITTING

Unfortunately, sitting is more popular than walking. Americans now sit more than they sleep, spending an average of 10 hours a day in a car or at work or at home—often in front of a computer screen or television set (Pope, 2012). Older adults are the most guilty, with the highest rates of sedentary behavior and the fewest hours of leisure-time physical activity. Research now shows that even daily exercise is not enough protection from the harmful effects of too much sitting.

The amount of time you sit, independent of a regular exercise routine, is a risk factor for a wide variety of health problems. Not only is ***prolonged sitting*** an independent risk factor, but some of the benefits of exercise appear to be offset by additional sitting on the days you exercise in comparison with the days you do not exercise (Matthews et al., 2018).

Prolonged daily sitting, even with a modest exercise program, is associated with insulin resistance, dyslipidemia, cardiac disease (Duvivier et al., 2018), weight gain (Saeidifard et al., 2018), early death (Diaz et al., 2017), arterial stiffening and hypertension (Morishima et al., 2016), and anxiety and depression (Lathia et al., 2017). Add to these health problems the effects of prolonged sitting on your brain.

Using brain imaging with low-fit persons aged 60 to 78, greater amounts of prolonged sitting revealed lower structural integrity in the white-matter tracts connecting the hippocampus, a structure that is crucial for learning and memory (Burzynska et al., 2014), reduced medial temporal lobe thickness (Siddarth et al., 2018), and reduced cerebral blood flow (Carter et al., 2018). The researchers concluded that these physiological effects of prolonged sitting, even if you still get exercise for a half hour a day, have a detrimental effect on your brain.

One interesting study reported that not all types of sitting are equally harmful. Sitting in front of a television set seems to be more hypnotic than other types of sitting, such as in front of a computer screen, reading, being on the telephone, sitting in a car, or sitting while doing paperwork (Whitaker et al., 2017). There is a positive correlation between television watching and the accumulation of visceral fat in the midsection (fat surrounding organs such as the liver, digestive tract, lungs, and heart).

To avoid or reduce these outcomes, engage in dynamic sitting—standing up every half hour for 2 minutes, or frequent fidgeting, that is, jiggling and tapping your feet every few minutes. Some researchers suggest that dynamic sitting or frequent standing and short strolls, or anything that reduces prolonged sitting, might be the best starting point for an exercise program for sedentary older adults, rather than beginning with a more formal exercise program with a much lower likelihood of success (Sardinha et al., 2015).

EXERCISE FOR DISEASE PREVENTION AND FUNCTIONAL IMPROVEMENT

As many gerontologists have noted, if exercise could be encapsulated in a pill, it would be the single most powerful medication a physician could prescribe.

In 2004, the CDC convened an expert panel to review evidence for the effects of exercise in older adults. The research team reviewed 2,334 studies published in peer-reviewed journals between 1980 and 2000. This review concluded that exercise was beneficial in all the areas that were reviewed: heart disease, ***arthritis***, chronic obstructive pulmonary disease (COPD), endurance, strength, mobility/balance, mortality, disability, and mental health.

Although this comprehensive evaluation was too detailed to adequately summarize here, I report in the following sections on studies showing evidence that exercise demonstrates considerable promise for older adults in a variety of areas of ***disease prevention*** and improved physical and cognitive function.

Cardiovascular Disease

For quite a while we have realized that inactivity is the most powerful predictor of death from cardiovascular disease among healthy persons, surpassing smoking, hypertension, and heart disease (Myers et al., 2002). But it does not take much physical activity to reduce the risk of cardiovascular disease among older men and women (Sparling et al., 2015). Brisk walking is enough, though greater intensity beyond brisk walking results in more benefit (Gebel et al., 2015).

Exercise is also a major prognostic factor in patients with existing cardiovascular disease. Patients who are physically active after a first heart attack had a 60% lower risk of a fatal heart attack or a second nonfatal heart attack than those who did not become active (Steffen-Batey et al., 2000). For a number of years, exercise was contraindicated for patients with chronic heart failure (CHF). Subsequently, exercise was recommended for CHF patients, provided the heart problem was stable (Gielen et al., 2001).

Though aerobic conditioning has been considered the exercise of choice for improved cardiorespiratory function, other forms of exercise have proved beneficial as well. Resistance exercise (Tanasescu et al., 2002; Vincent et al., 2002a), for example, provides cardiorespiratory benefits by reducing blood pressure (Kelley & Kelley, 2000) and cholesterol (Kraus et al., 2002). Previously, it was believed that only aerobic exercise was beneficial for improved cardiovascular health. The American Heart Association and the American College of Sports Medicine recommend combining aerobic exercise with resistance training (such as weight lifting; https://www.heart.org/en/healthy-living/fitness/fitness-basics/aha-recs-for-physical-activity-in-adults; https://www.acsm.org/education-resources/trending-topics-resources/physical-activity-guidelines).

A study of peripheral vascular disease (PVD) reported what may seem incongruous to some—that an effective treatment for clogged or narrowed arteries of the legs is aerobic walking (Stewart et al., 2002). Walking increases muscle metabolism and may improve circulation to the legs, allowing more oxygen to get to tissues otherwise starved by blockages. The two caveats to walking interventions for PVD are to avoid extreme pain and to avoid exercise if pain continues when legs are at rest.

In the Framingham Heart Study, people who participated in moderate physical activity starting at age 50 lived 1.1 years longer free of heart disease and 1.3 years longer overall; people who participated in high levels of physical activity lived 3.2 years longer free of heart disease and 3.5 years longer overall (Franco et al., 2005). These gains were similar for both men and women.

Cancer

Epidemiological findings have established an association between the risk of cancer and physical activity or exercise. A meta-analysis of 26 types of cancer involving more than a million Europeans and Americans reported that physical activity and exercise lower the risk of 13 types of cancer (Moore et al., 2016). Higher levels of adult physical activity, for example, appear to afford modest protection against breast cancer or enhance survival after breast cancer (Holmes et al., 2005), perhaps by reducing body fat where carcinogens accumulate (Dirx et al., 2001), or by lowering the level of estrogen in the blood (McTiernan, 2002).

Also, women with substantial leisure-time physical activity had a 27% lower incidence of ovarian cancer (Cottreau et al., 2000). In comparison with more sedentary men, those who exercised had a 24% reduction in the risk of prostate cancer and a 62% reduction in the risk of upper digestive and stomach cancer (Wannamethee et al., 2001).

A high activity level is also associated with a substantial reduction, up to 50%, in colon cancer risk (Zhang et al., 2006). Although the mechanisms by which exercise protects against colon cancer are not known, exercise may speed food through the bowel and shorten the time carcinogens in fecal matter spend in contact with cells that line the colon. Constipation is associated with cancer risk but only for gastrointestinal cancers other than colorectal cancer (Sundbøll, 2019).

Correlation does not equal causation, and the evidence for the impact of exercise or physical activity on cancer is not as strong as it is for heart disease. One of the challenges is the lack of agreement on a single biological theory with any specific cancer, much less for all the varying types of cancer. The theories that do exist on the impact of exercise range broadly and include its effect on the immune, nervous, or endocrine systems. A further complication is the effect of obesity on cancer risk apart from physical activity.

Diabetes

Exercise appears to have an impact on type 2 diabetes, in terms of both prevention of the disease and the risk of death among those who already have it. The onset of diabetes may be delayed or prevented when high-risk persons make lifestyle changes that include increased exercise. Patients with type 2 diabetes who fail to exercise regularly show a 70% greater risk for cardiovascular death than those who exercise at least three times a week (Zethelius et al., 2014). The American Diabetes Association recommends structured lifestyle interventions that include at least 150 minutes per week of physical activity and dietary changes resulting in weight loss of 5% to 7% for preventing or delaying the onset of type 2 diabetes in high-risk populations and people with prediabetes (Colberg et al., 2016).

Finnish researchers investigated a population over a 4-year period and found that the incidence of diabetes was 11% among those who received exercise instruction and other counseling, and 23% among control subjects—a significant difference (Tuomilehto et al., 2001). A study of 70,000 female nurses who did not have diabetes at baseline documented almost 1,500 incidents of type 2 diabetes over an 8-year period. There was a substantially reduced risk of obtaining it, however, among those who exercised regularly—even among those who only engaged in brisk walking (Hu et al., 1999).

High-intensity resistance training also improves glycemic control in older patients with type 2 diabetes (Dunstan et al., 2002). The study's authors were surprised at the magnitude of the effects, as they equaled those typically seen with drugs for diabetes. They noted that muscles are major clearance sites for circulating glucose. The Diabetes Prevention Program showed that lifestyle interventions (exercise and diet for weight loss) were more effective than standard pharmacotherapy (metformin) in preventing or delaying diabetes for people at high risk. Benefits persist even after 15 years (https://www.niddk.nih.gov/about-niddk/research-areas/diabetes/diabetes-prevention-program-dpp).

Depression

A review of 30 large studies found a significant relationship between physical activity and development of depression (Mammen & Faulkner, 2013). Exercise may be just as effective as antidepressant medication in treating some cases of depression (Lawlor & Hopker, 2001). Those who stop exercising, though, lose the long-term mood-enhancing effects (Kritz-Silverstein et al., 2001).

An analysis of 33 studies reported that weight training was associated with feeling less anxious and nervous (Gordon et al., 2018). A study by Singh et al. (2001) reported that supervised weight lifting exercises significantly benefited depressed older adults.

Control group persons who attended health lectures did not benefit. (This was not a good control group activity, in my opinion. I would argue that if the weight lifters had been subjected to boring health lectures as well, both groups would have remained depressed! Placebos can also cause harm.) What was interesting about this study was that the antidepressant benefits were sustained even after exercise supervision was terminated and the participants were on their own. After 26 months, one third of the elderly exercisers were still regularly weight lifting.

Even a single exercise session can boost the mood of mildly to moderately depressed persons (Bartholomew et al., 2005). Just 30 minutes of brisk walking can immediately boost one's mood, providing a benefit that reaches near-normal mood levels comparable to alternatives such as cigarette smoking, consuming caffeine, or binge eating, which have harmful long-term effects.

A weekly ***tai chi*** class combined with an antidepressant produced significant outcomes when compared with those who completed a health education class and took the same antidepressant (Lavretsky et al., 2011). The tai chi participants, however, also demonstrated better memory and cognition, and reported a higher overall level of energy.

Cognition

Studies of physical activity or exercise among older adults report that those with higher physical activity or exercise levels were less likely to experience cognitive decline. The American College of Sports Medicine and the UK Alzheimer's Society have endorsed physical activity as a modifiable risk factor (https://www.acsm.org/blog-detail/acsm-certified-blog/2023/06/28/alzheimer-s-and-exercise-what-do-we-know-and-what-can-we-do; https://www.alzheimers.org.uk/get-support/daily-living/exercise). The Lancet Commission on Dementia identified obesity in midlife and lack of physical activity in old age as remediable risk factors for preventing dementia (Livingston et al., 2020).

Unlike prior studies that found positive results but relied on participant recall on how often they exercised, one study used a more objective measure of fitness (Wendell et al., 2014). The Baltimore Longitudinal Study on Aging measured VO2 max, the maximal amount of oxygen used by your lungs during 1 minute of strenuous exercise. The more oxygen your lungs are able to use, the fitter you are. It found that 80-year-olds with high VO2 max and who were therefore more fit made about 25% fewer errors on a test of memory and concentration than their less-fit age peers.

Greater leisure-time physical activity at midlife is associated with a decreased risk of dementia later in life, even with a modest amount of exercise—as little as 15 minutes, three times weekly. This was associated with a 32% reduced risk for developing dementia over the next 6 years (Larson et al., 2006). Another study of physical fitness in midlife produced more dramatic results: a 90% reduction in dementia risk and a delayed onset—age 90 among the most fit compared to age 80 for the least fit (Horder et al., 2018).

One study examined the relationship between aerobic fitness and in vivo brain tissue density. High-resolution MRIs from 55 older adults revealed that declines in brain tissue densities, as a function of age, were substantially reduced by fitness level (Colcombe et al., 2003).

Exercise may not just stem a decline in cognitive functioning, it may improve functioning as well. Researchers found that older men and women who engaged in aerobic exercise improved the higher mental processes of memory and executive functioning—such as planning and organizational abilities—that are based in the frontal and prefrontal regions of the brain (Khatri et al., 2001).

A randomized controlled research study found that 12 months of once-weekly or twice-weekly resistance training improved executive cognitive function, that is, an improved ability to make accurate decisions quickly, in community-dwelling older women (Liu-Ambrose et al., 2010). A later study conducted by some of the same researchers focused on a sample of women with mild cognitive impairment and reported, unexpectedly, that resistance training led to even more improvement in brain function than those who performed aerobics (Nagamatsu et al., 2012). Imaging studies suggest increases in brain hippocampal volume with exercise (Erickson et al., 2022).

Bone Density

A review of 24 studies that examined aerobic exercise and bone mineral density in women reported bone mass gain among exercisers versus nonexercisers and that walking was the most common form of exercise performed in these studies (Kelley, 2001). The Nurses' Health Study of 61,200 postmenopausal women concluded that moderate activity, including walking, is associated with substantially lower risk of hip fractures (Feskanich et al., 2002). The National Osteoporosis Foundation endorses high or low impact weight-bearing and muscle-strengthening exercises to prevent osteoporosis (https://www.bonehealthandosteoporosis.org/patients/treatment/exercisesafe-movement/osteoporosis-exercise-for-strong-bones/).

A study of healthy older persons who engaged in 6 months of resistance training showed greater bone density in the hip area, and showed signs that bone metabolism had shifted toward generating more bone than was being lost (Vincent & Braith, 2002). Another study reported that resistive back-strengthening exercises reduced the incidence of vertebral fractures among postmenopausal women (Sinaki et al., 2002).

Fall Prevention

While earlier studies suggested about one third of people age 65+ fall at least once each year, newer estimates from the U.S. Preventive Services Task Force (USPSTF) suggest a lower prevalence of about 27.5%, with 10.2% resulting in serious injury such as a hip fracture. In 2021, fall-related injuries resulted in 38,742 deaths (https://www.uspreventiveservicestaskforce.org/uspstf/recommendation/falls-prevention-community-dwelling-older-adults-interventions). One meta-analysis of 17 studies reported that older adults who exercise regularly are less likely to fall, and are 37% less likely to be injured after a fall (El-Khoury et al., 2013).

An individually tailored exercise program in the home reduced falls and decreased injuries in a sample of women aged 80 years and older. Over a 1-year period, older persons in the exercise program reduced falls by 46%, compared with a control group that received an equal number of social visits (Campbell et al., 1997). Another home-based exercise program with older adults reported significant fall reduction in comparison with groups that received home hazard management and treatment of poor vision (Day et al., 2002).

A meta-analysis of seven research trials titled Frailty and Injuries: Cooperative Studies of Intervention Techniques (FIC-SIT) revealed that a variety of exercise interventions—examined by way of randomized controlled clinical trials—led to a reduction in falls among older patients (Province et al., 1995). The exercise interventions were successful even though they varied in duration, frequency, intensity, and content—including endurance training, resistance training, flexibility training, and tai chi.

Not only can starting an exercise program lower an older woman's risk of falling, but the benefit can be lasting. Women aged 75 to 85 with low bone mass participated in one of three types of group-based exercise programs—strength training, agility exercise, or stretching exercise—and reduced their risk of falls about 40% (Liu-Ambrose et al., 2005). Apparently these interventions acted as a catalyst for ongoing physical activity, because the reduction in fall risk was maintained for at least 18 months.

Osteoarthritis

People with ***osteoarthritis*** of the knee often experience progressive deterioration in the cartilage of the knee joint until they reach the point of being disabled. Both aerobic and resistance exercise with patients who have osteoarthritis of the knee reduced the incidence of disability by about 50% (Penninx et al., 2001). Another sample of older adults with knee osteoarthritis experienced significant improvement in physical function and reduced pain as a consequence of a strength-training program (Baker et al., 2001).

A simple home-based exercise program significantly reduced knee pain from osteoarthritis (Thomas et al., 2002), and an exercise program combined with medication for knee osteoarthritis was more effective than medication alone for improving physical function and reducing activity-related pain in a sample of older persons (Petrella & Bartha, 2000). Systematic reviews support the benefits of exercise for managing pain and disability from osteoarthritis (Raposo et al., 2021).

Even a modest amount of exercise—fewer than 30 minutes per day of moderate activity—may prevent disability from arthritis, and those with arthritis show improvements in mobility with modest exercise (Feinglass et al., 2005).

Sleep

Older adults with sleep complaints improved self-rated sleep quality by completing a moderate-intensity exercise program. Exercising subjects reported significant improvement in subjective sleep quality, reduced sleep latency (average time in minutes needed to fall asleep), and increased sleep duration (average number of hours of actual sleep per night; King et al., 1997).

A sample of healthy older adult caregivers who had not initially reported sleep complaints, but who engaged in stressful caregiving with family members, reported improvements in subjective sleep quality after they completed a moderate-intensity exercise program (King et al., 2002).

Another study focused on older residents in assisted living facilities. The researchers concluded that regular yoga practice over several months improved the quality of sleep compared with residents who did not participate (Chen et al., 2010). Similar results were found in the community (Newton et al., 2014).

Other Conditions

Exercise appears to be beneficial for a wide range of other medical and functional conditions. Some examples follow: There is evidence to suggest that exercise *prolongs life* (Moholdt et al., 2018) by 3 years (Lee et al., 2017), *strengthens the immune system* (Duggal et al., 2018), *slows the progression of peripheral neuropathy* (Dixit et al., 2014), *lowers the likelihood of vision problems* (Klein et al., 2014), *reduces stress* among older female caregivers (King et al., 2002), *reduces symptoms of chronic fatigue syndrome* (Powell et al., 2001), *increases function in COPD patients* (Hernandez et al., 2000), *reduces stroke risk* (Hu et al., 2005), *improves motor function among stroke survivors* (Duncan et al., 1998), *improves mental health status* (Cheng et al., 2009), *relieves lower back pain and dysfunction* (Sherman et al., 2005), *relieves musculoskeletal pain* (Bruce et al., 2005), and *accelerates wound healing* among older adults (Emery et al., 2005).

Caution

It takes an act of supreme skepticism to deny the overwhelming evidence supporting the benefits of exercise. Nonetheless, I have met such skeptics who disparage the rigor with which most exercise research studies are conducted. Though I most happily do not side with these cynics, the evidence on the benefits of exercise does have to be viewed with a degree of caution. Many studies, for instance, are epidemiological in nature and reveal correlation rather than causality. In other words, exercise may be more the product of being in good health than a cause of it. Some of these observational studies attempt to compensate for this limitation by employing analytical controls on several baseline variables.

Other methodological limitations are also common among exercise studies. Many of these studies utilize unrepresentative samples, often relying on volunteers; lack randomization between treatment and control groups; are unblinded (i.e., do not restrict awareness of who is a treatment group member vs. a control group member); employ inadequate measurement tools, especially a reliance on self-reports; and report high dropout rates or do not include dropouts in the data analysis (this would be a more rigorous type of study called intention-to-treat analysis). Some of the exercise in these studies, therefore, may not be producing the miraculous results reported.

Nonetheless, the breadth and depth of research on exercise interventions with older adults—including more than 200 rigorous randomized clinical trials that were included in the CDC meta-analysis that I referred to earlier—can only lead one to conclude that exercise is an astonishing health intervention, and no amount of methodological nitpicking will seriously challenge its credibility.

QUESTION: What has been *your* major barrier when it comes to engaging in a well-rounded exercise program on a regular basis, and have you attempted to overcome it? If so, how?

EXERCISE FOR WEIGHT MANAGEMENT, NOT FOR WEIGHT LOSS

It has been said that man does not live by bread alone. It can also be said that man does not control weight by diet alone. Restricting the number of calories consumed without exercising can result in quick, dramatic weight loss. Unfortunately, it can also result in quick, dramatic regain. About half the initial weight loss from diet will be water, which will be regained, and muscle, which will make one weaker. Dieting without exercise also lowers the metabolic rate (the amount of energy used for physiological processes), causing a reduction in fat-burning capacity. This not only slows weight loss, but also, when the dieting ends, weight is gained back faster than ever.

Exercise, in contrast, ensures that weight loss will come primarily from reduction in fat, not water and muscle. Exercise may also increase the metabolic rate so that the body burns calories more efficiently and over a longer duration. Because muscle tissue is metabolically more active than fat, it burns more calories.

A study of more than 8,000 dieters who lost 10% of their starting weight and kept it off for at least a year reported that their number one successful weight loss maintenance strategy, cited by 81% of respondents, was exercise (Dieting, 2002). The most common form of exercise was walking, followed by increasing physical activity in their daily routine. A surprising finding from this study was that an unexpectedly high 29% of respondents reported that they added weight lifting to their exercise regimen.

The vital role of exercise has its limits, though. It appears to apply more to the maintenance of weight loss than to losing weight in the first place. Whereas energy intake comes 100% from food and drink, only 20% of energy expenditure is, on average, from exercise and physical activity. The other 80% is unaffected by exercise and constitutes the energy it takes to keep your body working (blood circulating, breathing, etc.). Thus, exercise for calorie expenditure is no match for eating for calorie intake. Thirty minutes of brisk walking is offset by four chocolate chip cookies and, if that is not cruel enough, exercise increases your appetite.

Lest we forget, exercise may not be great for losing weight, but it is great for improving strength, endurance, flexibility, balance, mood, disease prevention, disease management, and weight maintenance.

Exercise as a weight maintenance strategy*, though, becomes less efficient as we age.* Researchers monitored the fat and carbohydrate breakdown for older and younger participants who pedaled 60 minutes on stationary bikes. Measurement of oxygen consumption indicated how hard they were able to exercise. Then the study subjects pedaled at speeds that made them consume identical amounts of oxygen. Older participants oxidized less than one third as much fat as their younger counterparts. In other words, older adults appeared to burn less fat than younger adults while doing equivalent exercise. Paul Williams of the Lawrence Berkeley National Laboratory concluded that runners would have to substantially increase the amount of mileage they run each decade in order to stay at the same weight.

If you are maintaining weight, but are overweight, can you still be fit? Yes, according to the research of Stephen Blair and his colleagues at the Cooper Institute for Aerobics Research. Their data reveal that exercise can reduce disease risk even if body weight remains high. There is lower cardiovascular as well as all-cause mortality risk among persons who are overweight and fit, versus those who are normal weight and unfit (Heroux et al., 2009).

However, a study by researchers from the Harvard School of Public Health qualified these findings. You are better off fit and overweight than just overweight, but fitness does not counter all the risk of excess weight. For instance, when it comes to diabetes, exercise may not fully counter the effects of excess body fat, because fat tissue may release substances that affect the metabolism of insulin (Weinstein et al., 2004).

The best exercises for weight control are a combination of aerobics and ***strength building***. The aerobic activity should involve the large muscle groups like the quadriceps. Also, longer duration and higher intensity accelerate progress, but are likely to increase the likelihood of dropping out of an exercise routine. Strength building will increase muscle mass and boost the metabolic rate, which may allow the person to burn calories longer, not just when exercising.

Unfortunately, many Americans believe you can get fit without much physical effort, as proclaimed on commercials and infomercials on television. Instead of accenting the physical effort it takes to lose or maintain weight, viewers learn that weight reduction or maintenance is the consequence of buying a particular product that does not require much physical exertion to use.

Over a period of several years, for instance, electrical muscle stimulators were a popular product purchased by consumers. By passing currents through electrodes applied to the skin you contract muscles and, allegedly, can either build them or reduce them. These devices tend to focus on the abdomen. By placing an electronic "exercise belt" around your waist and pushing a button, you can develop "washboard abs." After more than $100 million worth of the devices were sold in 2002, the Federal Trade Commission took three of these companies to court.

Adults spend about $3 billion a year on exercise equipment for home use! However, for a large but unknown percentage of persons who purchase exercise equipment to use while watching television, television viewing rather than exercising continues to be the leisure activity of choice.

THE FOUR COMPONENTS OF MY EXERCISE CLASS

The four components of a community exercise class that I coordinated for about a quarter century were aerobics, strength building, ***flexibility*** and ***balance***, and health education. In a typical 60-minute class, I began with 25 minutes of aerobic exercise, warming up for the first few minutes and cooling down the last few minutes. I start with low-intensity aerobics in order to warm up the muscles for higher intensity aerobics, which, in turn, warms up the muscles for subsequent periods of strength building (15 minutes) and flexibility and balance (10 minutes). These three components—aerobics, strength building, and flexibility and balance—typically lasted 50 minutes; the final 10 minutes of class was devoted to health education.

With the aid of students in health science classes, I implemented this exercise class for about 25 years, continually refining it during this time (Figure 4.2). This exercise program was selected for the Best Practices in Health Promotion and Aging directory, compiled by the Health Promotion Institute of the National Council on Aging (NCOA).

The Aerobics Component

Aerobics has been defined as a series of strenuous exercises that help convert fats, sugars, and starches into aches, pains, and cramps. A more conventional definition is that aerobic means "with oxygen." An aerobic activity moves large volumes of oxygen, employs large muscle groups like the arms and legs, and is sustained at a certain level of intensity over a period of time. Aerobic exercise is rhythmic, repetitive, and continuous, and includes such popular activities as brisk walking (about twice one's normal speed), swimming, dancing, and bicycling.

FIGURE 4.2 The end-of-the-semester photograph of exercise class, taught by occupational therapy students.

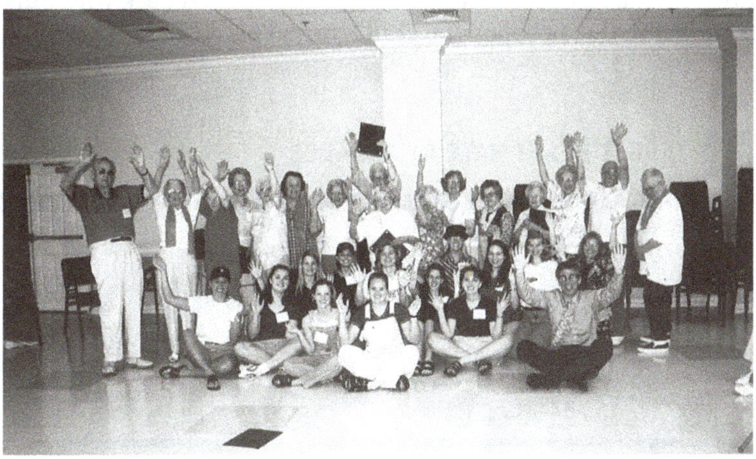

Aerobic activity can be contrasted to anaerobic ("without oxygen") activity, which depends on short bursts of energy (like a 50-meter sprint or barbell press), quickly depletes energy resources, and has limited cardiovascular benefit. This type of activity is, however, essential for strength-building purposes.

Aerobic capacity, or maximum oxygen uptake (VO2 max), is the maximum amount of oxygen that a person can utilize during strenuous exertion. Aerobic capacity is considered to be the best measure of cardiorespiratory fitness, and although it tends to decrease with age, aerobic capacity can be increased through a regularly practiced aerobic regimen.

Most aerobic exercise programs are designed to stimulate the heart and lungs for a sufficient period of time to produce an increased and sustained heart rate. Traditional programs encouraged participants to sustain exercise for a minimum of 20 to 25 minutes and to gradually raise the normal heartbeat (which is about 60 to 80 beats a minute) to the "target zone" of the person, the upper and lower limits of which are based on age (Table 4.1).

The ***target heart rate zone*** typically refers to between 50% and 85% of the estimated maximum heart rate, which is calculated by subtracting a person's age from 220 and multiplying the remainder first by 50% and then by 85%. The target for the beginning exerciser should be near the 60% level (or less if the person leads a sedentary lifestyle), and gradually increases to the higher level over succeeding months. Persons can assess the intensity of their aerobic exercise program by counting their pulse beats for a 10-second period and multiplying by 6. Before the invention of personal devices, aerobics instructors would ask their students to conduct this assessment at periodic intervals.

The advantage to calculating target heart rates for some older adults is that they believe this is a scientific approach and like this method. The disadvantages are (a) a significant percentage of older adults have difficulty obtaining a pulse count, (b) medications like beta-blockers can limit maximum heart rate intensity, and (c) there is controversy in the literature over whether the commonly used equation to estimate maximal heart rate (220 minus age) is valid for older adults (Tanaka et al., 2001). The formula for the target heart rate may be inappropriate for 30% to 40% of adults. These persons have hearts that beat faster or slower than the age-predicted maximum.

Older adults may appreciate a comment by Fries (1989): "... this whole heart rate business [is] a bit of a bother and somewhat artificial. There really are not good medical data to justify particular target heart rates. You may wish to check your pulse rate a few times to get a feel for what is happening, but it doesn't have to be something you watch extremely carefully" (p. 69).

TABLE 4.1 TARGET HEART RATE BY DECADES

AGE	TARGET HEART RATE[a] (60%–75% OF MAXIMUM)	MAXIMUM HEART RATE[a] (220 – AGE)
50	102–128	170
60	96–120	160
70	90–113	150
80	84–105	140

[a]Beats/minute.

Most older adults prefer the ***Borg perceived exertion*** technique. It has the advantage of being easy to gauge, and serves another purpose: It encourages older adults to become more aware of their bodies and how they feel (Table 4.2). One study of more than 7,000 men (mean age 66 years) reported that the person's perceived level of exertion is a better predictor of risk of coronary heart disease than whether they meet the current activity recommendations (Lee et al., 2003).

Ideally, the inactive older adult should seek an intensity level of very light, about 1 on the modified Borg scale, or less than 50% of maximum heart rate. The active older person should be about 7 on the scale, or approximately 65% of the maximum heart rate. Older participants were told that the exercise level should be of sufficient duration and intensity for them to be aware of more rapid breathing or a rising internal body temperature, but not so intense that they are unable to conduct a brief conversation (if desired) while exercising. Regardless of whether target heart rates or perceived intensity levels are utilized, exercise should be discontinued immediately in the case of shortness of breath, chest pain, dizziness, lightheadedness, confusion, or pain.

One option is exercise classes taught by health science students after they completed a brief period of training. Regarding the aerobics component of the class, we offered the students and the older adults two options, with the second option used periodically to boost interest.

- A series of arm and leg movements that gradually increase, and then decrease, intensity level. If students run out of movement ideas, students can draw ideas from one of several memory-jarring techniques; for example, playing one of a number of imaginary musical instruments (drums, trombone, violin, etc.) and pretending to generate the music that is playing in the background; or mimicking an activity of daily living (drying one's back with a towel, vacuuming the rug, weeding the garden, etc.); or mimicking a movement in a sport (boxing, throwing a baseball, or swinging a bat—ambidextrously, etc.).

TABLE 4.2 MODIFIED BORG SCALE OF PERCEIVED EXERTION

LEVEL	PERCEIVED EXERTION	PHYSICAL SIGNS
1	Very light	None
2		
3	Fairly light	Breathing rate increased
4		
5	Somewhat hard	Warmth, slight sweat, breathing rate increased
6		
7		
8	Hard	Sweat, heavy breathing
9		
10	Very hard	Heavy sweat, difficult to talk

- An imaginary trip is acted out, perhaps a cruise to Spain, or attendance at a local baseball game. The cruise might include climbing up the boat (taking big steps in place with knees raised high), putting away clothes in one's cabin, dancing that evening with an imaginary heartthrob, getting off the boat (more big steps), visiting a bullfight, becoming the matador, and so forth. The baseball game may entail fans walking to the stadium (walking around the room, sometimes in a haphazard fashion to promote social interaction), doing the wave, being unexpectedly called upon by the manager to pinch hit (swinging an imaginary bat in both directions), or to do some relief pitching (using right and left arms).

Exercise need not be targeted to fit older adults; some participants may be wheelchair bound (or walker dependent) as long as movements are individualized for those with special needs like Parkinson disease, stroke, an orthopedic condition, or mild confusion. Particular attention must be given to helping these adults keep movements simple, avoid quick action, and encourage caution with twisting movements.

Deconditioned older adults are encouraged to perform at 1 or 2 on the modified Borg scale, or at 50% or less of the maximum heart rate for their age. Fit older adults are encouraged to perform at 7 or 8 on the Borg scale, or at 70% of the maximum heart rate. People tended to be reliable self-raters using the Borg scale.

The emphasis, however, should be on having fun, and only secondarily on moving up the scale to higher intensity levels. Studies have supported the Surgeon General's findings that even activities of low- to moderate-intensity level not only improve the aerobic capacity of older adults, but also are less likely than more vigorous activities to result in injury, and are more likely to be maintained as a routine over time. And although low- to moderate-intensity activity does not provide the fitness benefits of higher intensity exercise, it can be sustained over a longer exercise period because it depletes only fat, the body's richest store of energy. Higher intensity exercise depletes carbohydrates, and cannot be sustained as long.

Older adults in classes that meet only two or three times a week need to be encouraged to comply with the Surgeon General's advice and engage in aerobic exercise on most of the other days of the week as well. On days when there was no class, therefore, older adults were encouraged to engage in longer sessions of walking, swimming, cycling, dancing, gardening, yard work, or other activities that could be performed at a low- or moderate-intensity level for a half hour.

Aerobic movement accompanied by music can promote better adherence to a regular exercise routine by adding to the enjoyment of the activity (Bauldoff et al., 2002). The power of music can not only motivate but also improve emotional and cognitive functioning. One study of stroke patients compared those who regularly listened to music with those in a control group who did not. The music listeners improved mood (e.g., reduced depression) and cognitive function (e.g., less confusion) in comparison with the control group (Sarkamo et al., 2008). Adding music to exercise sessions improves attendance, increases maintenance of physical activity after interventions, increases perceived exertion and exercise capacity and thus heart rate during exercise, and improves mood and cognitive performance (Chair et al., 2021).

The Muscular Strength or Endurance Component

Experts did not always believe that strengthening exercises were as important for older adults as other components of exercise (Fries, 1989, p. 66), and many geriatric exercise manuals ignored strengthening exercises altogether. Now, experts and community health leaders realize the importance of strength building for maintaining an independent lifestyle with age.

A report from the CDC noted that almost one in five Americans age 80+ had weak muscular strength, defined by such measures as difficulty with rising unaided from an armless chair (Looker & Wang, 2015). Preserving leg strength allows an older adult not only to get up from a chair in a restaurant, but to regain balance before falling. Preserving arm strength allows an older adult to carry groceries, pick up household items, twist off jar lids, and make minor repairs.

There is a condition referred to as ***sarcopenia***, the gradual loss of muscle mass with age, which is replaced by fat. This loss of muscle is generally about 0.5% to 1% a year after the age of 50, though it can begin as early as age 30. Sarcopenia is associated with insulin resistance, fatigue, falls, and premature death. The primary risk factor is lack of exercise, and a regular practice of strength building can prevent much of this deterioration. Sarcopenia is not entirely reversed through intervention, and even fitness buffs experience it, though to a much lesser degree.

For those who are reducing calories in an attempt to lose weight without significant loss of muscle mass, weight training is more effective than aerobic exercise. While losing about 17 pounds of fat, dieters who weight-trained lost 2 pounds of muscle while those who did aerobics lost 4 pounds of muscle (Beavers et al., 2017).

Organizations like the American College of Sports Medicine have developed training guidelines for weight lifting past age 50. And though strength-building exercise programs are still the exception rather than the norm, the popularity of including a strength-building component in an aerobics exercise class has grown quickly over the past two decades. Overall, however, a 2013 review of national data suggests that only 19.2% to 22.8% of people age 65 to 74, 15.0% to 19.9% of people age 75 to 84, and 9.0% of people age 85+ meet strength training recommendations two or more times per week (Keadle et al., 2016).

Muscular strength or endurance is the ability of the muscle to exert force (strength) or to repeat actions over time without fatigue (endurance). As people age, lean muscle tissue tends to decrease, and the percentage of body fat increases. Thus, muscle strength and endurance tend to decline with age, and bones tend to weaken. Strength training, however, will increase muscle mass, functioning ability, and bone density. When the skeletal frame is strengthened, the likelihood of bone fractures resulting from osteoporosis is reduced (Vincent & Braith, 2002).

In the spring of 1990, attitudes toward strength building for older adults began to change. A strength-exercise program captured the media headlines, which previously had been dominated by popular aerobic activities or unusual aerobic accomplishments—such as the exploits of Johnny Kelley, who completed the Boston Marathon race 58 times and ran his last one as an octogenarian.

This highly publicized strength-exercise program, however, captured attention because it involved 10 (including one dropout) frail, very old nursing home residents who, after completing an 8-week training program, almost tripled their leg strength, expanded their thigh muscles by more than 10%, and were able to walk 50% faster (Fiatarone et al., 1990). The participants ranged in age from 87 to 96 years!

One 93-year-old participant reported, "I feel as though I were 50 again. Now, I get up in the middle of the night and I can get around without using my walker or turning on the light. The program gave me strength I didn't have before. Every day I feel better, more optimistic. Pills won't do for you what exercise does!" Another resident who at first could not rise from a chair without using his arms was able to do so after the training, and two others no longer needed canes for walking.

Less dramatic results are found in community-dwelling octogenarians, however, because they begin with higher baseline strength levels than institutionalized elders, and have less potential for improvement (Slivka et al., 2008).

Most community exercise classes do not have the luxury of providing weights or exercise machines to older participants. That was the case with my exercise class as well. I found the most affordable and perhaps safest option for strength building to be elastic bands, and gravity-resisting exercises like modified push-ups, raising arms to shoulder level and making circles, half-squats, toe raises, and others.

Elastic bands are a good alternative to ***free weights***, which are associated with more injuries, and to resistance machines, which are less accessible. In addition to being safe and portable, they are inexpensive. By buying elastic bands in large rolls and cutting off 4-foot strips, I provided bands to older students at low cost.

I typically included four or five different upper extremity exercises to strengthen different muscles such as the triceps (Figure 4.3), biceps, deltoids, trapezius, pectoralis, and latissimus. I followed up with three or four lower extremity exercises to strengthen the quadriceps, hamstrings, and/or gastrocnemius. The elastic band manufacturers provided illustrated exercises and useful tips such as warming up, practicing smooth and slow movements in both eccentric and concentric directions, breathing while exercising, and emphasizing technically correct movements over quantity of movements.

Elastic bands come in increasing resistance levels. Typically, I started the lower resistance level and increased repetitions and sets before moving up to the next intensity level. Although the bands can be utilized at increasing levels of intensity, they are less precise than free weights or weight machines for measuring improvement.

The resistance level should allow the participants to perform about 12 to 15 repetitions of an exercise. A larger number of repetitions—such as 20 to 25 repetitions per set at 30% to 50% of maximum resistance—would place greater emphasis on endurance; while a smaller number of repetitions—such as 8 to 12 repetitions per set at 75% to 90% of maximum resistance—would emphasize strength. When it comes to repetitions, most older persons should err on the side of endurance over strength, as it is likely to lead to fewer injuries. Moreover, researchers report that muscle strength results are the same with high versus low repetitions, provided muscles are exhausted (Morton et al., 2016). It is unclear what interval between sets is optimal.

FIGURE 4.3 Horizontal triceps press.

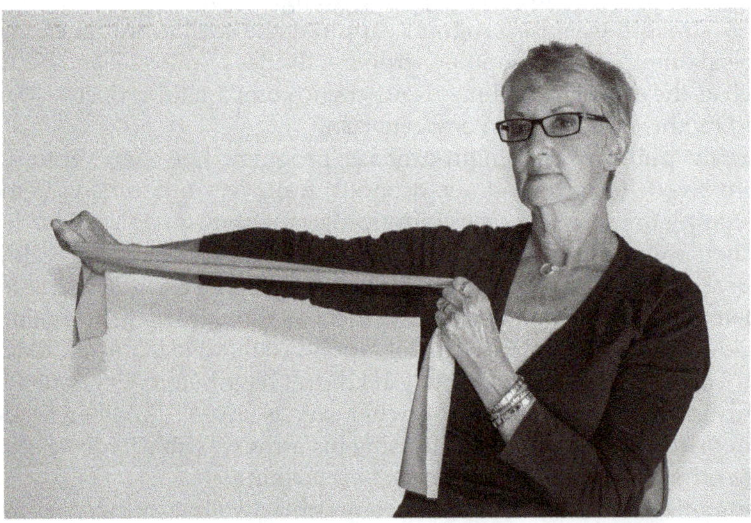

The elastic band fits easily into a pocket and is convenient to take to class, or anywhere else for that matter. A potential disadvantage is that it can be hard to grip with arthritic fingers. This limitation can be overcome by buying handles, or tying the band into a circle and exerting power through wrists or forearms. Another disadvantage to the band is that eventually it will break (which can be startling, to say the least, when it occurs midexercise), and it needs to be kept out of sunlight and replaced in a regular and timely fashion.

The preferred schedule of activity for improving or sustaining strength or endurance for older adults is 2 or 3 days a week, with at least 1 day of rest between workouts. One study reported that muscle strength gains achieved during a 12-week progressive resistance training program can be maintained by resistance training of only once per week thereafter (Trappe et al., 2002). Another study reported that even light resistance can help older adults get stronger while simultaneously reducing the possibility for injury (Vincent et al., 2002b). Yet another study reported that super slow movements combined with fewer repetitions may increase muscle mass more than normal-speed movements (Ring-Dimitriou et al., 2009).

A good alternative exercise for increasing strength in older adults with painful arthritic joints is isometrics, the contraction of a muscle without movement at the joint. The typical way to engage in isometrics is to pull or push against a stationary object, usually against a wall or against another body part. Each contraction should be held for about 5 seconds, and repeated three times. Many exercise physiologists are reluctant to recommend isometric exercise for heart patients because of the increased likelihood of performing the ***Valsalva maneuver*** (i.e., holding one's breath), and raising one's blood pressure level. It is possible, however, to avoid this when doing isometrics.

Because there is no movement and no equipment, you can do ***isometrics*** any place, any time, and at no cost. The muscle that you select tightens but does not change length; thus, there is no movement of the joint or the bone to which the muscle is attached. Isometrics, therefore, has the advantage of allowing you to build muscle at a fixed angle, avoiding those joint positions that may be affected by arthritic pain. However, unless you systematically alter the angle (about 20 degrees each time), you do not develop strength over the entire range of motion.

There are several problems to avoid with all strength-building techniques, but they can be especially problematic with isometrics. To avoid the unhealthy Valsalva maneuver, for instance, focus on inhalation and exhalation. To improve range of motion, it is not only important to vary the isometric angle but also to develop opposing muscle groups (e.g., quadriceps and hamstrings). Finally, the Borg scale for estimating appropriate aerobic intensity level can also be used with isometric exercise.

A good isometric exercise to avoid knee pain is as follows: In a seated position, the adult places the palms of both hands on one leg, about 2 or 3 inches above the knee, pushing down with the hands and up with the knee. The angle of the knee is altered by raising it slightly off the ground, and then raising it slightly higher two more times (see Figure 4.4). Repeat with the other leg. This exercise targets the important quadriceps muscle, the largest muscle in the body. It is an alternative to leg squats, which can exacerbate knee pain.

In addition to building strength and endurance, resistance training component included safety tips on how to lift objects and how to move one's body to avoid muscle strain, backaches, hernias, and the like. Injuries from weight lifting are not uncommon, and they increased by 300% from 1978 to 1998 for middle-aged women and men (More

FIGURE 4.4 Isometric exercise for quadriceps that avoids knee pain.

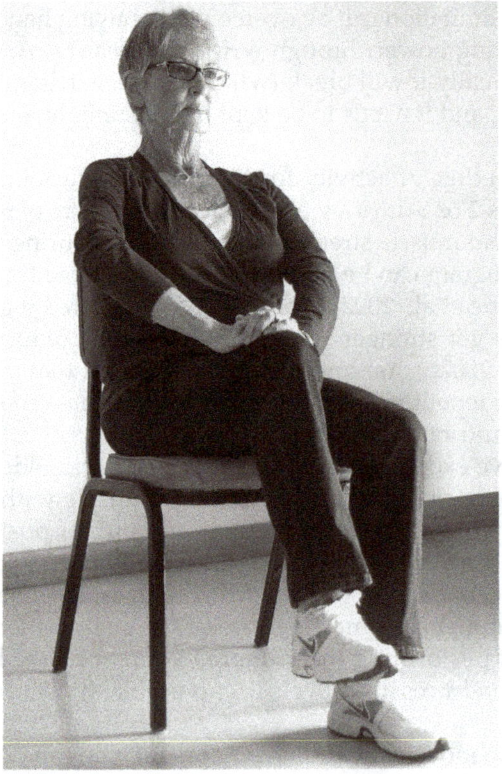

People Lifting Weights—and Getting Injured, 2000). In weight rooms around the country, you can frequently observe examples of incorrect techniques that lead to injury. Men and, less frequently, women are hoisting too heavy weights, arching their backs, holding their breath, swinging the weights or otherwise using momentum, and dropping the weights (in this case, both free weights and machine weights) when done.

Instead, manageable weights and proper technique should be used. Lift slowly and smoothly and return the weights under full control, maintain the natural curve of your back, exhale on exertion, and inhale as you relax. If you break form, the weights are too heavy. Weight lifters who use correct form reduce injuries by strengthening joints and ligaments. ***Machine weights*** are safer than free weights because they help foster proper technique and prevent the weight from falling on you.

Seventy percent of weight lifters are males, down from 80% two decades ago. Women have learned that they need not fear building bulging muscles, because they have less testosterone and fewer cells that make up muscle fiber. In addition to working toward a better appearance, female weight lifters enjoy the benefits of improving strength and balance and preventing or postponing osteoporosis.

Two research leaders who extol the benefits of resistance exercise (free weights, machines, isometrics, and rubber tubing), exercise physiologist William Evans and physician/researcher Maria Fiatarone, believe that strength building may be even more important for older adults than aerobic exercise. Although many physicians recommend walking because they think it is the safest activity for people who are weak, have poor balance, and are more subject to falling, prescribing resistance exercise can give older adults the strength and confidence they need prior to beginning a systematic program of aerobic activity.

Examples of strength and exercise programming include Growing Stronger: Strength Training for Older Adults (https://strongpeopleprogram.org/about-us/#our-director) and Enhance®Fitness (https://www.ncoa.org/article/evidence-based-program-enhancefitness).

The Flexibility and Balance Component

Different types of exercise activities for older adults result in different types of benefits. Programs emphasizing aerobics and strength building provide an array of benefits for older adults, but flexibility exercises are particularly well suited for improving range of motion and reducing arthritic and other types of pain among older adults. It should be noted, though, that stretching as a method for preventing injury or soreness has not been supported by research (Afonso et al., 2021; Thacker et al., 2004).

Ballistic stretching, using quick and bouncy movements, works against the protective reflex contraction and can result in muscle tears, soreness, and injury. Static stretching involves the slow and smooth advancement through a muscle's full range of movement until resistance or the beginning of discomfort was felt. The maximum position was then held 10 to 15 seconds, which allowed for reduction of the protective reflex contraction and additional range of movement.

Stretching should always be preceded by a brief aerobic warm-up to increase heart rate, blood flow, and the temperature of the muscles, ligaments, and tendons. Conversely, stretching while muscles are cold may sprain or tear them. Aerobics should always precede stretching.

A good way to develop different flexibility routines for older adults is to complete the Arthritis Foundation's 2-day PACE (People with Arthritis Can Exercise) training program to teach stretching to older adults. In addition, you receive the PACE manual, which includes a brief description of the purpose of each of the 72 movements, an illustration that demonstrates how to do each stretching movement, an explanation of the functional benefits of each movement, and the identification of special precautions—particularly for persons with arthritis or osteoporosis. There is also a separate section on teaching tips. To find out more information about the training program or the manual, contact the Arthritis Foundation, https://www.arthritis.org/about-us/contact-us.

Tai Chi

Tai chi consists of slow, graceful movements that are derived from a martial arts form in Asian cultures. It is gentle in nature and well suited to both young and old. In addition to improving flexibility, tai chi is conducted with a lowered center of gravity (knees and hips held in flexion) and can contribute to lower extremity strength building, body awareness, and balance control. Though not as popular as yoga in the United States, tai chi has increased in popularity over the past 20 years.

In terms of balance control, rigorously controlled studies—part of a 3-year exercise research project sponsored by the National Institutes on Aging and the National Institute for Nursing Research—supported the contention that tai chi has favorable effects upon the prevention of falls (Wolfson et al., 1996), and one tai chi group went without falls 48% longer than a comparison group before a first fall (Wolf et al., 1996). Older participants learn to stabilize their balance or regain it as they begin to fall. Other studies reported that tai chi decreased fibromyalgia symptoms (Wang et al., 2018), improved sleep quality among older adults with moderate sleep complaints (Irwin et al., 2008), and augmented the immune response in older adults to fight off zoster infection (shingles; Irwin et al., 2007).

A meta-review of 35 systematic reviews of tai chi reported that there was no benefit of this type of exercise for treating cancer, Parkinson disease, rheumatoid arthritis, or cardiovascular disease (Lee & Ernst, 2011). However, three of the four reviews for fall prevention demonstrated positive benefits, and four of the five reviews for psychological well-being also demonstrated positive benefits. These studies mostly focused on older adults. An updated systematic review confirms benefit (Leung et al., 2022).

Yoga

A 2016 Yoga in America Study (Yoga Journal & Yoga Alliance, 2016) reported that there were almost 37 million Americans who had engaged in some type of ***yoga*** practice, more than double the number in 2008. Twenty-one percent of these participants were age 60 or over. In 2022, the U.S. National Health Interview Survey found an age-adjusted percentage of 16.9% for adults age 18 and older who practiced yoga in the past 12 months. Eight percent of people 65+ years old practiced yoga in the prior year mostly to benefit overall health or to treat or manage pain (Elgaddal & Weeks, 2022).

To demonstrate the popularity of yoga among older adults in the United States consider Sadie Delany. She reported in her book that she began her yoga practice in her 60s and continued it for 40 years, the last several of which she followed a yoga program on television (Delany et al., 1993). Sadie died in 1999 at the age of 109. She noted in her book that when her sister Bessie turned 80, she decided that Sadie looked better than she did, and Bessie then began doing yoga too. Bessie, however, probably started too late to reap the same longevity benefits as did Sadie. Her life ended prematurely in 1995, at the tender age of 104.

The most popular yoga activity is hatha yoga, a sequence of stretching, bending, and twisting movements that cause each joint to move slowly through its maximum range of motion, held for several seconds, and then repeated (Figure 4.5). These practices improve body awareness, reduce stress, improve balance and coordination, and increase the maximum range of motion by expanding joint mobility.

Hatha yoga and other types of stretching, twisting, and bending exercise programs possess two characteristics that make them highly desirable for older adults: (a) They are well suited to all adults, even the very frail elderly (Haber, 1988), and (b) they are exceptionally easy to incorporate into a daily routine. The movements of a stretching program, for instance, can be performed while one is watching television or talking on the telephone (not ideal for the specific practice of yoga, though, for which the attention should be on one's body and breath). Also, for people who engage in regular aerobic or strength-building activity, a brief flexibility or yoga routine can be added at the end.

One research study focused on yoga with stressed-out caregivers ranging in age from 45 to 91 years old. The researchers reported that a group that performed daily yoga practice for 12 minutes over 8 weeks showed significantly lower levels of depressive symptoms and greater improvement in mental health and cognitive functioning when compared with a relaxation group (Lavretsky et al., 2012). The researchers also looked at the cellular level and found increased telomerase activity, which slows cellular aging. Insomnia symptoms may be reduced through a regular practice of yoga (Newton et al., 2014), as well as reductions in the levels of blood pressure, cholesterol, and triglycerides (Chu et al., 2014).

QUESTION: What is the primary difference between flexibility exercises and yoga movements?

For those interested in practicing yoga for therapeutic purposes, the International Association of Yoga Therapists will locate therapeutic yoga instructors in local areas

FIGURE 4.5 Shoulder roll to improve body awareness, reduce stress, and increase the range of motion.

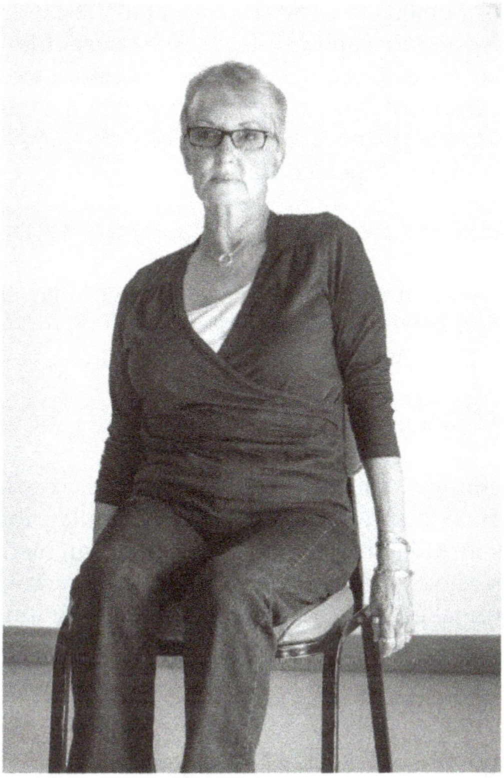

(https://www.iayt.org/). It should be noted, though, that there is no regulatory body for yoga therapy, and yoga instructors are unlicensed. There is no such thing as a certified or registered yoga instructor. It is crucial that a person, particularly a vulnerable older adult, choose an instructor carefully. Older adults may have to be guided into making changes in the moves that they are attempting.

For an interesting and important book on the frequency and ease with which many yoga participants injure themselves, ranging from ruptured discs to leg paralysis to strokes, read *The Science of Yoga* by Broad (2012).

Dance and Other Balance Exercises

An alternative to yoga and tai chi is the tango. In one study, the tango produced the most positive effects on balance and movement control in persons with Parkinson disease, followed by the waltz and foxtrot.

The treatment group in this randomized trial included 58 participants with mild to moderate Parkinson disease. They improved significantly on the Berg Balance scale, 6-minute-walk distance, and backward stride length in comparison with a control group (Hackney & Earhart, 2009). Even if the effects of dance on balance and mobility were not so promising, this would still be a fun option to insert into an exercise routine.

Several other studies report on the benefits of ***dance*** with older adults. One such study was focused on creative dance and its impact on physical function (Cruz-Ferreira et al., 2015) and another on ballroom dance and its effect on balance and functional autonomy (Borges et al., 2012).

Balance issues emerge slowly and subtly over the life cycle, beginning in the mid-40s and becoming more obvious by the mid-60s. Loss of balance is a major contributor to falling, and each year about one quarter of persons 65 and older experience a fall, as do about half of persons over 80 (Kakara et al., 2023). Even the fear of losing one's balance can curtail activity, and this fear can be particularly counterproductive. Less activity due to fear leads to more weakness, and more weakness to more falls.

Regarding ***balance exercises***, I included one or more of the following exercises at the tail end of some of my classes. All the exercisers stood next to a wall, chair, or something else that could be grabbed onto when needed.

- Toe raise: Rise to tiptoes 10 times, reaching for support only if necessary. Repeat with eyes closed.
- One-legged stand: Stand on one leg, flexing the other knee slightly. Balance on one foot for 10 seconds. Repeat with eyes closed.
- Tandem walk: Walk across the floor, heel-to-toe, remaining next to a wall for support if necessary.
- Sitting upside down (Figure 4.6). (Just kidding).

It is important to remind older adults that loss of balance can be caused by a number of conditions in addition to the physical losses that accumulate through a sedentary lifestyle. These conditions include problems with the inner ear, medications, poor posture resulting from arthritis or osteoporosis, poor vision, and muscle weakness. To rule out these problems, nothing takes the place of an evaluation by a health professional. Innovative ideas to improve balance—such as vibrating insoles (Priplata et al., 2006) and cobblestone mat walking (Li et al., 2005b)—appear on a regular basis, though some are of questionable value.

FIGURE 4.6 A photograph of two fellows with pretty good balance.

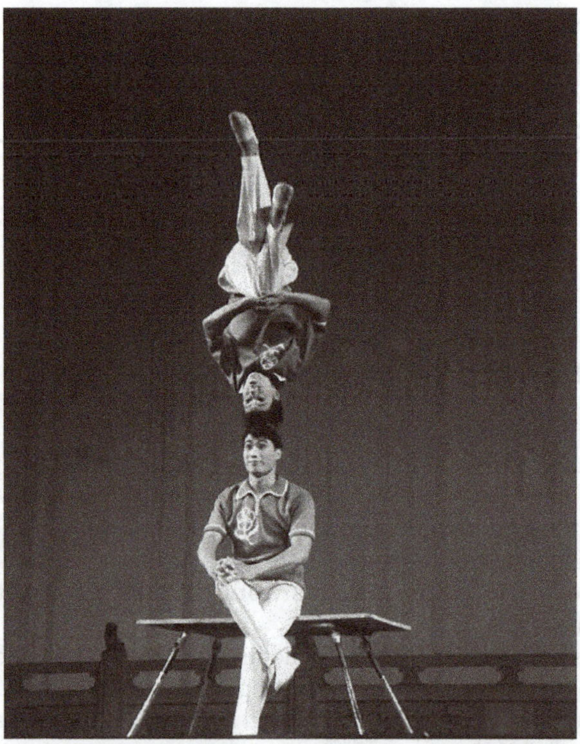

The Health Education Component

During the final minutes of a class, an instructor or one of the participating older adults would facilitate the health education topic. There are an endless number of subjects: describing an experience with a complementary medicine technique, providing a brief description of another health-promoting class in the community, sharing a healthy recipe, discussing fall prevention ideas, sharing a list of sleep hygiene techniques, discussing tips for improving memory, and so forth. The topic may also be presented as a demonstration, rather than pedagogically, such as leading a stress management exercise like deep breathing or progressive muscle relaxation (see Box 4.1). A standard curriculum using only recommendations supported by evidence from clinical trials and epidemiological studies is the *10 Keys to Healthy Aging* (Newman et al., 2010).

LESS CONVENTIONAL EXERCISES

Power yoga (an Americanized version of ashtanga yoga) is a blend of flexibility and strength building that has become popular mostly in New York and California. It was introduced into America by the aptly named Birch (1995). Power yoga differs from traditional stretching programs; the latter encourages relaxation into a pose while stretching, while the former advocates for isometrically tensing specific muscles while relaxing the opposing muscles.

QUESTION: How would you improve upon my community-based exercise class?

Vinyasa krama is another yoga variant that blends flexibility with aerobics instead of strength building. Rather than holding postures for a long time, students do a series of yoga movements without pause, synchronized with deep yoga breathing.

According to Andrew Weil, there is also disco yoga, tribal yoga (to the beat of African drums), aqua yoga, *hot yoga*, and iron yoga (with light hand weights). A uniquely American version is beer yoga. As blasphemous as it may seem (or is), there are also

BOX 4.1 Best Practice for an Exercise Program With Older Adults

Leading exercise and aging specialists list five key practices in order for exercise programs to be effective with older adults (Cress et al., 2005): (a) Implement a multidimensional program that includes endurance, strength, balance, and flexibility training. (b) Utilize principles of behavior change, including social support, self-efficacy, active choices, health contracts, assurance of safety, and positive reinforcement. (c) Manage risk by beginning at a low intensity level and gradually increasing to a moderate intensity level. (d) Have an emergency procedure plan in place. (e) Monitor aerobic and strength-building intensity to ensure motivation and to encourage progression.

Chances are quite good that the exercise programs for older adults in your local community fall short of this model. Perhaps an alternative set of criteria can be useful: (a) Is it safe? (b) Is it fun? If yes to both, it may not be a "best practice," but it is certainly good enough for promoting health.

yoga competitions in which participants are judged on the precision, appearance, and grace of their movements.

There are other hybrids like Yogilates, a blend of yoga and Pilates. Pilates (pronounced pi-LA-tees) is a technique that uses specially made exercise equipment with pulleys and springs to stretch and to strengthen your midsection. Trained instructors guide you through breathing exercises and a routine to help you move in a balanced way.

The Alexander technique also attempts to promote balance and to retrain your body to carry itself properly, with particular attention to head, neck, and spine alignment. The technique combines good posture with simple movements to reduce muscle tension (https://amsatonline.org/aws/AMSAT/pt/sp/find_a_teacher).

The Feldenkrais method is another alternative to train your body to move with efficiency and ease. A trained practitioner gently manipulates your muscles and joints to find the most comfortable ways to use your body (https://www.feldenkraisguild.com/page/certified-trainers). The Sit and Be Fit program was developed by a registered nurse, Mary Ann Wilson (born 1938!). Her program has been shown on public television for many years and is available online (https://www.youtube.com/SitandBeFitTVshow; www.sitandbefit.org).

The Body Recall program was created by Dorothy Chrisman in 1979 for persons age 50 and older. Ms. Chrisman died in 2011 at age 86, but there are still instructors who offer Body Recall classes around the country, but her book, *Body Recall: A Program of Physical Fitness for the Adult* (Lafayette Printing Company, 2001, [Chrisman, 2001]) is no longer in print.

For those readers who have found no modality of exercise to their liking, there is always the promise of the work of Dr. Sanders Williams, former dean of the Duke University School of Medicine. Dr. Williams was working on chemical pathways that muscle cells use to build strength and endurance. This could, theoretically, lead to the development of a medication that will let people get the health benefits of regular exercise by just taking a pill! If you run out of patience waiting for this pill, try obtaining one of these patented products, some fanciful:

#6,024,678: Vacuum cleaner leg exerciser: This invention consists of shoes with bellows, so that when you walk around your house, you create suction that pulls dirt into a cleaning wand and then into a tank strapped on your back.

#6,042,508: Remote-control dumbbell. This remote is built into a contoured weight that you lift up and down to switch television stations. It also calculates your pulse rate.

#5,984,841: Shower step master. This device makes you pedal in order to shower, with elastic bands that provide resistance. A side benefit is that you won't even know when you are sweating.

#7,037,243: Cordless jump-rope. A jump-rope minus the rope; all that's left is two handles (with moving weights inside that simulate the feel of a rope moving) and a pretend rope. The truly lazy can pretend to jump over the pretend rope.

Special thanks to WellnessLetter.com for alerting me about these patented gems.

Finally, we discuss an exercise that is not a "less conventional exercise"—swimming. This is a particularly relevant exercise for older adults, especially those with joint problems such as arthritis of the knee or hip. ***Swimming*** helps attain and preserve stamina and flexibility, as well as cardiac and respiratory function. There are more than 10 million residential pools and 300,000 public pools in the United States, but

TABLE 4.3 DIFFERENT EXERCISES AND BENEFITS

EXERCISE	ENDURANCE	STRENGTH	FLEXIBILITY
Swimming	High	Low	Medium
Brisk walking/jogging	High	Low	Low
Yoga	Low	Low	High
Tai chi	Medium	Medium	Medium
Weight lifting	Medium	High	Low

that does not necessarily mean they are conveniently located or affordable to every older adult.

One small study with 43 older persons reported that swimming three or four times a week lowered systolic blood pressure (Nualnim et al., 2012). Over a 3-month period, the swimmers reduced their systolic blood pressure nine points on average in contrast to no change in the relaxation control group.

Different Strokes for Different Folks

Table 4.3 shows variation in benefits that accrue from different exercise activities. Because the activities offer considerable variation in the types of benefits, engaging in a balanced approach to exercise is ideal. While no exercise provides maximal benefit in all three domains, each of the exercises can be performed in such a way as to improve its ranking (e.g., power yoga increases strength, high-repetition weight lifting improves endurance).

THE ACTIVITY PYRAMID

Most people have heard of the U.S. Department of Agriculture's food guide pyramid. Now several organizations have developed an ***activity pyramid***. Not having seen one that I like without modification, here is our contribution, shown in Figure 4.7.

Sedentary behaviors—like eating the junk food at the top of the food pyramid—should be done sparingly. It is acceptable to watch television and play computer games, and even to eat junk food while doing it, but doing it to excess is dangerous to your health. In contrast, slothfulness every now and then is an excellent antidote for "wellness self-righteousness."

Two to three "servings" of structured strength-building exercises per week are recommended. Medium or vigorous aerobic intensity, such as jogging and some recreational activities, is recommended three or four times a week for those who have left the ranks of the sedentary far behind. Light to moderate exercise, such as brisk walking, stretching, and finding additional activity bouts in the course of the day, can be done every day.

Incorporating additional activity bouts into your everyday routine can be done in a variety of ways. Park your car farther away from the store, use stairs instead of escalators, walk the dog, work in your garden, and, perhaps most torturous of all, do not use the remote control when watching television—and change channels frequently.

FIGURE 4.7 Activity pyramid.

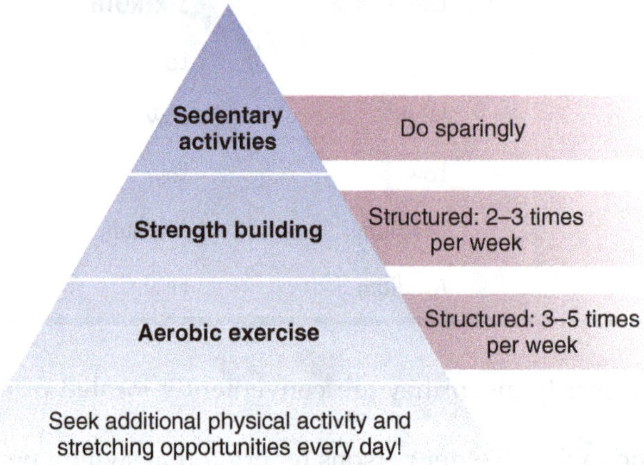

People who are sedentary need to focus their attention on the base of the pyramid. The everyday activity at the base is different from the exercises above it. Activity can be defined as any body movement produced by skeletal muscles that results in energy expenditure. It is in the lower sector of the pyramid that we can emphasize the healthy pleasures of spontaneity and enjoyment. Activities can be enjoyable, for instance, when they are turned into social occasions with family and friends.

Or you can take advantage of spontaneity in the lower sector of the pyramid by stepping up the intensity level of, say, vacuuming. You not only get your housecleaning done, but you also obtain a free bout of exercise in your home using your vacuum cleaner (or your duster, mop, or other household exercise tool).

Exercise, in contrast, is planned, structured, and emphasizes repetitive body movement. It is in these upper sectors of the pyramid where maintaining a routine, rather than spontaneity, is desirable. Routine exercise can be enjoyable too, though for me, the highlight is when I am done with it and can savor the way my body feels for several hours afterward.

ARTHRITIS: A BARRIER TO EXERCISE AND ACTIVITY

This story, entitled "The Joys of Aging," has been circulating anonymously for years. It goes like this: "I have become quite a frivolous old gal. I'm seeing five gentlemen every day. As soon as I awake, Will Power helps me get out of bed. When he leaves, I go see John. Then Charley Horse comes along, and when he is here, he takes a lot of my attention. When he leaves, Arthur Ritis shows up and stays the rest of the day. He doesn't like to stay in one place very long, so he takes me from joint to joint. After such a busy day, I'm really tired and ready to go to bed with Ben Gay. What a day!"

One of the major ***barriers*** to performing resistance training, yoga, aerobics, and other types of exercise is arthritic stiffness and pain. The 2017 Profile of Older Americans (Administration for Community Living & Administration on Aging, 2018) reported that about half of Americans over age 65 suffered from ***arthritis***. The National Health Interview Survey 2019 to 2021 noted that 47.3% of adults 65+ have diagnosed arthritis (Fallon et al., 2023). These percentages may even be higher than reported, depending on how you define "suffer from." Also, the likelihood of experiencing, and suffering the consequences of, arthritis steadily rises with age.

Osteoarthritis (degenerative joint disease) is the most common type found among older people, and ranges in intensity from occasional stiffness and joint pain to disability. This disease is affected by aging, genetics, obesity, injuries, and overuse of joint movement. Typically, the cartilage that acts like a cushion between bones breaks down over time, and bone rubs against bone. (Rheumatoid arthritis is less common, but can be more disabling. Although the cause is unknown, scientists believe it may result from a breakdown in the immune system.)

Many people with osteoarthritis think that any type of exercise will be uncomfortable—that is, cause joint or muscle pain or swelling of the extremities—or be downright harmful and lead to decreased functional abilities. These indicators of exercise intolerance, however, will typically not take place if exercise is performed properly. In fact, it is more likely that the joints will stiffen, the muscles will weaken, and the ability to function will decline if regular flexibility and other types of exercises are not performed.

To counteract arthritic stiffness, it may be necessary to briefly engage in flexibility exercises several times a day. It is also helpful to engage in strength-building exercise to strengthen the muscles that surround and support the joints and to force lubricating fluid into the cartilage that helps keep it nourished and healthy. The advice of a physical therapist, occupational therapist, or nurse can be especially helpful when developing an individualized exercise program that balances exercise and rest. One way to minimize aches and pains is to relax joints and muscles prior to exercise by applying heat (or soaking in a warm bath), or to gently massage muscles or apply ice packs. Weight control can also help keep unnecessary stress from joints.

Another technique for conquering the challenge of aches and pains in order to exercise is to choose a time of day when one is subject to the least amount of discomfort, stiffness, and fatigue. People who are on medication may find that their optimal time coincides with the period during which their medicine is having its maximum effect. Many persons with arthritis depend on antiinflammatory drugs to alleviate aches and pains and to allow them to exercise.

Many others hold out hope for a miracle medication that will not only alleviate their arthritic pain, but also reverse the disease process. One prospect in this regard, discovered by the public more than 20 years ago, coincided with the publication of *The Arthritis Cure* (Theodosakis, 1997). The book touted two supplements, glucosamine and chondroitin sulfate, to stimulate the growth of cartilage and keep it from wearing down. Although many arthritis sufferers are convinced of the benefit of these supplements, a multicenter, randomized controlled trial was equivocal, at best, on these two supplements.

Over 1,500 patients with symptomatic knee osteoarthritis were randomly assigned to glucosamine and chondroitin (individually and in combination) or to placebo, with no significant differences in the reduction of knee pain among groups (Clegg et al., 2006). A subgroup of patients with moderate to severe knee pain did receive benefit from the combination of supplements, but subgroup analysis is unreliable and can only be considered exploratory. The good press generated by these supplements has been fueled mostly by suspect manufacturer-funded studies, especially from a company in Italy that makes glucosamine. Many adults, though, have not given up hope on these two dietary supplements, despite a subsequent systematic review showing that neither glucosamine, chondroitin, or their combination had a positive effect overall on pain and range of motion and that the combination did not improve knee pain (Simental-Mendia et al., 2018).

Another option for avoiding arthritic discomfort is finding a more appropriate exercise routine, such as water aerobics. An older adult who believes they are aggravating an arthritic knee during a walking program may find an aquatic program more desirable. Water provides buoyancy, which can relieve some of the stress and strain of other exercise, where gravity and weight are greater influences. Body weight in water is less than 10% of its weight on the ground. Also, if the water is sufficiently warm, it will allow greater range of motion given that muscles stretch better when they are warm.

A free brochure from the Arthritis Foundation explains how to set safe exercise limits and includes tips for easing into exercises, such as taking a warm shower before engaging in exercise in order to loosen up. To obtain one, contact the Foundation at its website (www.arthritis.org). The Foundation also provides guidance on aquatic exercise.

Other Barriers and Cautions

There are several barriers to exercise besides arthritis and the belief that exercise will be painful, unenjoyable, or perhaps even harmful. Some older adults engage in a level of exercise that is inadequate or that lacks the proper intensity to meet their needs, yet are under the mistaken belief that they are sufficiently active. Others have a problem with overexuberance, tackling an exercise program too strenuously and too quickly, and suffering from the consequences of injury.

It is necessary to begin and end an exercise routine with adequate warm-up and cool-down periods consisting of gentle aerobics. It is important that the warm-up period begin with aerobics (walking or a slow version of the exercise to be engaged in) and not stretching, as the latter can create damage to the muscles and joints if the body is not warmed up first. The cool-down period prevents blood from pooling in lower muscles, which reduces blood flow to the heart and brain and can cause faintness or worse. Cooling down may also prevent muscle stiffness and soreness by restretching muscles that are shortened during exercise. One meta-analysis of randomized research trials, however, reported no significant effect of stretching on either muscle soreness or injury (Afonso et al., 2021; Herbert & Gabriel, 2002).

Another inhibitor of activity is the fear of falling. As noted earlier, one quarter of community-dwelling elderly persons fall each year. The potential for falling has been used as a justification for physical restraints in the nursing home. Fear of falling, reinforced by a caregiving spouse, may be a significant barrier to exercising. Some risk may have to be tolerated; however, the risk may be reduced by exercising in a seated or lying position or by a change in medication.

Medication usage can contribute to falling. Medications may require that exercise participants modify their exercise routine by decreasing the duration and intensity of an exercise, increasing fluid intake, or foregoing exercise for a period of time. One should be alert for dizziness, faintness, and fatigue that may result from a wide variety of medications, especially ones that belong in these categories: antiarthritic, psychotropic, antihypertensive, antiarrhythmic, antiparkinsonism, antihistamine, decongestant, and barbiturates (de Vries et al., 2018; Seppala et al., 2018a, 2018b).

To treat injury to a muscle or ligament in the form of a strain, sprain, or tear, and keep it from becoming worse, the most commonly recommended guideline is the acronym RICE, which stands for *r*est, *i*ce, *c*ompression, and *e*levation. Rest the injured area immediately to cut down on blood circulation to that part of the body. Apply ice immediately, which shrinks blood vessels and reduces swelling. Compress the injured area with an elastic bandage or cloth to also help reduce swelling. Elevate the damaged part to a level higher than the heart. For those who are prevention oriented, the acronym PRICE is preferred, with the *p* standing for *p*rotection prior to and during exercise.

Other barriers to exercise may include lack of transportation to an exercise facility, limited financial resources for joining a program, medical concerns, lack of access to consultation with a health professional, lethargy, inability to identify a pleasurable exercise that can sustain one's interest over time, and lack of time. Creative problem-solving can overcome most barriers.

Some health professionals erroneously believe that older adults have considerably more discretionary time than younger adults. A perceived lack of time, however, may be as likely a problem among older adults as among younger adults. In fact, a common response among older adults is that they lack the time for exercise because they provide care for a family member who is frail. Other older adults may also have a busy schedule that consists of sedentary hobbies, family events, and volunteer obligations.

In general, exercise is a safe activity. Research into exercise with older adults rarely reports serious cardiovascular or musculoskeletal complications in published trials. This is not to suggest that exercise is hazard free. Walkers and joggers often share a path with persons on bicycles, and rare collisions do occur. Overexertion in hot weather can lead to heat exhaustion (with symptoms of dizziness and a rapid or weak pulse) or potentially fatal heat strokes. High humidity is dangerous because the air is saturated with moisture, which prevents heat from leaving the body through perspiration.

Occasionally, older persons with unsuspected heart problems embark on exercise programs. To address this problem, they may be referred to an exercise stress test prior to beginning an exercise program. This test—consisting of treadmills, cycle ergometers, and steps—is designed to identify those persons without symptoms who may be at high risk of suffering a medical complication during exercise because of undetected heart disease. A review of several studies on stress tests, however, found that they are expensive, are of unproven benefit to low-risk adults without symptoms, and may serve as a deterrent to persons who delay (perhaps permanently) exercise until they get one (Firestone, 2000).

The USPSTF continues to recommend against stress-testing in low risk adults without symptoms of heart disease. Persons with known or suspected heart disease, however, should consider the test. Abnormal responses to a stress test may consist of a failure of the blood pressure level to increase as work intensity increases, a slow recovery of ventilation and heart rate, an excessive shortness of breath, chest pain, or electrocardiogram changes such as dysrhythmias. There are, however, an unusually high percentage of false positives (abnormal stress test results for people who can exercise) and false negatives (normal results for persons who should not exercise). False-positive tests can lead to additional psychological stress and invasive tests; false-negative tests can lead to delayed treatment.

SELECTED TOPICS

How to Respond to an Excuse

AARP's Staying Healthy After Fifty program (SHAF; now defunct) listed the most common *excuses* for not exercising: fatigue, fear of heart attack or hypertension, trouble catching breath, need to relax, too old, bad back, and arthritis. Each excuse was examined during the SHAF program and exposed as a myth or a general misunderstanding that can keep an older adult inactive.

Some examples of responses to these excuses are, respectively: improved strength makes daily tasks easier and less tiring; an exercised heart is stronger, works easier, and can lower blood pressure; heart, lungs, and muscles become more efficient through exercise and may make breathing easier; exercise can help relaxation; it is never too late to exercise—even nonagenarians benefit; bad backs are commonly caused by inadequate exercise, improper lifting, and poor posture; and exercise can alleviate the pain and stiffness of arthritis.

Benefits

A negative attitude also can be a barrier to exercise. When motivating someone to exercise, it is important to shift the emphasis from the negative—what will happen if you do not exercise—to the positive—how you will benefit if you do. The SHAF program listed ***benefits of exercise*** that are likely to motivate old and young alike: having fun; sleeping better; feeling more energetic; controlling body weight; feeling more relaxed; feeling stronger; increased joint flexibility; maintaining an independent lifestyle; improving heart, arteries, and lungs; new social contacts; improved morale and confidence; and enhanced agility and mobility.

QUESTION: Role play with a partner. Can you counter every excuse that your partner offers for not exercising by suggesting an idea that will encourage your partner to exercise?

If these benefits are not appealing, the humorist Erma Bombeck offered a particularly unique advantage to those who exercise: "The only reason I would take up jogging is so that I can hear heavy breathing again."

Health Club, Home, or Religious Setting

Membership in health clubs has risen steadily over the past two decades in the United States (https://www.statista.com/statistics/246984/obstacles-to-joining-a-health-club/). About 25% of health club members are over age 55, with baby boomers the fastest growing segment of the health club population. Bally Total Fitness centers (which amassed 440 facilities before it went defunct in 2016 due to financial shenanigans) and Gold's Gyms frequently included older adults in their advertisements for new members. Curves, which targets middle-aged, female fitness novices, developed a 30-minute circuit workout that led to the launching of 8,000 health clubs worldwide. Medicare Advantage plans often include gym memberships and access to exercise programs geared to older adults, such as Silver Sneakers.

There are many advantages to membership in a health club. Most clubs offer at least one free session from a qualified trainer as part of the membership fee. Weight machines are excellent for beginners because they are easy to use, and they reduce injury by controlling your form and preventing a weight from falling on you. Most health clubs arrange machines in a logical order to promote a balanced approach to strength building. Free weights are offered as an alternative; although more likely to produce injury, they involve stabilizing muscles that help you progress faster. Finally, aerobic and yoga classes are commonly offered at health facilities.

The downside is that fees often surpass $1,200 a year per individual. The more resources (including classes) in the fitness facility and the greater your access to them, the higher the fee. Also, many older adults may feel shy or inadequate in a health club with a preponderance of young, fit participants. Finally, if motivation is marginal, sometimes all it takes is the prospect of a 15-minute drive, or longer, to the health facility to put someone off.

Before joining a health club, it is wise to visit more than one, to go the same time of day that you intend to exercise, determine whether the classes are reasonable for your level of fitness, and find out whether a staff person is certified by a nationally recognized senior fitness organization to work with people who have age-related health issues. A number of organizations have developed certifications for senior fitness instructors, including the International Sports Science Association (ISSA), National Academy of Sports Medicine (NASM), American Fitness Professionals Association (AFPA), and American Council on Exercise (ACE; https://www.ptpioneer.com/best-senior-fitness-certification/).

Additional questions for assessing whether the health club is age-friendly or suitable to beginners, are as follows:

- If there is music, is it acceptable to you and is the volume set at a reasonable level?
- Are the display panels on the equipment easy to read, change, and understand?
- Do the treadmills start slowly, at 0.5 mph?
- Are there recumbent bikes, and do they have comfortable seats?
- Does the strength-building equipment have low starting resistance, about 5 pounds?

Welcyon gyms was founded by boomers Suzy and Tom Boerboom; the average age of the members in their several fitness centers in Minnesota and South Dakota is 62. For safety reasons, it has no treadmills (in 2015, for instance, the well-known tech guru, Dave Goldberg, age 47, fell off one at a Mexican resort and died—the primary cause of death may have been a heart condition, but the fall did not help). Instead, they use recumbent stair steppers. Many of their fitness instructors are boomers, 20+ years older than the average age of those trained by the American Council on Exercise. And they are continually coming up with new ideas to compete with the growing number of other fitness centers, like Nifty After Fifty, that also target older customers.

Exercising in the home setting is as convenient as it gets. You do not have to worry about how you look, and you do not have to adapt to other people's musical tastes. The investment is a one-time expense consisting of weights, weight machine, treadmill, stair stepper, or other preferred equipment. If money is a barrier, an excellent exercise routine can be devised from using the floor, wall, chair, and your own body weight; using household items as weights; or using a jump rope in a way that allows for a low- or medium-intensity level.

The downside is that you may be distracted by your television set, computer, or a family member. You may also lack the peer support of an aerobics class or role models doing strength building. Home exercise equipment typically does not include the variety found in a health club.

If you are going to buy a piece of exercise equipment for your home, consider the low-tech treadmill. One study reported that the walking or jogging machine outperforms a rowing machine, a cross-country skiing simulator, a stationary bicycle, and a stair stepper when it comes to burning calories (Prieto-González & Yagin, 2024; Zeni et al., 1996). Regardless of the home exercise equipment you purchase, check a consumer magazine for recommendations; try out the equipment before you buy; and remember that flimsy, uncomfortable, or noisy equipment is likely to wind up as a clothes rack.

An interesting alternative to the health club or home setting is the faith-based fitness movement. Synagogues and churches are hosting a growing number of fitness programs. A fitness and nutrition program called First Place has been tried in 12,000 churches. Faith-based fitness is more likely to focus on fellowship and community, and less likely to be competitive or appearance conscious. Sometimes an exercise session may end with a meditation or a prayer. Whether religious or not, however, two messages can easily apply to all exercisers regardless of setting: (a) Treat your body as your temple. (b) Focus on both inner and outer health.

Personal Trainer

Is it worth $80 an hour for a ***personal trainer***? If you can afford it, the answer is probably yes, both in terms of expertise and motivation. Want to make sure that your instructor is certified? Ask about their certification and call to check on their credentials. Most qualified trainers have been certified by a national fitness organization, such as the following:

- American College of Sports Medicine
- National Strength and Conditioning Association
- American Council on Exercise
- Aerobics and Fitness Association of America
- International Association of Fitness Professionals
- Cooper Institute for Aerobics Research

Most exercise certifications are not specific for exercises with older adults. Make sure that the organization and its instructors are experienced with working with older persons, and that the content of the training program addresses the preferences, needs, ***cautions***, and health of older adults.

There are also a number of online fitness trainer sites that match your personal health statistics and goals with a predesigned training program. Some sites send the user a daily text or e-mail prescribing that day's exercises; others display an exercise regimen on a personal monthly calendar that can be accessed by smartphone. Online sites produced by a single trainer tend to be less sophisticated and may merely consist of a training plan with illustrated exercises that are sent to you. Evidence for the effectiveness of these programs is now available (Solis-Navarro et al., 2022).

One study reported on older participants who received an instructional session and a handheld computer that was programmed to monitor their physical activity levels twice per day, and provide them with daily and weekly individualized feedback, goal setting, and support. In comparison with a control group that received age-appropriate educational materials on physical activity, the treatment group of previously underactive adults reported significantly greater physical activity levels (King et al., 2008).

Virtual Reality in Rehabilitation for Degenerative Diseases

When Nintendo's Wii gaming system was released in November 2006, more than 19 million consoles were sold over the next 2 years in the United States alone. Unlike traditional video game systems controlled by a player's thumbs and fingers, Wii games respond to a player's whole body movement.

The Wii-Fit games—referred to by some therapists as *Wiihabilitation*, or ***Wii-hab***—appeal to not only young and old alike but also to therapists working with clients who have Parkinson disease and other degenerative diseases. Players wave a wireless controller that directs the actions of animated athletes on a screen. The Wii features simulated movements such as swinging a tennis racket, throwing a bowling ball, or engaging in golf, baseball, or boxing. Some of the movements are similar to traditional therapy exercises. Newer "exergaming" digital applications are increasingly available and allow competition, group participation, and a mix of cognitive and physical challenges.

Significant improvements in rigidity, fine motor skills, energy level, endurance, reflexes, balance, and coordination have been recorded (Hinely, 2009). Although studies have focused on older adults in nursing homes, senior centers, and retirement communities, they tend to be clinical case studies rather than more rigorous random assignment to treatment or control group (Clark & Kraemer, 2009).

Video games may also improve memory and other cognitive functions (Pacheco et al., 2020; Stojan & Voelcker-Rehage, 2019). In an early study, adults aged 55 to 75 were assigned to play Super Mario 64 for 30 minutes a day, 5 days a week; take piano lessons for the first time for comparable minutes and days per week; or participate in the nonactive control group. After 6 months, only participants in the video game group increased gray matter volume in the cerebellum and hippocampus, the regions of the brain primarily associated with spatial and episodic memory. Their short-term memory also improved (West et al., 2018). The researchers speculated that video games may delay mild cognitive impairment or certain types of dementia.

Absence of the Health Educator in the Medical Clinic

The percentage of active older adults would likely increase if physicians were more inclined to recommend the health benefits of exercise. A Harris poll reported that 85% of adult respondents believe a physician's recommendation would help motivate them to engage in regular exercise.

Yet over the past quarter century, physicians have not been so inclined. Periodic surveys report that, on average, less than half of primary care physicians routinely ask patients about their exercise habits. Other surveys note that an estimated 30% to 50% of all sedentary patients reported that they received counseling about exercise. As mentioned previously, physicians are even less likely to ask patients age 65+ to change a health behavior than their younger patients.

The barriers to physician counseling of older patients include a lack of time, training, teaching materials, knowledge, reimbursement, and confidence in getting adherence from their older patients. Perhaps some of these barriers can be avoided by using other health professionals in the clinic. There have been examples of nurses being effective with reaching out to patients and encouraging them to exercise. A nurse in one clinic, for instance, posted signs by the elevator giving directions to the nearest stairs to promote physical activity (Colangelo et al., 1997).

A trained receptionist can distribute exercise materials to patients, answer questions, follow up on whether patients are pursuing exercise goals, answer additional questions, and offer further encouragement. Perhaps the ideal solution for health promotion is for each clinic with a sufficient number of patients to hire a health educator, a cost that can be shared among providers (and justified by the goodwill and additional referrals this will generate). A more fiscally conservative approach would be to require patients who accept the services of a health educator to bear some or all of the costs involved.

A Farewell to Jack

Jack LaLanne, the father of the fitness movement, died at the age of 96 in 2011. He started working out with weights in 1936 when it was an oddity. Shortly thereafter, he opened the first fitness facility in an old office building in Oakland, California. He had limited business, as people at the time thought there was a risk of heart attack with the use of weights. Things began to change with *The Jack LaLanne Show*, which made its TV debut in 1951 in the San Francisco area. His strength-building and aerobics routine quickly reached a national audience and lasted almost 35 years, with over 3,000 shows.

Jack invented leg extension and pulley devices, marketed juicers to blend vegetables and fruits, and sold exercise videos and fitness books long before Jane Fonda (who, by the way, is close to 90 as I write this) offered "prime time" fitness videos. At age 60, Jack swam from Alcatraz Island to Fisherman's Wharf while handcuffed and towing a 1,000-pound boat. At age 70, handcuffed again, he towed 70 boats and 70 people for a mile and a half.

Jack worked out 2 hours a day and his diet was equally rigorous. He maintained his health routine into his 90s, along with his 150-pound frame on his 5-foot-6-inch body.

I admired Jack LaLanne and his unbelievable fitness and eating routine, and particularly appreciated the sentiment that he expressed: He hated to work out, but loved the results. I have to confess, though: The few times I saw him on television he was a turnoff—a hectoring, badgering, guilt-inducing presence. Eventually, I learned for myself how to tolerate an exercise routine and, like Jack, loved the moment I stopped each day and could then start to feel good, a feeling that lasts the rest of the day.

It was Jack LaLanne who launched the American fitness movement.

SUMMARY

Surprisingly, perhaps the most important content in this chapter on exercise is not, technically, exercise. It is body movement that does not rise to the intensity level of exercise. As we age, sedentary behavior increases and the likelihood of contracting the "sitting disease" increases as well. One way to combat this disease is through dynamic sitting—yes, there is such a thing. Who knew?

Environmental factors are important as some neighborhoods invite walking while others discourage it. There is also an abundance of different types of exercise classes in the community and many comply with best practices for older adults. Exercise is, unfortunately, often equated only with aerobics, ignoring the importance of strength building, flexibility, and balance, which are especially important concerns for older adults.

Most barriers for older adults, particularly the barrier of arthritis, can be overcome with advice from a geriatrics-informed health provider. Moreover, healthcare in the United States would be well served by the placement of a health educator in every medical clinic to supplement the knowledge of clinicians and to compensate for their lack of time. Finally, with tech-savvy baby boomers taking over the ranks of older adults, more consideration should be given to ever-more-sophisticated technologies that can impact on the physical, cognitive, and emotional health of older adults.

We have come a long way since Jack LaLanne, the father of the fitness movement, began doing aerobics and strength building in 1936 when it was considered an oddity at best, and dangerous at worst. The acceptance of the importance of exercise is now universal, including all age groups; however, the practice of exercise does not match the knowledge of its worth, and it becomes increasingly challenging with age.

SPRINGER PUBLISHING CONNECT™ | **A robust set of instructor resources designed to supplement this text is located at http://connect.springerpub.com/content/book/978-0-8261-8386-6. Qualifying instructors may request access by emailing textbook@springerpub.com.**

REFERENCES

Only key references appear in the print edition. The full reference list can be accessed by visiting www.springerpub.com/courseconnect. See inside front cover and tear-out card for CourseConnect details.

Channa, A., Popescu, N., Skibinska, J., & Burget, R. (2021). The rise of wearable devices during the COVID-19 pandemic: A systematic review. *Sensors, 21*(17), 5787. https://doi.org/10.3390/s21175787

Chrisman, D. C. (2001). *Body recall: A program of physical fitness for the adult.* (9th ed.). Lafayette Printing Co.

Colberg, S. R., Sigal, R. J., Yardley, J. E., Riddell, M. C., Dunstan, D. W., Dempsey, P. C., Horton, E. S., Castorino, K., & Tate, D. F. (2016). Physical activity/exercise and diabetes: A position statement of the American Diabetes Association. *Diabetes Care, 39*(11), 2065–2079. https://doi.org/10.2337/dc16-1728

de Vries, M., Seppala, L. J., Daams, J. G., van de Glind, E. M., Masud, T., & van der Velde, N. (2018). Fall-risk-increasing drugs: A systematic review and meta-analysis: I. Cardiovascular drugs. *Journal of the American Medical Directors Association, 19*(4), 371-e1.

Duijvestijn, M., de Wit, G. A., van Gils, P. F., & Wendel-Vos, G. C. W. (2023, June 3). Impact of physical activity on healthcare costs: A systematic review. *BMC Health Services Research, 23*(1), 572. https://doi.org/10.1186/s12913-023-09556-8

El-Khoury, F., Cassou, B., Charles, M., & Dargent-Molina, P. (2013). The effect of fall prevention exercise programmes on fall-induced injuries in community-dwelling older adults: Systematic review and meta-analysis of randomised controlled trials. *British Medical Journal, 347*, f6234. https://doi.org/10.1136/bmj.f6234

Erickson, K. I., Donofry, S. D., Sewell, K. R., Brown, B. M., & Stillman, C. M. (2022). Cognitive aging and the promise of physical activity. *Annual Review of Clinical Psychology, 18*, 417–442. https://doi.org/10.1146/annurev-clinpsy-072720-014213

Fallon, E. A., Boring, M. A., Foster, A. L., Stowe, E. W., Lites, T. D., Odom, E. L., & Seth, P. (2023). Prevalence of diagnosed arthritis—United States, 2019–2021. *MMWR Morbidity and Mortality Weekly Report, 72*(41), 1101–1107. https://doi.org/10.15585/mmwr.mm7241a1

Harris, T., Kerry, S. M., Limb, E. S., Furness, C., Wahlich, C., Victor, C. R., Iliffe, S., Whincup, P. H., Ussher, M., Ekelund, U., Fox-Rushby, J., Ibison, J., DeWilde, S., McKay, C., & Cook, D. G. (2018). Physical activity levels in adults and older adults 3–4 years after pedometer-based walking interventions: Long-term follow-up of participants from two randomised controlled trials in UK primary care. *PLoS Medicine, 15*(3), e1002526. https://doi.org/10.1371/journal.pmed.1002526

Kakara, R., Bergen, G., Burns, E., & Stevens, M. (2023). Nonfatal and fatal falls among adults aged ≥65 years—United States, 2020–2021. *MMWR Morbidity and Mortality Weekly Report, 72*, 938–943. https://doi.org/10.15585/mmwr.mm7235a1

Keadle, S. K., McKinnon, R., Graubard, B. I., & Troiano, R. P. (2016). Prevalence and trends in physical activity among older adults in the United States: A comparison across three national surveys. *Preventive Medicine, 89*, 37–43. https://doi.org/10.1016/j.ypmed.2016.05.009

Livingston, G., Huntley, J., Sommerlad, A., Ames, D., Ballard, C., Banerjee, S., Brayne, C., Burns, A., Cohen-Mansfield, J., Cooper, C., Costafreda, S. G., Dias, A., Fox, N., Gitlin, L. N., Howard, R., Kales, H. C., Kivimäki, M., Larson, E. B., Ogunniyi, A., & Mukadam, N. (2020). Dementia prevention, intervention, and care: 2020 report of the Lancet Commission. *Lancet, 396*(10248), 413–446. https://doi.org/10.1016/S0140-6736(20)30367-6

Looker, A. C., & Wang, C. Y. (2015). *Prevalence of reduced muscle strength in older U.S. adults: United States 2011–2012*. NCHS Data Brief, No. 179. National Center for Health Statistics.

Newman, A. B., Bayles, C. M., Milas, C. N., McTigue, K., Williams, K., Robare, J. F., Taylor, C. A., Albert, S. M., & Kuller, L. H. (2010). The 10 keys to healthy aging: Findings from an innovative prevention program in the community. *Journal of Aging and Health, 22*(5), 547–566. https://doi.org/10.1177/0898264310363772

Pacheco, T. B. F., de Medeiros, C. S. P., de Oliveira, V. H. B., Vieira, E. R., & De Cavalcanti, F. A. C. (2020). Effectiveness of exergames for improving mobility and balance in older adults:

A systematic review and meta-analysis. *Systematic Reviews*, *9*, 1–14. https://doi.org/10.1186/s13643-020-01421-7

Paluch, A. E., Bajpai, S., Ballin, M., Bassett, D. R., Buford, T. W., Carnethon, M. R., Chernofsky, A., Dooley, E. E., Ekelund, U., Evenson, K. R., Galuska, D. A., Jefferis, B. J., Kong, L., Kraus, W. E., Larson, M. G., Lee, I. M., Matthews, C. E., Newton, R. L., Jr., Nordström, A., . . . Steps for Health Collaborative. (2023). Prospective association of daily steps with cardiovascular disease: A harmonized meta-analysis. *Circulation*, *147*(2), 122–131. https://doi.org/10.1161/CIRCULATIONAHA.122.061288

Simental-Mendia, M., Sanchez-Garcia, A., Vilchez-Cavazos, F., Acosta-Olivo, C. A., Pena-Martinez, V. M., & Simental-Mendia, L. E. (2018). Effect of glucosamine and chondroitin sulfate in symptomatic knee osteoarthritis: A systematic review and meta-analysis of randomized placebo-controlled trials. *Rheumatology International*, *38*(8), 1413–1428. https://doi.org/10.1007/s00296-018-4077-2

Van Dyke, M. E., Chen, T. J., Nakayama, J. Y., Moore, L. V., & Whitfield, G. P. (2023). Changes in physical inactivity among US adults overall and by sociodemographic characteristics, behavioral risk factor surveillance system, 2020 versus 2018. *Preventing Chronic Disease*, *20*, E65. https://doi.org/10.5888/pcd20.230012

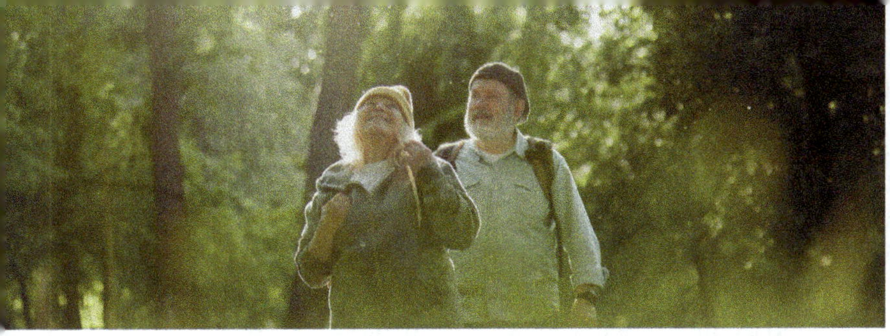

5

NUTRITION, WEIGHT MANAGEMENT, AND AGING

KEY TERMS

10 tips for weight loss and maintenance
age recommended dietary allowances
bariatric surgery
body composition
body mass index
calorie restriction
coffee
competitive eating
diet drugs
diets
fats: monounsaturated, polyunsaturated omega-3 and omega-6, saturated, and trans fat
Food Guide Pyramid versus nutrition bull's-eye
genetics versus lifestyle versus environment
malnutrition
Mediterranean and DASH diets
National Weight Control Registry
nutrients versus nutritionism
nutrients: carbohydrates, fiber, sugars, proteins, water, vitamins, and minerals
nutrition labels and food rating system
nutritional advocacy
organic foods
overweight and obesity
sensory decline
set-point theory
sodium
waist-to-hip ratio
weight-loss counseling

LEARNING OBJECTIVES

- Evaluate the *food guide pyramids*, MyPlate, and the *nutrition bull's-eye.*
- Contrast *nutrients* and *nutritionism.*
- Distinguish among fats, and examine the role of fat in the diet.
- Analyze the Mediterranean diet and its effectiveness.
- Contrast complex and simple *carbohydrates.*
- Explain the importance of *fiber* in the diet.
- Analyze the consequences of added *sugar* in food and drink.
- Explain why socioeconomic status relates to obesity.
- Examine the role of *protein* in the diet.
- Explain the importance of *hydration* in older adults.
- Identify the *vitamins and minerals* that have age-based recommendations.
- Identify the clinical manifestations of nutritional deficiencies.
- Analyze the influence of *sodium* on the blood pressure of older adults.
- Evaluate *nutrition labels and food rating systems.*
- Identify the risk factors for *malnutrition.*
- Identify the relevance for baby boomers of *organic* food consumption.
- Identify nutritional consequences of *sensory decline* with aging.
- Review the advocacy accomplishments of the Center for Science in the Public Interest.
- Analyze weight-gain trends in America over the past half century.
- Examine weight gain over the individual life cycle.
- Calculate *body mass index* and *waist-to-hip ratio.*
- Examine the relationship between *overweight and obesity,* and morbidity and mortality.
- Differentiate the contributions of *genetics, lifestyle, and environment* toward weight gain.
- Identify environmental changes in response to obesity in America.
- Critically evaluate whether we should gain weight with age.
- Identify measures of *body composition,* and the influence of sex and aging.
- Compare the effectiveness of weight-loss programs.
- Describe *bariatric surgery,* its coverage by Medicare, and outcomes of surgery.
- Summarize Medicare coverage for *weight-loss counseling.*
- Identify and describe *10 tips for weight loss and maintenance.*
- Analyze the effectiveness of *diet drugs.*
- Discuss *competitive eating* and its significance, if any.

Healthy eating is a cause that is extremely close to my heart.

—*Marcus Samuelsson*

A dietitian was making a presentation to a group of older adults at a senior citizens center. She began her talk by asking, "Over the long term, what is the single worst food that you can eat?" Immediately, a feisty older woman in the audience stood up and declared, "Wedding cake!" She probably was not referring to the *calories*.

Older adults may have a sense of humor about their eating habits, but they most definitely take the topic seriously as well. Studies report that older people are more conscientious about managing their ***diets*** than the middle aged. About two thirds of those over age 65 versus one half of those in their 40s report "trying a lot" to limit sodium, fat, and sugar; eat enough fiber; and consume sufficient vitamins and minerals.

If older adults are paying more attention to their nutritional habits, one can only speculate that they may be motivated by more immediate feedback (heartburn, constipation, etc.) or feelings of greater vulnerability (higher risk of impairment from disease and loss of independence). The emerging cohort of older adults—the baby boomers—bring more than motivation to the table. They also bring a higher level of formal education, including a strong interest in health education.

Advertisers took notice of the aging boomers several years ago when a series of clever television commercials targeted the Kellogg's Frosted Flakes that boomers used to eat when they were kids. Sales of this product increased appreciably as boomers decided their love of this sugary cereal trumped their skepticism about the statement on the cereal, proclaiming: "This product meets the American Heart Association's (AHA) food criteria for healthy people over age 2 when used as part of a balanced diet."

Apparently, the boomers and the AHA were not paying attention to the high sugar content on the nutritional label. Mysteriously, the criteria for the AHA's stamp of approval only included limits on fat, cholesterol, and sodium content. The AHA did have one more criterion: the willingness of the food manufacturer to pay for that stamp of approval—$7,500 per product the first year, and $4,500 annually thereafter. Many healthy products made by small manufacturers did not get this stamp because their manufacturers were unwilling to pay the fee.

Middle-aged boomers and older adults are influenced by earlier eating habits and clever advertising, but they do not typically ignore the nutritional content of what they eat. They can be manipulated, though, by the food industry's strategy of isolating nutrients such as fiber, fat, sugar, carbohydrates, and then declaring their importance—either their presence or absence—for preventing cancer, heart disease, stroke, cognitive decline, and so forth. This narrow-minded "nutritionism" is examined later.

The frequent nutritional controversies can be confusing and sometimes amusing, but they should not detract from the sensible and simple advice that guides most educated adults. *The best recipe for healthy nutrition is moderation and balance, including ample fiber in the diet and avoiding excessive fat, sugar, sodium, and calories.* This sentence could serve as the summary sentence for this chapter, but it raises questions: What's excessive when it comes to fat, and what kinds of fat are we talking about? What are the exceptions to this sensible advice? How are the nutritional needs of older adults different from younger adults?

THE FOOD GUIDE PYRAMID AND VARIATIONS

Let us begin with a little politics, because science does not always prevail in the world of nutrition. After years of study, the government finally replaced the long-standing circle that depicted the four food groups in 1991. This was not merely a question of aesthetics; the equally divided circle implied that the four food groups—bread/cereal, vegetable/fruit, milk, and meat—were equal in value, without other considerations.

The ***Food Guide Pyramid,*** however, better portrayed the desirable balance of foods we needed to eat—greater space for complex carbohydrates, fruits, and vegetables on the bottom of the pyramid (and in our diet), and less space for fat and protein at the top. At the narrow apex were the sinful ***fats,*** oils, and sweets (Figure 5.1).

In 1991, after briefly implementing the pyramid, the U.S. Department of Agriculture (USDA) quickly dropped it and returned to the circle format. Many accused the agency of caving in to the dairy and meat industries. Supporters of the retraction denied the political pressure, though not very convincingly (Nestle, 2002). They claimed the pyramid concept

FIGURE 5.1 Food guide pyramid.

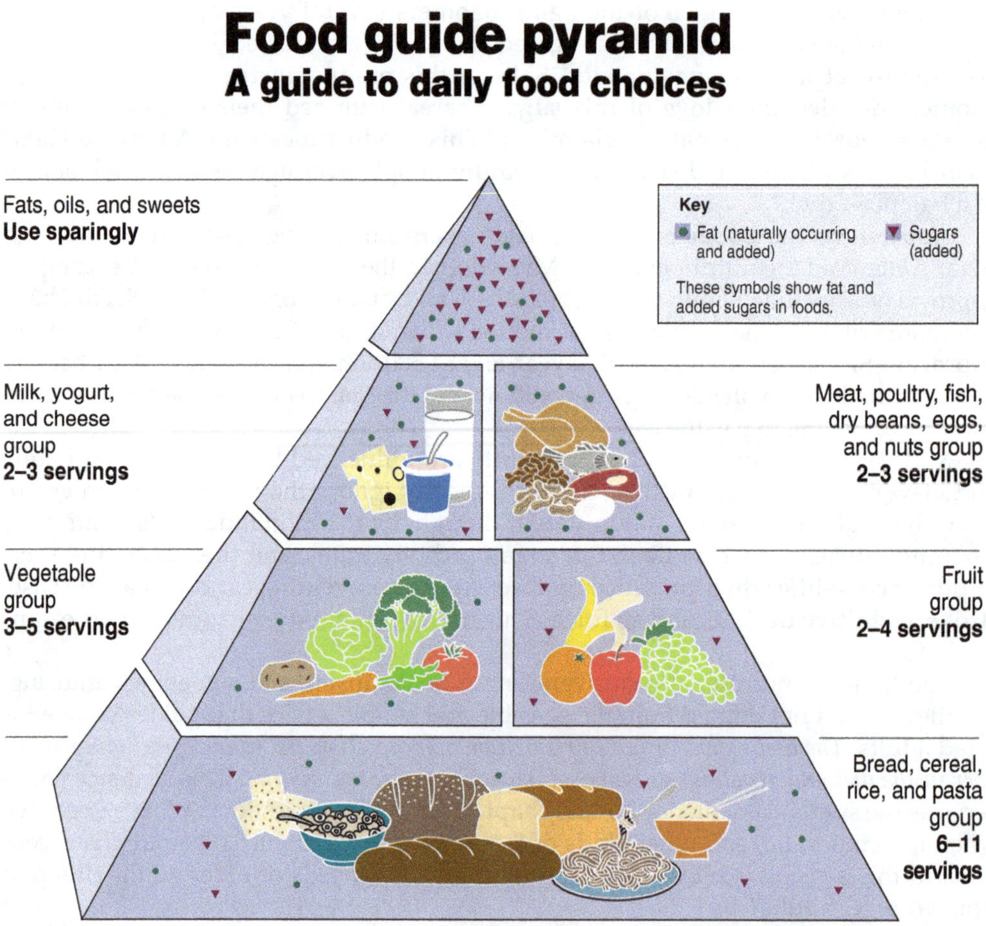

Source: U.S. Department of Agriculture. Retrieved from https://health.gov/sites/default/files/2020-01/DGA2000.pdf.

overlooked the recent surge of low-fat dairy products and leaner meats that made these foods more acceptable. Also, because we still have to worry about anemia, malnutrition, and calcium deficiency, the claim was made that we should not cut back on milk and meat.

One year later in 1992, the pyramid concept overcame the dairy and meat industry lobbyists and became the accepted illustration of good nutrition. Registered dietitians and nutritionists could point to it and recommend more daily selections from the bread and cereal group (6–11 servings) and the vegetable and fruit group (5–9), and fewer daily selections from the milk (2–4) and meat (2–3) groups than they previously did.

Most Americans, however, fell short of achieving the recommended number of servings in the important bottom parts of the pyramid, particularly whole grains, vegetables, and fruit. Even worse, as far as the pyramid goes, it was widely ignored by students in the classroom; grocery shoppers, despite the pyramid portrayed on their shopping bags; and older adults in general, who were not particularly interested.

Modified Food Guide Pyramids

Lack of interest was one huge problem, but lack of accuracy and utility was even worse. The carbohydrates at the base of the pyramid did not differentiate between complex and refined food products; the protein categories did not differentiate between products that had high ***saturated*** fat content such as red meat, and healthy products like fatty fish, beans, and nuts; and the fat category at the top of the pyramid did not differentiate among monounsaturated, polyunsaturated, saturated, and partially hydrogenated fats.

Thus, some carbohydrates, proteins, and fats should have shifted either upward or downward in the pyramid, depending on recommended amounts to be consumed.

Another line of criticism had to do with not targeting the Food Guide Pyramid to different age groups, particularly to older adults who had either not been identified as a separate category or had been lumped into an overly broad 50+ category by nutritionists. Did older adults have different needs regarding hydration, vitamins and minerals, and caloric intake?

As a consequence, modified pyramids began to be developed, such as the *Modified Food Pyramid for Mature (70+) Adults* (Russell et al., 1999) and the *New Healthy Eating Pyramid* (Willett, 2008). More recently, the U.S. Department of Agriculture has developed *MyPlate*, which is based on the *Dietary Guidelines for Americans, 2020 to 2025* (myplate.gov), which replaces the pyramid entirely.

The federal government's 2005 Dietary Guidelines for Americans, redrafted every 5 years by the USDA and the Department of Health and Human Services (DHHS), produced not only a 70-page blueprint for nutritional policy but also a revised Food Guide Pyramid, dubbed MyPyramid (www.foodpyramid.com/mypyramid). The Food Guide Pyramid had not been updated for quite some time, and the website was a new initiative. The entire update had been billed as an interactive food guidance system rather than a one-size-fits-all initiative.

The MyPyramid update engendered a whole host of positive and negative reactions. On the bright side, the content of the dietary guidelines appeared to reflect more of the thinking of the scientific community than in the past, and the USDA which represented the food industry and its lobbyists appeared to have had less influence than in years past. The guidelines basically encouraged Americans once again to eat fruits, vegetables, whole grains, and low-fat or fat-free dairy products, but there was much more detail on the consumption of these foods than was provided by previous guidelines.

Fruit and vegetable serving recommendations were increased; salt guidelines were made specific for the first time, limiting it to 1 level teaspoon a day; trans fat was identified, and the advice was to keep it as low as possible; saturated fat limitations were specific, keeping it to 10% of calories or less; cholesterol level was to be less than 300 mg; added sugars or sweeteners were discouraged for the first time, particularly in drinks; whole grains were differentiated from the broad category of carbohydrates; and the recommendation was that half the grains should be whole grains.

The old pyramid used ambiguous serving sizes, whereas the new one switched to cups, ounces, and other (allegedly) easier-to-grasp household measures. The old pyramid ignored exercise, whereas the new one advised one-half hour a day. As school lunches and programs that provided meals to seniors had to follow the guidelines, these constituencies would receive more whole grains, fruits, and vegetables, and less salty foods and sugary drinks.

Finally, on the good side of the ledger, the website lets people assess their diet and exercise habits. Depending on a person's age, gender, and activity level, the new pyramid comes in 12 versions. The user will get specific dietary recommendations on grain, vegetable, fruit, milk, meat/beans, total fat, saturated fat, cholesterol, sodium, oils, and fats/sugars. Type and duration of each physical activity are assessed as well, with specific recommendations. The website is interesting and informative.

Now for the dark side. There was no budget for mass media or other educational initiatives, so the new icon was ignored as much as the old one (though perhaps a huge media budget would not have mattered much). Also, while the website is very good, only the most motivated and educated—those least likely to need guidance—are likely to access it. Finally, the new pyramid symbol was confusing, with six colorful vertical stripes of differing widths, a stair-climbing stick figure, and no text attached to it.

> **QUESTION:** Review the website, www.foodpyramid.com/mypyramid. What did you learn from it?

Perhaps any effort is doomed to failure because much of the salt, fat, and sugar in processed and prepared foods do not penetrate the consciousness of the consumer (or only briefly, before purchase), and the food and drink industry spends billions of dollars in advertisements to promote these products.

MyPlate

After two decades of various USDA food pyramid diagrams, on June 2, 2011, the "plate" took over. The MyPlate icon (see www.choosemyplate.gov) depicted a place setting with a plate divided into four food groups unequally divided (Figure 5.2). The plate was approximately 30% grains, 30% vegetables, 20% fruits, and 20% protein. This was accompanied by a smaller circle representing dairy, preferably low fat. The associated slogans that are easy to visualize and remember: "Make half your plate fruits and vegetables." "Make at least half your grains whole."

The Personalized Nutrition Bull's-Eye

The nutritionist Covert Bailey created an icon called the ***nutrition bull's-eye*** (Bailey, 1996). The goal of the bull's-eye is for people to consume the nutritious foods that are listed in the center of it. These foods are low in saturated fat, sugar, and sodium,

FIGURE 5.2 MyPlate.

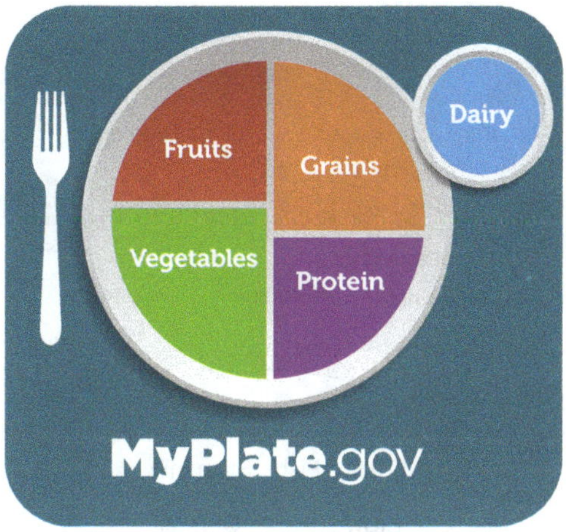

Source: U.S. Department of Agriculture. Retrieved from https://www.myplate.gov/.

and high in fiber. They include skim milk, nonfat yogurt, most fruits and vegetables, whole grains, beans and legumes, and water-packed tuna.

As you progress farther away from the center of the bull's-eye, less nutritionally desirable foods are listed (more saturated fat, sugar, sodium, and low-fiber foods). In the outermost ring of the bull's-eye, therefore, are the least desirable—cheeses, ice cream, butter, whole milk, beef, cake, cookies, potato chips, and mayonnaise.

Unlike the Food Guide Pyramid, Bailey's bull's-eye makes important distinctions *within* food categories. Whole-wheat products, for instance, are in the middle circle of the bull's-eye, whereas products from refined white flour or with added sugar are placed in the outer circles. Fresh fruits and vegetables are in the bull's-eye, but juiced vegetables and fruit with low fiber and concentrated sugars are placed in a ring just outside the bull's-eye. Skim and low-fat milk, nonfat cottage cheese, and part-skim mozzarella are in the center ring, whereas whole milk and most cheeses are in the outer circles of the target.

In a one-to-one setting focusing on the specific foods and drinks that a person consumes, this technique is easy to understand and practical as well, when older adults are encouraged to bring a list of bull's-eye foods with them to the supermarket.

Patients can create a personalized version of the bull's-eye: Have the patient Begin with blank concentric circles, and then add food and drink products usually consumed to each of the rings. The foods and drinks in the bull's-eye (Figure 5.3) are clearly superior; the second ring is not quite as nutrient dense or are neutral products that are not particularly harmful or helpful; and the outer ring includes the least nutritious foods and drinks that should be consumed sparingly.

QUESTION: Create your own nutrition bull's-eye, filling in the foods and drinks that you consume or might consider consuming. Use it for a week to guide your eating choices. Take a list of the food products listed in the center of your bull's-eye to the supermarket with you. Did you find this technique to be helpful?

FIGURE 5.3 The personalized nutrition bull's-eye.

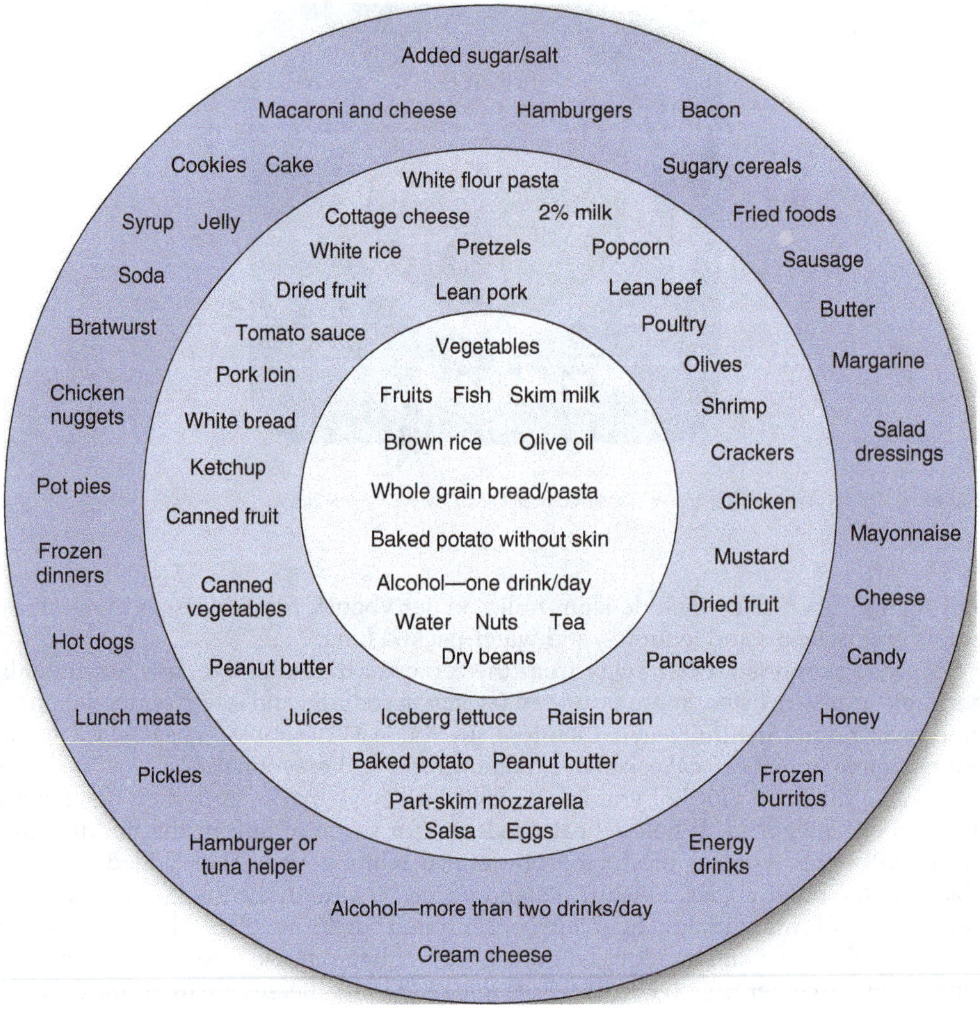

GOOD NUTRITIONAL HABITS

The principles of moderation, selectivity, variety, and balance are widely believed to be the key to healthy eating. Reduce portion sizes; consume less sugar, saturated fats, and salt; and consume more fiber, including a balance of vegetables, fruits, and whole-grain breads and cereals. *Interestingly, these recommendations are not too different from what the USDA first proposed by way of dietary recommendations more than a century ago in 1917* (Nestle, 2002)!

Although educated Americans believe good nutrition is based on these principles, they find them easier to endorse than to practice. Americans rightly believe that diet is only one component in the development and exacerbation of disease—heredity, environment, medical care, social circumstances, and other lifestyle risk factors also play a part.

Yet ignoring good eating and drinking habits also ignores that fact that nutrition has been implicated in five of the leading causes of death—heart disease, cancer, stroke, diabetes, and liver disease—as well as in several debilitating disorders, such as osteoporosis and diverticulosis.

Basic Nutrients

Nutrients are substances in food that build and maintain body tissues and are necessary for bodily function. Nutrition education helps us learn how to provide our bodies with the more than 40 nutrients they need. Good dietary habits help us feel energetic and avoid obesity and other health problems, whereas poor nutrition contributes to feelings of fatigue and weakness and to health problems.

The basic categories of nutrients are carbohydrates, fats, proteins, fiber, water, vitamins, and minerals. Carbohydrates—sugars (simple carbohydrates) and starches (complex carbohydrates)—are our main source of energy. Fats provide a reserve of energy. Proteins are needed for the growth and repair of tissues. Fiber aids in the regulation of bowel function. Water—the main ingredient in the body—provides the proper environment for the body's processes, which vitamins and minerals help to control and regulate. Large quantities of fats, carbohydrates, protein, fiber, and water, and small quantities of vitamins and minerals are needed by the body.

Nutrients Versus Nutritionalism

Almost everything written to this point has been long-standing mainstream nutritional thinking. But another approach to good nutrition was captured in Michael Pollan's book (2008), *In Defense of Food*. Pollan's idea can be summarized into one caution: We have been seduced by ***nutritionism***, the belief that what matters most is not the food but the nutrient.

This nutritional reductionism began several decades ago when members of Congress criticized certain foods, such as meat and whole milk, and the food manufacturers, through large political donations, made sure that these congresspersons were not reelected. Nutrients, however, were allowed to be criticized by these and other government representatives with impunity, just as long as specific foods were not identified. The industry was more agreeable with allowing the consumer to be cautioned about eating less desirable nutrients, such as fats and simple carbohydrates in moderation.

Pollan's advice? Let's get back to talking about food and less about nutrients, and in particular let us differentiate between whole fresh foods and processed food products. The former consist primarily of fruits and vegetables, which are even better if they are homegrown or from a nearby farmer's market. The latter have ingredients that are unfamiliar and unpronounceable, and these edible *food-like products* have taken over the supermarket, often proudly proclaiming some aspect of nutritionism: This product is "low in fat," "high in antioxidants," or "low in carbs."

Instead, Pollan's "Eater's Manifesto" is stated in the first line of his book: *Eat food. Not too much. Mostly plants.*

FAT

Since the early 1990s, fat supplanted cholesterol as our greatest dietary concern. And today? Surprisingly, neither one is considered a primary concern by the cutting-edge research community.

In 2015, the Dietary Guidelines Advisory Committee no longer deemed *dietary cholesterol* a nutrient of concern. The expert panel concluded that dietary cholesterol does not significantly impact cholesterol blood levels or increase the risk of heart disease in healthy adults. Thus, the long-standing recommendation of consuming less than 300 mg/day of dietary cholesterol (about the amount in one egg) was replaced by no limits.

And fat in the diet? Well, it too is no longer a major concern by some research experts in the field of nutrition. Remember that fat is an essential part of our diet and a major source of energy. It is the most concentrated energy source, with each gram of fat supplying nine calories to the body.

But when nutritionism came along, fat in general got painted with a broad brush of negativity: "We eat too much and we need to reduce it." But it is not that simple. What foods are the fats in? If fish or nuts, there is no concern other than the calories being consumed. And what kind of fat are we talking about? On a goodness/badness scale, it ranges from monounsaturated fat to trans fat. And except for trans fat and saturated fat, every other fat has a major beneficial component to it. And even the reduction of saturated fat in our diet has its detractors. For a couple of decades, research has reported that reducing saturated fat in our diet is typically replaced by refined carbohydrates. This does not lower our weight or improve our health, and some researchers suggest it probably makes things worse (Bazzano et al., 2014).

The low-fat-diet trial of the Women's Health Initiative (Howard et al., 2006) was a landmark study that raised the emerging questions involving fat into widespread doubt in the research field. This study involved a sample of 49,000 women over an 8-year period. Women joined one of two groups: (a) those who reduced their fat intake to 20% of daily calories, increased their vegetable and fruit intake to five servings per day, and increased their intake of grains to six servings per day; or (b) those who continued to eat their normal diet. The results were consistent: Reducing fat in your diet did not lower your weight or make you healthier in terms of heart disease or cancer.

The size of the study and the resources that went into it were impressive, though the results, as is the case with all research, were not without flaws. The low-fat diet proved to be difficult for the average woman to follow. The women in the experimental group, despite ongoing support from nutritional counseling, were unable to reach the dietary goal of 20% of calories from fat (though they lowered the fat content considerably). As the study progressed, their fat intake rose, though it never reached baseline. And, finally, the study did not differentiate among fats. The AHA, however, still cautions against "intakes of cholesterol that exceed current average levels" because of their association "with elevated total or low-density lipoprotein cholesterol concentrations." The AHA recommends diets low in cholesterol compared to current U.S. intake, such as the ***Mediterranean*** diet and the ***DASH*** (Dietary Approaches to Stop Hypertension) diet (Carson et al., 2020).

But the study got people thinking: Is fat the culprit for heart disease and other health problems? Only for one type of fat can we definitively say yes.

Trans Fat

Trans fat (also referred to as partially hydrogenated fat or trans fatty acid) naturally occurs in small amounts in some meat and dairy products. But most of it is formed through an industrial process that adds hydrogen to vegetable oil. This hydrogenation process causes the oil to become artificially solid at room temperature and extends the shelf life of many food products considerably, such as crackers, cookies, pastries, deep-fried products, candy, cakes, and frozen dinners.

The only way to have determined whether this kind of fat was in a food product prior to 2006—when trans fat was finally required to be on the food label—was through a chemist in a laboratory. Yet as far back as 1993, advocacy agencies called for the Food and Drug Administration (FDA) to expose trans fat and add it to the nutrition label. Why was this important? Epidemiological studies have consistently shown that it increases the risk of heart disease and diabetes.

Thirteen years after the Center for Science in the Public Interest (CSPI) petitioned the FDA to require trans fat on nutrition labels, the FDA finally required it. Just before trans fat had to be listed on the food label, many food manufacturers chose to eliminate it from their products. There was an estimated 78% decline in consumption of trans fat from 2005 to 2012, but still it persisted in a variety of products. Finally, in 2015, a ban on trans fat in restaurants and grocery stores was announced and implemented by the FDA on June 18, 2018.

This ban did not affect the Indiana State Fair, which had already banned the sale of products with trans fats in the summer of 2007. Ever health conscious, this state fair found required a trans fat–free frying oil for the battered and deep-fried Snickers bar, Oreo cookie, and Reese's Peanut Butter Cup. Outside the booths that were selling these concoctions were proudly posted signs: Trans-fat free!

The Mediterranean Diet

The first academic article on what would become the ***Mediterranean diet*** was published in 1953 by a social scientist named Leland Allbaugh. His initial positive findings derived from the eating habits and health outcomes of the residents of the isolated Greek island of Crete have stood fast over the decades. This diet started to become popular in America more than 40 years later, in 1997, as we discovered that the countries along the Mediterranean Sea had low rates of coronary heart disease and many common cancers found in the Western world. This near-vegetarian diet was high in unrefined grains, potatoes, fruit, vegetables, fish, wine, and olive oil, and low in meat, cheese, refined sugar or flour, butter, and margarine.

Although the Mediterranean diet is more expensive than most Western diets (Lopez et al., 2009), research reports that it reduces brain atrophy (Luciano et al., 2017) and delays cognitive decline (Rainey-Smith et al., 2018). It also reduces risk of cardiovascular disease (Estruch et al., 2013) and stroke (Sherzai et al., 2012) and overall mortality (Levitan et al., 2013). Moreover, these diets do not place limits on calories, which has long been a barrier to success with low-fat approaches (Estruch et al., 2013).

Another potential health benefit of the Mediterranean diet is its association with greater telomere length, a biomarker of aging. *Telomeres* are DNA sequences at the ends of chromosomes that progressively shorten with age, and are associated with age-related diseases and cancers. The fruits, vegetables, olive oil, and nuts of the Mediterranean diet have antioxidant and antiinflammatory effects that are associated with telomere length (Crous-Bou et al., 2014).

Ironically, as it has gained in popularity in the United States, the Mediterranean diet was in full retreat in Greece and other countries along the Mediterranean (Rosenthal, 2008). Two thirds of the children were overweight, and longevity was likely to be reduced in comparison with their parents. The increasing percentage of working mothers and the spread of supermarkets and highly processed convenience foods may have accounted for this change.

Surprisingly, the diet is not low in fat, with about 37% of calories coming from the diet (versus the 30% or lower recommended by the AHA)—primarily from olive oil, which consists mostly of ***monounsaturated*** fat. Thus, Americans began to extol the virtues of olive oil and other mostly monounsaturated and polyunsaturated fats like canola, safflower, and peanut oils.

The only other diet besides the Mediterranean diet that receives universal acclaim is the ***DASH diet*** (Dietary Approaches to Stop Hypertension). This eating pattern found its audience with the publication of a landmark study (Appel et al., 1997) that reported it lowered high blood pressure. Neither the DASH nor the Mediterranean diet is primarily for weight loss. The differences between the DASH and the Mediterranean diets, however, are minor. As you might suspect with hypertension, the DASH diet emphasizes sodium reduction, and the Mediterranean diet is more liberal with the percentage of fat allowed—in fact, fat is recommended—as most of it is not saturated, but the type found in healthy oils, nuts, fatty fish, and avocado. A Chinese variant, the Jiangnan diet, is growing in popularity (Wang et al., 2020).

Not All Fats Are Created Equal

All fats are a mixture of *saturated fats*, which are solid at room temperature, and *monounsaturated and polyunsaturated fats*, which are liquid at room temperature. What makes a fat healthy is the proportion of good fats contained within. Most nutritionists rank monounsaturated fat as the healthiest fat, followed by ***polyunsaturated omega-3***, then ***polyunsaturated omega-6***, with saturated fats and trans fatty acid bringing up the rear. The good fats lower unhealthy low-density lipoprotein (LDL) levels, while the less desirable fats do the reverse and may clog arteries or increase inflammation.

The healthy sources of fat include fish oils that come from fatty fish—salmon, sardines, cod, and so forth—and oils that come from seeds, nuts, and fruits—flaxseeds, cashews, walnuts, peanuts, olives, avocados, and so forth. There are a variety of other foods that contain a small amount of healthy fats, including such unexpected sources as green leafy vegetables and tofu.

The unhealthy sources of fat come mainly from snack foods and fast foods, which are processed foods that often contain unhealthy amounts of sugar or salt as well. The cooking oils to avoid are palm oil and coconut oil and the ones to consume are olive oil and canola oil. Saturated fats, solid at room temperature, are not desirable, and are found in high amounts in butter, cheese, and red meats. Coconut oil may be less harmful than once thought (Teng et al., 2020).

Saturated fats in particular have been singled out through controversies. How bad are they? And what is an acceptable level? They are a negative factor in the diet in that they raise the LDL level. However, many experts also argue that a focus on reducing saturated fat in the diet is often counterproductive, because most people replace it with refined carbohydrates, which may be more unhealthy, and we don't know the acceptable level for saturated fat in the diet, which is complicated by the fact that there are different kinds of saturated fats and some are less healthy (butter) than others (dark chocolate).

In short, teasing out the effects of a particular fat is difficult, and what the Mediterranean diet has taught us is the same message that Michael Pollan succinctly summarized: Shift the focus from a particular nutrient like fat, to thinking about eating real foods: fruits, vegetables, whole grains, fish, legumes, and lean meat. (Pollan is wary about meat, though, particularly given how animals are raised.)

Thus, the 1977 guidelines from the U.S. Select Committee on Nutrition and Human Needs accepted as gospel for about 40 years—limit overall fat intake to less than 30% of daily calories and saturated fat to less than 10% of daily energy intake—is now challenged by researchers (Chowdhury et al., 2014; Harcombe et al., 2015; Lawrence, 2013).

As stated by two respected experts in the field, these limits on fat consumption are "an outdated concept, an obstacle to sensible change that promotes harmful low-fat foods, undermines efforts to limit refined grains and added sugars, and discourages the food industry from developing products higher in healthy fats" (Mozzafarian & Ludwig, 2015, p. 8).

COMPLEX CARBOHYDRATES AND FIBER

Carbohydrates are complex (starches) or simple (sugars) and involve fiber (indigestible plant matter). Complex carbohydrates are most commonly found in breads, dry beans, potatoes, grains, pasta, carrots, peas, and corn. Many older adults have subscribed for years to the myth that all carbohydrates, especially bread and pasta, are fattening. In fact, when carbohydrates are whole grain, they are moderate in calories and rich in fiber and nutrients.

Grains are the seed-bearing fruits of edible grasses. Each kernel of grain has a nutritionally dense "germ" or seed at its core and a layer of bran that surrounds the kernel itself. When grains are refined into white flour, white rice, and so forth, a process that began in the 1940s, the bran and germ of the whole-wheat kernel are removed through the milling process, losing fiber, vitamins, and minerals, but not fat content.

The term *whole grain* means that the kernels are unrefined, still containing the germ and the protective bran coating. The germ provides fiber, B vitamins, and vitamin E; the bran contains fiber. The most familiar whole grains are wheat, barley, oats, rye, rice, and corn. When whole grains are a regular part of the diet, the risk for a variety of disease and mortality declines.

A meta-analysis of 14 prospective studies with 786,000 participants reported that those who ate the most whole grains had a 16% reduction in all-cause mortality and an 18% reduction in cardiovascular mortality, compared with those who ate the least amount of whole grains (Zong et al., 2016). Other studies report that the consumption of whole grains is associated with significant reductions in late-onset diabetes, several cancers, respiratory diseases, and infectious diseases.

However, when grains are refined and ingested exclusively in the form of mashed potatoes, white rice, and other processed foods that have little of their fiber left, the starch converts quickly to sugar. Thus, it is important to pay attention to the nutritional bull's-eye, mentioned earlier. Just as all fats are not created equal, the same holds true for carbohydrates and other nutrients, which can be situated in the middle of the bull's-eye or in an outer ring.

Vegetables and fruits are complex carbohydrates that are low in fat and high in fiber, vitamins, and minerals. The exceptions regarding fat are items like olives and avocados, which are considered by nutritionists to be healthy, versus salads doused with added high-fat dressing and vegetables that are fried or seasoned with margarine or butter, which are not considered to be healthy. Unfortunately, the most popular vegetable is the fried potato, that is, French fries. Not counting the dubious and ubiquitous French fry, Americans of all ages tend to eat less than half of the recommended amount of fruits and vegetables. A diet rich in fruits and vegetables protects against cardiovascular disease, cancers, and other morbidities.

Fiber is the indigestible residue of food (e.g., the husk, seeds, skin, stems, cell walls) that passes through the bowel and is eliminated in the stool. It appears to have a positive effect on cholesterol reduction, though scientists do not know exactly how this works. A diet that is high in fiber is especially important in later years, when constipation is likely to be a problem. Fiber is a natural laxative that promotes regularity, adds bulk to stool, absorbs water, and reduces the amount of time that stool is in the bowels.

Among persons age 65+, a diet high in fiber will lower the risk of cardiovascular disease. However, only about 5% of American adults follow the National Cancer Institute's recommendation to eat at least 20 grams of fiber a day. Moreover, some Americans are eating *fake fiber*, which are processed fibers extracted from plants or made in a laboratory. These types of fibers may not have all of the benefits of intact fibers, such as curbing food intake, improving regularity, or lowering cholesterol or blood sugar levels (Liebman, 2018).

Fiber supplements like Metamucil do not contain the essential nutrients found in high-fiber foods, and their nutritional benefits are questionable. Some older adults rely on laxatives that are costly and, in the long run, self-defeating because they create a "lazy bowel." Although laxatives and supplements are not effective complements to fiber, fluid intake is. In fact, fiber needs fluid to be effective, and about 64 ounces of water daily is recommended.

SUGAR

Sugars (also referred to as fructose, glucose, dextrose, maltose, lactose, honey, syrup, molasses, etc.) are carbohydrates. Some are naturally present in nutritious foods, such as fruit and milk, but a good many are added to foods. Added sugar provides calories that have no nutritional value (i.e., "empty calories") while increasing the likelihood of dental caries, excess weight, and diseases. Natural sugar in fruit, vegetables, and dairy products differs from added sugar in that it is accompanied by vitamins, minerals, and fiber.

The nonprofit Environmental Working Group examined 80,000 items sold in grocery stores across the nation, and 60% of the products contained added sugars. The figure increases to 75% when examining packaged foods purchased in the United States. Americans consume, on average, between a quarter pound and a half pound of sugar a day (DiNicolantonio et al., 2014). It is so addictive that if given the choice, rats will choose sugar over cocaine in laboratory settings.

Much of the sugar we ingest is hidden: Almost one third of Heinz tomato ketchup and Wish-Bone Russian salad dressing is sugar. Sugar also makes up two thirds of Coffee-Mate nondairy creamer; one half of Shake 'n Bake; and a high percentage of processed soups, spaghetti sauces, frozen dinners, yogurts, and breads.

The American population consumes more than double the recommended amount of sugar, and the amount of sugar consumed by the public has steadily increased over the past 25 years. The movement toward low-fat foods worsened the trend, as many of the products used sweeteners to make up for the lost fat flavor. Many low-fat foods, therefore, resulted in only a small caloric reduction—or no caloric reduction—from their full-fat counterparts.

The CSPI petitioned the FDA to change nutrition labels so that sugar can also be included in the percentage of the daily value it represents. At the present time, however, it is listed in grams (not helpful to most consumers) as a subset of carbohydrates (also not helpful), and exempted from the percentage-of-daily-value category (particularly unhelpful). The FDA approved a revised food label that includes sugars in the nutrition facts label (https://www.fda.gov/food/nutrition-facts-label/added-sugars-nutrition-facts-label). It states, for example, that "this product has 15 g of total sugar, or 30% of daily-value; and has 10 g of added sugar, or 40% of daily-value."

A nutritionally sound diet overall should probably derive no more than 10% of its calories from added sugar, a percentage that is almost half of what is consumed by the average American. https://www.fda.gov/food/nutrition-facts-label/added-sugars-nutrition-facts-label).

Nutrition advocates strongly urge that food and drinks with added sugar be taxed (penny per teaspoon, as proposed in the 2015 SWEET Act that was not enacted by

Congress) to offset the increased medical costs associated with high-sugar diets. Other suggestions are to remove sugar-sweetened beverages (i.e., liquid candy) from schools and hospitals, regulate sugar-added products as we do with alcohol and tobacco, place restrictions on advertising of sugary products, or require warning labels on high sugar-added products.

PROTEIN

Proteins are organic molecules that form antibodies, which help the body resist disease and enable the growth and repair of body cells: organs, muscles, skin, bones, blood, and hair. Amino acids, the units from which proteins are constructed, are the end products of protein digestion. Complete protein foods contain, in proper amounts for adults, eight essential amino acids that must be available for the body to properly synthesize protein. Fish, dairy products, and eggs—complete protein foods—contain all the essential amino acids.

Proteins obtained from vegetables are low in some of the essential amino acids. Previously, it was believed that complete, or complementing, protein needed to be present within a single vegetarian meal, but that theory has been discredited. Moreover, proteins obtained from vegetables may have the added benefit of decreasing bone loss and the risk of hip fracture more than proteins obtained from meat and cheese (Sellmeyer et al., 2001). The theory behind this research is that, unlike plant protein, animal protein produces an overflow of sulfuric acid into the bloodstream, and in order for the body to neutralize this excess, it must leech calcium from bones.

Protein should account for an estimated 12% to 20% of the total calories in the diet, and Americans tend to get at least that much. Older adults who are ill, however, are the most likely segment of society to experience protein deficiency. They suffer loss of appetite and often eat very little if any meat because of the cost, denture problems, lack of ability or desire to cook, or for ethical reasons. Protein deficiency in older adults can result in a lack of vigor or stamina, depression, poor resistance to infection, impaired healing of wounds, and slow recovery from disease (Box 5.1).

BOX 5.1 The Low Cost of Eating Poorly

We get five to nine times the amount of calories for the buck when we choose energy-dense (junk) foods rather than nutrient-dense foods (Monsivais & Drewnowski, 2007). Why is that? The $75-billion-a-year Farm Bill subsidizes crops like corn and soy, which are used for added sugar and fats in our food (Pollan, 2007), but not fruits and vegetables. Given the perverse incentives, farmers produce ever-increasing amounts of corn and soy, so the price of soda, for example (which has plenty of liquid corn syrup), stays low, but the cost of fresh produce continues to rise.

If you eat on a limited budget, the most rational *economic* strategy to get sufficient calories is to eat junk food. This helps explain why a much higher percentage of poor people are overweight or obese than those who are economically better off. And obesity among low-income Americans has been costly in terms of Medicaid expenditures and emergency department utilization.

Nonetheless, the Farm Bill does not generate a debate on health, just an economic debate—and this mostly occurs between congresspersons and lobbyists. These two groups value agribusiness profits over the quality of food accessible to all socioeconomic levels. Do you have any suggestions for correcting this?

WATER

Although we can get by without most nutrients for several *weeks* at a stretch, we cannot survive for more than several days without ***water***. Water is the medium in which all the reactions in cells take place. Water lubricates joints; transports nutrients and salts throughout the body; hydrates the skin; promotes adequate blood volume; moistens the mucosa in eyes, nose, and mouth; carries waste; and regulates body temperature. Nevertheless, older adults tend to drink only about three cups a day, less than what they need. This is due in part to *reduced thirst perception with age*.

Inadequate hydration can have many deleterious effects, beginning with constipation and fatigue and moving on to hypotension, hyperthermia, dizziness, breathing difficulties, and irregular heartbeats. Prolonged dehydration can lead to a variety of diseases. It is important, therefore, that older adults with inadequate fluid intake build up gradually to eight cups of fluids per day (including that which is found in food), regardless of thirst. Rising temperatures globally increase the risk of dehydration and make water intake even more important.

It should be noted, though, that researchers have been unable to find a single study that supports the need for the widely circulated recommendation to drink an *additional* eight glasses of water a day (Valtin, 2008). Much of the water we need exists in the food we eat, and the additional amount of water that any one person needs is not particularly challenging to achieve, with the exception of older adults and their declining thirst mechanism. For most Americans, "schlepping water bottles around all day long" is unnecessary for hydration (Negoianu & Goldfarb, 2008), though it is an excellent alternative to consuming snacks or sugary drinks.

Dehydration in the elderly is responsible for a substantial number of additional days of hospital care, at a significant cost to Medicare. The American Medical Association's (AMA) Council of Scientific Affairs recommended that undergraduate, graduate, and continuing education programs for nurses, allied health professionals, and physicians include the importance of hydration in older adults.

Water, juice, and milk meet hydration needs. More than 80% of many fruits and vegetables, about 50% of meat, and about one third of bread consists of water. Alcohol, caffeinated tea and coffee, and soft drinks raise the fluid level more modestly because of their diuretic effect. One study, however, reported that caffeinated drinks do not dehydrate the body more than noncaffeinated drinks (Grandjean et al., 2000).

Alcohol consumption is not effective for hydration purposes. For several years, though, research has supported the practice of moderate alcohol consumption of one to two drinks per day, which may lower cardiovascular risk (Mukamal et al., 2003), dementia risk (Ruitenberg et al., 2002), or the all-cause mortality rate (Lee et al., 2009). However, a much publicized study calls into question these prior research efforts. Light alcohol consumption, about one drink per day, may not offer any protective effects when it comes to disease. A slightly lower risk for heart disease is offset by a slightly higher risk for several cancers. Moderate alcohol consumption, two drinks per day, is associated with hippocampal atrophy and cognitive decline (Topiwala et al., 2017) and perhaps a slight increase in breast cancer risk (Rabin, 2018). The purported benefit of light-to-moderate alcohol consumption reported in research likely reflects a healthy survivor effect, in that people suffering negative effects are less likely to participate in research and people in poorer health reduce alcohol consumption.

Should we discard the repeated prior research findings that reported one drink per day is protective against disease? A cautious approach would suggest that it is *not a good idea to start drinking* one drink per day in order to protect your health. Finally, one disturbing trend that has come to light is that some allegedly "unbiased" alcohol studies were supported by the liquor industry and not powered sufficiently to even detect negative health effects (Rabin, 2018).

VITAMINS AND MINERALS

Vitamins in the right amounts are needed for normal growth, digestion, mental alertness, and resistance to infection. The body also needs 15 ***minerals*** that help regulate cell function and provide structure for cells. The vitamins include A, C, D, E, and K and B (thiamin B_1, riboflavin B_2, niacin B_3, pantothenic acid B_5, pyridoxine B_6, cobalamin B_{12}, biotin, and folate/folic acid). Key minerals essential for health include calcium, phosphorus, potassium, sodium, chloride, magnesium, iron, zinc, iodine, sulfur, cobalt, copper, fluoride, manganese, and selenium (https://www.nccih.nih.gov/health/vitamins-and-minerals).

Since 1941, the Food and Nutrition Board of the National Academy of Sciences has published the *Recommended Dietary Allowances* (RDAs) for the majority of vitamins, minerals, and protein that we require and has updated these recommendations every few years based on research findings. The RDA is the average daily dietary intake level that is sufficient to meet the nutrient requirement of nearly all healthy individuals (97%–98%) in a particular life stage and sex category.

In 1998, *Dietary Reference Intakes* were developed that added additional guidelines, such as Tolerable Upper Intake Level (highest safe intake level) to warn against the potential for adverse effects. Although the surplus *water-soluble* vitamins (C and eight of the B vitamins) are excreted in urine, adverse effects can still result from exceeding the upper level recommendations. The surplus *fat-soluble* vitamins (A, D, E, and K) are stored in body tissue and excessive amounts can become toxic.

Age recommended dietary allowances (RDAs) have been difficult to establish, especially for older adults who have been broadly, and inadequately, defined for the past several decades as persons age 51 and over. Although we know that increasing age alters nutritional requirements, the Food and Nutrition Board had delayed for many years the establishment of separate categories for adults over 50 based on insufficient research data.

The insufficient data stemmed from such research problems as inadequate numbers of older adults in studies, higher nonresponse rates from older adults, and the confounding influence of greater sample mortality. In addition, vitamin, mineral, and protein requirements for older adults in particular are complicated by age diversity in physiological changes over time, living arrangements, transportation access, and disability (Wakimoto & Block, 2001).

As the research base has improved over the past decade, RDAs are being expanded into a broader range of categories (Table 5.1). The most important change regarding older adults has been to create a separate category for people age 50+ (vitamin B_6, calcium, iron) and to differentiate adults age 51 to 70 versus adults older than age 70 (vitamin D).

A meta-analysis of studies focused on nutrition and age reported that nutritional intake declines with age (Wakimoto & Block, 2001). This is not surprising, as energy output and muscle mass decline with age as well. Along with nutritional intake decline, though, potentially important declines in protein, zinc, calcium, folate, thiamine, riboflavin, and vitamins D, E, B_6, and B_{12} were observed (Table 5.2). This raises two questions that require further research: Which nutrient intakes should decline with age,

TABLE 5.1 AGE-RELATED RECOMMENDED DIETARY ALLOWANCES (RDA), 2020 TO 2025, BY THE NATIONAL ACADEMY OF SCIENCES

NUTRIENT	AGE GROUP	RDA	SOURCES
Vitamin B_6	Women 51+	1.3 mg	Meat, poultry, seafood, liver, and fortified foods
	Men 51+	1.7 mg	
Vitamin D	Ages 51–70	600 IU	Sunlight, fatty fish, and fortified foods
	Ages 70+	800 IU	
Calcium	Ages 51–70		Dairy, fortified foods, leafy green vegetables, canned fish
	Women	1,200 mg	
	Men	1,000 mg	
	Ages 70+		
	Women	1,200	
	Men	1,200	
Iron	Women 50+	8 mg	Red meat, poultry, seafood, whole-grain flour
	Men 50+	8 mg	

Source: https://www.dietaryguidelines.gov/sites/default/files/2020-12/Dietary_Guidelines_for_Americans_2020-2025.pdf.

TABLE 5.2 NUTRIENTS AND CLINICAL MANIFESTATION OF DEFICIENCY IN OLDER ADULTS

Protein	Inability to cope with metabolic stress like infection or broken bone
Zinc	Impaired immune function, delayed wound healing, lethargy
Calcium	Increased risk of fracture
Folate	Increased risk of stroke, anemia, appetite loss, fatigue
Vitamin B_1 (thiamine)	Compromised nervous system, weight loss, fatigue, decreased reflexes
Vitamin B_2 (riboflavin)	Problems with lips and tongue
Vitamin D	Bone pain, fatigue, gait disturbances
Vitamin E	Uncertain; perhaps reduction in antioxidant effect
Vitamin B_6	Nausea, dizziness, confusion, depression, fatigue
Vitamin B_{12}	Nausea, fatigue, depression, memory problems, anemia, neurological disease

given that energy output declines as well? Which should increase with age, given that absorption and utilization efficiency decrease with age?

On the positive side, fruit and vegetable consumption appears to increase with age, especially among older women, along with vitamin A, vitamin C, and potassium intake. Older persons—again, particularly women—are more likely to consume vitamin

TABLE 5.3 GOOD SOURCES OF NUTRITION FOR OLDER ADULTS

TO INCREASE SOURCE OF	EAT MORE
Protein, iron, vitamin B_3 (niacin), vitamin B_{12}	Meats
Calcium, vitamin B_2 (riboflavin), protein	Milk products
B vitamins	Breads and cereals
Vitamins C and A, potassium	Fruits and vegetables
Vitamin D	Fatty fish

supplements (Wakimoto & Block, 2001). To improve the intake of important nutrients, Table 5.3 identifies some of the best food group sources for older adults.

One mineral that is of particular nutritional importance—and potential danger—for the aging body is salt or sodium chloride. It is the sodium component that has important health consequences.

SODIUM

Sodium keeps muscles and nerves working properly and attracts water, thereby helping us retain the proper amount of body fluid. Too much sodium in the system, however, causes the body to retain excess water, increases the blood pressure level, and makes the heart work harder.

The current average sodium consumption in the United States is 3,400 mg/day, about 1.5 teaspoons of salt. The dietary guideline endorsed by both the American government and leading nutritionists is 2,300 mg/day, or 1 teaspoon daily. According to the National Health and Nutrition Examination Survey (NHANES), in 2009 to 2012 85% of adults age 51+ had excess sodium intake, and the mean sodium intake of adults age 19+ was 3,552 mg/day (Jackson et al., 2016).

There is disagreement whether at-risk groups, including adults age 50+ (and Blacks, diabetics, hypertensives, and those with congestive heart failure or chronic kidney disease), should aim for a lower target of 1,500 mg. This latter goal is strongly endorsed by the AHA, even though it is the rare American who can achieve this level (less than 1% of the population, according to the Centers for Disease Control and Prevention [CDC]).

Moreover, there are no studies to suggest that the lower target reduces heart disease, stroke, or all-cause mortality rate. The Institute of Medicine surveyed the existing research and released a report in 2013 that discouraged limiting most people to sodium levels below 2,000 mg (or recommending above 2,400 mg).

This goal is challenging enough. Processed and restaurant foods rely heavily on salt as a cheap way to enhance flavor and texture and preserve food. Many foods contain high levels of sodium, such as potato chips, processed meats, frozen dinners, processed lunch meat, ketchup, most sauces, and canned foods, but many more foods have a high level unbeknownst to the consumer—did you know most blueberry muffins have more than double the salt of a serving of potato chips?

If for some reason you insist on a high-sodium diet, may we recommend Applebee's quesadilla chicken salad, which contains 4,890 mg sodium per dish (https://www.applebees.com/en/nutrition/info). Until removed from the menu, Appelbee's lemon shrimp fettuccine offered 5,300 mg of sodium in a single entrée!

Most Americans rightly associate high sodium intake in the diet with high blood pressure, but there is an absence of research assessing what percentage of the population is salt sensitive and needs to be most concerned. A person can assess this informally by alternately restricting salt and then removing salt restrictions for specified periods of time, while assessing the impact on one's blood pressure levels. Of course, the likelihood of such mass monitoring is null.

Hollenberg (2006) of Harvard Medical School recognized that reduced salt intake could make a substantial contribution to reducing hypertension, particularly among older adults—sodium sensitivity tends to increase with age, among Blacks, and in people with obesity, diabetes, and hypertension. But he also believed it was premature to invoke mandatory reductions in salt content that affected all people because some might be harmed by this approach, such as people receiving aggressive treatment for congestive heart failure.

These compromised patients, though, are aware of their unique medical conditions and likely aware of their salt needs as well. The few shabby research studies that concluded sodium intake below 1,500 mg/day leads to sickness probably came to a "reverse causation" conclusion. More likely, sick people eat less and, therefore, consume low levels of sodium (Brody, 2017). Consequently, the AMA has stuck to its position of promoting salt reduction on a general basis and has advocated that American food makers and restaurants reduce salt content. Salt substitutes have proven to be more effective in blood pressure control than salt restriction (Yuan et al., 2023; Zhang et al., 2024).

In January 2010, New York City set voluntary guidelines recommending maximum amounts of salt for a variety of restaurant and store-bought foods, with the (unrealized) goal of reducing salt levels in food by an average of 25% over 5 years. Restaurants and food manufacturers were encouraged to lower salt content gradually so consumers would not notice.

This innovative project, called the *National Salt Reduction Initiative*, had attracted the endorsements of 25 other city and state health agencies; 17 national health organizations; and 28 national food companies, retailers, and supermarket chains. The suggested salt reductions in products ranged from a 20% drop in peanut butter to a 40% decline in canned vegetables.

Food industry representatives reacted cautiously, stating they would take this initiative under consideration. Consequently, the initiative was not successful. Nor were prior efforts by food manufacturers between 2005 and 2011, when volunteer initiatives only lowered sodium in processed foods 3.5% and in restaurants only 2.6% (Jacobson et al., 2013).

In contrast to the United States's voluntary effort, England implemented, through its Food Standards Agency, a government-coordinated salt reduction program. From 2001 to 2011, sodium consumption decreased 15%, accompanied by a substantial reduction in blood pressure, a 40% drop in death from heart attacks, and a 42% decline in deaths from strokes (He et al., 2014). Similar large-scale government efforts were successful in Japan and Finland.

NUTRITION LABELS

The Nutrition Labeling and Education Act, implemented in 1993, required the FDA to enforce food ***nutrition labels*** that were more educational and less confusing. The initial confrontation pitted consumer advocates against the food industry, which only wanted ingredient amounts on the label. Advocates preferred percentages, like "this ingredient contained 25% of the total you should consume in a single day." After substantial debate and controversy, consumers won out over the food industry.

But a quarter century later, the food label had undergone only minimal change—adding trans fat in 2006 and sugar content in 2016. Why so stingy with food label revisions over the years, while science has made many discoveries about the impact of nutrients and calories on our health? Primarily because there has been an ongoing battle between the FDA and the food and drink industry, and those administrations that side with industry deregulations.

Finally, though, we seem to be entering a period of revising and improving the food label. Why is this important? Because most people often read labels (54%) and people age 68+ rely on them even more (57%), according to the FDA's Health and Diet Survey. Regardless of whether consumers make decisions based on the label content, the additional information allows for more informed choices.

Labels are not just placed on products. Part of the Affordable Care Act of 2010 was to require the listing of calories on menus. It took 8 years of war before the FDA finally won a single battle in 2018. On May 7, calories on menus were finally implemented in restaurant chains with 20 or more locations. (McDonald's, with its 14,000 locations in the United States, got a head start by posting calorie counts on its menus in 2012.) In addition, on that date, caloric information for consumers was required for supermarkets, convenience stores, movie theaters (for popcorn), and drinks in bars. Also starting on that date was a requirement to provide consumer information about sodium, saturated fat, and other nutrients at the same type of locations—though not necessarily on menus.

Some other major changes proposed for the Nutrition Labeling and Education Act were for food and drink labels to include added sugars; to display calories in larger, bolder type; and to use more realistic serving sizes. Unsurprisingly, these rules have been delayed multiple times by intense lobbying efforts. Fast-food chains have also joined the fray. For example. Domino's pizza spearheaded legislation that would allow retailers to use serving sizes that make their calorie counts look deceptively low. The bill (H.R.772—Common Sense Nutrition Disclosure Act of 2017) died in committee. How would this sleight-of-hand work? Most people drinking a 16-ounce soda, for example, do not stop at the 8-ounce mark. Instead, they consume what is in the container and do not consider that the one serving listed discreetly on the label is accurate only if you stopped halfway through the full bottle. Consumers typically do not realize that the amount of sugar they drink in such a situation is actually twice the number listed on the container. If a container of any sort, for instance a small package of chips, can be reasonably expected to be consumed in one sitting, then it should be labeled one serving—thereby doubling the amount of sodium in a bag of chips that might otherwise be listed.

Another label proposal is to do away with "calories from fat" because, as we noted earlier, a focus on fat can inappropriately encourage "nutritionism," not to mention the failure to differentiate among the types of fat. Also, vitamins A and C are not common deficiencies in this country, so there is a proposal to replace them with vitamin D and potassium.

An unlikely improvement for nutrition labels would differentiate added sugars from naturally occurring ones and identify when the percentage of added sugar is excessive—to be determined by government researchers. This ideally would be noted in red on the label. Evidence suggests this approach is effective (Song et al., 2021).

This idea relates to another idealistic proposal, which is actually taking place in some grocery stores. The ***food rating system*** provides either numerical ratings, star ratings, or letter grades that are posted on the shelf next to each product in a grocery store. Assigning value to foods, though, requires considerable judgment. How much value should be earned for a product that provides whole grains, fiber, vitamins, or minerals? How much value should be deducted for added sugars, saturated fat, sodium, or calories?

Without federal guidelines, nine large U.S. food manufacturers (with the input of academic nutrition professors) developed the Smart Choices Food Labeling Program in 2009. This rating system allowed processed foods high in sugar, such as Froot Loops cereal and Cracker Jack snack food, to be rated as "smart choices." After several months of bad publicity, it was terminated by federal regulators because it was deemed misleading.

To understand how food companies have influenced not only this food labeling attempt, but nutrition conferences, nutrition research initiatives, nutritional professional societies (e.g., the American Society for Nutrition), and advisory panels that influence government guidelines, read Marion Nestle's *Unsavory Truth: How Food Companies Skew the Science of What We Eat* (Hatchette, 2018).

One final deception in nutrition labeling is ground beef, which accounts for about half of the meat sold in the United States and adds more saturated fat to the average American's diet than any other single food. Yet a package of ground beef which can provide 14 grams of fat in a single serving can legally have an "85% *lean*" label placed on it.

Does labeling work? One national survey reported that 83% of restaurant diners wanted nutritional information posted. Studies show, however, that when given this type of information, only 10% to 20% of diners would choose lower calorie options (Rabin, 2007). On the plus side, that is much better than zero. And there is another unexpected benefit. In January 2009, Seattle, for example, was one of the first cities to require chain restaurants to post calories, and not coincidentally, at the same time many Seattle restaurants began using lower calorie ingredients.

MALNUTRITION

Americans are no longer dying of pellagra, rickets, beriberi, or scurvy—caused by deficiencies in vitamin B3 niacin, vitamin D, vitamin B_1 thiamine, and vitamin C, respectively—thanks largely to the fortification and enrichment of our foods. Nonetheless, ***malnutrition*** remains a serious problem, particularly among those over age 75. Malnutrition includes "undernutrition (wasting, stunting, underweight), inadequate vitamins or minerals, overweight, obesity, and resulting diet-related noncommunicable diseases" (https://www.who.int/news-room/fact-sheets/detail/malnutrition).

Malnutrition has severe health consequences for adults, not just children. One study used the 2018 Healthcare Cost and Utilization Project (HCUP) to examine health outcomes among people with discharge diagnoses that included malnutrition. Nearly 9% of all U.S. nonmaternal, nonneonatal hospital discharges had a coded diagnosis of malnutrition; these people were older, had longer lengths of stay, and incurred higher costs, as compared with those without a malnutrition diagnosis (Guenter et al., 2021).

Advanced age is a risk factor for malnutrition. For older adults, it is typically defined as being *under*nourished, though for some an excess of calories and obesity leads to *mal*nourishment. The prevalence of malnutrition varies according to the health and functional status of older people. A 2016 meta-analysis using the Mini Nutritional Assessment (MNA, the most commonly used nutritional assessment tool in older adults) determined that the prevalence of malnutrition overall was

3.1% among community-dwelling older adults. Among older people with disabilities receiving home care services, the prevalence was 8.7%; in older adults receiving hospital care, 22.0% met malnutrition criteria; and among older people residing in long-term care facilities the prevalence reached 28.7% (Cereda et al., 2016). Still, recent research suggests nutritional status may be improving among older people (Burman et al., 2022).

Which is worse for hospital patients: malnutrition or obesity? A chart review of 300,000 patients consecutively admitted to hospitals in Spain with chronic obstructive pulmonary diseases revealed that patients with malnutrition had a much higher risk of hospital death or readmittance within 30 days of discharge than those diagnosed with obesity (Zapatero et al., 2013). In this population, obesity may reduce mortality (Viasus et al., 2022).

There are many risk factors for malnourishment in older adults (Table 5.4). The link between malnutrition and social isolation is particularly strong, and suggests that encouraging participation in clubs and the sharing of meals with friends or neighbors may be far more effective in improving dietary intake than providing nutrition education.

Older adults living alone consume fewer fruits and vegetables and have a much greater propensity for selecting easy-to-prepare foods, which are high in fat and low in complex carbohydrates, than do those who have companions. Men living alone are at greater risk of less desirable intakes than women (Hanna & Collins, 2015). Loneliness, bereavement, and social isolation are associated with poor dietary intake in later life. An increasing percentage of older adults report difficulty in preparing meals, particularly after age 85.

Many older people depend on meals prepared at a congregate nutrition site or *Meals-on-Wheels* program (www.mealsonwheelsamerica.org). The demand for services of this type continues to increase along with the number of very old, frail adults. That the supply of such services will meet the increasing need is unlikely based on funding trends. Malnutrition is therefore likely to increase.

Nutrition screenings examine characteristics known to be associated with dietary and nutritional problems in order to identify high-risk persons. One such screening initiative, a collaborative project by the American Academy of Family Physicians, the American Dietetic Association, and the National Council on Aging, resulted in the production of a manual that begins with a checklist, "Determine Your Nutritional Health,"

TABLE 5.4 RISK FACTORS FOR MALNOURISHMENT IN OLDER ADULTS

Inappropriate food	Loss of appetite	Decreased thirst	Dental problems
Social isolation	Poverty	Dementing illness	Medical disease
Physical condition	Alcoholism	Endurance problems	Balance problems
Depression	Medication usage	Medication withdrawal	Dysphagia and other swallowing disorders
Food insecurity	Loss of taste and olfaction	Hospital- and nursing-home-acquired malnutrition	Inability to open packages and containers

shown in Exhibit 5.1. The manual includes a variety of screening tools on nutrition and related topics, including body mass index (BMI), eating habits, functional status, cognitive status, and depression.

When older clients lose their appetite, the following is recommended: Eat smaller and more frequent meals; take advantage of when you feel good and are hungry, regardless of the time; eat higher calorie foods or consider taking a nutritional supplement; postpone beverages toward the end of a meal; create a pleasant eating atmosphere and find company with whom to enjoy the meal; and see a physician to either change a medication that is affecting appetite, or add a medication that may relieve nausea, heartburn, or other symptoms.

EXHIBIT 5.1 DETERMINE YOUR NUTRITIONAL HEALTH

Determine your nutritional health

The Warning Signs of poor nutritional health are often overlooked. Use this Checklist to find out if you or someone you know is at nutritional risk.

Read the statements below. Circle the number in the yes column for those that apply to you or someone you know. For each yes answer, score the number in the box. Total your nutritional score.

	YES
I have an illness or condition that made me change the kind and/or amount of food I eat.	2
I eat fewer than 2 meals per day.	3
I eat few fruits or vegetables, or milk products.	2
I have 3 or more drinks of beer, liquor, or wine almost every day.	2
I have tooth or mouth problems that make it hard for me to eat.	2
I don't always have enough money to buy the food I need.	4
I eat alone most of the time.	1
I take 3 or more different prescribed or over-the-counter drugs a day.	1
Without wanting to, I have lost or gained 10 pounds in the last 6 months.	2
I am not always physically able to shop, cook, and/or feed myself.	2
Total	

Total your nutritional score. If it's –

0–2 **Good!** Recheck your nutritional score in 6 months.

3–5 **You are at moderate nutritional risk.** See what can be done to improve your eating habits and lifestyle. Your office on aging, senior nutrition program, senior citizens center, or health department can help. Recheck your nutritional score in 3 months.

6 or more **You are at high nutritional risk.** Bring this checklist the next time you see your doctor, dietitian, or other qualified health or social service professional. Talk with them about any problems you may have. Ask for help to improve your nutritional health.

These materials developed and distributed by the Nutrition Screening Initiative, a project of:

AMERICAN ACADEMY OF FAMILY PHYSICIANS

THE AMERICAN DIETETIC ASSOCIATION

NATIONAL COUNCIL ON THE AGING, INC.

Remember that warning signs suggest risk, but do not represent diagnosis of any condition. Turn the page to learn more about the warning signs of poor nutritional health.

(*continued*)

EXHIBIT 5.1 DETERMINE YOUR NUTRITIONAL HEALTH (*CONTINUED*)

The nutrition checklist is based on the warning signs described below. Use the word determine to remind you of the warning signs.

Disease

Any disease, illness, or chronic condition which causes you to change the way you eat, or makes it hard for you to eat, puts your nutritional health at risk. Four out of five adults have chronic diseases that are affected by diet. Confusion or memory loss that keeps getting worse is estimated to affect one out of five or more of older adults. This can make it hard to remember what, when, or if you've eaten. Feeling sad or depressed, which happens to about one in eight older adults, can cause big changes in appetite, digestion, energy level, weight, and well-being.

Eating poorly

Eating too little and eating too much both lead to poor health. Eating the same foods day after day or not eating fruit, vegetables, and milk products daily will also cause poor nutritional health. One in five adults skip meals daily. Only 13% of adults eat the minimum amount of fruit and vegetables needed. One in four older adults drink too much alcohol. Many health problems become worse if you drink more than one or two alcoholic beverages per day.

Tooth loss/mouth pain

A healthy mouth, teeth, and gums are needed to eat. Missing, loose, or rotten teeth or dentures which don't fit well or cause mouth sores make it hard to eat.

Economic hardship

As many as 40% of older Americans have incomes of less than $6,000 per year. Having less—or choosing to spend less—than $25–30 per week for food makes it very hard to get the foods you need to stay healthy.

Reduced social contact

One-third of all older people live alone. Being with people daily has a positive effect on morale, well-being, and eating.

Multiple medicines

Many older Americans must take medicines for health problems. Almost half of older Americans take multiple medicines daily. Growing old may change the way we respond to drugs. The more medicines you take, the greater the chance for side effects such as increased or decreased appetite, change in taste, constipation, weakness, drowsiness, diarrhea, nausea, and others. Vitamins or minerals, when taken in large doses, act like drugs and can cause harm. Alert your doctor to everything you take.

Involuntary weight loss/gain

Losing or gaining a lot of weight when you are not trying to do so is an important warning sign that must not be ignored. Being overweight or underweight also increases your chance of poor health.

Needs assistance in self-care

Although most older people are able to eat, one out of every five have trouble walking, shopping, buying, and cooking food, especially as they get older.

Elder years above age 80

Most older people lead full and productive lives. But as age increases, risk of frailty and health problems increase. Checking your nutritional health regularly makes good sense.

The Nutrition Screening Initiative, 2626 Pennsylvania Avenue, NW, Suite 301, Washington, DC 20037

The Nutrition Screening Initiative is funded in part by a grant from Ross Laboratories, a division of Abbott Laboratories.

Source: Determine Your Nutritional Health developed and distributed by Nutrition Screening Initiative, a project of the American Academy of Family Physicians, the American Dietetic Association, and the National Council on Aging, Inc. http://www.dhs.gov.vi/wp-content/uploads/2023/02/SCA_DetermineNutritionChecklist.pdf.

SELECTED NUTRITION TOPICS

Organic Foods

As supermarket chains that cater to consumers interested in ***organic foods*** expand throughout the country, their marketing executives have noticed that their typical customer is increasingly a well-educated female baby boomer. This sentiment has been shared by the Organic Trade Association, which believes that the buying trend of the past decade has been led by the health-conscious baby boomers.

One of these boomers was Michelle Obama (she just made it—born in 1964), who seized upon an opportunity in 2009 to organically grow vegetables and assorted herbs on the White House grounds. Boomers, though, need to be vigilant about a variety of issues that extend beyond the effort in one's own garden. The integrity of the organic movement depends on resisting the softening of rules in regard to pesticides, hormones, chemical fertilizers, antibiotics, irradiation, bioengineering, artificial preservatives, flavors, synthetic ingredients, conservation of soil and water, and humane treatment of animals.

Apparently there has been some success in maintaining standards for organic foods, as a meta-analysis of 340 studies found that organically grown crops contain more antioxidants and fewer pesticides than conventional foods (Baranski et al., 2014).

Walmart has offered organic foods in its nearly 4,000 stores for quite some time, and the consequences have been positive. In the Walmart tradition, cost is a factor, and they have vowed to keep costs to only 10% over conventional food, instead of the additional 25% or more charged elsewhere. The good news is that many more people will be able to afford organic food.

There is more possible good news. Critics were concerned that Walmart would look for large-scale producers to keep prices low and begin the decline of local organic farming. Instead, Walmart announced an initiative to double the amount of *locally* grown fruits and vegetables it sells. The shorter travel distances would help to reduce air pollution. Now let's see if Walmart follows through—a big if—and whether it launches more green initiatives (https://corporate.walmart.com/content/corporate/en_us.html).

Coffee

Boomers in particular like their ***coffee***, even though it has been cast as a vice on and off for centuries. As far back as 1600, for instance, a few monarchs destroyed coffeehouses, believing that coffee incited gossip and rebellion. Yet research over the last few years has leaned more toward coffee being a virtue that may promote longevity (Barrea et al., 2023).

Researchers analyzed the coffee-drinking habits of 400,000 people ages 50 to 71. Whether caffeinated or not, they found that controlling for risk factors (smoking, diet, exercise, etc.), the more coffee a person consumed (within limits), the less likely that person was to die from a number of health problems, including diabetes, heart disease, respiratory disease, stroke, and injuries or accidents (Freedman et al., 2012). A later study reported that coffee drinkers who consume one to three cups of coffee a day will attain a 15% reduction in their mortality rate compared with nondrinkers (Park et al., 2017).

Researchers have also found that those who consumed up to six cups of coffee a day were almost 20% less likely to develop prostate cancer over a two-decade period than those who drank none, and 60% less likely to develop a lethal form of the disease (Wilson et al., 2011). Other researchers report that coffee is a major source of dietary antioxidants, and that coffee consumption is associated with reduced risk of death from inflammatory and cardiovascular diseases (Andersen et al., 2006), diabetes (Salazar-Martinez et al., 2004), and cirrhosis (Klatsky et al., 2006).

A cautionary note is in order for the coffee-drinking reader of this section. Some studies continue to associate coffee drinking with heart disease and other health problems. Why the conflicting research results? Some theorists suggest that the answer is in the genes. A specific gene can cause the liver to metabolize four times faster than those without the gene. Because caffeine persists longer in a slow metabolizer, it has more time to act as a trigger of heart attacks, according to Ahmed El-Sohemy, a professor in nutritional sciences at the University of Toronto.

Regardless which side of the research divide you stand, coffee can be counted toward one's recommended fluid intake as, contrary to popular belief, it is only slightly more of a diuretic than water.

Sensory Decline

An age-related ***sensory decline*** in smell—rather than taste—directly affects a person's ability to taste or enjoy food. As many as half of persons between the ages of 70 and 80, and three quarters of persons over age 80, experience problems with their sense of smell (Doty & Kamath, 2014). African Americans are more likely to experience olfactory decline, consistent with other indicators of accelerated aging among this subgroup (Motter et al., 2023). Declines in olfaction are also harbingers of neurological disease, such as Alzheimer and Parkinson diseases. Older persons have more trouble identifying pureed foods, for instance, than do younger persons. If younger persons held their noses while eating, their ability to identify foods would drop to the level of older adults.

Because some people try to compensate for the loss of smell and taste, they may add too much sugar or salt to make food taste better, which can affect their risk for heart disease, stroke, diabetes, and other diseases. To enhance food aromas for older adults, herbs and spices are encouraged. Adding flavors and sweeteners can also enhance taste. Another technique for stimulating appetite is a combination of different textures; for example, adding granola to yogurt.

Food Films

The great Mexican movie *Like Water for Chocolate* is about a young woman who transfers her feelings of forbidden love into cooking. Her passion is channeled into her food preparation, and those who subsequently dine on her creations experience her emotions as well.

There are other films in which people pour their love into the preparation of food. *Babette's Feast* is about a group of quarreling people who become transformed by a magnificent feast and end the meal by forgiving and blessing one another. *Eat Drink Man Woman* is about a famous Chinese chef concerned about his daughters, but only able to communicate through loving meal preparations. *Big Night* is about two Italian brothers trying to save their restaurant through the feast of a lifetime. In all these films, the food is fresh and delicious, and prepared slowly and lovingly. (Interested in the slow food movement? Visit www.slowfood.com.)

At the other end of the continuum is the movie about fast food, called *Super Size Me*. Morgan Spurlock was a healthy young man who became fascinated by two young people who sued McDonald's for making them fat. Spurlock then decided to make a movie about eating at McDonald's for three meals a day, for 30 straight days. Spurlock at first found the meals to be tasty, but eventually he sustained liver damage, stomach pains, vomiting, weight gain, depression, and impaired sexuality (though perhaps the attitude of his girlfriend—a vegan chef—toward his project contributed to the last problem).

Just before *Super Size Me* began appearing in movie theaters in 2004, McDonald's (they claimed coincidentally) eliminated the supersize option and also announced the introduction of a new, healthier menu.

Advocacy

CPSI (https://www.cspinet.org/) is an educational and advocacy organization. Its educational component consists primarily of *NutritionAction*, a newsletter published monthly, which informs more than 800,000 subscribers (https://www.cspinet.org/page/nutrition-action-archive).

CSPI staff have led the fight for nutrition labels on food items in the supermarket; for exposing the hidden fat in Chinese, Mexican, Italian, and delicatessen foods; for pressuring movie theaters to stop cooking popcorn in artery-clogging coconut oil; for warning labels on Procter & Gamble's fake fat, Olean, which may interfere with the absorption of nutrients and cause loose stools and cramping; and for more accurate labeling of ground beef in supermarkets.

This ***nutritional advocacy*** group also successfully lobbied for the listing of trans fat on nutrition labels, then went one step further—getting the substance banned altogether. For more information on the *Nutrition Action Health Letter*, contact the Center for Science in the Public Interest, 1250 I Street NW, Suite 500, Washington, DC 20005; or visit its website, www.cspinet.org.

Woody and *Sleeper*

You may be familiar with the 1973 science fiction comedy movie *Sleeper*, in which a character played by Woody Allen is frozen in time and comes back to life centuries later where deep-fried fat, hot-fudge sundaes, and steaks are the real health foods. Products like wheat germ and organic honey have long been exposed as worthless. This parody provides a cautionary tale on recommendations that often do change as better studies force us to revise our thinking.

Fast-Food Restaurants

Over the past four decades, consumers have doubled the percentage of their food dollars spent at restaurants to about 46% of their food budget—a majority of which takes place at fast-food restaurants. Some Americans, therefore, may be theoretically starting off their day with the Cheesecake Factory's Breakfast Burrito, which has 2,730 calories (more than a day's worth of calories), 4,630 mg of sodium (2 days' worth), and 73 grams of saturated fat (more than 3 days' worth). For lunch, our hypothetical American is feeling guilty and decides to skip the Double Quarter Pounder with Cheese at McDonald's for the seemingly healthier choice of the Southwest Salad with Crispy Chicken. Alas, the salad has 10 more calories than the super-duper cheeseburger.

Results from NHANES 2017 to 2018 data show that more than half of adults age 20+ obtain food from restaurants on a given day. However, the percentage who reported eating food from a restaurant daily decreases with age (Hoy et al., 2022).

Fueled in part by recourse to calorie-rich restaurant and prepared foods, obesity has more than doubled over the past four decades in America. Obesity is defined as body mass index (BMI), calculated as weight (kg)/height (m)^2, of 30 and above, and overweight, defined as BMI 25 to 30, is driven by the ubiquity of food (vending machines everywhere); escalating advertising budgets; subsidized production of high-calorie foods (mainly from corn and soybean oil); and an ever-increasing consumption of fast food, junk food, and high-calorie restaurant food, with the average adult eating about 250 to 300 more calories a day in 2018 than in the 1970s (Hall, 2018). Increasingly sedentary lifestyles compound the problem.

Why the concern? Obesity leads to higher rates of disease and death among middle-age and older adults. It is associated with shorter life expectancy; overweight is associated with heart disease and other diseases at a much earlier age and for a longer period of time as life expectancy has increased among those who are overweight (Khan et al., 2018b).

TRENDS IN WEIGHT GAIN

The U.S. Preventive Services Task Force (USPSTF) recommends that clinicians screen all adults for obesity and offer intensive behavioral counseling to obese adults (Grade B: https://www.uspreventiveservicestaskforce.org/uspstf/recommendation/obesity-in-adults-interventions). This decision was based not so much on the effectiveness of clinician counsel, which is questionable, but rather on the evidence that overweight and obesity have become epidemics in America.

A comparison between 1960 and 2000 is instructive. In 1960, with weight relatively stable over the previous years, American women age 40 to 49 averaged 140 lbs. By 2000, though, the average weight of women in their 40s jumped to 169 lbs (Kessler, 2009), more than 7 lbs gained for each decade. Age 40 to 49 was not even the heaviest age group; that distinction went to adults ages 50 to 69, followed by those ages 70 to 75. After age 75, there begins to be a tendency to lose weight. Unfortunately, this weight loss is due more to loss of muscle mass than fat, so older persons not only become thinner, but weaker and less functionally independent as well. The increase in obesity continues. The age-adjusted mean BMI increased from 28.7 (95% Confidence Interval 28.2–29.1) in 2011 to 12 to 29.8 (29.2–30.4) in 2017 to 18 (Liu et al., 2021).

Obesity is most prevalent among low-income minority women. Regarding *income*, 25% of women above the poverty level are obese compared to 37% of women with incomes below the poverty level. Regarding *sex and ethnicity*, Mexican American women are 40% obese, compared with 29% for Mexican American men; African American women are 50% obese compared with 28% for African American men (Flegal et al., 2002; Squires, 2002). More than 80% of African American women age 40 or older were overweight or obese (Flegal et al., 2002).

In 2016, data from the NHANES concluded that about 70% of American adults are overweight or obese, and the percentage of obese adults (39.8%) continues to rise so rapidly that it has widened the gap with those who are merely overweight (about 30%). This epidemic has escalated despite the fact that Americans spend about $90 billion a year on diet products and programs, including the new and expensive GLP-1 medications (https://blog.marketresearch.com/u.s.-weight-loss-industry-grows-to-90-billion-fueled-by-obesity-drugs-demand); excess weight is widely known to be a risk factor for disease and death; obesity is a social stigma in our society and continues to offend most people's personal vanity; and a health revolution had supposedly occurred in America over the past few decades.

Over more than four decades, cigarette smoking declined significantly; alcohol abuse was identified as a common risk factor and steps were taken to curtail it, especially among automobile drivers; seatbelt use rose steadily; brisk walking, jogging, aerobic dancing, and other exercises had attracted millions of new participants; and the use of low-fat food alternatives had proliferated. How could the nation have grown fat while all of this was happening?

Some health analysts believe that the fitness revolution was limited to only a segment of the population, perhaps 20%, with the majority of Americans still sedentary and consuming more calories than ever. Others theorize that significant numbers of Americans have been relying on their computers rather than physical activities for entertainment as well as work. Another theory is that many people in this highly stressful era have been using food as a coping device to combat the anxiety and depression caused by violence, dramatic reduction in good-paying union jobs, increased divorce, and so forth, and of course COVID. Yet another theory is that legions of exsmokers have turned to overeating. Obesity has also become more acceptable to some as it becomes normative.

Each of these ideas contains some element of truth, but perhaps none more than the fact that our society is aging. The familiar population pyramid, with a few old people at its top and many young people at its base, is fast becoming a rectangle. This population rectangle, which has been taking shape over the past 40 years, will complete its metamorphosis over the next decade. In 1980, nearly three times as many persons were under age 18 as were over age 65 (28% vs. 11%). By 2030, the percentages will be equivalent (20%).

As we age, our *metabolism*—the chemical processes that build and destroy tissue—gradually slows. When it comes to eating, our fat oxidation, or fat-burning rate, slows by about 30% with age. The metabolism that breaks down food components releases them in the form of energy and heat more slowly.

Thus, the number of calories that were required to maintain our weight when we were young no longer maintains our weight, but increases it. Also, chronic conditions—most notably arthritis—that accompany the aging process can place limitations on our ability to stay active. Activity is a crucial factor in long-term weight management.

MEASURING OVERWEIGHT AND OBESITY

The ***body mass index*** has been the standard gauge of weight status. It provides a simple and roughly accurate method for determining population (but not individual) ***overweight*** and ***obesity.*** BMI can be calculated by multiplying weight in pounds by 700, divided by height in inches, and then divided by height in inches again; or if you prefer metric, divide body weight (kg) by height squared (m^2).

Adults who have a BMI between 25 and 29.9 are *overweight* (about 30% of American adults), between 30 and 39.9 are *obese* (39.8%); within this category of obese Americans are those with a BMI of 40 or over who are extremely or *morbidly obese* (7.7%). Of U.S. adults aged 60+, 42.2% are obese (Hales et al., 2020).

The BMI is a useful and sufficiently accurate tool for screening the general population, but, similar to height/weight charts, it fails to differentiate fat from lean body mass. Also, centrally obese apple-shaped bodies are more of a heart risk factor than pear-shaped bodies. The two shortcomings of this tool associated with age are:

1. Excess body fat in older adults may be underestimated by a BMI score because it is counteracted by a loss of muscle mass with age. The net result can be a BMI under 25 for an older person, but with excess body fat.
2. It is not uncommon for older adults to lose about 2 to 3 inches in height as they age, and there is no consensus on whether to use the new or old height (or an in-between height) in determining BMI.

A ***waist-to-hip ratio*** is a better predictor of heart attack than BMI (Yusuf et al., 2005). This ratio refers to waist measurement divided by hip measurement. A score above 0.85

in women, or 0.9 in men, shows a risk for heart disease. The higher the ratio, the greater the risk of a heart attack. (A cruder measure of the visceral fat that accumulates around abdominal organs is to just measure your waist—if over 35 inches for women or over 40 inches for men, problems lie ahead.) BMI is useful for predicting disease but probably not ideal for assessing metabolic status.

Morbidity and Mortality

One study reported that even being modestly overweight increases the chances of developing heart failure. This study of almost 6,000 adults reported that although the risk of heart failure is double in obese people, it is still a substantial 34% higher in those who are only overweight (Kenchaiah et al., 2002). For each increment of one unit on the BMI scale, the risk increased 5% for men and 7% for women.

QUESTION: Some people argue that, despite the amount of overweight and obesity in old age, the bigger geriatric concern is malnutrition. What is your opinion on this? Why?

Obesity, however, is the major risk factor. It is associated not only with heart disease, diabetes, breast cancer, colon cancer, prostate cancer, osteoarthritis, and gallbladder disease, but premature death (Peeters et al., 2003). Obesity is associated with a 2- to 3-year shorter life expectancy; overweight does not shorten life expectancy but does expand the years of living with morbidity in middle and old age (Khan et al., 2018a).

Costs

Obesity is associated not only with a wide range of diseases but also with increased expenses—Medicare costs accrue with these diseases. Obese Medicare recipients accumulate $170,000 more in Medicare charges than normal-weight patients (Raebel et al., 2004). The higher the BMI in middle age, the greater the accumulated Medicare charges later on. Health economists have calculated that nearly 10% of health spending in 2008—$147 billion—was related to obesity, nearly double the total of a decade prior (Finkelstein et al., 2009).

The incremental cost of overweight and obesity far exceeds that of smoking. Not only are smokers considerably fewer in number, but a 7-year study reported that smokers do not live as long as the overweight and obese because the latter are being kept alive with drugs for heart disease, diabetes, and other diseases (Moriarity et al., 2012). The extra costs for long-term prescriptions as well as additional hospitalizations add up over time.

GENETICS, LIFESTYLE, AND ENVIRONMENT

Genetics

Although genes do not destine you to become fat, a family history of obesity increases your chances of becoming obese by about 25% to 30%. Moreover, if you are genetically inclined to carry the extra weight primarily around your waist (apple shaped), you are at higher risk for heart disease, hypertension, stroke, and diabetes than the noncentrally obese (pear shaped).

There may also be a genetic thermostat for body fat. ***Set-point theory*** states that a genetic thermostat for body fat maintains a fairly constant weight. If body weight decreases through dieting, the set-point either triggers appetite or makes the body conserve energy (i.e., lowers the basal metabolic rate) to maintain the fat cells and a set weight. The body burns calories more slowly than normal when weight is lost, a useful compensation in olden times when sources of food were more unpredictable.

Even more disheartening is that if weight is regained over time after major weight loss through dieting, the genetic thermostat is permanently lowered. Your metabolic rate does not go back up to its previous level. So, if you eat the same amount of calories after regaining your weight that you once consumed to maintain your weight, it will now increase your weight. The hormone *leptin* which decreases appetite is permanently weakened, and the hormone *ghrelin* which increases appetite is permanently strengthened. In short, the number of calories you want to eat is greater than before you lost weight, while your body burns calories more slowly.

Lifestyle

Although ***genetics*** is a contributor to the development of obesity, a more important reason that a person becomes overweight or obese—in terms of being able to take action—relates to ***lifestyle***. By limiting the types and quantity of food and increasing daily energy expenditure through physical activity and exercise, one has the ability to make a significant impact on body weight.

The ***National Weight Control Registry*** was a landmark study of 800 persons, average age 45, who had shed at least 30 lbs and kept the weight off for at least 5 years (Klem et al., 1997). Weight loss was confirmed in a variety of ways, including documentation from physicians, interviews with family members or friends, and photographs. The researchers concluded that *persistence* was one of the most important components of successful weight loss. The average person failed half a dozen times before success was obtained.

Moreover, there was no single magical way to achieve success, unless you count modifying eating and exercise habits as magical. About 44% limited their food portions, 40% counted calories, 33% limited fat intake, 25% kept track of fat grams, and 4% relied on diet drugs.

Most of the registry's participants had been overweight since childhood, nearly half had at least one overweight parent, and more than a quarter had two overweight parents. Genes may predispose some toward obesity, but apparently lifestyle changes can initiate and sustain weight loss. On average, the participants reduced their body weight by 29% and successfully moved into the normal weight range.

A similar study with a smaller sample size ($n = 160$) was conducted earlier by Fletcher (1994), a registered dietitian, and the results were reported in her book *Thin for Life*. Fletcher distilled her strategies for success from persons who kept off at least 20 lbs (average weight loss was 63 lbs) for a minimum of 3 years and most for more than 5 years. The successful strategies employed by this sample of adults included the following:

- Focus on what you can eat, not on what you cannot eat.
- Do not deny yourself your favorite foods and do not worry about periodic slipups.
- Identify and then avoid high-risk situations and emotional eating.
- Find a way to incorporate exercise into your weekly routine.
- Identify when you need to seek outside help.

What about the vast majority of overweight and obese people who try to lose weight and fail? The ones who diet repeatedly and are frequently losing and then gaining weight are engaging in "yo-yo dieting." This may increase one's risk for heart attacks, strokes, new-onset diabetes, and mortality (Bangalore et al., 2017). The best lifestyle approach to weight loss is to go slow, be modest in your weight-loss goals, and eventually discover a strategy that you can maintain in the long run.

Environment

Perhaps it is not our genes or our lack of willpower that is the major contributor to overweight and obesity, but our ***environment***. Our society produces an abundance of food: food that is high in fat, sugar, and salt, much of it processed and packaged for our convenience; food that is heavily advertised; and food that is available everywhere—gas stations, drugstores, food courts in shopping malls, and the ubiquitous vending machines.

Also, during the last 30 years, Americans have doubled the frequency with which they eat at restaurants, and when they eat out, they eat more. In a busy society, consumers seek the convenience that restaurants provide. Consumers also have been seeking greater value at restaurants. Profit-seeking restaurant owners have come to the realization that the food itself is the least costly ingredient of a food product compared to the costs of labor, packaging, and marketing. Thus, restaurant owners are providing ever-larger portion sizes, with little increase in cost.

QUESTION: Regarding weight management, which do you believe is more important: lifestyle counseling or environmental change? Explain your answer.

Food is low cost and overproduced in the United States. According to Marion Nestle, professor emerita in nutrition and health at New York University, there are 3,800 calories produced per person per day in the United States, and we only need about half of that (Nestle, 2002). Food wastage is estimated at between 30% and 40% of the food supply (https://www.usda.gov/foodwaste/faqs). Food is abundant, ubiquitous, cheap, and fattening, and it is promoted everywhere, all the time.

Environmental Change to Accommodate Obese Americans

Given how difficult it has been for people to lose weight, it is not surprising that businesses are focused on a complementary challenge: adjusting the environment for bigger people. Restaurants provide larger chairs for obese customers or switch to armless chairs and reinforced seats. Airlines have allowed—and charged for—obese customers to take up two adjoining seats. Some obese customers request seatbelt extenders.

Men's slacks formerly labeled "regular" are now "slim cut." Larger sizes are "easy fit," "loose fit," or "baggy fit." Larger sized women's clothing now has smaller sized numbers: What used to be a size 12 is now labeled a size 8. The petite health writer Jane Brody, who believes she is at best a size 4, was thrilled to find a pair of size 0 slacks that fit perfectly.

Hospitals use larger beds and bigger wheelchairs. To avoid the embarrassment of taking a patient down to the loading dock for the use of a scale, human scales have been developed to accommodate up to 1,000 lbs. Rear ends are so large that extra-length needles are necessary for an injection to pass through the fat and reach the buttocks muscles. Medical clinics add loveseats to the waiting room. Open MRI machines are not just for claustrophobic patients, but for obese ones as well. Blood pressure cuffs, body fat calipers, and patient gowns are super-sized.

Examination tables have been anchored into the floor to prevent obese patients from flipping them as they sit on the end. Floor-mounting of commodes prevents them from being pulled out of the wall. Doorways have been widened from 36 to 52 inches. Portable hoists are placed by bedsides to prevent worker injuries. Hospital suppliers have developed more than 1,000 items specifically for obese patients, including a wider body bag, which leads to a final comment: Funeral homes now offer extra-large coffins that accommodate up to 700 lbs. Sales are brisk.

SHOULD WE GAIN WEIGHT WITH AGE?

Many argue that gaining a few extra pounds with age may be not only common in America, but healthy. Dr. Reubin Andres, former clinical director of the National Institute on Aging, conducted a series of long-term studies and found that people in their 60s who were somewhat overweight (according to the Metropolitan Life Insurance charts), but not obese, had a better chance of living into their 80s and 90s than those whose weight was normal. Thus, he created age-specific weight tables that generally had upper weight limits that were 10 to 20 lbs higher than the insurance-based tables.

A study by the Cooper Institute for Aerobics Research (Lee et al., 1999) appeared to support Andres's contention that we need to be more lenient with recommended weight ranges, especially among persons who maintain their fitness. Men who gained significant amounts of weight over time but remained moderately or very fit had lower death rates than men who were in the average weight range for their group but were unfit.

The chief opponent of Dr. Andres's theory was Dr. Roy Walford of the UCLA School of Medicine, who died at age 79, 41 years short of his goal to live to 120. Dr. Walford practiced what he preached, which was to maintain reduced caloric intake, and placed himself on a lifelong diet in adulthood of 1,500 calories a day. His animal research had shown that underfed rats lived one-third longer than well-fed rats. Other studies have reported that a caloric intake decreased by 30% in young or middle-aged laboratory animals prolonged longevity (Colman et al., 2009; Masoro, 2005).

Critics of Dr. Walford's research, however, were concerned not only with his extrapolation from rodents to humans, but also with whether longer life on an "eat less" diet, even among the rats being studied, is associated with stunted growth, lower energy levels, and greater irritability. Comedians are also critical of Dr. Walford's diet, lamenting that eating less may not really lengthen life; it may just make life *seem* longer.

In a 25-year study funded by the National Institute on Aging, Rhesus monkeys fed a calorie-restricted diet (30% reduction in calories) lived no longer than monkeys fed a normal-calorie diet (Mattison et al., 2012). The response to this study, conducted by well-respected researchers, some of whom were calorie restrictors themselves, was surprise and disappointment.

The extra-weight theory has also generated its critics, who noted, for instance, that Dr. Andres's sample was biased toward the affluent elderly who could pass life insurance medical examinations and had the resources to effectively manage diabetes, hypertension, and hyperlipidemia.

Also, the Nurses' Health Study suggested that the increasingly permissive weight guidelines may be unjustified. The researchers tracked the health status of 115,000 female nurses for 16 years and discovered a direct correlation between weight and susceptibility to stroke (Rexrode et al., 1997). Women whose BMI score rose into the 27 to 31 range during the 16-year period were 1.7 times more at risk for stroke; women who rose to a BMI of at least 32 more than doubled their risk.

The controversy over "extra weight versus underweight" was heightened by the results of a major study conducted by researchers at the CDC and the National Cancer

Institute. The researchers concluded that people who were overweight had a lower death risk than people of normal weight (Flegal et al., 2005), and the study's methodology was applauded for its rigor. Others argued, however, that if overweight is strongly associated with hypertension, heart disease, diabetes, hyperlipidemia, and sleep apnea, the results of the study appeared to be biologically implausible.

Despite the seemingly contradictory findings, there are studies that help to make sense of the controversy (Corrada et al., 2006; Dahl et al., 2010; Lenz et al., 2009; Reynolds et al., 2005). Being overweight in midlife increases morbidity and physical and mental decline in late life, but it may have no effect on longevity, or may even extend longevity a bit. This may be due to:

- improved medications and surgical procedures that are able to extend life for overweight adults,
- extra weight lowering the risk of hip and other types of fractures that can shorten longevity, and
- the cushion extra weight provides against debilitating weight loss that accompanies many major diseases.

In short, overweight probably does not shorten life expectancy, but it does impact quality of life as people live longer with major diseases. Obesity, though, is not controversial in terms of longevity. It increases death rates by 20%, and for those with extreme obesity, by 200%. Likewise, the graphed relationship between body mass and negative health outcomes is likely to be u- or j-shaped, with increased risk at extremes of both underweight and overweight (Prospective Studies Collaboration, 2009).

BODY COMPOSITION

Body composition is a better measure of health and fitness than body weight. Improving your fat-to-muscle ratio helps protect you from serious ailments and improves your fitness. No one, however, has been able to evaluate the ideal percentage of body weight that should be fat versus lean tissue. Researchers have attempted, though, to develop broad guidelines for body fat ranges for men and women (Table 5.5).

While the relationship between *age and body fat* is less strong than *sex* differences, it is, for both sexes, susceptible to lifestyle intervention. This is important because one study reported that middle-aged and older men with more than 24% body fat, and middle-aged and older women with more than 35% body fat, are at increased risk for heart disease, stroke, various cancers, high blood pressure, diabetes, and degenerative joint disease (Howley & Franks, 1997).

TABLE 5.5 AGE AND RECOMMENDED BODY FAT RANGES

AGE (YEARS)	MEN	WOMEN
18–39	9%–19%	22%–32%
40–59	12%–21%	24%–33%
60–79	14%–24%	25%–35%

Source: From Gallagher, D., Heymsfield, S. B., Heo, M., Jebb, S. A., Murgatroyd, P. R., & Sakamoto, Y. (2000). Healthy percentage body fat ranges: An approach for developing guidelines based on body mass index. American Journal of Clinical Nutrition, *72*, 694–701. https://doi.org/10.1093/ajcn/72.3.694.

There are several ways to measure body fat:

Hydrodensitometry, or underwater weighing, is the gold standard for measuring body fat. It is based on the principle that fat is less dense than water and that overweight persons weigh less in water.

Skinfold caliper is quick and reasonably accurate. Fat is pinched and measured in several areas, including the triceps, suprailium, and thigh for women; and chest, abdomen, and thigh for men. This technique, though, came into use in the 1950s, when people were leaner. A half-century later, nearly 25% of women in their 50s had too much body fat to be measured with the traditional 2-inch calipers, and were being excluded from research samples (Himes, 2001).

Bioelectrical impedance is another way to measure body fat. One electrode is attached to a foot and another to the hand, and a weak electrical current (that is safe and painless) is sent from one electrode to the other. The technique is based on the premise that the signal will travel faster through muscle than fat, because water conducts electricity and muscle is 70% water. Fat, in contrast, is about 9% water.

The *Bod Pod* works on the premise that a muscular body is denser and takes up less space than one that has more fat. The pod chamber has a built-in computer that uses your weight and how much space you take up, and then converts it into a percentage of your body that is fat.

Today there are *apps* that calculate body fat using factors such as weight, height, age, and waist circumference.

There is not only a direct relationship between age and body fat, but an inverse relationship between age and lean muscle mass. This condition is referred to as *sarcopenia*, a gradual loss of muscle mass with age that affects all aging persons regardless of their fitness routine. However, sarcopenia is amenable to intervention through a regular exercise practice, particularly strength building. Women have a greater challenge with sarcopenia due to greater muscle atrophy and higher levels of body fat over time.

DIETS

As mentioned earlier, Americans spend around $90 billion a year on ***diets*** and related attempts to lose weight. Despite this investment, 95% of people who lose weight regain the weight in 5 years, and the percentage of overweight American adults continues to increase. Diets tend to reduce weight in the short run—primarily due to loss of water and high short-term motivation—but invariably prove ineffective in the long run. But they still do not lose their popularity, because along comes another one that this time "really works!"

The *low-carbohydrate, high-protein, and high-fat* diet has been around since the early 1970s, and resurfaced years later as *Dr. Atkins' New Diet Revolution* (1992). Variations of this diet have been developed by Sears, *Entering the Zone* and *Mastering the Zone* (1995, 1997); Steward et al., *Sugar Busters* (1998); Agatston, *South Beach Diet* (2003); and the latest one, the *Keto Diet* (which used to be for specific medical conditions like epilepsy) that recommends even higher levels of fat intake and lower levels of carbohydrates and protein than previous diets. These high-fat types of diets are unique in their popularity and in the number of research studies that support them—much to the surprise of many experts. But after a year or two, the weight loss is typically partially or fully regained (Atallah et al., 2014).

Dr. Jules Hirsch, former emeritus professor and physician in chief at Rockefeller University, had been researching obesity for nearly 60 years, cautioned dieters about low-carbohydrate, high-protein, and high-fat diets: "When carbohydrate levels are low in a diet and fat content is high, people lose water" (Kolata, 2012). I suspect most people prefer to lose fat rather than water.

High-fat foods and protein do promote satiety. In order to satisfy hunger, though, one need not engage in an Atkins or similar diet programs, but just greater consumption of high-fiber complex carbohydrates, lean protein, monounsaturated fats, and polyunsaturated omega-3 fats. Sound familiar? This is similar to the well-known *Mediterranean diet*.

There are problems not only with high-fat diets, but low-fat diets as well. Low-fat diets have not been particularly effective (Tobias et al., 2015). Moreover, there is a major concern with removing fat from your diet, one of which was voiced by the Irish dramatist George Bernard Shaw: "No diet should attempt to remove all the fat from your body, because the brain is entirely fat; without a brain, you might still look good, but all you could do is run for public office."

On a positive note, one meta-analysis (Atallah et al., 2014) that focused on the gold standard of research design—randomized controlled trials—found that *Weight Watchers*, a calorie-restricted diet with a behavior modification plan, achieved more long-term success compared with a control group. It encourages participation in a weekly support group meeting and a nutritional strategy that assigns a point value based on calories, fat, and fiber content. Dieters are allocated a preferred number of total points each day, which they can spend any way they like. Adding exercise to one's daily routine allows for additional points to be spent. It has done well in other controlled studies (Heshka et al., 2003; Tsai & Wadden, 2005).

The latest word on diets that focus on reducing fat or carbohydrates is that they can work if you focus on food quality and not calorie counting—which is more typical of these diets. Healthy fats and complex carbohydrates can help prevent heart disease, diabetes, and other diseases, as evidenced by one expensive, $8 million study funded by the National Institutes of Health (Gardner et al., 2018). The participants were divided between low-fat and low-carbohydrate diets, and the ones who lost weight on both diets ignored calories and focused on quality foods (again, similar to the Mediterranean diet).

And now a few thoughts on religion-based diets. *Christian weight-loss programs* began in 1957 when Presbyterian minister Charlie Shedd urged his readers to pray their weight away. During the 1990s, Christian diet books and church-based weight-loss programs began to proliferate, combining evangelical theology, psychology, and nutrition education. Critics have expressed concern about the accuracy of the nutritional advice and the questionable association between losing weight and gaining God's approval (Box 5.2).

One of the more successful Christian diet books was Shamblin's (1997) *The Weigh Down Diet*. This book sold more than a million copies and was followed up with a second book, *Rise Above* (Shamblin, 2000). One concern with her advice is that despite her background as a registered dietitian, Shamblin advocated that even people with serious weight problems should turn to God rather than to medical professionals. "Trust God, not exercise. The only exercise you need is getting down on your knees to pray."

About 4,000 overweight people each year undertake a pilgrimage to Durham, North Carolina, in order to participate in weight-loss and nutrition programs, as well as to transfer $51 million into the city's economy. These programs are effective, with one caveat: When you return home, the weight returns as well. The programs provide group support, a supportive culture, personal attention, and medical care associated with weight problems—none of which are brought back home.

A surprising intervention for keeping off extra weight is yoga, despite the fact that it doesn't burn off much in the way of calories. Researchers found that people in their 50s who regularly practiced yoga lost about 5 lbs over 10 years, whereas a comparison

BOX 5.2 You Need Divine Intervention to Choose Among Religion-Based Diet Programs

The religion-based diet programs are, to state the obvious, mostly unscientific, and some are a bit eccentric as well. The Hallelujah Diet by Rev. George Malkmus was inspired by the Bible's Book of Genesis, chapter 1, verse 29: "And God said, 'Behold, I have given you every plant yielding seed which is upon the face of all the earth, and every tree with seed in its fruit; you shall have them for food'." Therefore, this vegan diet basically consists of fruits and vegetables, and 80% of what is eaten must be raw.

The Maker's Diet was created by Jordan Rubin, a Messianic Jew, who drew his inspiration from the book of Leviticus, and discourages readers away from the vegan regimen of the Hallelujah Diet. Instead, it promotes organic meat and nonpasteurized dairy products. Another program called Bod4God relies on God and low carbohydrates. Pastor Steve Reynolds leads this program in Baptist churches across America, and he has his work cut out for him, as Baptists have the highest rates of obesity among several denominations studied (Salmon, 2007).

It is unclear whether incorporating any type of religious ideology into a weight-loss or weight-management program is helpful to participants in terms of guidance, motivation, or other factors. Regardless of the ideological content, however, program participants in synagogues and churches that follow nutritiously sound diets—a major qualifier—can take advantage of the fellowship, trust, and support that typifies these settings.

Do you know older adults who are open to change in their own eating patterns? Do you think the persons you have in mind would be more or less motivated to attend a program located in their religious institution? Would they be more or less motivated to attend if there were dietary practices linked to religious ideology compatible with their own beliefs?

QUESTION: If you had developed your own weight-loss program and you wanted to pilot-test this program with older adults in your community, which of these three sites would you choose: a physician's office, a religious institution, or a shopping mall? Why?

group, controlled for physical activity and diet and didn't practice yoga, gained more than 13 lbs (Kristal et al., 2005). The researchers believed that yoga helped people cultivate awareness of their emotions that make them more likely to overeat (Caldwell et al., 2022).

Ridiculous Diets

Some of the previously described diets were ridiculous, but in this section I up the ante. The most unique weight-loss program is "fidgeting," or what researchers so eloquently refer to as *nonexercise-induced thermogenesis* (Levine et al., 2005). Spontaneous fidgeting can make a significant contribution to daily energy expenditure, whereas nonfidgeters may experience a 10% additional weight gain. Fidgeting is likely to be genetically based, however, and it is unlikely that patients can be successfully counseled to fidget more.

Along this same vein was a purported study (no reference provided) in *Health* magazine that reported on gum chewing. Chomping for an hour on a big wad of sugarless gum raises the metabolic rate 19% and burns 11 extra calories. The researchers alleged that chewing gum every waking hour can knock off 10 lbs a year. It would seem to me that chewing gum every waking hour and missing three meals a day would result in a weight loss of more than 10 lbs a *week*—until there was no more you. (See Exhibit 5.2 for a similar fanciful diet—author unknown.)

The *Imaginary Diet* was reported in the prestigious journal *Science* (Morewedge et al., 2010). People who first imagined themselves eating several pieces of a specific food became less likely to gorge on that specific food afterward. The imagining habituates you to the real thing and lessens your desire to eat as much of it. The best part of this diet is the—imaginary for the time being—cookbook. It would be all pictures, the first diet flip book.

Perhaps the most preposterous diet was practiced by the *Breatharians*, who allegedly lived off the air and the energy from sunlight. This fasting to the extreme led to several recruits dying of starvation or dehydration, as well as lawsuits (LaGesse, 2002). ***Calorie restriction***, intermittent fasting, and elimination of various components of diet have all been proposed for enhancing longevity (and supported in some animal model studies), but the jury is still out for effects on human aging.

This suggests that the last word on diets should be given to the late comedian and quasi-nutritionist Art Buchwald, who said the word *diet* comes from the verb *to die*.

EXHIBIT 5.2 THE 10-CALORIE DIET

MONDAY	Breakfast:	Weak tea
	Lunch:	1 Bouillon cube in ½ cup of diluted water
	Dinner:	1 Pigeon thigh and 30 oz. of prune juice (gargle only)
TUESDAY	Breakfast:	Crumbs scraped from burned toast
	Lunch:	½ dozen doughnut holes
	Dinner:	2 Jellyfish skins
WEDNESDAY	Breakfast:	Boiled out tablecloth stains
	Lunch:	½ dozen poppy seeds
	Dinner:	Bee knees and mosquitoes sautéed in vinegar
THURSDAY	Breakfast:	Shredded eggshell skin
	Lunch:	Belly buttons from navel oranges
	Dinner:	2 Eyes from Irish potatoes
FRIDAY	Breakfast:	2 Lobster antennae
	Lunch:	1 Guppy fin
	Dinner:	1 Filet of softshell crab claw
SATURDAY	Breakfast:	4 Chopped banana seeds
	Lunch:	Broiled butterfly liver
	Dinner:	Jellyfish vertebrae
SUNDAY	Breakfast:	Pickled hummingbird tongue
	Lunch:	Prime rib of tadpoles
	Dinner:	Aroma of empty custard pie plate, tossed with paprika, and 1 cloverleaf

The first week you lose 50 lb, the second week you lose another 50 lb, and the third week we lose you.

Happy Holiday!

The good news is that many Americans gain only four fifths of a pound during the mid-November to mid-January holiday period. The bad news is that this gain may not be reversed during the rest of the year, and this translates to a 24-lb weight gain over 30 years of celebrating the end-of-year holidays (Yanovski et al., 2000).

BARIATRIC SURGERY

Bariatric surgery is the surgical modification of the gastrointestinal tract for the purpose of initiating substantial weight loss. Common types of bariatric surgery include sleeve gastrectomy, gastric bypass, and adjustable gastric banding. In sleeve gastrectomy, surgeons remove up to 80% of the stomach using a stapling device. Gastric bypass (Roux-en-Y) reduces the size of the stomach and changes its connection to the small intestine. Gastric banding slows passage of food into the stomach. Owing to the possibility of complications, subsequent dietary restrictions, and expense, this technique is often reserved for clients with extreme obesity—those with a BMI of 40 or more, or a BMI of 35 or more for Medicare patients—who have attempted nonsurgical weight loss without success.

There is continuing controversy over whether obesity is a disease or just a failure in individual willpower. Perhaps the best argument for the former—that it is not just a disease, but an epidemic—is that the prevalence of overweight and obesity has increased dramatically rather quickly in the United States and has spread to all developed and some developing countries. At the same time, the food and drink industry has marketed their products relentlessly, vending machines are ubiquitous, calorie-dense foods have been government subsidized, fast-food restaurants have proliferated, and so forth. One person's willpower is no match for this societal onslaught.

In 2002, the Internal Revenue Service designated *obesity as a disease*, allowing eligible taxpayers who spend over 7.5% of adjusted gross income on medical care because of obesity to deduct expenses for bariatric surgery (as well as weight-loss drugs and nutritional counseling). In 2004, the Centers for Medicare & Medicaid Services (CMS) followed suit, reversing a long-standing policy and opening the door for Medicare reimbursement for bariatric surgery. Declaring obesity a disease was necessary because Medicare is limited to treatments for illness and injury based on the 1965 law that created it. (The AMA, tardy as usual, declared obesity a disease in 2013.) A similar process is at work for approval of the current generation of GLP-1 drugs, first approved in 2021, which are effective for weight loss (losses of 15%–20% of body weight compared to 5% for lifestyle interventions) and offer many other health benefits but which unfortunately are expensive (Ard et al., 2024).

In 2006, the CMS began to cover bariatric surgery for older adults, provided they had a BMI of 35 or more, at least one obesity-related condition, and unsuccessfully attempted weight loss without surgery. Just prior to this Medicare policy change, bariatric surgeries overall rose from 47,000 in 2001 to an almost fourfold increase in 4 years—to 170,000 in 2005. Given the high percentage of obese baby boomers becoming eligible for Medicare in the coming years, the number of bariatric surgeries is expected to increase accordingly. In 2021, over 280,000 bariatric operations were performed, according to the American Society for Bariatric and Metabolic Surgery (Clapp et al., 2022). With increasing use of GLP-1 receptor agonist medications (semaglutide and liraglutide) for control of obesity, bariatric surgery has begun to decline in 2023 (Lin, Mehrotra, & Tsai, 2024). Going forward, the most likely scenario is a combination of GLP-1 use and bariatric surgery, as patients may take the medication before surgery and also use it for weight management following surgery.

A major concern with bariatric surgery has been complications. Complications increased costs by 20% and included vomiting, diarrhea, hernias, infections, pneumonia, respiratory failure, and fistulas.

Improved surgical techniques have lowered the complication rate by two thirds (Chang et al., 2014). By 2015, though, longer term studies revealed that women (but not men) who had undergone bariatric surgery were at increased risk of developing fractures and osteoporosis. Malabsorption and possibly endocrine effects in women may play a role in the reduction of bone-mineral density in the femur a year after surgery.

When bariatric surgery was first approved by Medicare, reimbursement was linked to having it done in accredited facilities that specialized in the procedure and were designated as "centers of excellence." About 750 U.S. inpatient and outpatient bariatric centers became accredited centers. Much to the consternation of surgical groups, Medicare dropped the accreditation requirement for bariatric surgery facilities in 2013. Nonetheless, complications from bariatric surgery appear to have declined and are roughly the same for persons age 60+ as for younger adults (Berger et al., 2018). Moreover, long-term results for weight loss are positive. A decade after surgery, more than 70% of patients kept more than 20% of their starting weight off (Maciejewski et al., 2016).

Surprisingly, bariatric surgery not only reduces weight but also places type 2 diabetes into remission 74% of the time after 1 year follow up (Madsen et al., 2019). Also unexpectedly, the effects of glycemic control *preceded* the substantial weight loss rather than the reverse (Saliba et al., 2009). One possible explanation for this phenomenon might have to do with changes in hormonal effects accompanying the surgery. Thus, the Medicare program is considering covering bariatric surgery for diabetes alone.

There is also evidence that the results of bariatric surgery for the severely obese, versus those who did not opt for surgery, are beneficial for not only weight loss and diabetes remission, but for the control of hypertension, cholesterol, sleep apnea, heart attacks, strokes, and death (Fisher et al., 2018).

Bariatric surgery can also lead to interesting interpersonal outcomes, according to one study. Adults who had undergone the procedure were twice as likely to marry as a control group that did not get the procedure. Also, if married, they are 40% more likely to get divorced, with an increase in jealousy and feelings of not being needed by the partner (Bruze et al., 2018). Bariatric surgery also improves work outcome, such as earnings, absenteeism, and presenteeism (Alfonso-Cristancho et al., 2016).

MEDICARE COVERAGE FOR WEIGHT-LOSS COUNSELING

If you have a BMI of 30 or higher, Medicare will pay for one ***weight-loss counseling*** session a week for the first month, then five more monthly sessions. If you have lost at least 6.6 lbs by the end of the sixth month, you can get six more monthly sessions. If you have not, you must wait six more months before Medicare will cover another weight-loss attempt. Weight-loss sessions are covered under Medicare Part B, with no copayment or deductible if they are conducted by a qualified practitioner in a primary care setting.

In 2014, the third full year of counseling coverage, less than 1% of eligible Medicare recipients took advantage of this benefit. Some attribute this extraordinarily slow adoption of coverage to the policy of limiting the service to primary care doctors' offices. The argument against allowing referrals to weight-loss counseling specialists in the community is the difficulty with assessing diverse credentials. Just about everyone in the weight-loss or fitness business would want to be able to bill Medicare for obesity counseling.

10 TIPS FOR WEIGHT LOSS OR MAINTENANCE

Here are ***10 tips for weight loss and maintenance***:

1. *Motivation*. Is the client motivated by functioning better, that is, more energy, better mood, and so forth? Or are they motivated by avoiding or alleviating the impact of heart disease, arthritis, and other age-related maladies? Or perhaps the client is primarily motivated by appearance? The challenge is to find out which motivation works best, and then encourage the client to be conscious of that motivation on a daily basis, perhaps through strategically placed written reminders.
2. *Modest*. Clearly, a loss of 1 lb each week is more achievable than a 40-lb weight-loss goal with no particular time frame in mind. An even more modest goal is to avoid a focus on poundage and to focus instead on improved nutrition and exercise; that is, establish a goal to eat one additional fruit and vegetable each day, to substitute one whole-grain product for a refined one each day, or to walk briskly an additional time or two each week.
3. *Measurable*. Make sure that the client's goal is measurable, and be sure to provide, at least at first, an end point. A 1-month time frame is a good first target after which reassessment takes place. Does the client's measurable goal modestly allow them to have days off during the week or an exemption during a holiday or special event?
4. *Memory*. Can clients place a subtle, or not-so-subtle, sign on the refrigerator? Can a list be prepared before going food shopping? Do clients need a friend to call regularly to remind and motivate them?
5. *Positive Thoughts*. It is hard to nurture positive thoughts when the average person has several failed attempts before succeeding at weight loss. Hard, but not impossible. Encourage clients to be persistent, until positive thoughts finally match positive deeds.
6. *Reinforcement*. Losing weight or maintaining a desired weight tends to be reinforcing in its own right. If clients need additional external reinforcement, just about any reinforcement not involving food will do.
7. *Environmental Support*. If at all possible, keep junk food out of the house. Have a jar of healthy snacks handy. Place health magazines around the house. Keep enjoyable activities (crossword puzzle, letter writing, organizing a photo album) at strategic locations in the house, as a substitute activity for snacking. Ban eating in front of the television/computer.
8. *Stress Management*. Emotional disturbances can lead to poor eating habits. One of the best stress managers is also the best technique for long-term maintenance of weight loss—exercise. For most people, timing exercise before meals decreases appetite; timing it between meals, when you are most likely to snack, can take your mind off eating. Deep breathing or progressive muscle relaxation may help with stress.
9. *Social Support*. Someone who used to be overweight and has kept the weight off makes for a particularly effective social support person. But just about any person who genuinely cares for the person will do. Multiple sources of support are preferable.
10. *Problem Solve*. Examine failed previous attempts at achieving a desired weight, or anticipate new problems likely to emerge in the near future. Keep a record of what is eaten, where it is eaten, and who it is eaten with, and try to reduce unhealthy eating patterns triggered by emotions.

DIET DRUGS

For the past several years, the FDA has approved about one new drug for weight loss per year. Yet the best-selling diet pill prescribed in America, phentermine, was approved in 1959, and still commands about 80% of the market, with over 2 million prescriptions annually (https://clincalc.com/DrugStats/Drugs/Phentermine). Its generic status allows it to be produced by several manufacturers, who compete in part by lowering the cost, often to about $30 a month.

The drug is considered relatively safe and effective for jump-starting diets, but can be misused. A particularly unfortunate case of misuse occurred in the 1990s when phentermine was combined with fenfluramine, to create fen-phen. Prescriptions for fen-phen increased by 6,390% in the 4 years before it was taken off the market in 1997. The drug worked by curbing people's appetites, and studies reported the average weight loss to be about 20 lbs in the first year. The drug, however, was linked to heart valve abnormalities, pulmonary hypertension, and brain cell damage.

Current misuse focuses on the drug intensifying existing heart problems or being abused by people with eating disorders, often at normal or below-normal weights. Also, it is only approved for short-term use, as persons often develop a tolerance and require higher doses. Many physicians, however, prescribe it for long-term use, fail to monitor blood pressure, or prescribe the drug for people who are of normal weight.

Defenders of ***diet drugs*** proclaim that the hazards from serious obesity are far greater risks, resulting in 300,000 deaths per year from heart disease, diabetes, kidney disease, and stroke. Proponents were successful in getting the first over-the-counter weight-loss pill, Alli, approved by the FDA in 2006. The drug has been associated with side effects such as diarrhea and oily stools.

An herbal mixture used at Nutrisystem weight-loss centers was called Herbal Phen-Fen, a combination of St. John's wort and ephedra. *Ephedra*, a herb that is also known as ma huang, is a major constituent in many herbal weight-loss products and appeared to work in the short run. Ephedra was also the likely culprit in approximately 800 health problems reported to the FDA, including more than 40 deaths.

In 2004, the FDA banned the sale of dietary supplements containing ephedra—the first time the FDA had banned a dietary supplement since the Dietary Supplement Health and Education Act, an industry-friendly piece of legislation, passed in 1994. In 2005, though, the ban was partially overturned to permit low-ephedra products, with fewer than 10 milligrams, to be sold.

A U.S. House Committee passed The Treat and Reduce Obesity Act of 2023, which allows Medicare Part D to cover the cost of weight-loss drugs. This change in Medicare policy was spurred by the success of the new GLP-1 medications such as Ozempic, Wegovy, and Zepbound. The change has not yet received full approval, however, which will be critical in determining whether other insurers follow.

COMPETITIVE EATING AND IMPLICATIONS FOR ADVOCACY

Given America's fixation on food and on competitive events, it was not surprising to find out that there is an International Federation of Competitive Eating, and most of the events take place in America. The most popular ***competitive eating*** event takes place in Coney Island, New York, on July 4 each year, and is hosted by Nathan's Famous, a fast-food restaurant known for its hot dogs. Nathan's has sponsored this annual event almost every year since 1916.

One dominant gurgitator (competitive eater) was a relatively slender Japanese man named Takeru Kobayashi, who won the contest every year from 2001 to 2006, capping it off with his record-breaking 53.75 dogs in 12 minutes on July 4, 2006. Kobayashi's technique was to separate the bun, dip it in water to condense it (yum!), and eat it separately from the hot dog. His 6-year reign was followed by a 9-year reign by the American Joey Chestnut—who lost in 2015. Apparently champion gurgitators eventually poop out (no pun intended).

Although Steve "the Terminator" Keiner ate only 20 hot dogs at one of Nathan's Annual Hot Dog Eating Contests, he was quite proud of his very American strategy—a pile-driver approach, keeping hot dog and bun together as he rammed them down his throat. When explaining his eating philosophy, the Terminator said he combines the American pile-driving strategy with a Zen philosophy: "I went down a path that the hot dog was one with me and I was one with the universe."

Aside from the fact that these competitions are too disgusting for most of us to watch, there is something sad and funny about this anecdote. Sad, because many Americans have an unhealthy relationship with food. Besides the excess weight, gorging on food can pose immediate health dangers. Funny, because Americans are a diverse and tolerant lot, and perhaps we do not need to get the Wellness Police to shut down a New York tradition into its ninth decade.

There is a similar conflict in the attitude regarding obesity. Most persons would argue that obesity is unhealthy and we need to do as much as possible to reduce this epidemic. Yet a growing number of health promoters advocate a more laissez-faire approach because some overweight Americans are fit and should be left alone, and others are not helped by the stigma and rejection that add to their burden.

A more laissez-faire approach toward overweight *people*, however, does not necessarily mean a do-nothing approach in *society*. The food industry spends more than $30 billion on marketing food each year, and the government spends only a tiny fraction of that amount on nutrition education ($907 million; https://www.gao.gov/products/gao-19-572). What should be done to address this imbalance? Unfortunately, most of the emphasis continues to be on what *people* should do, not changes in society.

THE END OF OVEREATING

In his book, *The End of Overeating*, Kessler (2009), former commissioner of the FDA, pointed out that the average weight of Americans grew by three quarters of a pound each and every year between 1960 and 2000. Something else happened beyond a sudden decline of individual willpower to instigate this multidecade epidemic.

Kessler argued that a major culprit is that food manufacturers have learned how to combine fat, sugar, and salt in order to stimulate dopamine in the brain, for an effect as powerful as drugs like cocaine or amphetamines. Then the manufacturers added on the emotional gloss of advertising, eating tasty foods with friends, and having a good time, and food products became addictive.

What to do about it? Kessler argued that we should limit the advertising of foods that have excessive combinations of fat, sugar, and salt, and increase the number of messages about the consequences of unhealthy foods. Also, practice these six tips:

1. Determine ahead of time what you will eat for meals and snacks.
2. Figure out how much food you need, and put it on your plate. No seconds.
3. Select foods that satisfy, rather than stimulate, such as whole grains, fruits, and vegetables, and combine them with lean protein and a small amount of fat.
4. Anticipate what to do when you encounter stimulating food, and rehearse your response.

5. Recognize emotions like sadness and anxiety that stimulate overeating.
6. Remove the image of a trigger food in your mind before you start to debate whether or not to eat it.

SUMMARY

Aging and physical vulnerability go hand in hand, so it is not surprising that older adults pay particular attention to what they eat and drink. Dehydration, constipation, hypertension, overweight, and malnourishment are just some of the age-related challenges facing older adults. Fortunately, much of what older adults need to know about nutrition has been around for more than a century. In 1917, the USDA declared that vegetables, fruits, and fibers were healthy, and sugar and salt need to be limited.

Since that time, researchers have been busy and we know that there is good fat and bad fat, that dietary cholesterol is not the big deal we once thought, that sodium sensitivity increases with age, that hydration becomes increasingly important as the thirst perception declines with age, that food has become more caloric and ubiquitous, and that the obesity epidemic shows no sign of relenting.

The good news is that the Mediterranean diet is becoming more popular, and research consistently demonstrates that it positively affects our health. The bad news is that the proliferation of less credible diets, the increasing prevalence of food and drink advertising, and the escalating spread of fast-food restaurants are not helpful in our quest for good health.

Medicare recognizes that not only is obesity a disease, but it is an epidemic in America. Funding weight-management counseling for older adults is a step in the right direction. It is an incredibly small step, however, when less than 1% of Medicare beneficiaries take advantage of this benefit. Approval of GLP-1 medications for Medicare Part D coverage may have a greater effect. But neither addresses the fundamental challenge of an industry and lifestyle that has turned food into a source of ill health.

Perhaps the best-known nutrition expert in the United States, Michael Pollan, states it best: "Eat food, not too much, mostly plants." Less credible, though more entertaining, is Jack LaLanne's maxim: "If it tastes good, spit it out."

SPRINGER PUBLISHING CONNECT™ | **A robust set of instructor resources designed to supplement this text is located at http://connect.springerpub.com/content/book/978-0-8261-8386-6. Qualifying instructors may request access by emailing textbook@springerpub.com.**

REFERENCES

Only key references appear in the print edition. The full reference list can be accessed by visiting www.springerpub.com/courseconnect. See inside front cover and tear-out card for CourseConnect details.

Ard, J. D., Lewis, K. H., & Moore, J. B. (2024). Lifestyle interventions for obesity in the era of GLP-1 receptor agonists. *Journal of the American Medical Association*, *332*(1), 16–18. https://doi.org/10.1001/Jama.2024.7062

Burman, M., Hörnsten, C., Öhlin, J., Olofsson, B., Nordström, P., & Gustafson, Y. (2022). Prevalence of obesity and malnutrition in four cohorts of very old adults, 2000–2017. *The Journal of Nutrition, Health and Aging*, *26*(7), 706–713. https://doi.org/10.1007/s12603-022-1820-x

Carson, J. A. S., Lichtenstein, A. H., Anderson, C. A., Appel, L. J., Kris-Etherton, P. M., Meyer, K. A., Petersen, K., Polonsky, T., & Van Horn, L. (2020). Dietary cholesterol and cardiovascular risk: A science advisory from the American Heart Association. *Circulation, 141*(3), e39–e53. https://doi.org/10.1161/CIR.0000000000000743

Hales, C. M., Carroll, M. D., Fryar, C. D., & Ogden, C. L. (2020). *Prevalence of obesity and severe obesity among adults: United States, 2017–2018*. NCHS Data Brief, No. 360. National Center for Health Statistics.

Jackson, S. L., King, S. M., Zhao, L., & Cogswell, M. E. (2016). Prevalence of excess sodium intake in the United States—NHANES, 2009–2012. *MMWR Morbidity and Mortality Weekly Report, 64*(52), 1393–1397. https://doi.org/10.15585/mmwr.mm6452a1

Liu, B., Du, Y., Wu, Y., Snetselaar, L. G., Wallace, R. B., & Bao, W. (2021). Trends in obesity and adiposity measures by race or ethnicity among adults in the United States 2011–18: Population based study. *British Medical Journal, 372*, n365. https://doi.org/10.1136/bmj.n365

Song, J., Brown, M. K., Tan, M., MacGregor, G. A., Webster, J., Campbell, N. R., Trieu, K., Ni Mhurchu, C., Cobb, L. K., & He, F. J. (2021). Impact of color-coded and warning nutrition labelling schemes: A systematic review and network meta-analysis. *PLoS Medicine, 18*(10), e1003765.

Yuan, Y., Jin, A., Neal, B., Feng, X., Qiao, Q., Wang, H., Zhang, R., Li, J., Duan, P., Cao, L., Zhang, H., Hu, S., Li, H., Gao, P., Xie, G., Yuan, J., Cheng, L., Wang, S., Zhang, H., Niu, W., Fang, H., Zhao, M., Gao, R., Chen, J., Elliott, P., Labarthe, D., & Wu, Y. (2023). Salt substitution and salt-supply restriction for lowering blood pressure in elderly care facilities: A cluster-randomized trial. *Nature Medicine, 29*(4), 973–981. https://doi.org/10.1038/s41591-023-02286-8

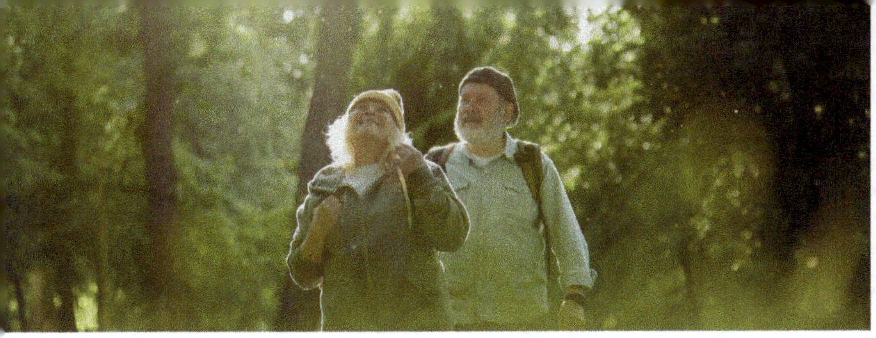

6

COMPLEMENTARY AND ALTERNATIVE MEDICINE AND AGING

KEY TERMS

antioxidant
biomedical model
ConsumerLab.com
Dietary Supplement Health and Education Act
Dietary Supplement Verification Program
dietary supplements
energy therapies
herbs
hormone supplement
manipulative and body-based therapies
mind–body therapies
National Center for Complementary and Integrative Medicine
naturopathy
nutraceuticals
nutritional drinks
vitamins and minerals

LEARNING OBJECTIVES

- Define complementary and alternative medicine (CAM).
- Review the history and accomplishments of the *National Center for Complementary and Integrative Medicine.*
- Contrast CAM and the *biomedical model.*
- Review the usage of CAM among Americans of different ages.
- Differentiate the categories of CAM.
- Describe and assess different types of CAM.
- Define *naturopathy.*
- List CAM techniques covered by medical insurance.
- Assess the accomplishments of Drs. Weil, Chopra, and Oz.
- Define *dietary supplement.*
- Critically evaluate the *Dietary Supplement Health and Education Act.*
- Evaluate the effectiveness of dietary supplements.
- Describe the strengths and limitations of *ConsumerLab.com* and the *Dietary Supplement Verification Program.*
- Define *nutraceuticals.*

Always laugh when you can. It is cheap medicine.

—*George Gordon Byron*

NATIONAL CENTER FOR COMPLEMENTARY AND INTEGRATIVE HEALTH

The Office of Alternative Medicine existed between 1992 and 1998 as the newest and smallest institute of the National Institutes of Health (NIH). In 1998, it was renamed as the National Center for Complementary and Alternative Medicine and, in 2014, renamed once again as the ***National Center for Complementary and Integrative Medicine*** (NCCIM). Its current name is the National Center for Complementary and Integrative Health (NCCIH), with a budget of under $200 million in 2023 (https://www.nccih.nih.gov/about/budget/nccih-funding-appropriations-history).

The name changes—from "complementary" to "alternative" to "integrative" and from "medicine" to "health"—show the challenges of recognizing the varieties of nonmainstream approaches to health. While *integrative* may be a more harmonious term, many of these nonmainstream therapies are used as alternatives to physician- or health professional–guided care (recognizing that health professionals may also recommend these alternative therapies). We use the popular acronym CAM to reflect complementary and alternative medicine.

While NCCIH is a small NIH institute, CAM has exploded in popularity among American consumers with no end in sight. The NIH status of CAM reinforces the need to assess the effectiveness of these practices using the scientific method (Box 6.1).

BOX 6.1 Complementary, Alternative, and Unimpressive?

NCIIH and its predecessors have very little to show for their investment. Large-scale, rigorous government studies have produced few positive findings. Distance prayer heals heart disease? Not a chance. Echinacea cures colds? No. Ginkgo biloba improves memory? Can't remember the findings—because they aren't worth remembering. In summary, almost two decades of increasingly funded CAM research has produced no big wins.

Proponents of CAM suggest that its content areas are hard to research. For example, there are multiple manufacturers of the same herb using different techniques for producing versions of the same product. Would the results be better if another manufacturer, technique, or version of the product were used? There are plants, such as Echinacea, that have nine different species, most of which have not yet been tested. One herbal brand might contain a plant's flowers, another its seeds, and another its stems and leaves, in varying amounts. There are also natural sources versus synthetic forms of some vitamins. Finally, although the government's outlay on CAM research has been growing, it is still a tiny overall investment relative to past and current spending on conventional medications and interventions.

Opponents argue that CAM techniques and products are running far ahead of the science, resulting in true believers/advocates who pressure funding agencies for more research dollars. Some of the studies seem downright foolish from a scientific perspective; for example, distant healing by anonymous prayer (supported by $1.5 million in NCIIH research funds), acupuncture results explained by body meridians, coffee enemas to treat pancreatic cancer, magnets to improve a whole host of bodily problems, lemon or lavender scents to improve arthritis—none of which are based on biological principles.

Where do you stand on this topic? Over the next few years, would you favor giving more, less, or the same funding to the NCIIH? Would you fund CAM studies even if they are not based on a scientific foundation? Would you require multiple successful pilot studies before approving a large-scale CAM grant?

See whether your opinion is strengthened or changed after you read this chapter.

The question of effectiveness is not unique to CAM, as the parallel movement toward more evidence-based medicine in mainstream medicine attests. Nor is the concern over the safety of CAM unique, as it is an issue for allopathic medicine as well. Medical error is the third leading cause of death in the United States (Makary & Daniel, 2016), and medication errors injure approximately 1.3 million people annually in the United States alone (World Health Organization [WHO], 2017).

Despite consistently unimpressive research findings, CAM remains a rapidly growing business, reaching $145 billion in 2023 (Grandview, 2023). This is due, in part, to grandiose, and potentially harmful, expectations. For example, 39% of adult Americans believed alternative medicine can cure cancer according to a 2018 national Harris Poll commissioned by the American Society of Clinical Oncology (2019).

PREVALENCE OF COMPLEMENTARY AND ALTERNATIVE MEDICINE

The majority of American adults participate in some type of complementary or alternative care each year, with 52% taking one or more ***dietary supplements*** (Kantor et al., 2016). This is not surprising, given the more attractive set of characteristics that describe CAM than allopathic medicine (referred to in Table 6.1 as the ***biomedical model***). An analysis of the 2007 National Health Interview Survey found that 38.1 million adults made an estimated 354.2 million visits to practitioners of CAM (Nahin et al., 2009).

The highest period of CAM usage is between the ages 50 and 59, followed by ages 60 to 69 and then ages 40 to 49 (Barnes et al., 2008). These decades include those in the baby boom cohort at the time of the survey (Figure 6.1), making the topic particularly relevant to a book on aging. This should not be surprising, given that CAM techniques are primarily utilized for chronic conditions—conditions that begin to increase in number and severity during the boomers' later years (Falci et al., 2016).

TABLE 6.1 CHARACTERISTICS OF COMPLEMENTARY AND ALTERNATIVE MEDICINE AND THE BIOMEDICAL MODEL

CAM/ALTERNATIVE MEDICINE	BIOMEDICAL MODEL
Patient responsibility	Health professional responsibility
Mind/body/spirit	Body and mind separate
Healer serves as guide	Physician in charge
Holistic	Specialized
Promoting health	Fighting disease

CAM, complementary and alternative medicine.

FIGURE 6.1 Complementary and alternative medicine use among adults and children: United States, 2007.

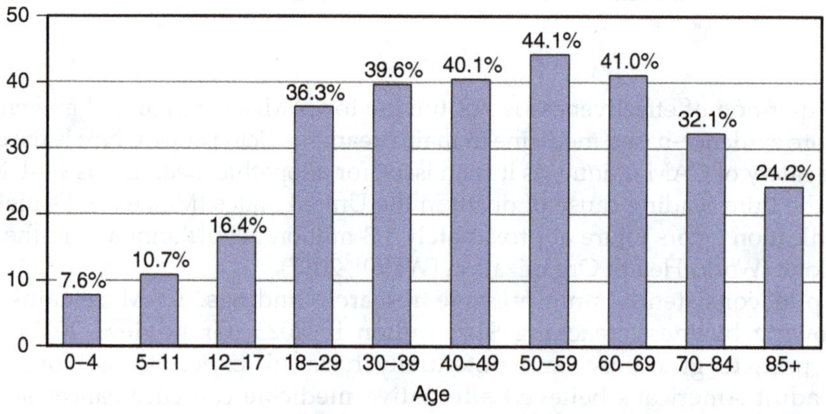

Source: Data from Barnes, P. M., Bloom, B., & Nahin, R. (2008, December). *Complementary and alternative medicine use among adults and children: United States, 2007* (National Health Statistics Report No.12). U.S. Department of Health and Human Services.

COMMUNICATION BARRIER BETWEEN COMPLEMENTARY AND ALTERNATIVE MEDICINE AND ALLOPATHIC MEDICINE

Surveys consistently report that more than half of the participants in CAM therapies neglect to communicate with their physicians about their usage of CAM (Jou & Jonson, 2016). This is true of 52% of older White Americans and 58% of older African Americans (Flaherty et al., 2001). Among Medicare recipients in another study, 58% did not discuss CAM use with their physicians (Astin et al., 2000). Regarding dietary supplement use, one study examined the medical charts of 182 older adults; only 35% of self-reported dietary supplements were documented in the medical charts (Cohen et al., 2002).

There are reasons CAM users may not want to communicate such participation with their physicians. They may believe that their physicians do not approve of their activities, do not understand their motivations, or do not have the expertise to contribute to their own CAM knowledge. The consequences of this lack of communication, however, can be serious.

For instance, over-the-counter herbal therapy—plant-derived preparations to improve function, prevent illness, or counteract pain—can diminish or exacerbate the effects of prescription drugs. CAM can also interfere with cancer treatment. One study of older cancer patients found that 26% used at least one type of CAM and some of these, like St. John's wort, have the potential to interfere with cancer therapy (Nightingale et al., 2015).

TYPES OF COMPLEMENTARY AND ALTERNATIVE MEDICINE

Exactly what constitutes CAM has never been clearly established. Reinforcing this assertion, a definition of CAM that describes what it is not, rather than what it is: "As medical interventions not taught widely at U.S. medical schools or generally available at U.S. hospitals (Eisenberg et al., 1993).

Despite the imprecision, some practices have been consistently associated with CAM, such as herbal medicine and other dietary supplements (Offit, 2012). Other CAM strategies are hard to categorize, such as *homeopathy* (treatment with highly diluted substances that have little or no active chemical content, but that leave an "energy signal") and *chelation therapy* (IV infusion of ethylenediaminetetraacetic acid to bind heavy metals in the bloodstream).

Much of CAM falls into one of the following categories:

Mind–body therapies: Meditation, visualization, prayer, humor, tai chi, yoga, and support groups;
Manipulative and body-based therapies: Chiropractic, massage therapy, postural restructuring, acupuncture, and osteopathic medicine;
Energy therapies: Healing touch, Reiki, magnetic field therapy, and laying-on of hands; and
Whole medical systems: Ayurvedic medicine, traditional Chinese medicine, and naturopathic medicine.

Nutrition and exercise are sometimes included in CAM but they are also claimed by practitioners of allopathic medicine. Providers in mainstream medicine may not be accomplished health educators, but none of them discount the importance of nutrition and exercise.

POPULAR COMPLEMENTARY AND ALTERNATIVE MEDICINE TECHNIQUES

Diaphragmatic Breathing

One symptom of stress is shallow and rapid breathing. A way to counteract this symptom is through diaphragmatic breathing, also called belly breathing, deep breathing, or yoga breathing. This technique is simple, convenient, and has face validity for most adherents. In other words, people feel better quickly.

From a research perspective, the technique's short- or long-term effect on stress management is largely untested, and the results with disease management are mixed (Cahalin et al., 2002; DeGuire et al., 1996). One study on slow breathing, that is, slowing respiration to six breaths/minute, reported a decrease in blood pressure in hypertensives (Joseph et al., 2005). Deep breathing improved exercise capacity and respiratory function in patients with chronic obstructive pulmonary disease (COPD; Hamasaki, 2020).

Progressive Muscle Relaxation

Another symptom of stress is muscle tension. Edmund Jacobson began his work on reducing muscle tension through progressive muscle relaxation in 1908. Jacobson believed that tension can manifest itself in any muscle in the body, and in order to relax, you must learn to differentiate between muscle tension and relaxation. There has been little scientific inquiry to produce evidence in support or refutation of this technique. One systematic review suggested benefit for stress reduction (Muhammad-Khir et al., 2024).

Caution must be observed with this relaxation technique for older people with painful arthritis or a heart condition. Older adults may choose to eliminate or just to imagine the tension phase of the technique, or focus exclusively on visualization, which tends to follow this technique.

Visualization

Relaxation can be further facilitated by following progressive muscle relaxation with 10 minutes of visualization or imagery. One popular image is to recall the warmth of the sun, the sensation of a gentle breeze, the sound and smell of the ocean, and the sight of a swaying palm tree. Just visualize and relax.

Interactive guided imagery is a component of visualization that typically involves guidance by a trained therapist. The therapist may focus on relaxation and visualization and then direct your attention to an ailing part of your body (including internal organs) and ask you to focus healing thoughts on it. One study using guided health imagery with former smokers found that after 24 months, abstinence rates were double for the guided-imagery group versus the placebo control group (Wynd, 2005). Guided imagery reduced symptoms for people approaching the end of life (Correa-Morales et al., 2024).

Relaxation Response, Meditation, and Mindfulness

The relaxation response is based on the technique of meditation, but without the Eastern spiritual overtones. It operates on the premise that the repetition of a sound (like *Om*, considered to be the sound of the universe) or a word (like *one* or *peace*) is equivalent to the repetition of an Eastern philosophy-derived mantra, a one- or two-syllable sound that is part of a meditation technique. (For more information on the relaxation response technique and theory, see Benson's 1984 landmark book, *Beyond the Relaxation Response*.) The repetition of either a Western word or Sanskrit mantra or sound produces the same effect: deep relaxation.

Researchers at the Maharishi University in Fairfield, Iowa, have reported in academic journals that the technique of transcendental meditation—first brought to the United States in the 1950s by Indian guru Maharishi Mahesh Yogi and later popularized by the Beatles—is an effective option for lowering high blood pressure. Through randomized and controlled single-blind trials, the researchers report that meditation lowers blood pressure as effectively as hypertension drugs but without the side effects (Castillo-Richmond et al., 2000; Paul-Labrador et al., 2006) and may decrease mortality in older persons (Schneider et al., 2005). A systematic review showed benefit for anxiety, depression, and pain but "no evidence that meditation programs were better than any active treatment" (Goyal et al., 2014).

Meditation may also be associated with changes in the brain's physical structure. Long-term meditators experienced less age-related gray matter loss compared with matched control persons who did not meditate (Fox et al., 2014; Luders et al., 2015). Also, the prefrontal cortical area—an area of the brain associated with attention—was thicker in meditation participants than in matched control subjects (Lazar et al., 2005). Differences were especially notable in older persons, suggesting that meditation may help reduce the cortical thinning that occurs with age.

Both the relaxation response and meditation are based on the technique of letting thoughts drift away from the mind as they arise. This generally is referred to as emptying one's mind, but in actuality the technique is better described as allowing thoughts to pass through the mind as they arise, while the participant keeps returning to the chosen repetitive sound. Although repeating a sound or word is the most popular meditative device, some people prefer to visually focus on the center of a yantra (a geometric form), or to imagine a peaceful scene (such as the beach or the woods), or to mindfully pay attention to their inhalation and exhalation patterns, or to chant.

Stress management techniques such as meditation are deceptively simple—the technique is easy to learn but difficult to sustain. To help develop a stress management habit, it is important to establish a consistent routine and it is helpful to have a partner to reinforce your practice.

One form of meditation, *mindfulness*, is defined as paying attention to one's immediate experience, whether it be breathing, eating a grape slowly, or walking (also referred to as a walking meditation). This technique is a focus on the present moment with curiosity, openness, and acceptance. One researcher argues that this technique is particularly relevant to older adults attempting to cope with chronic disease, pain, and disability (Rejeski, 2008).

Older adults who were assigned mindfulness meditation improved their sleep quality and had fewer symptoms of insomnia and fatigue than those who had received standard care for sleep problems (Black et al., 2015). Mindfulness also appeared to mediate the association between age and negative affect (Raes et al., 2015). Finally, a mindfulness program decreased chronic low back pain and improved function. Six months later, though, when sessions were reduced to monthly, the function returned to baseline (Morone et al., 2016). Positive results with reducing chronic low pain were similar between mindfulness and cognitive behavioral therapy in another study (Turner et al., 2016). Meta-analyses and systematic reviews of clinical trials present small or null effects for cognition (Sanchez-Lara et al., 2021), anxiety (Li & Bressington, 2019), and pain (Hilton et al., 2017).

Acupuncture

One major source of stress is having to cope with chronic physical pain. In 1997, a committee of independent physicians and scientists at the NIH reviewed a wide range of research findings and concluded that acupuncture treatment—the 2,500-year-old Chinese needle therapy that has been on the fringe of American medicine for years—is effective for pain control and nausea and has promise to be beneficial in other areas as well. Efforts to assess the benefits of acupuncture continue (Lu et al., 2022).

The NIH committee encouraged insurers, both public and private, to cover acupuncture services for nausea caused by anesthesia, chemotherapy, and pregnancy, as well as for postoperative dental pain (NIH Consensus Development Panel on Acupuncture, 1998). Only 19% of health plans provide acupuncture benefits, however, and Medicare is not one of them. According to 2010 to 2019 Medical Expenditure Panel Survey data, about half of acupuncture visits were covered by health insurance (Candon et al., 2022). Medicare Part B began reimbursement for acupuncture in 2020.

The Chinese theory behind acupuncture—that the body is made up of channels of energy flow called qi (pronounced *chee*) and that inserting needles into specific points on the body relieves energy blockages along these channels—has not received support from Western science. Research does support the idea, though, that acupuncture needles inserted into specific nerve junction points on the body and rotated or electrically stimulated will increase the production of the body's own natural painkilling chemicals (Lin et al., 2022).

Currently, all but three states have licensed or regulated the practice of acupuncture by nonphysicians and provided training standards for certification (https://www.nccaom.org/state-licensure/). The Food and Drug Administration (FDA) regulates the needles as part of its medical device authority. The number of acupuncturists in the United States numbers at about 10,000 (https://www.bls.gov/oes/current/oes291291.htm), including physicians who are members of the American Academy of Medical Acupuncture. To find a licensed or certified specialist, contact the National Certification Commission for Acupuncture and Oriental Medicine (www.nccaom.org) or the American Academy of Medical Acupuncturists (www.medicalacupuncture.org).

Research into the effects of acupuncture on cocaine addiction, rheumatoid arthritis, low back pain, asthma, emesis, and myocardial disease has been mostly negative (Berman et al., 2004; Margolin et al., 2002; Shen et al., 2000; Vickers et al., 2004; Witt et al., 2005). However, women with moderate to severe menopausal symptoms reported significant symptom relief from an acupuncture treatment (Lund et al., 2019). Also, the placebo effect—sham acupuncture, which consists of needles placed superficially at nonacupuncture sites—can have a positive impact on participants with tension headaches or knee pain (Melchart et al., 2005; Witt et al., 2005). Older adults have seen improvements in sleep and pain after acupuncture (Chen et al., 2020).

To find information about *acupressure*—pressure applied by hands rather than needles—consult the American Organization for Bodywork Therapies of Asia, at www.aobta.org. One randomized, double-blind study with patients in six dementia units in Taiwan reported that acupressure applied to older residents with dementia decreased agitation and aggressive behaviors in comparison with a control group (Lin et al., 2009).

Therapeutic Massage

Chances are you will feel better after a good massage. In addition, some studies suggest that a therapeutic massage has a greater impact on lower back pain than does acupuncture (Cherkin et al., 2001) and produces migraine relief as well (Field, 2016; Hernandez-Reif, 2001; Hernandez-Reif et al., 2001). For a listing of licensed professionals in your area, contact the American Massage Therapy Association (www.amtamassage.org).

Chiropractic

Chiropractors focus on spinal and extremity manipulation, physical medicine modalities, rehabilitation, and nutrition. They are licensed in all 50 states and can become board certified in such subspecialties as orthopedics, sports medicine, and nutrition.

Patients seek chiropractic doctors for musculoskeletal disorders, with low back pain being the most likely referral. Several studies report that, compared with medical treatment for low back pain, manipulation by chiropractors provided as much or more pain relief, higher activity levels, and greater patient satisfaction (Hurwitz et al., 2002; Sierpina, 2001), but systematic reviews have questioned these results (Parkinson et al., 2013).

One study reported that chiropractors spent more time with their patients than physicians, explaining their treatment for low back pain and advising them about self-care once they get home (Hertzman-Miller et al., 2002). Consequently, chiropractic patients were more satisfied with their care than with physicians' care. Differences in satisfaction disappeared, however, when equal time was spent by the two types of professionals on explanations about their technique and the offering of advice about self-care. It should also be noted that chiropractic manipulation is not without risk (Gouveia et al., 2009).

Hypnosis

A committee of independent physicians and scientists at the NIH reported that hypnosis may be effective for treating some types of pain. Hypnosis is a deep state of relaxation, accompanied by inertia, passivity, and a narrowing of consciousness. This technique has considerable potential for reducing anxiety and has been used with patients undergoing coronary angioplasty (Kanji et al., 2004) and other medical procedures (Häuser et al., 2016).

Guides are available to help clients learn self-hypnosis (Davis et al., 2000), and there is a professional society that focuses on hypnosis research (Society for Clinical and Experimental Hypnosis, http://www.sceh.us; American Society of Clinical Hypnosis, https://asch.net/).

Biofeedback

The NIH committee recommended biofeedback for tension headaches. The biofeedback practitioner hooks you up to a machine to make you aware of bodily processes that you do not ordinarily notice—muscle tension, skin surface temperature, brain wave activity, skin conductivity or moisture, blood pressure, and heart rate—so that you can bring them under voluntary control (Kennedy & Parker, 2019).

Magnet Therapy

A few poorly controlled studies with positive results generated substantial publicity for the healing power of magnets and has led to over $700 million in sales of magnets in

2022 (https://www.linkedin.com/pulse/magnetic-therapy-devices-market-2023-fastest-growing/). When studies began to use control groups and participants proved to be unsure who was wearing real versus sham magnets (Collacott et al., 2000), or ionized versus placebo bracelets (Bratton et al., 2002), no differences in pain relief were found. Failure of blinding and placebo effects may be responsible for positive results (Hinman et al., 2002).

Aromatherapy

Evidence of the use of aromatherapy dates back thousands of years. The technique is based on the practice of treating people with essential oils extracted from plants. There is speculation that beyond the effects of the treatment's pleasant smell, the oils may affect the nervous system when inhaled or absorbed by the skin.

One study found that 60% of severely demented patients who had lemon balm rubbed into their faces and arms twice a day for 4 weeks reported a significant reduction in their symptoms of agitation, compared with only 14% of those treated with a placebo lotion (Ballard et al., 2002), but systematic reviews do not support benefit (Taslim et al., 2024).

Other studies have utilized the lavender scent for easing anxiety. One interesting study involved linalool, an alcohol component with a lavender odor. Researchers observed anxious behavior among mice, which were then administered the lavender odor which produced a sedative impact on mice brain. The researchers concluded that the olfactory system (sense of smell) gave relief from the anxious behavior of the mice similar to the effects of valium, but without the motor impairment that the drug would have induced (Harada et al., 2018; Malloggi et al., 2022).

Laughter

There are organizations that certify people as laughter leaders, and there are laughter clubs worldwide. There is also an International Laughter Day each year on May 6—mark your calendar! Or try the International Moment of Laughter Day (https://izzyg.com/international-moment-of-laughter/).

One study reported an inverse relationship between laughter and heart disease (Clark et al., 2001). The difficulty of investigating laughter has not stopped researchers from designing clinical trials (Kramer & Leitao, 2023) or developing training in therapeutic humor (Association for Applied and Therapeutic Humor, www.aath.org).

COMPLEMENTARY AND ALTERNATIVE MEDICINE AND MEDICAL EDUCATION

Most medical schools and residency programs in the United States are teaching CAM content or practices in one or more required or elective courses, usually in a department of family practice or internal medicine. This interest in CAM in medical education, however, does not necessarily amount to an endorsement.

Some medical schools and residency programs offer CAM courses and lectures in order to better inform physicians and students about what patients are doing. One large Midwestern medical school reported that most first-year medical students (84%) were interested in learning about CAM because they believed this knowledge will be important to them when they become physicians and discover that some of their patients are using it (Greiner et al., 2000). However, medical students are more skeptical of CAM than the general population (Frass et al., 2012).

SELECTED COMPLEMENTARY AND ALTERNATIVE MEDICINE TOPICS AND RESOURCES

Complementary and Alternative Medicine Insurance

About two thirds of health maintenance organizations (HMOs) offer coverage for at least one form of CAM, usually chiropractic (65%) or acupuncture treatments (19%), followed in single-digit percentages by massage therapy, biofeedback, and homeopathy (Institute of Medicine, 2005). Coverage of chiropractic treatment is mandated by 42 states, acupuncture by seven states, and massage therapy by two states. The state of Washington requires that insurers cover all categories of providers, including acupuncturists, massage therapists, and naturopaths.

Chiropractic coverage is endorsed by some insurers because there are studies reporting that this type of treatment is as successful at treating patients with chronic low back pain as allopathic care, although costing substantially less. One study, however, reported that chiropractic care is more expensive than medical care for the treatment of low back pain (Kominski et al., 2005).

CAM coverage is endorsed by some insurers in the hope of attracting better educated consumers with higher incomes and above-average health. In general, though, CAM coverage is quite limited, with insurers waiting for research results on clinical efficacy and cost-effectiveness (Herman et al., 2005). When insurers do cover a CAM therapy, it must be deemed medically necessary, visits are limited, and deductibles and copayments are high.

Oxford Health Plans in Connecticut became the first major U.S. healthcare plan to offer comprehensive coverage for a wide range of CAM services. Its network of 2,000 alternative providers include licensed practitioners of acupuncture, chiropractic, ***naturopathy***, massage therapy, nutrition, and other specialties such as yoga and tai chi.

In 2006, Medicare made a breakthrough by approving participation in two demonstration prevention programs developed by physicians Dean Ornish and Herbert Benson, though the first patients did not begin their participation until 2011. These comprehensive health promotion programs—nutrition education, exercise, cognitive restructuring, and others—also include CAM activities such as yoga, meditation, deep breathing, and support groups. Ornish's program is offered at eight sites in Pennsylvania and at five medical centers in West Virginia; Benson's program is available in Indiana, Rhode Island, Tennessee, Washington, and Virginia.

This marked the first time that the federal government had reimbursed Medicare beneficiaries for lifestyle intervention programs. These two programs have prompted a shift from an exclusive focus on the biomedical model to a regimen also including complementary medicine. There is coverage for 36 sessions within an 18-week period, with a possible extension to 72 sessions in 36 weeks.

QUESTION: What CAM services would you like to see generally covered by health insurance? Why?

As of 2020, Medicare covers acupuncture, chiropractic, and some alternative treatments within the setting of traditional medical care (https://www.healthline.com/health/medicare/does-medicare-cover-acupuncture#finding-coverage).

Complementary and Alternative Medicine Rock Stars and Organizations

Andrew Weil is on the medical school faculty at the University of Arizona in Tucson, where he developed a 2-year residency program that integrates traditional medicine and other disciplines, such as meditation, nutrition, herbal medicine, acupuncture, and osteopathic manipulation. He has published several books, such as *Spontaneous Healing*, *Eight Weeks to Optimum Health*, and *Healthy Aging*, and he reports receiving thousands of questions a week online at www.drweil.com.

Dr. Weil is an influential purveyor of CAM. His opinions have become more mainstream over the years, and he has regularly appeared on the covers of national magazines and on television shows. Dr. Weil appears to take the generally more supportive and less rigorously conducted European studies on dietary supplements at face value and, as a consequence, prematurely recommends an astonishingly broad array of supplements.

While also a physician, Deepak Chopra's ideas lie more in the mystical realm, and mainstream medicine is more critical of him than of Dr. Weil. He writes books and a monthly newsletter; records spiritual lyrics and poetry; delivers lectures and seminars; sells tapes, ***herbs***, and aromatic oils; and has plans—yet unrealized—for a nationwide chain of healing centers.

Popular physicians who are active in the media have the potential for serving a useful societal purpose by expanding our strategies for improving health, but some appear to be primarily raking in every last buck from a gullible public. The mainstream consensus in healthcare is that an increasing number of medical gurus are enriching their bank accounts more than our health knowledge. "Lifestyle medicine" faces similar temptations.

There is no shortage of organizations promoting CAM. Here are a few of the most prominent:

American Holistic Health Association, www.ahha.org
Academy of Integrative Health & Medicine, www.aihm.org
American Holistic Nurses Association, www.ahna.org
The *Center for Mind-Body Medicine*, www.cmbm.org
Commonweal (cancer patients and health professionals who treat them), www.commonweal.org
Ayurvedic medicine, www.nccih.nih.gov/health/ayurveda
Herb Research Foundation, www.herbs.org
The *National Wellness Institute*; www.nationalwellness.org
Alternative Therapies in Health and Medicine, www.alternative-therapies.com
Journal of Alternative and Complementary Medicine, www.liebertpub.com/acm

DIETARY SUPPLEMENTS

The traditional wisdom in the nutritional sciences has been that it is best to rely on the variety of good foods provided by nature to meet our nutritional goals. Over the years, though, an increasing number of researchers have found evidence of the need for specific dietary supplements.

For example, the research supporting folate as a supplement was so persuasive that the FDA required manufacturers of breads, cereals, pasta, and other grain products to fortify their products with it. The American public, however, has gone one giant step further, finding the need to buy a wide range of dietary, nutritional, or food supplements containing vitamins, minerals, herbs, or other ingredients.

This perceived need is so strong that one study reported that 71% of regular patrons of dietary supplements would continue to use them even if research proved them to be ineffective (Blendon et al., 2001)! The benefit of supplements for people without medical conditions is dubious (Wierzejska, 2021).

As many as 70% of Americans age 60+ have taken one or more dietary supplements in the past 30 days, according to one survey (Gahche et al., 2017). That is pervasive! And a substantial minority, 29%, was taking four or more dietary supplements. The most popular supplements consumed by the American public are multivitamins or minerals (39%), vitamin D (37%), omega-3 fatty acids (22%), vitamin B_{12} (12%), and calcium (19%; Mishra et al., 2021). Women are almost twice as likely to be taking a dietary supplement as men.

Cautions

There are good reasons to be more cautious in taking dietary supplements. It is not clear, for example, if dietary supplements are adequate substitutes for the nutrients in foods. Most dietary supplements are narrowly targeted, whereas the nutrients in foods work in synergy.

Phytochemicals show this distinction well. These chemical compounds are found in abundance in fruits and vegetables and seem to exert a synergistic effect in cancer prevention. The compounds, however, are impossible to replicate in pill form. Adults who eat a poor diet and try to compensate with a variety of specific supplements will not derive the same benefits they would from healthy eating.

Another caution with taking supplements is that they can be dangerous. An *overdose of vitamin A* can cause headaches, nausea, diarrhea, liver problems, and hip fracture. *Excessive vitamin D* intake can cause appetite loss, fatigue, nausea, and constipation; can lead to abnormal calcium deposits in the body; and can adversely affect the kidneys. An *overdose of bran* can lead to seriously reduced calcium absorption. *Excess vitamin* B_6 can cause numbness, *vitamin E* can cause bleeding, and *niacin* can lead to gastric problems and liver damage.

In addition, people on medication need to be careful about taking dietary supplements. For instance, a person taking Coumadin, a blood-thinning medication, should avoid vitamin K, which can negate the effect of this medication, and also avoid several herbs (including ginkgo biloba) that can unsafely exacerbate the effects of blood-thinning medication.

Finally, people need to be cautious about the proclaimed benefits of dietary supplements, which are often exaggerated. If consumers acquire a false sense of security regarding supplements, it may contribute to failure to pay sufficient attention to the nutritive value of the foods they eat.

Dietary Supplement Health and Education Act

In 1994, the federal government passed the ***Dietary Supplement Health and Education Act*** (DSHEA), which eliminated premarket safety evaluations for a wide variety of dietary supplements, including many herbs, vitamins, minerals, and hormones. Through this law, the FDA can only intervene after consumers complain about illnesses from supplements.

Even then, the FDA can restrict the product only if it can be proved that the specific supplement caused the harm. Proof is difficult to accomplish because it is hard to separate out people who did not take the supplement as directed, or who exceeded the recommended dose, or who took different types of supplements simultaneously, or who engaged in some other confounding practice.

Though the lay public remained bullish on the prospects of dietary supplements, after the 1994 legislation passed, the FDA quickly logged more than 2,500 reports of side effects associated with dietary supplements, including 79 deaths (Neergaard, 1998). Because the government decided to take a *caveat emptor*, or "buyer beware," approach to regulating supplements, there has been insufficient consumer guidance about what works, what does not work, and what the potential side effects are.

The 1994 legislation also allowed advertisers to make unproven claims for their products—for instance, that their product reverses aging—as long as the product is not being sold at the same time (i.e., the advertisements are physically separated from the items being promoted). Even the placement of false claims on product labels, which is illegal, is often not punished because government agencies lack the resources for enforcement. Moreover, the unprotected consumer has to contend with the lack of regulation over product purity, as well as the amount of active ingredient in a supplement. Two packages of the same product may contain vastly dissimilar amounts of the active ingredient(s).

Even worse, researchers who analyzed dietary supplements that had been recalled between January 1, 2009 and December 31, 2012 found that two thirds of them were still available for purchase on the shelves of health food stores and elsewhere after 3 years (Cohen et al., 2014).

In 2015, six herbal supplements being sold at GNC, Target, Walmart, and Walgreens were investigated by the New York State Attorney General's office. They found that 80% of the many samples examined contained little or none of the medicinal herbs being advertised on their labels. In many cases, cheap fillers and contaminants were substituted. Owing to inadequate FDA enforcement, many mislabeled or contaminated dietary supplements were back on the shelves a few years later.

The FDA conducted a survey of dietary supplements and found 776 separate products were tainted or had unapproved pharmaceutical ingredients in them (Tucker et al., 2018). Moreover, these supplements came from 146 different manufacturers. The worst offenders were products for sexual performance, weight loss, and muscle building.

Despite the lack of quality or proven effectiveness of most supplements, the DSHEA provided few safeguards against grandiose advertisement claims. Not surprisingly, the growth of the dietary supplement business has been steady and spectacular. Dietary supplement sales in the United States went from $9 billion in 1995, to $16 billion in 2000, $21 billion in 2005, $23 billion in 2009, $40 billion in 2017, and $45 in 2023 (https://www.statista.com/statistics/828481/total-dietary-supplements-market-size-in-the-us/).

Utilizing herbs, vitamins, minerals, hormones, enzymes, and many other "natural" products, Americans have attempted to improve mood, ease achy joints, enhance memory, strengthen immune function, increase intelligence, boost stamina, improve sleep, relieve stress, prevent wrinkles, or reverse the aging process. All such claims are being allowed on the labels of dietary supplements without evidence to support them, again thanks to the DSHEA.

It took a whole decade for this legislative act to ban even a single supplement—ephedra—and even then the ban was partially rescinded to allow small amounts of this product. Ephedra products claimed to promote weight loss and increase energy, but they also drove up blood pressure and were linked to many cases of heart attack and stroke. The FDA finally banned sales of most ephedra products in 2004, after more than 18,000 adverse events and an estimated 100 deaths had been tied to this weight-loss product, which contains an amphetamine-like herb.

In 2008, 14 years after the passage of the DSHEA, things had gotten so out of hand that even the dietary supplement industry backed federal legislation to require supplement manufacturers to report to the FDA serious adverse events linked to their products. Previously, as was the case with ephedra, a manufacturer would sit on a large number of adverse-event reports it had received over the years, as it was not obligated to pass them on to the FDA.

But lack of reporting is not the only problem. As the New York Attorney General's office found out, there are more than 40,000 products on the market and the FDA has limited resources to ensure compliance. Thus, the decision whether to test and how to test the safety and purity of a new dietary supplement is pretty much left up to the manufacturers.

One final comment: A study led by the FDA and the Centers for Disease Control and Prevention concluded that dietary supplements cause 20,000 emergency department visits each year (Geller et al., 2015).

QUESTION: How would you change the Dietary Supplement Health and Education Act so that it provides as much consumer freedom as possible while protecting the safety of the public?

VITAMIN AND MINERAL SUPPLEMENTS

Multivitamins

Taking a daily multivitamin did not seem like a good idea at first, an unnecessary rip-off, in fact, for the late Robert Butler, Pulitzer Prize-winning author and former chair of the Department of Geriatrics and Adult Development at New York's Mount Sinai Medical Center. Later, though, Dr. Butler supported the practice of routine multivitamin use. He had changed his mind after studying the methods of food production and processing in the United States, which led him to recommend that older adults consume an inexpensive multivitamin supplement daily. Other influential leaders followed suit.

Fraud

One such leader was Dr. Ranjit Chandra. In an essay in the *Journal of the American Medical Association*, Chandra (1997)—a physician twice nominated for the Nobel Prize in medicine—reported that deficiencies in vitamins and trace elements have been observed in almost one third of sampled older adults. He further observed that because it was expensive and impractical to analyze the blood levels of various nutrients in people on a periodic basis, all older adults should take a multivitamin containing modest amounts of ***vitamins*** and ***minerals*** as good preventive medicine practice.

A review of studies that were published between 1966 and 2002 concluded that all adults, and especially older adults, should take a daily multivitamin (Fletcher & Fairfield, 2002). Another review of nutritional interventions involving older adults in clinical trials found that nutritional supplements boost immunity among older adults (High, 2001). Chandra (2001) conducted a placebo-controlled, double-blind study with 86 older adults and concluded that those who took a multivitamin supplement showed significant improvement in short-term memory, problem-solving ability, abstract thinking, and attention, and a decline in infection-related illnesses relative to placebo.

What has happened since then? The research of the internationally recognized Dr. Chandra on the strengthened immune response of older adults who took daily multivitamins has been discredited! Independent statisticians concluded that his methods and statistical findings were so dubious that it was unlikely that he actually conducted the studies!

An independent panel convened by Dr. Chandra's university concluded that he had pretended to recruit participants and then fabricated results. When asked for his raw data, Dr. Chandra reported that they had mysteriously disappeared. The editor of *Nutrition* wrote an editorial acknowledging serious statistical flaws in an article by Chandra that the journal had published, regretting that their peer-review process had failed to identify the flaws before publication of the article.

Dr. Chandra's research, from the time he contributed to *Lancet* in 1992 (Chandra, 1992) to the printing of the *Nutrition* article in 2001, had been lauded as a landmark contribution to the fields of nutrition and immunity. During that time, Dr. Chandra formulated and then patented a supplement based on his "findings" and licensed the rights to his daughter, who founded a company that sold the multivitamin, called Javaan 50. Experts denounced not only the validity of Dr. Chandra's findings but also the link of his research to the sale of this profitable dietary supplement. According to a statement in Dr. Chandra's divorce proceedings, he was living off $2 million (Canadian) held in 120 bank accounts located in tax havens around the world.

Evidence

A study released since then reported that regular use of commonly available multivitamin and multimineral supplements is *not* likely to reduce infections or use of health services (Avenell et al., 2005). A panel of nutritionists, biostatisticians, and epidemiologists met at the NIH in May 2006 and concluded that there was no evidence to support the regular use of multivitamins. Moreover, given that 65% of Americans consume fortified foods or beverages, they may be unknowingly exceeding the upper safe limits of some vitamins. After an 8-year follow-up period in the Women's Health Initiative clinical trials, multivitamin use was found to have little or no influence on the risk of cancer, heart disease, or total mortality in postmenopausal women (Neuhouser et al., 2009).

A review of almost 50 years of research studies on multivitamins and minerals reported that there was no association between the supplements and the risk of cardiovascular disease, stroke incidence, or mortality rate (Kim et al., 2018). And even though multivitamins rarely cause harm, they are not completely safe either. Some of their many ingredients can interact with medications and cause side effects, distort laboratory test results, cause gastrointestinal symptoms, and raise the amount of a specific substance to an unsafe level.

Multivitamins are advertised in effective—they are consumed more than any other supplement—but sometimes tricky ways. Ritual, a company that sells multivitamins to women, pays for positive articles on websites, then takes content from these paid-for articles and uses them for positive quotes on Facebook and Instagram. Then, when *The New York Times* and other reputable outlets merely cite the presence of these (paid) endorsements, Ritual (falsely) reports that these reputable outlets endorsed the benefits of their multivitamins (Maheshwari, 2018). The United States Preventive Services Task Force (USPSTF) has given use of multivitamin supplements for the prevention of cardiovascular disease or cancer an "I" rating, indicating lack of conclusive evidence of benefit (https://www.uspreventiveservicestaskforce.org/uspstf/recommendation/vitamin-supplementation-to-prevent-cvd-and-cancer-preventive-medication).

Calcium and Vitamin D

Calcium is essential for maintaining bone strength. If the amount of calcium contained in the diets of older adults is inadequate, the body takes calcium from the bones and uses it for other purposes. When people lose calcium from their bones, or their body's ability to absorb calcium is reduced (an aging process exacerbated by the excess use of such products as mineral oil laxatives, caffeine, alcohol, and so forth), bones become more brittle and fragile.

Vitamin D is also essential in that it helps bones to absorb calcium. Many consumers purchase these two supplements in combination. However, most vitamin D, about 85%, is obtained through exposure to sunlight. About 10 minutes of daily exposure is thought to prevent deficiency.

Let's cut to the chase: The USPSTF recommends against routine use of calcium or vitamin D supplementation for the primary prevention of fractures among postmenopausal women (Grade D) and finds insufficient evidence to justify such supplementation among men and premenopausal women (Grade I) (https://www.uspreventiveservicestaskforce.org/uspstf/recommendation/vitamin-d-calcium-or-combined-supplementation-for-the-primary-prevention-of-fractures-in-adults preventive-medication).

What's relatively new about calcium and vitamin D? The problem with routine use of these supplements, as we now know, is the greater likelihood of kidney stones.

The Recommended Dietary Allowance for women is 1,200 mg of calcium after menopause and 600 IU (age 51–70) to 800 IU (beyond age 70) of vitamin D. If women are getting close to that in their diet, a substantial supplement may do more harm than good, particularly regarding the increased risk for kidney stones. Thus, routine supplementation is no longer recommended. The USPSTF now recommends against supplementation even for women who experience fractures.

Ideally, postmenopausal women should get their calcium needs met through their food sources and take advantage of screening for blood and urine calcium levels and bone density. The most common sources of calcium are dairy products, fortified foods, and dark green leafy vegetables—kale and broccoli, but not spinach.

Vitamin D is more difficult to get in sufficient amounts from food and drink, though it is found in fatty fish, eggs, dairy products, and added to some cereals and breads. Many older adults have digestive issues that can cause their bodies to absorb less vitamin D than younger adults.

Weight-bearing exercise helps to maintain strong bones by increasing bone mineral density and reducing calcium loss. The positive effect of exercise on bone strength, however, appears to be lost within a relatively short period of time if the weight-bearing exercise program is discontinued.

A final point about vitamin D supplementation. As noted by Marion Nestle, "Entire organizations are devoted to convincing people to take high-dose vitamin D" (via an email to Reuters Health in 2013), and they have been wildly successful. Vitamin D sales in 2017 rose to $930 million, with more than 10 million laboratory tests conducted for vitamin D deficiency—a ninefold increase in 10 years. Celebrities like Gwyneth Paltrow, Oprah Winfrey, and Dr. Oz proclaim without evidence that vitamin D supplements will help you avoid heart disease, depression, obesity, memory loss, and cancer. The USPSTF, which does not recommend routine vitamin D supplements, is no match for these celebrities.

Primary care physicians also contribute to "magical thinking" about vitamin D by routinely testing patient levels, using a deficiency threshold that was probably set too high, and advising supplements (Rabin, 2018). Although 30 ng/mL is commonly used as the low end of the recommended range, most experts believe it should be set at 20 ng.

As noted in the opening section of this section, about one in four adults over age 60 are taking a vitamin D supplement—the second most popular supplement (amassing $1.4 billion in sales in 2023, https://www.marketsandmarkets.com/Market-Reports/vitamin-d-market-22034298.html). This occurs despite the research which reports that *routine* vitamin D supplementation does not help prevent fractures, increase bone mineral density, or prevent falls (Bolland et al., 2018) even in persons with levels as low as 20 ng/mL.

Vitamin E

Many areas of nutritional research start out with positive findings, and then subsequent, more rigorously conducted studies fail to support the early research. This is certainly true for vitamin E. At first, promising observational studies associated high intakes of vitamin E with protection against cancer and heart disease. Studies of older adults taking vitamin E supplements of 200 IU/day (significantly higher than the 30 IU/d currently recommended) reported improvements in T-cell and other immune functions (Meydani et al., 1997). This is noteworthy because with age we produce fewer T cells and antibodies that help us attack viruses, cancers, and infection.

Vitamin E also appeared to be important in reducing the risk of heart disease. It seemed to be a potent ***antioxidant*** that attaches directly to low-density lipoprotein (LDL) cholesterol to prevent damage from free radicals. One study (Stephens et al., 1996) reported that adults who were given 400 or 800 IU of vitamin E a day for 18 months had a 77% lower risk of heart attacks.

Vitamin E supplementation appeared to reduce prostate cancer incidence and mortality rate in male smokers in Finland and provided some protection against colorectal and lung cancers (Heinonen et al., 1998). Yet another study reported that 1,000 IU of vitamin E twice a day slowed the progression of Alzheimer disease, though it did not stop or reverse it (Sano et al., 1997).

The next generation of research studies, however, was more rigorously conducted, and the results were *not* positive. The effects of long-term vitamin E supplementation were not significant in comparison with a placebo in terms of cancer incidence, cancer deaths, myocardial infarction, stroke, or cardiovascular deaths (HOPE and HOPE-TOO Trial Investigators, 2005; Lee et al., 2005). In fact, the risk of heart failure was *higher* in the vitamin E group than in the placebo group (HOPE and HOPE-TOO Trial Investigators, 2005). A meta-analysis of 19 randomized, placebo-controlled trials reported that vitamin E *increased* the risk of all-cause mortality, and this dose-dependent increase began as low as the 150 IU/day level of supplementation (Miller et al., 2005). Yet another study reported that vitamin E supplementation was significantly correlated with increased risk for prostate cancer in men (Klein et al., 2011).

A study of 9,500 patients at high risk for cardiovascular events reported that treatment with vitamin E for 4.5 years had no apparent effect on cardiovascular outcome in comparison with a randomly assigned control group (Heart Outcomes Prevention

Evaluation Study Investigators, 2000). Another study reported that vitamin E supplements did not reduce the risk of cardiovascular disease over a 3-year period (Hodis et al., 2002) and yet another study reported that vitamin E provided no benefit for age-related cataracts (Christen et al., 2008).

What *was* promising was food intake. Vitamin E in food (green, leafy vegetables; corn; whole grains; nuts; olives; and vegetable oils) slows decline in mental function among older adults, whereas a vitamin E supplement does not (Morris et al., 2002). Another study conducted with 5,395 residents in the Netherlands, age 55 and older, reported that vitamin E intake from food may reduce the risk of developing Alzheimer disease, whereas vitamin E from supplements does not (Engelhart et al., 2002). A study in the *New England Journal of Medicine* (Kushi et al., 1996) reported that older women who ate more *foods* rich in vitamin E reduced their chances of getting heart disease by almost two thirds.

When the more recent wave of studies reported that daily vitamin E doses of 400 IU or more can increase the risk of heart failure, and even 150 to 400 IU/day may have a detrimental effect, U.S. sales of vitamin E supplements declined 25% in 2005. For those who choose to continue to take a vitamin E supplement, it is not clear what the recommended amount should be, though less than 150 IU/d seems prudent. Vitamin E supplementation is not recommended for patients on anticoagulant therapy, as vitamin E is itself an anticoagulant.

Vitamin C

For almost 30 years, millions of people followed the lead of Nobel laureate Linus Pauling and consumed vitamin C pills to fight the common cold and cancer. The late Pauling earned his laurels for work in molecular structure, however, not vitamin C research, and most scientists rejected his theory that vitamin C is an antioxidant that fights disease-causing free radicals. One study reported that vitamin C supplementation failed to reduce the incidence of the common cold in the population, with the possible exception of people who are exposed to brief periods of severe physical stress (Cerullo et al., 2020; Douglas et al., 2007).

Nonetheless, studies on the positive effects of vitamin C still appear from time to time. The most promising of these studies suggest that vitamin C supplementation may prevent cataracts. Cataracts are thought to result from the oxidation of lens protein, and vitamin C may prevent this oxidation. One study found that long-term vitamin C supplement use among 492 nondiabetic women over a 15-year period was associated with a 60% reduction in the risk of cataracts, compared with no supplement use (Taylor et al., 2002).

Most nutritionists argue that the recommended five daily servings of vitamin C–rich fruits and vegetables would easily meet the minimum daily recommendation. Unfortunately, only 12% of Americans eat the recommended minimum (Lee, 2022).

Antioxidant Cocktail

The *antioxidant vitamins* are vitamin E, vitamin C, and beta-carotene. Advocates of antioxidant vitamins once recommended a cocktail of all three.

Antioxidants stabilize *free radicals*, which are unstable forms of oxygen. Oxygen is used during metabolism to change carbohydrates and fats into energy. During this process, oxygen is converted into stable forms of water and carbon dioxide, but some oxygen (i.e., free radicals) ends up in an unstable form with a normal proton nucleus but a single unpaired electron. The unpaired electron seeks to steal a second electron from a stable molecule, and in so doing damages proteins and lipids in a process that likely contributes to heart disease, cancer, and other diseases. This chain reaction among unpaired electrons continues until antioxidants become available to help stabilize the free radicals.

Antioxidants are found in foods, especially fruits and vegetables. As mentioned, though, few Americans get adequate servings of fruits and vegetables in their daily diets. Thus, many nutritionists for several years in the 1990s recommended the antioxidant cocktail. The typical cocktail guidelines ranged from 250 to 1,000 mg of vitamin C, 200 to 800 IU of vitamin E, and 10,000 to 25,000 IU of beta-carotene.

Nutritional leaders no longer recommend the cocktail. Antioxidant supplements do not delay death. A meta-analysis of 67 randomized clinical trials with a total of 230,000 participants reported no evidence that antioxidant supplements decrease mortality; in fact, some studies report that vitamin A, beta-carotene, or vitamin E may increase it (Bjelakovic et al., 2008).

One ray of hope for the antioxidant cocktail lies with macular degeneration. A modified version of the original cocktail—400 mg of vitamin E, 500 mg of vitamin C, but only 15 mg of beta-caroteneplus 80 mg of zinc and 2 mg of copper—provided the first effective treatment for this particular type of vision loss among older adults. Studies among persons with macular degeneration who have not yet lost the central portion of their vision to the disease have shown reductions of vision loss by 20% (Jampol, 2001) and 35% (van Leeuwen et al., 2005). However, other studies are less positive (Chong et al., 2007).

Vitamin B_{12}

Vitamin B_{12} (cobalamin) helps maintain red blood cells, nerve function, and the synthesis of DNA. It is found naturally in animal foods such as meat, poultry, fish, eggs, and dairy products. The prevalence of vitamin B_{12} deficiency is age related (two thirds of the cases), primarily because of decreased secretion of hydrochloric acid in the stomach over time which makes it difficult to absorb vitamin B_{12}. Also, older adults are the most susceptible to taking antacids or multiple medications. In addition, many older adults have gastrointestinal problems, such as celiac disease or Crohn disease, or have had bariatric surgery.

A deficiency in vitamin B_{12} can lead to fatigue, memory loss, balance problems, constipation, and depression. Close to 80% of older adults who have a vitamin B_{12} deficiency do not know it, according to Dr. David Spence, a neurologist at the Robarts Research Institute in London, Ontario, and are in danger of acquiring permanent neurological damage.

The National Academy of Sciences, Engineering, and Medicine, which advises the federal government on nutrition, urged people over age 50 to take a vitamin B_{12} supplement or to eat cereals fortified with vitamin B_{12}. The Academy's review concluded that up to 30% of persons over age 50 (with the percentage increasing with advancing age) cannot absorb vitamin B_{12} in foods, primarily due to the onset of *atrophic gastritis*—insufficient stomach acid to separate vitamin B_{12} from the protein in food and thereby utilize it.

The Framingham Offspring Study reported that 39% of their national sample had low vitamin B_{12} levels. Some participants had a primarily vegetarian diet and failed to get enough of the vitamin in their foods. Others did get sufficient amounts of meat, poultry, and fish but had difficulty with absorption. The authors speculated that an increased use of antacids may contribute to the absorption problem (Tucker et al., 2000).

Researchers are beginning to suggest that persons over age 50 consider increasing the recommended daily allowance of vitamin B_{12} in their diets from 2.4 mcg to 25 mcg. Though most multivitamin supplements have only 6 mcg, Centrum Silver and other supplements designed for older adults typically have 25 mcg. An option to dietary supplementation that is nearly as effective is to eat vitamin B_{12}—fortified cereals and dairy products five or more times a week (Tucker et al., 2000).

Some researchers argue that vitamin B_{12} is water soluble, likely safe even in large doses, and should be added to flour as is now done with another B vitamin, folate. Others maintain that vitamin B_{12} supplements have not been adequately tested in randomized clinical trials, and even if safe, it is likely to be an insufficient amount for correcting even a mild deficiency.

HERBS

The medicinal benefits of plants are undeniable. Herbs are the basis for aspirin, morphine, digitalis, and other medicines. Most of the millions of dollars that consumers spend on herbal remedies do not produce beneficial outcomes, however, and some carry health risks. Even among products that appear to be helpful, the consistency of ingredients is unregulated and uncertain.

The regulation of herbs in Europe, where they are treated almost like drugs, sharply contrasts with the situation in America. In Europe, herbal labels warn people with diseases or conditions of potential dangers. Germany's Commission E of the Federal Department of Health has tested hundreds of herbs, approving those with absolute or some proof of efficacy (though nowhere near the research standard for efficacy that is used in the United States). These clearly labeled herbal medicines outsell prescription drugs in most European countries.

In contrast, Americans can access herbs over the counter, but they must rely on books for safety and efficacy information or they need to contact the nonprofit educational and research organization, the American Botanical Council (www.herbalgram.org).

Ginkgo Biloba

Ginkgo biloba is an extract from the leaves of the ginkgo biloba tree, and it is believed by many consumers to be a memory enhancer. It is the most studied and popular herbal medicine in Europe. It is also the most popular herb used by older adults in the United States, many of whom are worried about loss of memory. Ginkgo biloba was, for a short period of time, popular with college students as well, for allegedly enhanced memory performance on tests. The theory is that ginkgo biloba dilates blood vessels and can improve blood flow in the brain.

At first, the theory seemed to translate into practical results. A placebo-controlled, double-blind randomized trial in the United States reported that ginkgo biloba was safe and appeared capable of stabilizing, and in some cases improving, the cognitive performance and social functioning of demented patients for 6 months to a year (Le Bars et al., 1997). This study, however, was limited by a high dropout rate. A team of Dutch researchers employed the same ginkgo preparation as did the U.S. study and did not find significant differences between ginkgo recipients and placebo recipients in a study with higher quality follow-up (van Dongen et al., 2000).

Another randomized controlled trial with 230 people over age 60 with no signs of memory impairment found that the ginkgo biloba supplement worked no better than a placebo on learning, memory, attention, concentration, naming, and verbal fluency outcomes (Solomon et al., 2002). Finally, over an 8-year period researchers at six universities across the United States studied more than 3,000 adults aged 72 to 96 with normal mental functioning or mild cognitive impairment. Compared with a placebo, the use of ginkgo biloba did not result in less cognitive decline (Snitz et al., 2009).

Given the well-controlled studies that refute claims of benefit for memory and related cognitive function, sales of ginkgo biloba, which had been steadily increasing in the United States through 2007, started to decline in 2008. This decline also occurred on college campuses, replaced in popularity by Adderall around 2010 even though that drug is not available over the counter.

If you are among the still-considerable number of Americans taking ginkgo biloba, there is more bad news. ***ConsumerLab.com***, a laboratory that analyzes dietary supplements, reported seven of nine tested ginkgo products flunked for quality in 2003, five out of seven in 2008, and six out of 10 in 2018 (Schardt, 2018). Results were even worse in London, with 33 of 35 ginkgo supplements declared adulterated in 2016. Real ginkgo extract is expensive, requiring 50 lbs of dried leaves to make 1 lb of extract. Turns out ginkgo is among the most adulterated herbs being sold throughout the world. It is also an anticoagulant and the older you get, the risk for internal bleeding increases.

The Other Gs

In addition to ginkgo biloba, there are other popular herbs that begin with the letter *g*—ginseng, garlic, and ginger—that are also anticoagulants and can increase the risk of bleeding problems. The risk is even worse when taken with aspirin, warfarin (Coumadin), and other over-the-counter and prescription blood-thinning medications.

Ginseng products are used as energy boosters and to cure a wide range of ills. The few well-designed studies of ginseng do not bear out the claims that it boosts energy (Engels & Wirth, 1997) or enhances psychological well-being (Cardinal & Engels, 2001) when compared with a placebo control group. Another problem is that authentic ginseng in standardized doses is difficult to find. *Consumer Reports* tested 10 ginseng products and found that one contained almost none of the active ingredient and the remainder varied by 1,000%.

The typical claim for garlic is that it lowers the cholesterol level and improves cardiovascular health. A panel of experts reviewed 1,800 studies on the potential health benefits of garlic and found little evidence that it lowers cholesterol, blood pressure, or blood sugar, or that it prevents heart attacks, cancer, or blood clots (Garlic: Case Unclosed, 2000). Commission E, the agency that advises the German public and health professionals on herbal medicines, no longer recommends garlic for cholesterol reduction. The small reductions in cholesterol in some of the short-term studies were no longer evident at 6 months or longer. A randomized clinical trial found that garlic had no significant effects on LDL, high-density lipoprotein (HDL), triglycerides, or total cholesterol level (Gardner et al., 2007). Other studies are more positive (Imaizumi et al., 2023)

Ginger is typically taken to relieve nausea associated with seasickness, motion sickness, and anesthesia. Studies of ginger extract and its effect on the lowering of cholesterol were promising, but focused on mice (Fuhrman et al., 2000), with no evidence that results can be generalized to human beings. Ginger, like the other "g" herbs, can exacerbate internal bleeding. Again, other studies are more positive (Anh et al., 2020), making it difficult for consensus to emerge on proper guidance to consumers. Still, the preponderance of studies of herbal supplements suggests unlikely benefit and the need for caution.

St. John's Wort

St. John's wort is a weed native to the western United States and parts of Europe. This weed is named for St. John the Baptist, whose birthday is celebrated on June 24, about the time the plant puts forth its yellow blooms.

St. John's wort is the second most popular herbal medicine (after ginkgo biloba) in the United States, but it is the most popular antidepressant in Germany, where it outsells Prozac four to one. St. John's wort was not effective in the treatment of moderate or severe depression in two separate studies (Hypericum Depression Trial Study Group, 2002; Shelton et al., 2001), but there was evidence that it was effective with milder depression in comparison with a prescription antidepressant (Philipp et al., 1999; Woelk, 2000). The studies of milder depression, however, have been criticized for the lack of rigor (Kupfer & Frank, 2002; Spira, 2001).

Prozac costs on average eight times more than a regimen of St. John's wort. Researchers warn, however, that the German studies supporting the efficacy of St. John's wort involved small numbers of patients, brief trial periods, nonstandardized diagnoses of depression, and varied potencies and dosages.

St. John's wort can interfere with drugs for depression, cancer, heart disease, asthma, and AIDS, as well as with antibiotics. Clinicians warn about the adverse effects of stopping prescribed antidepressants without direction of a medical professional or taking St. John's wort while taking prescription antidepressants such as Prozac. Older adults are particularly susceptible to the hazards of combining the herb with prescription antidepressants and are likely to experience dizziness, confusion, headaches, and anxiety.

Finally, several organizations have analyzed dozens of brands of St. John's wort and found serious deficiencies in a majority of the products (Nutrition Action Healthletter, 2000; https://www.consumerlab.com/reviews/st-johns-wort/stjohnswort/.

Saw Palmetto

Extracts of the berries of saw palmetto, a small palm tree native to the southeastern United States, are used widely to improve urinary flow in men with noncancerous enlarged prostate or benign prostatic hypertrophy (BPH). A review of 18 randomized controlled trials examining saw palmetto extracts for the treatment of BPH was, at first, generally positive (Wilt et al., 1998). The *United States Pharmacopeia* (USP), published by a quasi-governmental agency that sets manufacturing standards for drugs and advises health professionals, reported in April 2000 that there was moderate evidence of effectiveness for saw palmetto in men with BPH (Schardt, 2000b).

However, an exceptionally well-designed government study found that men randomly assigned to a saw palmetto did not differ in symptoms, prostate size, urinary flow, or quality of life from placebo (Bent et al., 2006). This study lasted 1 year and was carefully blinded: The placebo had a similarly strong taste and smell as saw palmetto, perhaps revealing a weakness in blinding in prior studies.

The potential market for saw palmetto extracts is huge, with half of all men over the age of 50 having enlarged prostates. Moreover, prescription prostate drugs have substantial side effects. Saw palmetto is definitely not a substitute for conventional medical prostate treatment. Some older men report that it relieves the symptoms of enlargement, such as the frequent urge to urinate, but this is probably a short-term placebo effect. Saw palmetto is also not effective when the dried berry or extract is made into a tea.

Echinacea

Extracts of the plant Echinacea, a purple coneflower, are widely used in the United States and some European countries for the treatment or prevention of common colds (upper respiratory tract infections). An initial review of 16 randomized and quasirandomized trials with 3,396 participants suggested that a few Echinacea preparations may be better than placebo (Melchart et al., 2000).

Subsequent studies, however, have not supported this herb's effectiveness. Compared with a placebo, Echinacea provided no detectable benefit in more rigorous randomized trials (Barrett et al., 2002; Sperber et al., 2004; Turner et al., 2005). Despite a growing number of clinical studies producing negative results, Echinacea retains its popularity.

Black Cohosh and Other Herbs for Menopausal Symptoms

After the publication of the results of the Women's Health Initiative on the risks of hormone replacement therapy, many women sought alternatives for the treatment of menopausal symptoms. As noted by one reviewer, dietary supplements for the relief of menopausal symptoms receive little scientific support for their efficacy despite their popularity (Albertazzi, 2006).

Most studies report that black cohosh, soy supplements, ginkgo biloba, ginseng, St. John's wort, and combination herbal remedies are *no* more effective than placebos for alleviating symptoms, though they all may be perceived as effective by up to 40% of women (comparable to placebos). Not surprisingly, two thirds of current users of these supplements believe they are effective in relieving symptoms, whereas 70% of former users believe they did not help (Ma et al., 2000; Franco et al., 2016).

In the general absence of support for dietary supplements, women who are no longer willing to take hormone replacements may want to consider exercise, relaxation techniques, improved sleep hygiene, and nutritional changes. The common side effect of these interventions is good health, with little additional out of pocket expense.

HORMONE SUPPLEMENTS

Human Growth Hormone

Human growth hormone (HGH) is secreted by the brain's pituitary gland and helps regulate growth during childhood and metabolism during adulthood. HGH levels begin declining by age 30 along with the body's muscle mass. By age 70, hormone levels are only 25% of the peak reached by most people between the ages of 18 and 30. An estimated 20,000 to 30,000 American adults take a synthetic version of HGH. Injecting HGH appears to boost lean body mass and improve physical function, and is promoted as an antiaging remedy. It allegedly improves strength, energy, and immunity and has been used as a treatment for heart disease, cancer, erectile dysfunction, and Alzheimer disease.

Although there is limited or no support for these claims, there is evidence that this ***hormone supplement*** is more harmful than beneficial. It can lead to carpal tunnel syndrome, edema, joint and muscle pain, high blood pressure, congestive heart failure, and tumor growth, and it can worsen the effects of arthritis and diabetes. Two studies have associated HGH with increased mortality rates (Demling, 1999; Maison et al., 1998). Benefits in muscle mass must be weighed against a variety of negative effects (Liu et al., 2007).

HGH does not yet translate into improved function for older adults, and the risk of adverse effects is substantial (Cassel, 2002). Researchers conclude that the participation of older persons in this therapy should be confined to controlled studies (Blackman et al., 2002). Moreover, buying pills or getting shots that can cost up to $15,000 a year and are not covered by insurance is a poor financial investment.

Nonetheless, there is a strong and growing black market demand for HGH, for both older and younger persons. For the former, the antiaging movement and, in particular, the American Academy of Anti-Aging Medicine tout HGH as a way to stop or reverse the aging process. Its appeal has been particularly strong among people age 40 to 60. Perhaps the lucky ones are only wasting their money. A recent analysis by ConsumerLab.com showed that that only a minuscule amount of HGH can be found in the supplements sold at health food stores or on the internet.

Testosterone

Testosterone is a sex hormone, popular with men for gaining muscle strength, energy, and sex drive. Experience with testosterone therapy to restore vitality in aging has been disappointing. Testosterone therapy appears to be beneficial only to those with an original deficit in the hormone (below 300 ng per deciliter of blood), regardless of age. From the perspective of the young athlete, however, high-quality and high-dose testosterone is a performance booster. One piece of evidence for this is the success of the disgraced cyclist Lance Armstrong, who took it along with a panoply of other performance-enhancing drugs.

Supplemental testosterone replacement may be more risky for men than hormone replacement therapy has been shown to be for women. There have been concerns that this therapy increases the risk for stroke and prostate cancer, but it was two federally funded trials, in 2009 and 2013, that reported a correlation with heart attacks that prompted the FDA to recommend a label change. In 2015, the FDA reported that manufacturers of testosterone drugs are required to change their labels to warn that the drugs could increase the risk of heart attacks and strokes. The label also states that it should not be prescribed to treat symptoms in men brought on by age, such as declining sexual drive.

Despite the warning, testosterone prescribing for age-related hypogonadism has increased in men, not decreased (Morden et al., 2018). Moreover, there is higher testosterone use among older men on Medicare with heart disease than those without heart disease, despite the greater risk for these men. Prescriptions for testosterone have increased from $150 million in 2000 to $1.8 billion in 2011, and a significant portion of men using the therapy do not meet the laboratory criteria for hypogonadism (Yabluchanskiy & Tsitouras, 2019).

A testosterone alternative, dehydroepiandrosterone (DHEA), is made by the adrenal glands and is converted into testosterone and estrogen in cells. Studies report that there were no differences after 2 years between those who took DHEA and those who were given a placebo, in terms of muscle mass and strength, exercise capacity, and quality of life.

Melatonin

Melatonin is a hormone produced in the brain by the pineal gland and is believed to set the body's sleep cycle. This hormone ramps up production in the evening as the light fades to encourage sleep and turns down production in the early morning hours. Melatonin became the first best-selling hormone supplement in the United States, with 20 million new users in 1995. Adults were using melatonin not only to induce sleep but also to reduce the effects of jet lag. It remains popular (Li et al., 2022).

These uses of melatonin have received some research support, but mostly the results have been disappointing, especially for older adults, the age group with the most sleep problems. Scientists are not convinced that there is an age-related decline in melatonin levels, or that sleep problems typical of older people occur because of a deficit in this hormone (Duffy et al., 2002). A meta-analysis of 25 controlled trials did not provide much support for the use of melatonin for sleep disorders (Buscemi et al., 2006). Valerian, a plant extract typically added to tea to induce sleep, also has not received support.

Melatonin might not be an effective jet lag antidote either. Traveling physicians randomly assigned to a melatonin treatment group or a placebo control group did not report differences in jet lag symptoms after a trip from Norway to New York (Spitzer et al., 1999).

One problem with melatonin supplements is that the label may not reflect what is in the product. In one study, 71% of the melatonin products examined varied more than 10% from what was stated on the label, and 26% included serotonin in the product but was not listed on the label (Erland & Saxeno, 2017).

OTHER DIETARY SUPPLEMENTS

Glucosamine and Chondroitin

Glucosamine and chondroitin in the human body are used to make cartilage and have been touted as a way to reverse the effects of arthritis since the publication of the best-selling book *The Arthritis Cure* (Theodosakis, 1997). In supplement form, these compounds come from crab shells, cow tracheae, and shark cartilage and appeared to ease arthritic aches and slow the loss of cartilage.

Studies of the two supplements published between 2000 and 2010 were encouraging, though far from definitive. Several studies reported positive results with one or the other supplement, or a combination of glucosamine and chondroitin. (Chondroitin is a more expensive supplement than glucosamine, and it is difficult to make. Twelve of 14 glucosamine samples had at least 90% of the ingredient amount listed on the label, but only five of 32 chondroitin samples contained the listed amount [Schardt, 2000a].)

In an NIH-supported multicenter trial, researchers examined glucosamine (1,500 mg) and chondroitin (1,200 mg) in 1,583 patients with knee arthritis. Of the patients who received the placebo, 60% reported at least a 20% reduction in pain, compared with 65% of patients taking one or the other supplement or both together (Clegg et al., 2006). The 5% difference, however, was not statistically significant. Only Celebrex (which was found to double the risk of heart attacks and was taken off the market in 2004), led to greater pain relief.

When researchers examined a subgroup of people with moderate to severe knee pain (eliminating those with mild pain), 79% taking the supplement combination reported pain relief, a significantly higher percentage than those taking a placebo (54%)

or Celebrex (69%). Subgroup analysis can be notoriously unreliable, though, and results are often not confirmed. Instead of waiting for follow-up studies, proponents inaccurately touted the benefits of these supplements allegedly supported by an NIH-funded study.

More rigorous double-blind, randomized clinical trials have not been kind to these supplements. Chondroitin and glucosamine have not outperformed placebo when it comes to reduction in joint pain or improved function. In one study, the opposite happened. People who took the supplements had a 19% reduction in pain scores after 6 months on the regimen, but those who took the placebo had a 33% reduction (Roman-Blas et al., 2017). There is still hope that the right combination of these two drugs, at the correct dosage, with consistent ingredients, and a reputable manufacturer, will someday produce an effective supplement.

Omega-3 Fatty Acids Versus Eicosapentaenoic Acid

The third most popular dietary supplement in the United States is commonly referred to as fish oil, or omega-3 fatty acids. Despite the enduring popularity of this supplement, it consistently fails to produce positive results when examined through rigorous randomized clinical trials (Grey & Bolland, 2014). In contrast, omega-3 fatty acids in foods, particularly fatty fish, is considered healthy. Salmon, trout, and sardines in particular—and to a lesser extent other fatty fish such as tuna, flounder, halibut, cod, haddock, and catfish—are recommended, while omega-3 supplements are not.

However, one strain of omega-3 fatty acids is being touted as the next big breakthrough. Instead of a small, nontherapeutic amount of eicosapentaenoic acid (EPA) found in your typical fish oil supplement, a concentrated dose of 4 grams daily of EPA may reduce the risk of ischemic stroke, heart attack, or death, according to presenters at the 2018 American Heart Association meeting in Chicago. When studied as a prescription drug, concentrated EPA reduced heart attacks and strokes by 25%, even when study participants were on statins (Bhatt et al., 2019).

In the meantime, though, most consumers will achieve higher blood levels of EPA from foods such as fatty fish that are associated with healthy aging (Lai et al., 2018), rather than a dietary supplement or a prescription drug with concentrated EPA.

Coenzyme Q10

With the increasing prevalence of statins, which are cholesterol-lowering drugs, there has been an increasing number of complaints of myopathy, or muscle aches and fatigue, particularly among those over age 70. Accompanying statin-induced myopathy is a reduced level of an enzyme that, theoretically, may be able to be corrected by taking a coenzyme Q10 supplement, also referred to as CoQ10.

Unfortunately, taking coenzyme Q10 for statin-associated myopathy has not alleviated myopathy symptoms (Marcoff & Thompson, 2007), nor has it helped with other health conditions such as heart failure, Parkinson disease, or Huntington disease.

Cannabidiol

Cannabidiol (CBD) is a component of cannabis, and popular it is—sales reached $4.2 billion in 2022 (https://www.statista.com/statistics/1067467/cbd-product-dollar-sales-us/). And no wonder! It allegedly helps with or cures anxiety, inflammatory diseases, depression, insomnia, addictions, and, well, most everything else.

CBD is taken in cocktails, coffee, tea, skin creams, pills, gummy bears, and edibles such as pastries—you name it. My favorite advertising promotion is Recess, a sparkling water spiked with CBD. A six pack sells for the bargain rate of $29.99 in your local health food store. It is alcohol free, caffeine free, and only a touch of sugar in its carbonation. Take your pick among three flavors: peach ginger, blackberry chai, or pom *Hibiscus*.

CBD has little effect on cannabinoid receptors in the brain, so unlike the tetrahydrocannabinol (THC) in marijuana, it does not have an intoxicating effect. It does alter the brain's serotonin receptors, but it is unclear what effect this might have. Research, unfortunately, does not support any beneficial effects of CBD, according to the National Academies of Sciences, Engineering and Medicine's expert panel, but rigorously conducted research studies have been scarce. As with other herbal products, people do not always get what they paid for (https://www.consumerlab.com/reviews/cbd-oil-hemp-review/cbd-oil/). For many people this may not matter as the placebo effect is alive and well.

Nutritional Drinks

Ensure, Sustacal, Nutrastart, and Boost are liquid meal supplements touted as energy increasers. The supplements were designed for older adults who have debilitating health conditions that make it difficult for them to eat or keep food down. Advertisers, though, are also promoting the products to baby boomers who are still in good health but are seeking more vitality; for them, these supplements may be expensive and ineffective. Sometimes the nutrients in these supplements are not fully absorbed by the body and provide only one third of the calories (about 240 vs. 750) of a meal if used as a substitute.

Consumers should be aware that these drinks are often laden with sugar. Boost has 28 grams of sugar in its 8-ounce bottle, more than Froot Loops and Lucky Charms. Some geriatricians refer to these supplements as "liquid candy."

Some ***nutritional drinks*** are advertised as protein drinks that are either energy boosters or meal replacements. These drinks are two thirds protein and are useful for the few adults who have a protein deficiency. But they lack vitamins, minerals, fiber, phytonutrients, fat, and carbohydrates found in whole foods. Protein bars are likely to be even less healthy than the drinks, as they tend to be high in saturated fat. Moreover, based on tests by ConsumerLab.com, protein bar products often failed to meet their labeling claims (https://www.consumerlab.com/reviews/protein-energy-fiber-meal-replacement-fruit-nut-bars/nutritionbars/).

DIETARY SUPPLEMENT VERIFICATION

As noted earlier, dietary supplements, unlike drugs, are not required to undergo premarket safety testing, which means that a brand may not contain the ingredients claimed on the label. The ingredients may also be unsafe, perhaps owing to contamination or to amounts that exceed safe limits.

In partial response to this challenge, ConsumerLab.com subjects different brands of dietary supplements to laboratory analysis. Similarly, the USP launched a ***Dietary Supplement Verification Program*** in 2002 (https://www.usp.org/verification-services/dietary-supplements-verification-program). The USP mark, which states "Dietary Supplement Verified," refers to the presence, quantity, and purity of a supplement's ingredient. If a bottle of ginseng pills bears the USP seal, it means that the product contains the amount of ginseng listed on the label and that the ingredient is free from contamination; it does not verify that ginseng provides additional energy or that it is safe.

These are at least steps in the right direction, and other organizations, including Consumers Union (www.consumersunion.org), are joining in. Unfortunately, efforts to regulate dietary supplements remain woefully inadequate overall, and caveat emptor (buyer beware) is an inadequate descriptor of the state of events in dietary supplements. Perhaps the situation was best described in *Is This the Right Way to Test Supplements?*: "Not since the early 1900s, when unregulated patent medicines were sold from circus wagons, has there been such a free-for-all" (Wellness Letter, 2000).

NUTRACEUTICALS OR FUNCTIONAL FOODS AND DRINKS

Americans have been eating fortified foods since 1924, when manufacturers added iodine to salt to prevent goiters. Since then, we have had vitamin D-fortified milk, calcium-fortified orange juice, flour enriched with B vitamins and iron, and other useful products.

Nutraceuticals represent a new pathway in the field of functional foods by exploiting nutritionally weak foods and marketing them as health products. Waffles with refined flour and orange drinks with sugar and water are now calcium fortified. Corn chips have kava to promote relaxation. Donuts are vitamin fortified and portrayed as healthy. A chocolate-chip cookie is laced with 500 mg of calcium and called Calci-cookie. Tortilla chips contain St. John's wort to boost your mood. And potato rings have ginkgo biloba to increase memory and alertness.

The bottom-line function of most functional foods and drinks is to make a profit for the manufacturer. At least with this function, they have been a success. Sales almost doubled between 2000 and 2008 to $31 billion. The global nutraceuticals market size was estimated at $317.22 billion in 2023 (https://www.grandviewresearch.com/industry-analysis/nutraceuticals-market).

Some foods are merely getting image makeovers. Ketchup is now more than a mere condiment; it is the richest dietary source of lycopene, which may ward off prostate cancer (though the evidence is questionable at best). So squirt a little ketchup on a supersized order of French fries and avoid cancer. Milk (calcium), tea (flavonoids), grapes (phenols), carrots (beta-carotene), broccoli (sulforaphane), and beef (linoleic acid) have also undergone image makeovers (Haney, 1999).

Some products may turn out to be useful, but manufacturers are unwilling to wait for the research to be completed. As previously mentioned, glucosamine and chondroitin are dietary supplements that may have promise in the area of reducing pain from arthritis. Rather than wait for definitive and consistent research results, though, Coca-Cola formed a partnership with Procter & Gamble to market the drink Elations, which has 1,500 mg of glucosamine and 1,200 mg of chondroitin added to it. The advertisers brazenly proclaim that you will receive joint comfort in 6 days, and significant improvement in only 3 days. Their motto: "The drink that brings 'Joy for Joints'." Funny, this product seems to have disappeared.

> **QUESTION:** Do you think there is too much skepticism in America about CAM? Why or why not?

The good news is that the herbal supplements added to most functional foods are in amounts so minuscule that they are quite safe. The bad news is that you are wasting your money. The additional bad news is that junk foods and drinks with a supplement added are still junk. The real bad news on top of that is that manufacturers could add unsafe dosages of herbs without premarket safety testing. Then it will be up to a sufficient number of sick consumers to demonstrate that it was the functional food and not some other factor that caused their health problem. There are safer ways to enjoy placebo effects or secure health.

SUMMARY

Boomers, now mostly in their 60s and early 70s, are the leading edge in the use of CAM. The NIH defines CAM as efforts to secure health outside the medical mainstream. This definition, while glib, nonetheless provides a framework for the status of a variety of treatments and practices.

Take exercise and nutrition, for instance. These two topics were outside the realm of mainstream medicine at one time, and now they are not. Hence, they are not discussed in this chapter on CAM. Same with yoga and tai chi: Once considered outside the mainstream, they are proven strategies for enhancing range of motion, balance, and fall prevention.

The reverse can also be true. At one time encouraging, the routine use of calcium and vitamin D supplements for older women was recommended by many mainstream healthcare providers, including geriatricians. Now, because of increased reporting of kidney stones, this combination of vitamin and mineral for those without deficiencies is considered questionable.

The sales of dietary supplements have been unleashed ever since the DSHEA stripped away much of the regulations. The three most popular dietary supplements in the United States—multivitamins, vitamin D, and omega-3 fatty acids—are supported by research only for special populations.

There is always initial fanfare for new supplements that are eventually demythologized by repeated research investigations. The list is long: ginkgo biloba, saw palmetto, St. John's wort, garlic, black cohosh, fish oil, CoQ10, glucosamine, chondroitin, and so forth. But there is always a new supplement to come along that starts off with a flourish.

SPRINGER PUBLISHING CONNECT™ | **A robust set of instructor resources designed to supplement this text is located at http://connect.springerpub.com/content/book/978-0-8261-8386-6. Qualifying instructors may request access by emailing textbook@springerpub.com.**

REFERENCES

Only key references appear in the print edition. The full reference list can be accessed by visiting www.springerpub.com/courseconnect. See inside front cover and tear-out card for Course-Connect details.

Falci, L., Shi, Z., & Greenlee, H. (2016). Multiple chronic conditions and use of complementary and alternative medicine among U.S. adults: Results from the 2012 National Health Interview Survey. *Preventing Chronic Disease, 13*, E61. https://pubmed.ncbi.nlm.nih.gov/27149072/

Franco, O. H., Chowdhury, R., Troup, J., Voortman, T., Kunutsor, S., Kavousi, M., Oliver-Williams, C., & Muka, T. (2016). Use of plant-based therapies and menopausal symptoms: A systematic review and meta-analysis. *Journal of the American Medical Association, 315*(23), 2554–2563. https://doi.org/10.1001/jama.2016.8012

Goyal, M., Singh, S., Sibinga, E. M., Gould, N. F., Rowland-Seymour, A., Sharma, R., Berger, Z., Sleicher, D., Maron, D. D., Shihab, H. M., Ranasinghe, P. D., Linn, S., Saha, S., Bass, E. B., &

Haythornthwaite, J. A. (2014). Meditation programs for psychological stress and well-being: A systematic review and meta-analysis. *JAMA Internal Medicine, 174*(3), 357–368. https://doi.org/10.1001/jamainternmed.2013.13018

Häuser, W., Hagl, M., Schmierer, A., & Hansen, E. (2016). The efficacy, safety and applications of medical hypnosis. *Deutsches Arzteblatt International, 113*(17), 289–296. https://doi.org/10.3238/arztebl.2016.0289

Hilton, L., Hempel, S., Ewing, B. A., Apaydin, E., Xenakis, L., Newberry, S., Colaiaco, B., Maher, A. R., Shanman, R. M., Sorbero, M. E., & Maglione, M. A. (2017). Mindfulness meditation for chronic pain: Systematic review and meta-analysis. *Annals of Behavioral Medicine, 51*(2), 199–213. https://doi.org/10.1007/s12160-016-9844-2

Institute of Medicine Committee on the Use of Complementary and Alternative Medicine by the American Public. (2005). *Complementary and alternative medicine in the United States.* National Academies Press. Available from: https://www.ncbi.nlm.nih.gov/books/NBK83799

Lee, S. H. (2022). *Adults meeting fruit and vegetable intake recommendations—United States, 2019.* MMWR. Morbidity and Mortality Weekly Report No. 71.

Makary, M. A., & Daniel, M. (2016). Medical error—the third leading cause of death in the U.S. *British Medical Journal, 353,* i2139. https://doi.org/10.1136/bmj.i2139

Mishra, S., Stierman, B., Gahche, J. J., & Potischman, N. (2021). Dietary supplement use among adults: United States, 2017–2018. NCHS Data Brief No. 399, 1–8. https://www.cdc.gov/nchs/data/databriefs/db399-H.pdf

Sanchez-Lara, E., Lozano-Ruiz, A., Perez-Garcia, M., & Caracuel, A. (2021). Efficacy of mindfulness-based interventions in cognitive function in the elderly people: A systematic review and meta-analysis. *Aging & Mental Health, 26*(9), 1699–1709. https://doi.org/10.1080/13607863.2021.1976724

Yabluchanskiy, A., & Tsitouras, P. D. (2019). Is testosterone replacement therapy in older men effective and safe? *Drugs & Aging, 36*(11), 981–989. https://doi.org/10.1007/s40266-019-00716-2

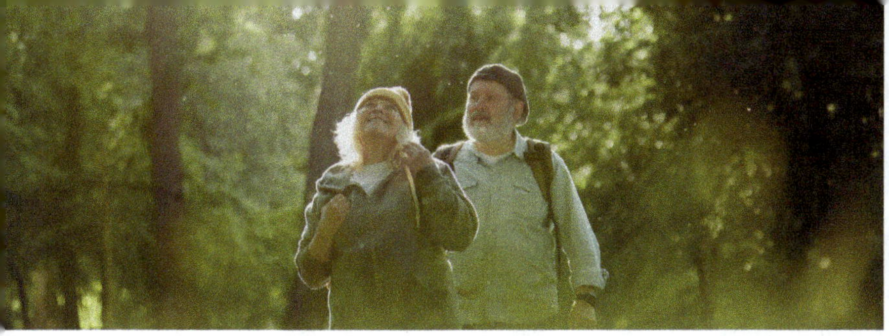

7

SELECTED TOPICS ON HEALTH EDUCATION AND AGING

KEY TERMS

accelerated driver screening
advertising of prescription medicines
alcohol use disorder
driverless cars
driving cessation
drug misuse
fall prevention
Family Smoking Prevention and Tobacco Control Act
Independent Transportation Network
Medicare smoking cessation coverage
motor vehicle safety
pedestrian safety
polypharmacy
secondhand smoke
sex in nursing homes
sexual intimacy and physical intimacy
sexuality
sexually transmitted infections
sleep disorders
sleep efficiency
smokers: age, gender, and education
smoking bans
smoking cessation
smoking prevalence and associated diseases
stages of sleep
universal design

LEARNING OBJECTIVES

- Describe the history of smoking prevalence in the United States.
- Review the diseases associated with smoking.
- Cite the smoking *quit ratio*.
- Examine age, gender, and educational/income differences among smokers.
- Compare *smoking cessation* interventions.
- Examine the impact of taxes on smoking.
- Review the history of secondhand tobacco smoke and the tobacco industry settlement.
- Review the history of *smoking bans* in public places.
- Summarize the Family Smoking Prevention and Tobacco Control Act.
- Describe the implications of the rise in e-cigarette use.
- Describe *Medicare smoking cessation coverage*.
- Define *alcohol use disorder*.
- Review alcohol assessment tools.
- Examine alcohol prevalence among older adults.
- Review diseases and problems associated with alcohol use disorder.
- Describe the positive effects of alcohol.
- Examine medication usage in the United States.
- List medication problems that are patient versus physician initiated.
- Explain the consequences of television advertising of prescription drugs.
- Review medication safety resources.
- Examine the prevalence of falls.
- Review *fall prevention* strategies and resources.
- Examine *motor vehicle safety* issues and interventions for older drivers.
- Review reexamination of older drivers.
- Identify the benefits of *driverless cars* and enhanced safety features for older adults.
- Analyze the consequences of older adults' quitting driving.
- Examine *pedestrian safety* issues.
- List resources for driving safety.
- Examine *sexual and physical intimacy* with age.
- Identify the challenges of sex in long-term care facilities.
- Describe changes in sleep as we age.
- Review medical sleep disorders and sleep hygiene issues.
- Contrast behavioral interventions and medications for sleep disorders.
- Cite sleep interventions and resources.

Health professionals and older adults need to be informed about a great many health education topics. In this chapter, we explore a few of these topics: smoking, alcohol, medication usage, injury prevention (***fall prevention***, ***motor vehicle safety***, and ***pedestrian safety***), sexuality and intimacy, and sleep.

SMOKING

Although most health providers proclaim the leading causes of death to be heart disease, cancer, and stroke, health educators view these diseases as pathological diagnoses rather than as causes. The latter group cites the leading causes of death as smoking, diet, inactivity, and alcohol. From the perspective of these analysts, the number one cause of death is smoking tobacco, and the Americans who are most likely to die as a result of smoking are over the age of 65.

Prevalence

Smoking prevalence (combustible cigarettes) in the United States declined between 1965 and 2022, from 44% of American adults age 18+ to 11.7%, according to the National Cancer Institute. As shown in Figure 7.1, this trend is accelerating and the prevalence of cigarette smoking continues to fall.

FIGURE 7.1 Percentage of adults aged 18 years and older who reported current cigarette use, 1965–2022.

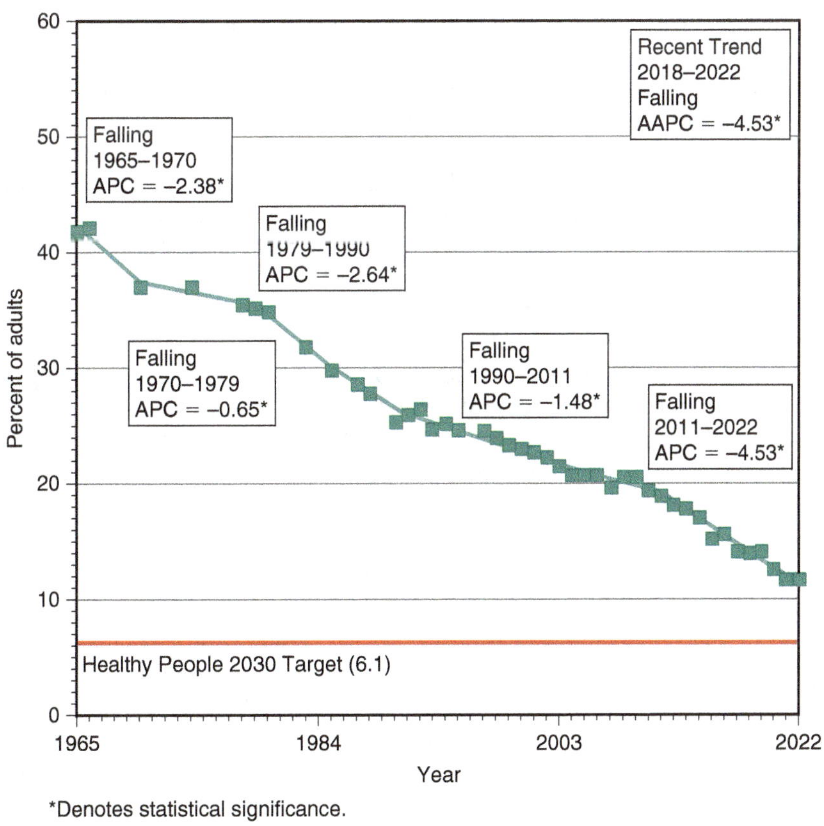

Source: Centers for Disease Control and Prevention, National Center for Health Statistics. National Health Interview Survey. https://progressreport.cancer.gov.

Thus, the *Healthy People 2030* goal of 6.1% prevalence may be within reach. However, the age-adjusted prevalence shown in Figure 7.1 masks a troubling trend for smoking in old age. A Centers for Disease Control and Prevention (CDC) analysis suggests that the number of cigarette ***smokers*** aged 65+ has increased (Le et al., 2024). Older smokers, who for the most part started smoking early in life, may be less likely to switch to electronic, noncombustible tobacco products. The figure suggests that declines in smoking are mainly driven by fewer people starting to smoke.

Worldwide ***smoking prevalence*** has also declined, from 22.7% in 2007 to 17% in 2021 (*Tobacco Atlas*, American Cancer Society and World Lung Foundation; https://tobaccoatlas.org/challenges/prevalence/). Still, because of the lag between the start of smoking and onset of smoking-related disease, deaths attributable to smoking continue to increase. While smoking is a leading cause of premature death in all developed countries, 70% of the deaths from cigarette smoking in the coming century will occur in developing countries. Since 1960, tobacco production has increased threefold in low- and middle-income countries, but in richer countries production has been cut in half. Major producers of cigarettes include China, India, and Brazil (https://www.statista.com/chart/30094/worlds-largest-tobacco-producers/).

Associated Diseases and Mortality

In 2014, on the 50th anniversary of the landmark Surgeon General's report titled *Smoking and Health*, which exposed the deadly effects of smoking, another Surgeon General's report was issued. Even after all these years of ongoing research and publicity, this new report contained shocking new information from just a few years ago. First, because of changes in design (e.g., ventilated filters) and composition of cigarettes (e.g., blended tobaccos with carcinogenic nitrosamines), cigarettes have become deadlier. Second, cigarette smoking kills many more Americans annually than previously estimated—about 480,000 people a year (https://www.cdc.gov/tobacco/data_statistics/fact_sheets/health_effects/effects_cig_smoking/index.htm). We will not see a decline in mortality associated with smoking in the United States until 2030. Third, the revised estimate for medical costs associated with smoking is more than $300 billion a year, rather than the previously estimated $200 billion. Fourth, lifetime smokers can expect to lose about 10 years of life expectancy. And fifth, the list of diseases linked to smoking has grown considerably.

Diseases associated with smoking include 14 different kinds of cancers; chronic obstructive pulmonary disease (COPD), pneumonia, and other respiratory diseases; cardiovascular and cerebrovascular disease; osteoporosis; peptic ulcers; reproductive diseases; cataracts; periodontitis; cognitive decline; and many others.

Focusing on respiratory diseases, more deaths occur from lung cancer than from any other type of cancer, yet lung cancer is rare among those who have never smoked. Smokers with a habit of two packs or more per day have lung cancer rates about 20 times greater than those who have never smoked. Cigarette smoking accounts for 80% of the deaths due to COPD. Moreover, death from COPD usually is preceded by an extended period of disability due, in most cases, to chronic bronchitis or emphysema.

Quit Ratio and Benefit

I phoned my dad to tell him I had stopped smoking. He called me a quitter.

—*Steven Pearl*

It's not that difficult to quit. I did it a thousand times.

—*Mark Twain*

Despite declines in prevalence, in 2020 the United States had about 30.7 million current smokers. This number would be much higher but for the number of people who have managed to stop smoking. Since 2002 former smokers outnumber current smokers, and most smokers are interested in quitting or have tried to quit (VanFrank, 2024).

About 61% of smokers age 65 and older report a desire to quit, but younger people are more successful with ***smoking cessation*** than older adults. Self-report data from the National Health Interview Survey, 2022 show that 15.3% of adults aged 18 to 24 quit but only 5.6% of adults aged 65+ did (VanFrank, 2024).

Many seniors now realize that they can reduce their risk of death from heart disease to close to that of nonsmokers within 2 to 3 years after quitting. A U.S. Surgeon General report (2020) noted that successfully quitting smoking can add as much as 10 years to life expectancy. For example, quitting smoking reduces the risk of coronary heart disease substantially 1 to 2 years after cessation but the risk continues to decrease over the longer term (U.S. Department of Health and Human Services [DHHS], 2020).

Age

The percentage of older adults who smoke (8.8% in 2020) is less than that of the adult population overall (11.7%–12.2% according to different estimates). Part of that is due to the mortality rate for smokers, a selection effect. Smoking is linked to a higher mortality rate, shortening lives about 10 years, and preventing some people from reaching old age.

Older smokers have a personal history of more unsuccessful quit attempts than do younger smokers. They contend with a longer smoking history, the tendency to be thoroughly addicted as a result of a heavy smoking habit, the likelihood of not being exposed to the nonsmoking norms and influences in the modern workplace, less knowledge than younger adults about the physical effects of smoking, and less likelihood of being told by their physician to quit than younger smokers. As mentioned, older smokers may also make less use of electronic cigarettes as an alternative. Quit success in all ages depends heavily on level of nicotine dependence (Arancini et al., 2021).

Two stereotypical attitudes about smokers who survive into old age are: (a) They must be resistant to the health hazards of smoking. (b) Because of their advanced age, they no longer have time to benefit from a reduction in risk by quitting. In fact, as mentioned, smokers who continue to smoke as older adults continue to increase their risk of morbidity and mortality. Those who quit smoking, even late in life, can improve their physical function and overall health in comparison with those who continue smoking.

A presentation by Virginia Reichert of the Center for Tobacco Control at the 2007 American College of Chest Physicians conference stated that smokers over age 65 reported that the most frequent motivations for quitting smoking were physician pressure and stress due to a major health problem. In contrast, younger smokers reported cigarette costs and tobacco odor as prime motivations for quitting.

Gender

Just as it took women longer to reach the same prevalence of smoking as men, achieving that in 2000, it is taking them longer to lower this prevalence. In fact, there was even a slight, though temporary, rise among female smokers who were age 65 and over in 2000. Rates of death from smoking among men and women are now roughly equal (Wensink et al., 2020).

Lung cancer death rates climb rapidly about 20 to 30 years after a large increase in the incidence of smoking. Men began smoking in large numbers after the turn of the previous century, and their death rate from smoking peaked during the first half of the century. Women's rapid rise in smoking began in the 1950s, and by 1986, lung cancer had surpassed breast cancer as the leading cause of cancer death among women.

Forty-five percent of women who have ever smoked have quit, versus 52% of men. Researchers believe that it is more difficult for women to quit smoking because many depend on cigarettes to control their weight. About a quarter century ago, a nationwide survey of adults over age 35 revealed that gaining weight was a more ardent concern for women smokers, and women who gave up smoking gained an average of 11 lbs (Flegal et al., 1995). An umbrella review (review of reviews) suggests that women may have more difficulty maintaining long-term abstinence than men (Smith et al., 2016).

Although from a health perspective a modest weight gain is much more desirable than continued cigarette smoking, it is probably still a difficult trade-off for many female American smokers to make because of the greater stigma for women associated with additional weight. One study, although a bit dated, reported that women who exercised while trying to quit smoking were twice as likely to quit and only gain half as much weight as those who did not exercise (Marcus et al., 1999). Mortality associated with current smoking is similar among men and women as are benefits of smoking cessation (Thomson et al., 2022).

Education and Income

Among Americans in 2020 who never graduated high school, 24.8% smoked. Of those who graduated high school, 24.2% smoked; those with undergraduate degrees, 11.7% smoked; and with graduate degrees, 8.6% smoked. A similar gradient is seen for annual household income: less than $35,000, 25.2%; $35,000 to $74,999, 20.3%; $75,000 to $99,999, 18.4%; $100,000 or more, 13.7% (Cornelius et al., 2022).

Smoking Cessation Legislation

The Affordable Care Act (ACA) requires insurance providers to cover tobacco cessation services with no copay from patients. Fully covered are two cessation attempts a year, each involving four counseling sessions and access (though not free) to all tobacco cessation drugs, over the counter and prescription, approved by the Food and Drug Administration (FDA). With this legislation, the prevalence of receiving advice to quit from a health professional increased from 51.4% to 60.6% between 2010 and 2015 (Tan et al., 2018).

Another weapon for smoking cessation was the 2009 law passed by Congress, the ***Family Smoking Prevention and Tobacco Control Act***, that gave the FDA authority for the first time to regulate tobacco products. So far, the FDA has used this power in a limited way, mainly by rejecting new tobacco products that it deems pose a public health risk above and beyond comparable products already on the market.

But the FDA has not yet even attempted to reduce the addictiveness and harmfulness of cigarettes by reversing the design changes that have made them more dangerous in the past few decades. In addition to not reducing nicotine content and regulating the chemicals in cigarette smoke, the law grants an unfortunate waiver to menthol in its ban on most tobacco flavorings.

The law does tighten restrictions on the marketing and advertising of tobacco products, replacing colorful advertisements and store displays with black-and-white-only text. All outdoor advertising of tobacco within 1,000 feet of schools and playgrounds is illegal. Terms such as "light" and "low tar" are banned. The tobacco industry has to disclose all its product ingredients along with research results and their health effects.

The major casualty to the legislation, until recently, was the watering down of the large, graphic health warnings that were to be placed on cigarette packages by 2012. A 2024 court ruling upheld the FDA's original mandate for graphic health warning labels on cigarette packaging and advertising, which was "a pivotal win for public health" (https://www.publichealthlawcenter.org/commentary/240328/3/28/24-triumph-public-health-affirmation-graphic-warning-labels).

Medicare Smoking Cessation Coverage

Initially, in 2005, ***Medicare offered coverage for smoking cessation*** counseling only for beneficiaries who had tobacco-related diseases (e.g., cardiovascular, cancer, respiratory, gastrointestinal, osteoporosis, cataracts, blood clots) or who were on drug regimens that were adversely affected by smoking (e.g., insulin, hypertensive medications, treatments for blood clots or depression). Thanks to the ACA and its emphasis on prevention, cessation services are now available to all Medicare-eligible people who want to quit smoking. The Centers for Medicare & Medicaid Services (CMS) estimates that 4 million seniors fit this profile.

Two quit attempts are covered per year, each consisting of up to four counseling sessions. Smoking counseling must be prescribed by and provided by a qualified doctor or a Medicare-recognized practitioner. The CMS, however, does not provide guidelines when it comes to qualifications, and encourages clinicians to become appropriately trained until a consensus on national credentialing emerges.

Smoking Cessation: Physicians and Nurses

About 70% of all adult smokers visit a physician each year, and the American Cancer Society reports that almost 80% of heavy smokers claim they would stop smoking if their doctors urged them to do so. Only half of all smokers, however, report having heard an antitobacco admonition from their physician. One problem is the training of physicians. A majority of U.S. medical school graduates are not adequately trained to treat tobacco dependence. Medical education increasingly recognizes the need for such training (Elfandi & Poudyal, 2023).

Even when patients receive a prescription for nicotine replacement therapy (NRT), physicians provide very low levels of smoking cessation assistance beyond how to use the replacement therapy (Bartsch et al., 2016; Solberg et al., 2005). Fewer than one quarter of the more than 1,000 patients surveyed reported that their physician followed up on their smoking cessation therapy.

When client readiness is combined with the authority of the physician, even brief smoking cessation counseling by primary care physicians—especially when reinforced by follow-up visits or telephone calls during the first 4 to 8 weeks—is effective in getting clients to quit (Kottke et al., 2000). An attempt to quit is at least twice as likely to occur among smokers who receive smoking cessation advice from their physicians compared with those who are not advised to quit (Milch et al., 2004).

Physicians either overestimate the percentage of smokers whom they counsel to stop smoking, or their patients do not hear them. In several studies, a much higher percentage of physicians reported that they counseled smokers compared with the percentage of smokers reporting that they received counseling from a physician.

Physicians are more likely to communicate effectively with smokers if they are well prepared for the task. One simple but effective smoking cessation intervention consists of asking whether patients smoke, motivating those who do to quit, setting a date, providing a written reminder or prescription, and using either a nicotine patch or gum as a supplement. These principles have been incorporated into the *Doctors Helping Smokers* (DHS) system, which was developed by Minnesota physicians Thomas Kottke, a cardiologist, and Leif Solberg, a family practitioner. The system was implemented in 31 Minnesota clinics and reimbursed through Blue Plus, a health maintenance organization.

DHS is based on the four As—which, in 2000, expanded to five: *Ask* if patients smoke. *Advise* them that smoking is harmful. *Assess* their readiness to quit. *Assist* them by providing self-help guides, education, and counseling. *Arrange* for a follow-up visit, mailing, or telephone call as the proposed quit date nears. Nurses and other staff assist the physician in counseling and follow-up duties.

Nursing interventions for smoking cessation appear to be effective, based on a meta-analysis of 16 studies. There were significant increases in patients' quitting rates due to nursing intervention compared to a control group or usual care. Moreover, there was no evidence that interventions classified as intensive had a larger effect on patients than less intensive ones, such as the offering of brief advice (Rice et al., 2017).

Nicotine Replacement

It is estimated that more than 95% of smokers relapse after their first attempt to quit (National Institute of Health State-of-the-Science Panel, 2006). Withdrawal symptoms, such as irritability, anxiety, restlessness, and a craving for nicotine, are the major causes of relapse.

The transdermal nicotine delivery system, commonly referred to as the *nicotine patch,* was developed to combat withdrawal symptoms. In the early 1990s, the tobacco industry was opposed to this type of NRT, but by 2016 it was marketing its own products. In addition to not being able to prevent the production of NRTs, they discovered that many smokers were using it to supplement their smoking habit rather than replacing it (Apollonio & Glantz, 2017). A recent review concluded that quit success did not differ by use of a nicotine patch versus other types of NRT, but a combination of NRT types increases odds of success (Theodoulou et al., 2023).

The E-Cigarette Debate

The electronic cigarette is a battery-powered device that delivers an odorless dose of nicotine and flavoring without tar or additives, and produces a vapor mist similar to tobacco smoke. Proponents argue that it is more effective than prior nicotine replacement devices and much less harmful than traditional cigarettes. Opponents argue that they do more harm than good, primarily by recruiting younger people to smoke and by providing a heavier dose of nicotine (and other additives).

One study reported that 55% of those who use e-cigarettes were also smoking cigarettes and another 15% had not smoked cigarettes in the first place. That leaves 30% who had quit smoking using e-cigarettes (Mirbolouk et al., 2018). While 30% is a high termination rate, it is unclear how many of those would have quit smoking using another technique and how many used vaping as a gateway to smoking.

Studies with laboratory mice demonstrated that nicotine vapor can cause damage to DNA, impede ability of cells to repair themselves, and possibly increase the risk of cancer and heart disease. Human studies have shown that e-cigarettes cause a unique innate immune response that can contribute to lung disease (Reidel et al., 2018), and another study reported a significant association with heart attacks (Alzahrani et al., 2018).

As smoking rates have declined, major tobacco companies view e-cigarettes as an important product for survival. They are not discouraged by a survey that found 24% of high school seniors reported vaping nearly daily and 45% have tried it (Zernike, 2018). In 2018, the FDA restricted access to flavored e-cigarettes that lured young people into vaping.

Given insufficient research, the U.S. Preventive Services Task Force (USPSTF) recommends that clinicians direct patients who smoke tobacco to cessation interventions other than vaping, and with established effectiveness and safety results. "Current evidence is insufficient to assess the balance of benefits and harms of electronic cigarettes (e-cigarettes) for tobacco cessation" (https://www.uspreventiveservicestaskforce.org/uspstf/recommendation/tobacco-use-in-adults-and-pregnant-women-counseling-and-interventions).

Other Interventions

In addition to NRTs, there is Zyban (also known as Wellbutrin), which was initially marketed exclusively as an antidepressant. In 2006, a nicotine-free antismoking pill, Chantix, which blocks nicotine receptors, was FDA approved after 22% of successful users remained smoke free after 1 year of a clinical trial (Klesges et al., 2006). Chantix is taken twice a day and has the effect of making smoking unpleasant while reducing withdrawal symptoms.

A problem with consuming either Chantix or Zyban is that in 2009 the FDA required these two smoking cessation drugs to carry the strongest "black box" warning. This warning was based on a substantial number of people who reported feelings of depression, suicidal thoughts, or other unwanted changes in behavior.

Other Tobacco Threats

A taxonomic approach to tobacco products suggests a wide variety of products and modes of delivery, with each requiring a potentially different intervention strategy. Tobacco-containing products include combustible products (cigarettes), heated products (vaping), and smokeless products (nasal snuff, chewing tobacco, and oral snuff; Cox et al., 2023). Smokeless tobacco has seen a rise in popularity, especially among younger people, in the form of nicotine pouches, which may carry new health risks.

History of Government Interventions

Since 1964, under the continued leadership of the federal government, the smoking rate has been lowered by two thirds; however, it has taken a half century to accomplish it. This is due to the tremendous power and resistance of the tobacco industry and the general reluctance of the public to support government involvement in regulating what is considered to be freedom of choice—no matter how deadly that choice may be.

The government's battle against smoking was initiated in 1964 when Surgeon General Luther Terry produced a report titled *Smoking and Health,* in which smoking was declared to be causally related to lung cancer. Since then, the two most powerful weapons at the disposal of the government have been *public bans*, such as television and radio advertising (1970), domestic airplane flights (1990), and government buildings (1997); and *taxes*, such as a huge increase in the federal excise tax on cigarettes (2009).

Let us begin with taxes.

Taxes

Do taxes affect behavior and health? The answer is yes. In 1988, the California Tobacco Control Program was initiated, increasing cigarette taxes by 25 cents a pack and requiring that 20% of the tax money be used for smoking cessation programs, especially for an antismoking television campaign. Subsequently, smoking rates declined and there was a 14% decrease in lung cancer in that state over the following decade, compared to less than 3% in the rest of the country (Tough Anti-Tobacco Effort, 2000), and a lower rate of death from heart disease during this same time period (Fichtenberg & Glantz, 2000).

Researchers followed 632 smokers over a decade, average age 58, and at the same time gathered data on taxes, ***smoking bans*** (to be examined later), and smoking habits. For every $1 increase in cigarette price during this time period, there was a reduction of 35% in the average number of cigarettes smoked by heavy smokers, and a 7% reduction in becoming a heavy smoker (Mayne et al., 2017).

There are smokers who will do whatever it takes, though, to minimize economic disincentives. A study of the effects of taxes on cigarette consumption from 1955 to 1994 reported that state taxes were less effective than federal taxes because smokers bootlegged cigarettes across state lines to avoid state taxes (Meier & Licari, 1997). Teenagers, however, have had fewer options in this regard. California raised its excise tax on cigarettes by 50 cents on January 1, 1999, and sales went down 29% over the next 6 months—particularly among teenagers—compared with the previous year (California Cigarette Sales, 1999).

In New York City, where the price of cigarettes escalated to $8 a pack and to $65 a carton in 2006, the percentage of public high school students who smoked dropped to 11%, compared with 23% in 1999. The biggest decline in youth smoking occurred among Black and Latinx students, who had smoked at a higher rate (29%) and were considerably poorer than White students. By 2024, a pack of cigarettes cost about $12 a pack in New York City, with taxes constituting more than half of the cost.

Many states struggling with budget deficits raised their cigarette taxes substantially, mostly for the purpose of raising revenue. As a consequence of the steep tax increases, many smokers abandoned the practice, but many also became creative at dodging them. Popular strategies included buying on American Indian reservations, in low-tax states like Virginia and Kentucky, from illegal sources, and over the internet. The effect of taxes on the choice to switch between combustible and smokeless products is complex (Abouk et al., 2023).

QUESTION: Do you think raising cigarette taxes in *your* state next year would lead to lower consumption rates? Why?

To fight the avoidance of state taxes through online cigarette purchases, some states have attempted to outlaw these purchases, or they have obtained the customer lists of internet cigarette vendors and sent tax bills to residents who purchased online.

Secondhand Smoke

In January 1993, an Environmental Protection Agency report that was widely publicized in the media declared that passive tobacco smoke is a human carcinogen responsible for

3,000 lung cancer deaths annually among U.S. *non*smokers and that there is an increased risk of cancer, lower respiratory tract infection, and severe asthma symptoms among children.

Subsequent research has also documented the link between ***secondhand smoke*** and lung cancer (Kreuzer et al., 2000), heart disease (Kawachi et al., 1997), stroke (Bonita et al., 1999), and respiratory symptoms (Janson et al., 2001). The mortality rate is about 15% higher among nonsmokers who are exposed to smoke at home than among those not exposed (Hill et al., 2004).

In the latter part of 1996, Michael T. Lewis, a personal injury lawyer from Clarksdale, Mississippi, developed a strategy for attacking the tobacco industry on the basis of secondhand tobacco smoke and tobacco-related illnesses. Realizing that smokers as plaintiffs had had little success winning conventional lawsuits (after all, the argument goes, it is a free country to do what you want), this small-town lawyer convinced the Mississippi Attorney General Michael Moore to sue the tobacco companies to recover money the state spent in Medicaid bills for *smoking-related* illness.

By April 1997, 25 states had filed copycat suits against the tobacco industry and eventually won a large Tobacco Master Settlement ($206 billion over 25 years). Over the years most states, however, either did not use the settlement monies for smoking cessation interventions or used a very low percentage of the settlement for such purposes.

Smoking Bans

Based on the successful legal arguments against secondhand smoke, in 1998 California became the first state to implement a smoking ban in bars, casinos, and even private clubs. The main motivator was not a clamor from the public, but the state's legal liability to wait staff and bartenders who were forced to inhale secondhand smoke during the workday.

After the ban took place, the respiratory health of bartenders improved dramatically with the establishment of smoke-free environments. Respiratory irritations to eyes, nose, and throat decreased from 77% to 19% among bartenders; coughing, wheezing, shortness of breath, and phlegm symptoms decreased from 74% to 32% (Eisner et al., 1998).

Since that time, the majority of states (including the two most prolific producers of tobacco, North Carolina and Virginia) have banned smoking in enclosed public places. Research has shown these bans to be effective public health practices. In Pueblo, Colorado, for instance, a ban on all workplace smoking sites led to a 41% reduction in the rate of heart attacks requiring hospitalization over a 3-year period. There was no such drop in two neighboring areas that did not enact this ban.

A review of 13 studies of public and workspace smoking bans revealed a 36% reduction in heart attacks over a 3-year period in communities in the United States, Canada, and Europe (Lightwood & Glantz, 2009). According to the authors of this meta-analysis, the data add to the already strong evidence that secondhand smoke causes heart attacks, and that passing 100% smoke-free laws in all workplaces and public places will produce substantial health benefits. A global analysis showed similar benefit (Akter et al., 2023).

In 2006, the Surgeon General issued a report on secondhand smoke, titled *The Health Consequences of Involuntary Exposure to Tobacco Smoke* (Samet et al., 2006). The report states that secondhand smoke is not a mere annoyance but a serious health hazard. The Surgeon General at that time, Richard Carmona, declared that smoking sections with the best ventilation systems were still not safe, and advocated for completely smoke-free buildings and public places throughout the United States.

The 670-page study reported that there was "overwhelming scientific evidence that secondhand smoke causes heart disease, lung cancer, and many other illnesses." The report helped to accelerate an already growing movement toward statewide smoking bans in public spaces. (It also accelerated the "retirement" of Surgeon General Richard Carmona by the Bush administration, which viewed the report as too antibusiness.)

Tertiary smoking, when traces of smoke remain for years on walls, furniture, and other surfaces, is also a concern. This residue persists even when there are no active smokers in the environment. It is unclear at this time how much damage may be done to people, particularly those with compromised immune systems.

Whole countries are now banning indoor smoking. Ireland began the trend in 2004, followed by Norway, New Zealand, England, Scotland, Puerto Rico, and others. In 2006, Latin Americans joined in when Uruguay banned smoking in the workplace, shopping malls, and many other public spaces. The president of Uruguay, who promoted the ban, also happened to be a practicing oncologist. In Cuba, you cannot even smoke a legendary Cuban cigar in most public places. In cigarette-friendly France, a ban on smoking in schools, offices, and other public buildings took effect in 2007, and was followed up in 2008 by including restaurants, dance clubs, and some bars.

In China, however, there has been resistance. A majority of Chinese men are smokers and the prevalence of current smoking overall is 26.6% (https://www.who.int/china/health-topics/tobacco). Smoking is permittec in hospitals, and hospital shops sell cigarettes. There are 300 million smokers in China, and thanks to China becoming a member of the World Trade Organization, Western tobacco companies are eagerly attempting to break into this lucrative market.

A 2005 survey reported that 90% of the Chinese population believed that smoking had little effect on their health, or that it was good for them. By 2011, though, the worldwide trend had an impact on the Chinese government. In 2020, about 60.2% of Chinese cities were covered by partial smoke-free policies and about 38.5% by comprehensive smoke-free policies (Wen et al., 2023). The same is true of Russia, the second-largest cigarette market in the world. Smoking bans in many public places have been slow to be enforced, along with proposed cigarette taxes and tobacco advertising restrictions.

ALCOHOL

Definition

No consensus exists among alcohol researchers and other experts regarding what constitutes moderate drinking and what constitutes alcoholism. The Department of Agriculture somewhat arbitrarily defined moderate drinking as no more than two drinks a day for men and one drink a day for women, with a drink defined as approximately 12 ounces of beer, 5 ounces of wine, or 1.5 ounces of spirits. Some researchers conclude, however, that given the substantial increase in the proportion of body fat with aging and the concomitant decrease in volume of total body water, a maximum of one drink a day may be advised for both older women and men. A review notes that older individuals experience higher blood alcohol concentrations in response to an equivalent dose of alcohol compared to younger adults; they also demonstrate less awareness of impairment (Yarnell et al., 2020).

It may be best, when attempting to define alcoholism, to avoid associating it with a specific number of drinks. The National Council on Alcoholism and Drug Dependence defines it as impaired control over drinking, preoccupation with alcohol, use of alcohol despite adverse consequences, and distortion in thinking.

The diagnostic criteria for alcohol dependence used in the fifth edition of the *Diagnostic and Statistical Manual of Mental Disorders* (American Psychiatric Association, 2013) dropped the term alcohol dependency, which was deemed confusing, and replaced it with ***Alcohol Use Disorder***. The manual lists 11 criteria, with the presence of one or two indicating mild disorder; four or five, moderate disorder; and six or more, severe disorder. Examples of such disorder criteria are persistent desire, recurrent problems, increased tolerance to an equivalent amount of alcohol, and withdrawal symptoms.

The National Institute on Alcohol Abuse and Alcoholism simplified the definition of *alcohol use disorder* as compulsive alcohol use and a negative emotional state when not using alcohol. The definition stops short of identifying chemical dependency. Using this definition, the fastest increase in alcohol use disorder is among older adults, with a 107% increase between 2001 and 2013 (Grant et al., 2017). Older adults also saw a large increase in binge drinking over this period (Han et al., 2017). One possible explanation is the aging of the baby boomers into the age 65+ category, and their higher levels of drinking and drug use than the prior generation of older adults.

Types of Alcohol Use Disorder

About one third of older adults with alcohol use disorders are late-onset, reactive problem drinkers (Emiliussen et al., 2017). *Late-onset al*cohol problems are likely to be the product of a life cycle crisis, such as the death of a spouse or the loss of a physical function. Once the precipitating event is identified and therapy is pursued, the condition may be reversible. A return to moderate drinking may be viable for older adults with late-onset alcohol use disorders.

Early-onset drinkers have had a drinking problem for many years and have either avoided treatment or undergone unsuccessful treatment. Although the prognosis for successful treatment of chronic, lifelong problem drinkers is poor, it is not impossible to treat.

Binge drinking is defined as four or more drinks on a single occasion for women, five or more for men. While binge drinking is highest among adults aged 18 to 24 (28%) about 1 in 10 older adults binge drink (Han et al., 2017). When older adults do binge drink, they do it more frequently, averaging six drinks, and increase their risk of health and social problems considerably.

Assessment

The USPSTF recommends that all adults be screened for alcohol misuse, with referral for counseling if necessary (Grade B, U.S. Preventive Services Task Force, 2018). The USPSTF summary recommendation reports that a few brief counseling sessions can help cut excessive drinking among people who do not have a resistant case of alcohol use disorder.

During the early stages of alcohol use disorder, no physical signs or symptoms signal the shift from health to disease. Often, behavioral problems such as repetitive accidents or injuries, or ongoing work and family problems, accompany alcohol misuse.

It may be especially difficult to detect alcohol problems among retired persons who have fewer opportunities to experience problems in the work or community setting. It appears to be particularly difficult for physicians to detect. When presented with early symptoms of alcohol use disorder, only 6% of 462 physicians mentioned substance misuse as a possible diagnosis (Schmid, 2000). It is estimated that physicians make the correct diagnosis of alcohol use disorder in older adults in only about one third of actual cases seen in emergency departments or during hospitalizations.

Even when alcohol use disorder is recognized, the physician is less likely to initiate or recommend treatment for older clients than for younger clients. Some physicians believe it is too late in their older patients' drinking lives to do anything constructive about their problems (Butler et al., 1998). Other physicians believe it is too difficult and time-consuming to accurately assess. One qualitative study of 14 primary care physicians at a Veterans Affairs General Internal Medicine Clinic revealed that providers often did not pursue disclosures from older patients about alcohol problems, or provided advice that was typically vague and tentative—particularly in contrast to alcohol- and smoking-related advice given to younger patients (McCormick et al., 2006).

One of the most popular assessment tools for busy health professionals and one that has been tested with older clients is the CAGE questionnaire. It has good sensitivity and specificity for alcohol misuse in general, though it is less sensitive to early problem or heavy drinking. The four questions in the CAGE questionnaire are

Have you ever:

Thought about	*C*utting down?
Felt	*A*nnoyed when others criticize your drinking?
Felt	*G*uilty about drinking?
Used alcohol as an	*E*ye opener?

Two or more affirmative responses to these questions suggest an alcohol problem.

Although the CAGE instrument is practical for the busy healthcare professional, more sensitivity and specificity can be obtained with longer questionnaires, especially the 25-item Michigan Alcohol Screening Test (MAST), which has been tested with older adults. The MAST, however, is too lengthy for routine screening. A 10-item version of the MAST targeted toward older adults—the Short Michigan Alcohol Screening Test–Geriatric Version—can be used in outpatient settings (Naegle, 2008). It appears to capture different aspects of unsafe drinking, however, and perhaps both it and the CAGE instrument should be used (Moore et al., 2002).

A third commonly used assessment tool is the Alcohol Use Disorders Identification Test (AUDIT). The AUDIT incorporates questions about quantity, frequency, and binge behavior but also focuses on drinking during the previous year and is less sensitive for past drinking problems that can help the clinician distinguish between late-onset versus long-term drinking problems.

QUESTION: Do you have any ideas on how we can better detect problems with alcohol among older adults?

Another assessment option is a biochemical test for diagnosing alcohol misuse. The *carbohydrate-deficient transferrin test* improved upon the specificity and sensitivity of previous biochemical tests and could help break through the denial and rationalization of a patient. However, certain medical conditions, particularly liver diseases, can confound the results.

Prevalence

Estimates of the percentage of Americans who are problem drinkers vary widely, with men having four times the rate of alcoholism as women. According to the 2023 National Survey on Drug Use and Health (NSDUH), 28.9 million people ages 12 and older (10.2% in this age group) suffered from alcohol use disorder in the past year (https://www.samhsa.gov/data/report/2023-nsduh-detailed-tables). The NSDUH survey of Medicare beneficiaries reported an alcohol use disorder prevalence of 4.6% among males and 1.7% among females (Parrish et al., 2022).

It is not easy to estimate the scope of problem drinking in late life because much of it may take place out of the glare of work and community life. Alcohol misuse and dependence in old age will likely increase in the coming decades, as baby boomers, who have a history of greater alcohol consumption than past cohorts of older adults, replace these cohorts.

Associated Diseases and Problems

Although problem drinking in late life is less common than in midlife, the risks of alcohol misuse for older drinkers are elevated in terms of falls and accidents, dementias, medical problems, reaction time, memory, and interactions with prescription and over-the-counter drugs. Nutritional deficiencies, particularly vitamin and protein deficiencies, are more common among older alcohol drinkers as well because of the decreased absorption of many nutrients caused by alcohol.

With age, the body absorbs a higher percentage of the alcohol consumed. This occurs because alcohol is more soluble in water than in fat and, as we age, the water content in our body declines. Lean body mass that is high in water content decreases, and body fat that is low in water content increases. Thus, alcohol reaches a higher concentration in the blood of an older person. Also, as we age, there is a decline in a stomach enzyme—alcohol dehydrogenase—that can break down alcohol before it reaches the bloodstream. This further increases the blood alcohol level and places an extra burden on the liver, where most alcohol metabolism takes place.

Moreover, as we age, blood flow through the liver declines, as does kidney function, which means that alcohol is eliminated more slowly from the blood. Consuming the same amount of alcohol as a younger person, the older person will have a blood alcohol level that is 30% to 40% higher.

Although alcohol adds calories to the diet, it adds almost no nutrients; therefore, malnutrition becomes a problem as well. Other problems of excess alcohol consumption are an increased risk of injury or accident, especially when driving and, along with excess caffeine and medications, an adverse effect on sleep. At least 100 of the most commonly prescribed medications interact negatively with alcohol.

Intervention and Referral

Most patients with suspected drinking problems receive no counseling from primary care physicians. Although physicians report having counseled patients on alcohol misuse, it is much less likely to appear on patients' medical records when they are examined. In 2014 to 2016, the National Ambulatory Medical Care Survey (NAMCS) noted low levels of alcohol screening with a validated questionnaire—just 2.6% of visits. Alcohol counseling, provided either by the physician or by referral, was documented in less than 1%. Screening was more likely if patients were seen by a primary care physician or if they had multiple chronic medical conditions (Chatterton et al., 2022).

Older adults often drink in response to depression and loneliness, whereas younger adults are likely to use multiple substances to assuage their anger, frustration, tension, interpersonal conflicts, and social pressure. If interventions are to be effective, most older adults with alcohol misuse problems will need to be referred by their health professionals to groups or specialists who recognize the different needs of older versus younger persons. Some 17,000 substance misuse programs are available nationally (https://www.statista.com/statistics/450281/total-number-of-substance-abuse-treatment-facilities-in-the-us/), but it is unclear how many offer specialized treatment for older adults (Box 7.1).

Some evidence indicates that persons referred to age-specific support groups remain in treatment longer and complete treatment more often than those in mixed-age groups. Problems such as widowhood and retirement may be particularly difficult for older people to share in support groups of mixed ages. Older adults tend to grapple with different health issues, want a more peaceful environment in which to share, and expect a different pace of verbal interaction than younger adults (Gross, 2008).

BOX 7.1 Gerontologizing Smoking Cessation and Alcohol Counseling

Among the health education topics discussed in this chapter, tobacco and alcohol are two problems likely to be associated with interventions that focus primarily on younger adults. Suppose, however, that an alcohol misuse specialist and a smoking cessation specialist, both of whom have had practices almost exclusively with young adults, are confronted with older clients. What advice would you give to each of them to help them become more responsive to the needs and interests of older clients? Think about topics that are unique to older adults, such as motivation for behavior change in late life, perceived stigma toward drinking or smoking, polypharmacy or comorbidity issues, responsiveness to group facilitation strategies, and so forth.

Alcohol and smoking misuse programs can be run by professionals who have had training with more of a clinical bent, such as nurses, clinical psychologists, or social workers, or by professionals with more of a health education perspective, such as graduates of health education departments or gerontology programs. The relative effectiveness of these professionals for health behavior change has yet to be studied, and it is hard to draw a distinct line between offering health education and providing counseling. Either way, an awareness of the issues impacting older adults is paramount.

About one third of those who attend Alcoholics Anonymous (AA) meetings are over age 50, and many communities launch groups specifically for older adults. The geriatrician Robert Butler suggested: "Because of the magnitude of drinking problems among older people, it would be useful to have AA programs set up especially for them" (Butler et al., 1998, p. 178).

AA employs a strategy that encourages public confession, intense social support, contrition, and a spiritual or philosophical awakening. Founded in the 1930s, AA has expanded to over 120,000 groups around the world, and over 2 million members. Companion organizations have been set up for spouses (Al-Anon), teenage children of alcoholics (Alateen), and adult children of alcoholics (ACA-Dysfunctional Families). AA Sober Seniors addresses the older population.

A Cochrane Review (2020) determined that AA interventions performed as well as established comparison treatments (such as cognitive behavioral therapy), and that AA-like programs were more effective for promoting abstinence (Kelly et al., 2020). Older persons with alcohol issues may raise a unique set of research questions when evaluating the effectiveness of AA groups. Are older adults prepared for the openness that characterizes these types of support groups? Do older adults have access to a support group with other older adults with alcohol problems to whom they can relate?

Professionally led programs should be viewed as complementary to AA and other peer support groups, rather than in competition with them. Professionally run treatment programs may be more effective than AA groups for some older adults, but they have disadvantages as well. They are typically costly and time-bound, in comparison with support groups that can and do meet frequently (some several times a week) and are ongoing.

The self-management strategies and vulnerability to relapse discussed for smoking cessation are applicable to alcohol addiction as well. Behavior management techniques may have to be reapplied on multiple occasions.

Positive Effects?

Early studies suggested that those who consume moderate amounts of alcohol may reduce their risk of heart failure and stroke and promote longevity. Red wine was thought to have particular benefit. More recent research suggests these claims are almost certainly wrong and reflect healthy survivor effects and other forms of confounding (Zhao et al., 2023). Cross-sectional studies do not capture people who die and are removed from populations as a result of heavy and even moderate alcohol use. The result is a spurious association between current drinking and age. Likewise, moderate drinking is a feature of higher socioeconomic status, and it is the greater income, education, and access to healthcare associated with this status that confers health benefit.

Resources

For written material and other resources on alcohol misuse, contact:

Alcoholics Anonymous, www.aa.org
Adult Children of Alcoholics/Dysfunctional Families, www.adultchildren.org
How Do You Talk to Older Adults Who May Be Addicted?" https://www.hazeldenbettyford.org/articles/how-to-talk-to-an-older-person-who-has-a-problem-with-alcohol-or-medications
National Institute on Alcohol Abuse and Alcoholism, www.niaaa.nih.gov

MEDICATION USAGE

In 2022, around 6.7 billion prescriptions were dispensed in the United States (https://www.statista.com/statistics/238702/us-total-medical-prescriptions-issued) with a value of about $634 billion (Tichy et al., 2023). It is not unreasonable to suggest that most Americans consider taking medications a normal part of life. In fact, about half of all adult Americans took at least one prescription drug in the past 30 days, according to 2015 to 2018 data from the CDC, increasing to almost 90% among those aged 65 and older. Americans buy more medicine per person than do citizens of any other country.

Because vulnerability to chronic disease increases over time, medication usage becomes more typical with age. Although adults aged 65+ make up 17% of the population (2023), they account for more than one third of outpatient prescription medications and a similar percentage of those purchased over the counter. To get a sense of how fast medication use is escalating, consider that between 1999 and 2012, the use of five or more prescription drugs increased from 10% to 15% among those age 40 to 64 and from 24% to 39% among those age 65 and over (Kantor et al., 2015).

Many diseases that used to be fatal, including some cancers and AIDS, have now turned into chronic conditions requiring consistent medications. Older persons rely on drugs to survive, to alleviate pain and discomfort, and to promote a sense of security and control in sometimes frightening health situations. Drugs, however, can make matters worse as well as better. The potential for inappropriate prescribing and serious adverse drug effects is great.

A Physician's Experience

Deprescribing refers to identifying problematic medications and carefully reducing inappropriate use. One geriatrician told me it is like removing weeds and debris from a garden. Although it is true that many new medications have been miraculous for the functioning of older adults, this observation remains timely: Many older adults clearly have suffered the consequences of drugs, or fear the consequences of drugs as well.

Research backs this up. If their doctor said it was possible, 92% would stop one or more of their medications (Reeve et al., 2018). If physicians are considering deprescribing, they should be reassured of a likely positive response.

Inappropriate Prescription Use

Potentially inappropriate prescribing is common, with about one third of patients prescribed a medication either not recommended for older people or recommended only in limited circumstances (Tian et al., 2023). Lists of potentially inappropriate medications, such as the Beers criteria (Rochon & Hilmer, 2024), are based on pharmacist assessment and are continually updated.

In the Medicare Part D prescription drug program, 7.3 billion doses of potentially inappropriate medications were dispensed in 2018. The most common medications were proton pump inhibitors, benzodiazepines, and tricyclic antidepressants; and the top five unique medications by reported spending were dexlansoprazole, esomeprazole, omeprazole, dronedarone, and conjugated estrogens (Fralick et al., 2020). Prescribing of benzodiazepines is still common, despite prolonged sedation that can lead to deadly falls and fractures (Maust et al., 2018).

To avoid potential misuse, patients need to understand their medication regimen, report possible side effects, and exercise caution with over-the-counter medications. Only 15% of older patients who visited an emergency department were able to accurately report on their medications, dosages, frequencies, and indications—even with patients who were disoriented or medically unstable excluded from this study (Chung & Barfield, 2002). Audiotaped office visits from 185 outpatient encounters revealed that physicians addressed adverse effects of new medications only one third of the time with patients (Tarn et al., 2006).

Physicians need to take a good drug history, carefully assess dosage, communicate the rationale for the drug treatment and the expected response and common side effects, and monitor patient reactions. The aging process complicates this course of action because it affects the absorption, distribution, metabolism, and excretion of medications.

Physicians must also consider the cost of medications. The Senate Special Committee on Aging issued a report in December 2016, stating that the cost of brand-name popular drugs had increased 10 times the rate of inflation between 2011 and 2016. In addition to the escalation of popular drug costs, in 2016, a new cancer drug Bavencio cost $156,000 a year; a new bladder cancer drug Tecentriq cost $150,000 a year; and a new muscular dystrophy drug cost $300,000 annually. In 2022, approximately one in five older adults reported cost-related nonadherence (Dusetzina et al., 2023).

Whenever possible, physicians need to emphasize the viability and effectiveness of lower cost generic drugs. At a societal level, Congress needs to intensify efforts to negotiate drug prices with pharmaceutical industries for Medicare-covered therapies. Canada, Britain, Germany, and other countries limit drug prices based on effectiveness, or based on the prevailing prices in other countries (Frakt, 2018).

Overprescribing is common as well. Even when nonpharmacologic treatments are suitable for a given condition, physicians often prescribe medications, sometimes encouraged by their patients. Predictably, the greater the number of drugs prescribed, the greater the risk of inadvertent or intentional misuse of drugs by the patient or caregiver.

Polypharmacy is the use of more medications than are clinically indicated. Older adults are particularly vulnerable to polypharmacy because most of the chronic conditions associated with aging are potentially responsive to medications. This leads to the increased risk of multiple drug use among older adults, complicated by the fact that many older patients see more than one healthcare provider. With more than one provider, prescription and over-the-counter drug usage may not be coordinated, and older clients are vulnerable to potential interactions—drug–drug, drug–allergy, drug–food, drug–drink, and drug–disease—and therapeutic duplication. Many pharmacies do not have complete computer records of all the medication usage of their customers.

Listed below are some of the factors that lead to ***drug misuse***:

Patient-Related Drug Misuse Factors

- expectation for the physician to prescribe medication for a problem;
- inadequate reporting of other medications being taken;
- failure to complain about medication-related symptoms;
- use of multiple, automatic refills without visiting a physician;
- hoarding and using prior medications;
- use of multiple pharmacies or multiple physicians;
- borrowing medications from family members or friends;
- self-medication with over-the-counter drugs;
- impaired cognition or vision, or depression;
- underuse of medications due to side effects or cost considerations;
- failure to understand how to take a medication;
- forgetfulness; and
- failure to fill the prescription, or self-determined need to discontinue the medication (due to lack of symptoms, fear of dependency, etc.).

Physician-Related Drug Misuse Factors

- presuming that patients expect a prescription to be written;
- treatment of symptoms with drugs without sufficient clinical evaluation;
- treatment of conditions without setting therapy goals;
- communicating instructions in an unclear, complex, or incomplete manner;
- failure to review medications and their possible adverse effects at regular intervals;
- use of automatic refills without adequate follow-up;
- lack of knowledge of geriatric clinical pharmacology, leading to inappropriate prescribing practices;
- failure to caution about medication interactions;
- failure to simplify drug regimens as often as possible; and
- failure to identify and adequately communicate the equivalency of cost-effective generics.

We can also anticipate greater use of *illicit drugs* among older adults as baby boomers continue to enter their ranks. Since 2000, deaths from opioid overdoses have nearly quadrupled, but for people ages 55 to 74, the increase has been more than sevenfold (*AARP Bulletin*, 2018, January–February issue, p. 4). According to CDC data, the rate of fatal drug overdoses among people 65 years and older was 3.0 per 100,000 population in 2002 and 12.0 per 100,000 in 2021. Rates were highest rates among non-Latinx African Americans (30.9 per 100,000; Humphreys & Shover, 2023).

Opioid use is also a concern for older adults. Prescribed for pain management, opioid use in older adults is associated with many adverse effects. These include impaired motor coordination and dizziness, which increase the risk of falls. "Hangover" effects are common because drug clearance is slower among older people. While opioid misuse appears to be rare in older people, affecting just 2.5% per year (Han et al., 2019), diagnosis of opioid use disorder in this population is likely underestimated because older adults are screened and treated less frequently than younger adults, and diagnostic criteria for the disorder reflect definitions of disability appropriate for younger populations.

Prevention

One of the most effective prevention strategies is to avoid unnecessary medication. Many Americans unthinkingly take pills to alleviate constipation, insomnia, indigestion, headache, and other types of pain or discomfort. Diet, exercise, and stress management, however, may be effective alternatives.

Older clients with high blood pressure, for instance, are susceptible to adverse drug reactions. Treating some patients with mild high blood pressure with nonpharmacologic alternatives, therefore, may be appropriate. Many older adults can be responsive to a reduction in sodium intake, or to exercise that positively affects blood pressure levels. Greater recognition of the high rates of adverse events and even mortality associated with medications may help in this effort (Kramarow &Tejada-Vera, 2022).

Advice From Pharmacists

Pharmacists are required to give patients advice about their prescription drugs. In addition to informing patients verbally and in writing, pharmacies must maintain files of patient information (including a list of the medicines and healthcare devices used by the patient). The pharmacist must provide specific information about each medication and its common side effects, potential interactions, and contraindications, and must instruct patients on how to monitor their responses, explain what to do if a dose is missed, and inform patients on how to store the medicine. Pharmacies are required to provide an area suitable for confidential patient counseling. This medication therapy review is valuable but can sometimes be pro forma in the busy setting of the chain pharmacy or in mail order settings.

The consumer who is most disadvantaged, especially in the way of monitoring potential interaction effects, is the one who pharmacy-hops for either financial purposes or convenience. It is not unusual for a patient to obtain prescription drugs from multiple sources, such as a community pharmacy, a hospital pharmacy, a mail-order pharmacy (some from abroad), and directly through samples from the physician. Patients should consider carrying a current prescription record with them to document medications.

Advertising

Only the United States and New Zealand permit ***advertising of prescription medicines*** to consumers. As the number of advertisements continues to rise, along with consumer spending on advertised prescription medications, this practice has become increasingly controversial. The 50 most-advertised prescription medicines in 2,000 contributed an additional $10 billion in spending on medications. The television messages are almost irresistible: After taking a medication, people with allergies are now able to romp happily in an open field, or those with painful heartburn are able to scarf down a pepperoni pizza.

In 2000, Merck & Company spent $161 million on advertising Vioxx, an arthritis drug, and sales of that one drug alone increased more than $1 billion. (Vioxx was voluntarily withdrawn from the market in 2004 because of its association with increased risk for heart attacks and stroke.) The amount spent on advertising for Vioxx that year was more than PepsiCo spent to advertise Pepsi or Budweiser spent to advertise beer.

Besides prescription arthritis drugs, the most heavily advertised medications were cholesterol-lowering drugs, antidepressants, allergy medicine, and heartburn medicine (Petersen, 2001). By 2007, drug advertising had reached $5 billion, generating untold billions of additional dollars spent on medications, and it remains high at over $6.6 billion in 2020 (https://healthpolicy.usc.edu/article/should-the-government-restrict-direct-to-consumer-prescription-drug-advertising-six-takeaways-from-research-on-the-effects-of-prescription-drug-advertising/). In 2015, the American Medical Association called for a ban on direct-to-consumer advertising of prescription drugs. Big Pharma, however, continues to be the victor in this battle.

Greater exposure to prescription drug advertising was significantly associated with a higher probability of patient requests for advertised drugs. Among older adults who were exposed to direct-to-consumer advertisements, 31% in one sample requested a prescription drug from their physician (Datti & Carter, 2006). Physicians grant about 75% of these requests for advertised drugs, and about half of these transactions result in drug prescriptions that physicians would not choose for a similar patient with the same condition (Mintzes et al., 2003).

Does television advertising increase overall awareness of drugs that might otherwise not be prescribed, or does it stimulate patient demand for unnecessary medication? You decide. My opinion, though, is in line with that of geriatrician John Morley: "Nancy Reagan's 'Just say no to drugs' campaign may have been more effective if it had been aimed at adults rather than teenagers" (Morley, 2002).

Resources

Many readily available booklets on medication are good sources of consumer safety advice for today's cohort of older adults. These booklets list important questions to ask physicians and pharmacists, offer ideas to improve daily compliance with prescription indications, identify generic equivalents, note commonly reported side effects of medications, and include blank charts for listing prescriptions and over-the-counter medications for the patient to take to an appointment with a physician.

AARP provides free materials on the safe use of medications. Contact AARP Publications, Program Resources, 601 E St. NW, Washington, DC 20049. For answers to questions about the drug approval process, drug reactions, and new and approved medications, contact the FDA, Center for Drug Evaluation and Research, 5600 Fishers Lane, Rockville, MD 29857. Tools and resources for addiction recovery are provided by Smart Recovery, www.smartrecovery.org. BeMedWise, launched by the National Council on Patient Information and Education, provides medication information and safety resources, www.bemedwise.org.

QUESTION: If you wanted to reduce polypharmacy and drug misuse through a grant proposal and could focus on only one group—older persons, physicians, or pharmacists—which one would it be? Why? What strategies would you recommend?

INJURY PREVENTION

Unintentional injuries were the third leading cause of death in the United States in 2019, accounting for about 7% of deaths. It is the seventh leading cause of death among older adults, reflecting the effects of chronic disease mortality. The mortality rate from unintentional injuries for older adults was more than twice that of other age groups. Major causes of these deaths involve falls and motor vehicle traffic accidents.

A number of physical and environmental factors contribute to the greater frequency and severity of injuries as well as death from both falls and motor vehicle accidents among older adults: diminished vision and hearing, poor coordination and balance, slower reaction time, and arthritis and neurologic disease. In addition, medication use, which increases with age, can produce drowsiness, confusion, and depression, increasing the likelihood of accidents.

Certain factors are extrinsic to the increased incidence of falls among older people. Homes age along with people; uneven floor surfaces and the absence of safety equipment, such as grab bars for bathtubs and showers, contribute to accidents. Other culprits in the home are throw rugs, inadequate lighting, steep stairs, and lack of handrails.

Accidents can also result when road repairs and improvements and law enforcement fail to keep pace with the increased demands of automobile traffic. Transportation systems and cars are not designed with older people's capacities in mind. For example, few cities acknowledge the need to extend the duration of walk signals at crosswalks to accommodate older pedestrians.

Falls Prevention

According to the CDC, between one quarter and one third of older adults seek medical care for a fall each year in the United States. Falls are the leading cause of death due to injury among older adults, and fall-related deaths among older adults have risen significantly this past decade as the older population increases in number and longevity (Cigolle et al., 2015) and the number of active older adults increases. Falls are also the most common cause of hospital admissions.

About 25% of older adults who fall suffer moderate to severe injuries that make it hard for them to get around or live independently. A majority of older adults who suffer a serious hip fracture—the most common fall-related fracture—never regain their previous function. Falls result not only in decreased physical functioning but also in decreased confidence and a heightened fear of falling. This fear can lead to a cycle of social isolation, further functional decline, and depression.

The older the person, the greater the fall risk. The incidence rate of fall injuries for adults age 85 and older is four times that of adults age 65 to 74. People who fall are more likely to be admitted to a long-term care facility for a year or longer.

Many fall risk factors are preventable. Studies of tai chi, starting over a quarter century ago (Wolf et al., 1996; Wolfson et al., 1996), consistently demonstrate that it improves balance and reduces falls. Weight-bearing and other types of exercise reduce the risk of hip fracture and falls (Robertson et al., 2001). Persons with osteoporosis—which can lead to falls—can be helped by treatment with medications that increase bone density. Footwear is important, with sneakers associated with the lowest risk of a fall, and going barefoot or in stocking feet associated with the highest risk (Koepsell et al., 2004). Environmental changes, such as adding night lights, adjusting placement of objects and furniture, removal of tripping hazards, use of nonslip floor mats, and installation of grab bars in the bathroom, can lead to a reduced incidence of falls by older adults.

An innovative exercise program combining balance training and strength training, and incorporating *spontaneously* into daily life, led to a significant reduction in falls in older adults compared to those who participated in a more structured exercise program (Clemson et al., 2012). Similarly, participants in the Lifestyle Integrated Functional Exercise (LIFE) program also sought spontaneous opportunities to exercise, such as standing on one leg while working at the kitchen counter or doing a squat to close a drawer, rather than adhering to a prescribed exercise routine. By doing these exercises opportunistically in the course of daily life, the participants not only increased their frequency of exercise compared to a more traditional exercise program, but had one-third fewer falls over a 12-month period.

A fall risk screening and prevention program significantly reduced fall-related hospitalizations for older adults who were at risk of falls (Johnston et al., 2018). This program was implemented out of a primary care clinic. Primary prevention, that is, mass screening of balance and gait deficits in people who receive aging services, followed by referral to medical and community services, may also reduce the incidence of falls (Albert et al., 2014).

Most falls occur within the home. It behooves the health professional, therefore, to recommend a home assessment to identify conditions that increase the risk for falling, to suggest environmental changes, and to educate clients to help reduce the risks. For example, in the homes of 1,000 persons age 72 and older, two or more environmental hazards were found in 59% of the bathrooms and in 23% to 42% of the remaining rooms (Gill et al., 1999).

Two thirds of all deaths due to falls in the home are preventable. The following is a list of 10 simple precautions that can reduce the risk of falls within the home:

1. Provide proper illumination and convenient light switches—by the bed, at the end of the hall, and at the top and bottom of stairs. Older persons generally need two to three times as much illumination as younger persons do.
2. Install handrails and place nonslip treads in strategic locations.
3. Tack down or remove loose throw rugs, and repair or replace torn carpet.
4. Install grab bars and place adhesive strips in shower and bath.
5. Eliminate such hazards as trailing electrical cords, sharp corners, slippery floors, and household items that require a step stool to reach.
6. Lower bed height for ease in getting in and out.
7. Wear footwear that provides adequate traction, such as supportive rubber-soled, low-heeled shoes.
8. Exercise to improve balance, flexibility, strength, and coordination.
9. Avoid the misuse of medications and alcohol.
10. Limit fluids after dinner, which can reduce the need for nighttime trips to the bathroom.

Several health conditions, listed in Table 7.1, place older adults at increased risk for falling. A multidisciplinary geriatric assessment can identify those at risk and help to prevent serious injuries from falls. An increasing number of internal medicine and family medicine departments at university medical schools, as well as private practitioners, provide multidisciplinary geriatric assessments. Teams typically include a physician and nurse, and one or more of the following health professionals: occupational therapist, physical therapist, counselor, social worker, health educator, and pharmacist.

TABLE 7.1 PRIMARY RISK FACTORS FOR FALLING

Balance abnormalities	Muscular weakness
Visual disorders	Gait abnormalities
Cardiovascular disease	Osteoporosis
Cognitive impairment	Alcohol
Antihypertensive, sedating analgesic, hypnotic, and antidepressant drugs	Environmental hazards

In 2011, the American Geriatrics Society and the British Geriatrics Society issued guidelines for health professionals on preventing falls in older persons. Health professionals should determine whether their older patients are at risk of falling by asking: "Have you fallen recently? Are you unsteady walking?" The CDC STEADI tool adds, "Are you afraid of falling?" (https://www.cdc.gov/steadi/media/pdfs/STEADI-Algorithm-508.pdf). A yes to any of the questions should trigger assessments for muscle weakness, poor balance, orthostatic changes in blood pressure, foot problems and footwear, and other factors.

About the same time, the USPSTF also came out with recommendations for older adults who are at high risk of falls. Older adults should be encouraged to see a physical therapist, to exercise, and to consider a supplement of 800 IU of vitamin D (Leipzig et al., 2010). The benefits from the first two interventions would reduce the risk of falling by 15%. Exercise received a Grade B recommendation and multifactorial geriatric assessment a C (https://www.uspreventiveservicestaskforce.org/uspstf/recommendation/falls-prevention-community-dwelling-older-adults-interventions). Vitamin D supplementation for falls prevention remains controversial, though a meta-analysis suggests benefit as part of broader supplementation strategies (Tan et al., 2024).

Several strategies are available to assist or protect older adults at risk of falls. An emergency alert system, for instance, uses a signaling device that is worn around the neck or on the belt of an older adult who has a tendency to fall. Anatomically designed external hip protectors reduced the risk of hip fracture among frail older adults in one study (Kannus et al., 2000), but not, however, in another (Kiel et al., 2007) and meta-analyses are equivocal (Da et al., 2024).

Universal design is an architectural philosophy for new homes, or the modification of existing ones, to make them safer for older persons and those with disabilities. Universally designed homes may include grab bars that look like towel racks, counters with stripes around the edge to enhance definition for people with poor vision, showers with pull-down seats, entrances with no steps, doorways that are wider to accommodate wheelchairs, and bedrooms and bathrooms on the same level as the main entrance so that stairs will not hinder access.

A guide that includes summaries of innovative programs to prevent falls, short descriptions of research findings on the topic, a home safety/fall prevention assessment tool, and educational strategies is provided by AARP. For a copy of *The Perfect Fit: Creative Ideas for a Safe and Livable Home* or *Fall Prevention Guide*, contact AARP/Program Resources, 601 E St. NW, Washington, DC 20049

QUESTION: Think about your classroom space, your neighborhood, or your home. What steps can you take to reduce the chances that an older person will have an accident in one of these locations?

or download from https://www.aarp.org/livable-communities/housing/info-2020/homefit-guide-download.html.

For an overview of evidence-based, effective fall prevention programs, the CDC has published two guides: *CDC Compendium of Effective Fall Interventions: What Works for Community-Dwelling Older Adults*, 4th ed., 2023; *Preventing Falls: A Guide to Implementing Effective Community-Based Fall Prevention Programs*, 2nd ed., 2015.

Motor Vehicle Safety

On July 16, 2003, an 86-year-old driver killed 10 people and injured 60 more when he plowed into a crowded farmer's market in Santa Monica, California. Apparently he thought his accelerator was the brake and he could not correct his mistake quickly.

Despite widely publicized tragedies like this one, older drivers kill fewer motorists and pedestrians than any other age group and have a lower crash rate than younger drivers. In 2022, 21.3% of all licensed drivers were age 65+, but only 19% of fatal accidents involved older drivers (https://www.marketwatch.com/guides/insurance-services/senior-driver-statistics-2024/; https://www.nhtsa.gov/book/countermeasures-that-work/older-drivers). Experts attribute this to self-imposed limitations, such as driving fewer miles; avoiding driving at night, in bad weather, and during rush hour; and driving primarily along familiar routes (Agimi et al., 2018). Still, the decision to stop driving, ***driving cessation***, is a complex decision for older people and often difficult for families to navigate.

There were nearly 50 million registered drivers over age 65 in 2021, and a sharp increase is expected in the next two decades as more baby boomers enter the ranks of the older adult. Therefore, older drivers will account for an increasing share of motor vehicle accidents each year. Once a person reaches age 75 and beyond, collision risk is nearly equal to that for drivers age 16 to 24. For older adults in a collision, however, the risk of serious injury and death is much higher.

A number of physiologic changes affect the driving of older adults. Arthritis makes it difficult to turn one's head and directly observe cars coming up from behind. Slower reflexes make emergencies more dangerous to contend with. Susceptibility to the blinding effects of glare, poor adaptation to the dark, and the need for additional light make night driving riskier. Cognitive impairment rises with age and has been linked to higher motor vehicle crash rates in older persons.

Some additional measures to prevent motor vehicle accidents among older drivers include:

- Enroll in a driver safety class designed for midlife and older motorists, such as a course available through AARP 55-Alive or the state motor vehicle department.
- Adjust to hearing and vision losses: Keep the radio, air conditioner, and heater noises low; crack windows to help you hear warning signals; wear good-quality sunglasses; and keep windows clean inside and out.
- Stop frequently to stretch muscles and rest eyes.
- Use seatbelts all the time, even on short trips and in cars with airbags, in order to prevent injury from side collision.
- Keep the car in good working condition.
- Avoid drinking before driving.
- Lobby for state policies that are more responsive to the functional abilities of older drivers.
- Lobby for state policies that require physicians to report motorists who have health problems that could affect their driving ability.

In regard to advocating for more responsive state policies, selected states have begun to make the following traffic improvements: wider highway lanes, larger road signs with bigger letters and numbers, more reflective pavement markers to better illuminate roads at night, traffic-calming efforts and reduced speed limits for local streets, and street names displayed well in advance of intersections.

Relating to more responsible physician reporting, six states—California, Delaware, Nevada, New Jersey, Oregon, and Pennsylvania—require physicians to report motorists who have health problems that could affect their driving ability. In the District of Columbia, physician certification of physical and mental driving competency, a vision test, and sometimes a reaction test are required for the person renewing a driver's license at age 75 or older (Tran & Lee, 2024).

Another study reported that people with early Alzheimer disease or mild dementia may initially be able to drive safely, but their driving skills predictably decline over a 1- to 2-year period to a level that often precludes safe driving (Ott et al., 2008). The researcher highlighted the need for valid screening tests of cognition and driving skills that can identify at-risk drivers in a timely fashion. Clinical assessments of cognition, vision, physical function, medical comorbidities, and medications, along with direct assessment of driving performance, are important for determining competency to drive safely (Hill et al., 2019).

There is no consensus on whether, or at what age, older drivers should be required to be screened more frequently. The earliest age for ***accelerated driver screening*** is 59 in Georgia, and the latest age is 85 in Texas. Illinois, however, has a frequent renewal cycle: every 2 years between ages 81 and 86, and every year for age 87 and older. Iowa drivers over age 70 can only receive driver licenses for 2 years before renewal is required. Overall, 17 states have adopted an accelerated renewal cycle for older drivers, 12 require that older drivers renew their licenses in person, 12 require additional vision tests for older drivers, and one requires additional road tests for older drivers (https://www.taosinjurylawyers.com/blog/elderly-driving-laws-by-state/).

Is this age discrimination? In the driving arena it may be appropriate to use age as a criterion for screening. This is less the result of discrimination than the physical and mental decline associated with aging. One study of older drivers in British Columbia reported that restricted licenses, limited to daylight driving plus a speed maximum, led to a lower crash risk among the restricted older drivers than among the unrestricted drivers (Nasvadi & Wister, 2009). Another study reported that states that mandate in-person license renewal for older adults had a 17% lower death rate among drivers 85 years and older compared with those states without such laws (Grabowski et al., 2004). Mandatory vision testing reduced fatality rates in Florida (McGwin et al., 2008). In an investigation of state-by-state policies, mandatory vision and road testing reduced the likelihood of crashes involving drivers with dementia, but mandatory physician reporting of dementia to motor vehicle bureaus did not have this effect (Agimi et al., 2018). More research is required because older people restrict driving to enhance safety as part of adaptation to sensory and cognitive challenges (Koppel et al., 2020).

Engineering solutions may avoid some of the ethical challenges to use of age as a criterion for license renewal. Cars are increasing age friendly, with error-detecting pedals, automatic emergency braking, sensors to track a vehicle's surroundings or whether a driver has depressed the wrong pedal, and movable seats that make it easy to enter and egress. Many safety features are becoming standard, including lane departure warnings, dashboard backup cameras, glare-reducing rearview and side mirrors, and so forth. Do you want to know if an older driver is even fit to drive a car? There is an online tool, fitnesstodrive.phhp.ufl.edu, that rates a driver's difficulty with 54 driving skills and classifies the driver as at-risk, routine, or accomplished.

All these safety factors may be superseded by ***driverless cars***. In 2017, there were about 200 Uber self-driving cars being tested on roads in Arizona, Pittsburgh, San Francisco, and Toronto. Unfortunately, in Tempe, Arizona, a woman was fatally struck at night by one of those cars, setting back the driverless car movement. Nonetheless, the cars are still being tested in traffic with human supervision, and will soon be operational in geographically limited areas. The long-term goal is to have unrestricted driverless cars throughout the country, with the even longer term goal of zero auto fatalities. Increasingly, rideshare services now cater to older adults, with drivers trained to help older people into and out of cars, and apps that allow others to order rides for older people.

Those Who Quit Driving

The stakes are high for those who give up driving, estimated at about 600,000 people age 70 or older each year, with about a threefold increase in driving cessation for each decade of age (Schouten et al., 2022), and do not find effective transportation alternatives. Some older adults do not need alternatives because they enter a long-term care institution, but most remain in their homes or in independent living facilities and live about 10 years beyond their driving days. During this time, they will need to rely on other forms of transportation. In many communities, public transportation is not available, and even when it is, older adults can find negotiating bus and subway schedules and multiple transfers confusing.

The 2011 Florida Aging Road User Survey asked older driver respondents about their plans for the day when they are no longer able to drive safely. Eighty-three percent reported that they had no postdriving plan. Many responded they had never thought about it, and a few said they would die before they needed to stop driving.

An innovative response to the challenge for older adults who have given up driving is the ***Independent Transportation Network***. If an older adult agrees to stop driving and trades in the car, its value is booked into an account from which the person can draw to receive rides. About $8 is deducted for each car ride given by a paid driver, and less when a ride is scheduled in advance or shared. The Independent Transportation Network program was started by Katherine Freund, whose 3-year-old son was hit by an older driver in Portland, Maine. (Her son recovered and eventually attended the University of Oregon.) Pilot programs are being started in several cities. For more information, contact www.itnportland.org, or one of the 27 affiliates nationwide.

To prepare professionals, family members, and concerned community members to engage in effective conversations about driver safety and community transportation issues with older adults, including alternatives to driving, there is a free publication titled *Driving Transitions Education: Tools, Scripts, and Practice Exercises* (https://www.nhtsa.gov/sites/nhtsa.gov/files/811152.pdf). It was developed by the American Society on Aging and the National Highway Traffic Safety Administration, www.nhtsa.dot.gov.

For a booklet on how to talk to an older family member who may need to consider giving up the driving privilege, *Safe Driving—Conversations With Older Drivers* (https://ewcstatic.thehartford.com/thehartford/the_hartford/files/CMME/we-need-to-talk.pdf) may be useful. In the same way that people prepare for retirement, older adults will also need to plan ahead for the resources they will need after they stop driving. If adequate attention is not paid to this challenge, social isolation and depression may result. The CDC now encourages older people to develop mobility plans that span both walking and other forms of transportation (https://www.cdc.gov/older-adult-drivers/mymobility/index.html).

QUESTION: Think of an older adult you know who has given up or will soon give up driving, and what you can do to reduce this person's chances of becoming isolated and depressed. What ideas can you suggest to enhance this person's ability to remain connected to the world?

Motorcycle Safety

An interesting ***motor vehicle safety*** issue for the future is motorcycle riding, a popular hobby for baby boomers. In 2021, 10% of motorcycle fatalities are people aged 65+ (https://crashstats.nhtsa.dot.gov/Api/Public/ViewPublication/813466.pdf#page=4.16). This percentage may rise, as the median age of motorcycle owners has been going up each year, from age 32 in 1990 to age 47 in 2017 (2017 Annual Report of the Motorcycle Industry Council). Some boomers do not realize that their skill levels and reflexes are not as good as they once were, and that today's motorcycles are heftier and more powerful (Figure 7.2).

Other boomers have begun to recognize their limitations, such as slowing reflexes, bad knees, and aching joints, and have started to "trike" it. Trikes are three-wheeled motorcycles and are popular not only with boomer men, but with women as well. Sales of trikes increased 45% in 2011. Three-wheelers do not require boomer riders to lean into curves or hold them steady at stoplights. Adapted golf carts are always becoming more popular.

Pedestrian Safety

On February 15, 2006, Mayvis Coyle, age 82, was given a $114 ticket for taking too long to cross a Los Angeles street. Ms. Coyle, who used a cane, was unable to make it to the

FIGURE 7.2 Motorcycle riding is not just for young adults and boomers. Motorcycle rider, Hazel Poole.

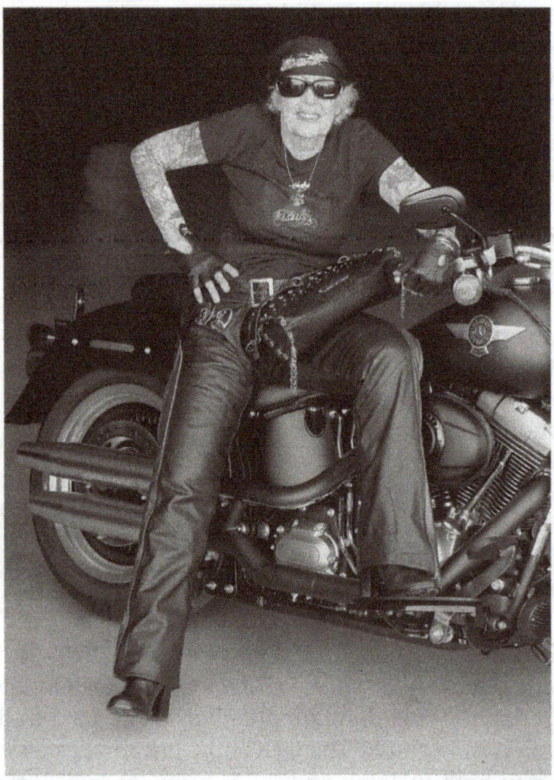

Source: *The Star Press*, Muncie, IN. Photographer, Jeri Reichanadter.

other side of the street before the light turned green for oncoming traffic. While Ms. Coyle was fighting city hall for receiving what she deemed to be an outrageous ticket, city council members acknowledged the error of their ways and voted to lengthen the walk light time at that intersection. They also waived her fine.

The National Highway Traffic Safety Administration reports a decline in pedestrian traffic deaths since 2022: 1.2 deaths per million miles driven despite a 1% increase in miles traveled (https://www.nhtsa.gov/press-releases/nhtsa-2023-traffic-fatalities-2024-estimates). Older adults are more likely than members of any other age group to be injured by motor vehicles while crossing a street and experience the highest death rate from pedestrian accidents. About 16% of vehicle–pedestrian crashes are related to pedestrians over 65 years of age (Toran Pour et al., 2018). A study of residents aged 72 or older from New Haven, Connecticut, revealed that less than 1% of these pedestrians had a walking speed sufficient to cross the street in the time typically allotted at signalized intersections (Langlois et al., 1997).

To find out how you can make your neighborhood safer, the Walk Audit Tool may be helpful (https://www.aarp.org/content/dam/aarp/livable-communities/getting-around/2022/AARP%20Walk%20Audit%20Tool%20Kit-singles-1302023.pdf). The Strollsafe program teaches older people safety strategies for outdoor ambulation (Chippendale et al., 2022).

Some other measures to prevent pedestrian accidents follow:

- Wear highly visible clothing, preferably light-colored or even fluorescent material.
- Do not assume that drivers in moving vehicles see pedestrians.
- Do not return to the curb if the "don't walk" sign begins to flash near the halfway point. Continue to walk at maximum comfortable speed, moving your arms to be more visible.
- Lobby local officials to install properly timed pedestrian traffic signals.

SEXUALITY AND INTIMACY

Older adults can share intimate support in many ways. Some older adults, for instance, cherish playing with grandchildren, watching a sunset with a companion, feeding ducks with children by a pond, walking with a friend in the woods, and enjoying ***sexual intimacy***. Playing, watching, feeding, and walking are not problematic for most older adults; sexual intimacy, however, may present more of a challenge.

A national survey of Americans aged 57 to 85 reported that the majority of older couples remain sexually active, but sexual practices decline with age. Seventy-three percent of Americans between ages 57 and 64 had sex, 53% between ages 65 and 75, and 26% for those aged 85 and over (Lindau et al., 2007). Sexual problems are common among older adults but are rarely discussed with physicians. Men are more likely than women to have a partner, to be sexually active with that partner, and to have more positive and permissive attitudes toward sex (Waite et al., 2009).

Although these surveys may be reassuring in that they report that sexual practices continue into late life, they ignore the more important topic of intimacy, and the warmth, sharing, touching, and intimate communication that is maintained in good relationships. As consumers of research, we might find it useful to pay more attention to the studies that give primacy to intimacy over intercourse.

We also need to pay attention to research biases that use aging American samples that are unnecessarily limited to heterosexual activities, Caucasians, and healthy older adults. Sexual function and aging vary by race and ethnicity (Huang et al., 2009), by sexual orientation (Jackson et al., 2008), and even by geography (Træen et al., 2019). Also, patient–provider communication about sexual health among unmarried, middle-aged, and older women can be problematic when providers make assumptions about marital status and sexual orientation, and when patients view questions and discussions as judgmental (Politi, 2009).

The sexual expression of aging Americans can get waylaid by psychological factors, such as depression, guilt, monotony, performance anxiety, and anger. Young and old alike can be hampered by negative attitudes that reveal hostility or disgust toward the expression of ***sexuality*** in late life. Physical limitations are yet another cause of sexual dysfunction. Arthritic pains, cardiovascular disorders, respiratory conditions, hormonal imbalances, and neurologic disorders can interfere not only with sexual performance but also with intimacy. In addition, various medications can lead to a loss of interest in sexuality and intimacy.

The most significant cause of sexual inactivity or lack of intimacy, particularly among women, is widowhood or lack of opportunity. This problem is exacerbated in older adults who are not accepting of alternative intimacy practices. Family members might try to expand the options of an older adult by arranging to have a respected health professional prescribe the reading of a book that was way ahead of its time in open-mindedness, *The Joy of Sex* (Comfort, 1972), in which the physician–author, Dr. Alex Comfort, presented a wide variety of ideas on sex and intimacy. Older women who have a sexual problem, though, are less likely than men—22% versus 38%—to consult a physician or other health professional (Lindau et al., 2007).

When talking about sex and aging, it would be remiss to ignore the CDC data that demonstrated that the topics of gerontology and ***sexually transmitted infections*** (STIs) have converged. This report notes that STIs had increased among older adults between 2007 and 2011 as rapidly as it had for the 20- to 24-year-old age group (Emanuel, 2014). Between 2014 and 2017, the age 60 and over group surpassed all other age groups with an increase of STIs of 23% (CDC, 2018). As more boomers surpass age 65 and above, the STI rate among the old is expected to increase.

Even more alarming is that condoms were used in 6% of sexual encounters among people age 60 and older, versus 40% among college-age Americans. Unconcerned about pregnancy and having grown up prior to the safe sex era, older adults may not give much thought to STIs. Not surprisingly, therefore, there has been an increase in the number of adults age 50+ with HIV/AIDS. Among newly diagnosed HIV cases, 2% to 4% involve people aged 65+ (https://www.cdc.gov/hiv/data-research/facts-stats/age.html#). Yet very little HIV prevention education has been targeted toward boomers or older adults. In fact, the CDC recommendation to test everyone between the ages of 14 and 64 for HIV/AIDS reinforces an implied irrelevancy of testing and prevention education for adults age 65 and over.

Sex in nursing homes has been a neglected topic as well. Most long-term care administrators prefer to ignore the topic and, if that is not possible, prevent it unless the couple is heterosexual, married, and cognitively intact. The Hebrew Home at Riverdale in New York, however, delved into this topic as early as 1995, and wrote a groundbreaking four-page policy statement accompanied by staff training on sexual situations. Their policy affirms the right of residents to seek out and engage in sexual expression, with staff sensitized to the issues involved on a case-by-case basis. But only about half of skilled nursing homes have policies on sexuality among residents (Lester et al., 2016).

Ever the groundbreaker, the Hebrew Home at Riverdale started a dating service called G-Date, which stands for Grandparent Date. More than a dozen of the 870 residents participated (Hu, 2016); while none found love that first year, several developed friendships. Charlotte Dell, the director of social services, proclaimed: "We're going to get a wedding out of this yet."

The topic of sex in nursing homes received national publicity when Henry Rayhons, age 78, a longtime Iowa lawmaker, went to trial for allegedly sexually abusing his wife, who had Alzheimer and was living in a nursing home. Staff members told him she was mentally unable to agree to sex, and he was arrested and pled not guilty. The jury was convinced of the loving relationship between the two, and acquitted Mr. Rayhons on April 22, 2015. The case highlights why this subject can no longer be neglected.

Intimacy is a universal need and few, if any, would deny older adults the opportunity for it. It is often as simple as touching. The importance of touching was clearly demonstrated when a yoga class, which had been enthusiastically received by older adults at senior centers and congregate living facilities (Haber, 1983, 1986), was presented at 10 nursing homes (Haber, 1988). After unsuccessful attempts to engage these nursing home residents were made during the first three classes, it was decided to begin each class with massage—mostly instructor-to-resident massage (with help from student assistants), but also resident-to-resident and self-massage (Figure 7.3).

QUESTION: The anecdote on the importance of touch should probably have included a cautionary note. What would that be?

As a consequence of this innovation, there was a dramatic increase in *fun* and *intimacy*. The nursing home residents enthusiastically awaited the remaining classes.

This demonstration of the need for touch and intimacy brought to mind a passage from a book by Ebersole and Hess (1990): "When a group of Boy Scouts completed their performance for [a group of nursing home] residents [an old woman] beckoned to the scout leader and said, 'Do you suppose I could hug one of those little boys?'"

FIGURE 7.3 Self-massage techniques for the knee, elbow, fingers, and neck.

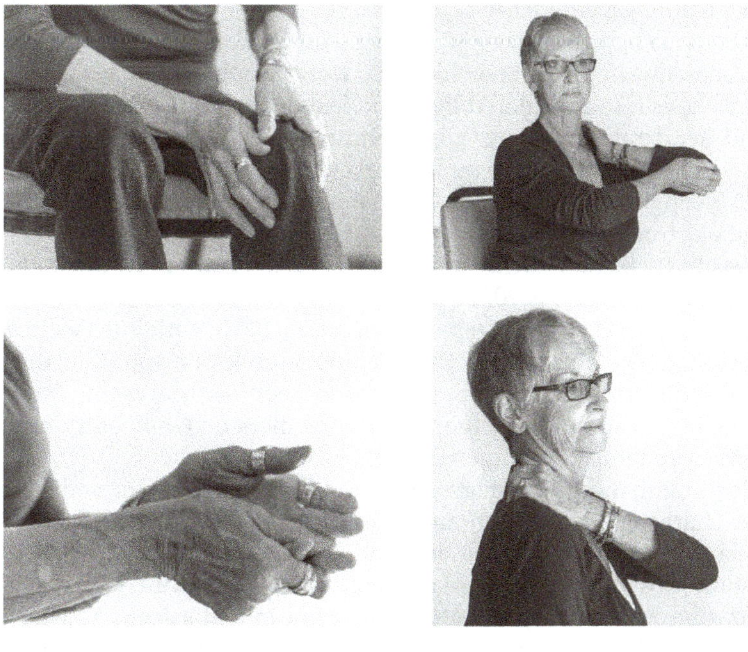

SLEEP

Normal aging is accompanied by lessened quality and quantity of sleep. There appears to be a measurable decrease in the ability of the healthy older adult to initiate and maintain sleep, accompanied by a decrease in the proportion of the deeper, more restorative sleep (Espiritu, 2008). But this does not mean that most older adults have *insomnia*, defined by the *Diagnostic and Statistical Manual of Mental Disorders* (5th ed.; *DSM-5*; American Psychiatric Association, 2013) as difficulty in initiating or maintaining sleep that occurs at least three times a week and persists over 3 or more months.

People require different amounts of sleep, so it is hard to give a definitive answer to the prevalence of sleep problems based on the number of hours of sleep a person gets. But based on self-reports, chronic, primary (not due to medical, psychiatric, or environmental causes) insomnia in older adults is estimated at 10%. About 50% of older adults, however, complain about sleep problems at least once a week that do not rise to the level of insomnia, according to the University of Michigan's National Poll on Healthy Aging.

Significant sleep disturbance is likely to impact quality of life. Insomniacs are 2.5 times more likely to have accidents than other drivers; are more likely to be anxious, depressed, or forgetful; and may recover more slowly from an illness. Inadequate sleep has also been associated with changes in the brain structure and cognitive functioning (Lo et al., 2014), hypertension (Gangwisch et al., 2006), and weight gain (Gangwisch et al., 2005).

A national survey conducted by the National Sleep Foundation reported that over half of Americans experienced one or more symptoms of sleep disturbance over the past week, including difficulty falling asleep, waking up during the night, waking up too early, and waking up feeling fatigued. Forty percent of the adults in this survey reported being so sleepy some days that it interfered with their daily activities. Yet only 4% were seeing a healthcare provider for advice or treatment.

Sleep Changes With Age

There are four ***stages of sleep***: three nonrapid eye movement (REM) sleep phases and one REM or dreaming sleep phase.

Stage 1: Sleep is light, lasts 5 or 10 minutes, and is considered a transitional period. If wakened, someone might not feel like they were sleeping at all.

Stage 2: Sleep is also considered light and lasts 20 or more minutes, with body temperature and heart rate declining. Older adults tend to spend more time in the two lighter stages of sleep and to have more awakenings.

Stage 3: Sleep is deep sleep and is defined by the presence of low-frequency, high-voltage electroencephalographic (EEG) waves, called *delta waves* or slow waves. We are not easily awakened during this stage of sleep. As we grow older, the time spent in deep sleep reduces (Vorona, 2009).

Stage 4: This is REM sleep, or *rapid eye movement sleep*, with intense dreaming. With the exception of our eye muscles and the principal muscle of respiration, the diaphragm, we are paralyzed during REM sleep, perhaps to keep us from acting out our dreams. REM sleep lasts up to an hour and there is disagreement on whether the amount of time spent in REM sleep tends to decline with age.

We cycle through these four stages, back and forth, around four or five times a night.

Another characteristic of sleep and aging is that the *circadian rhythm*—roughly a 24-hour cycle that responds to light and dark—shifts earlier over the lifecycle for unknown reasons. Most older adults are not disturbed by this shift.

Sleep efficiency is the proportion of time spent in bed asleep. As we age, sleep efficiency typically declines from 90% to about 70%. Does this mean that the *typical* older adult has significant sleep problems? Most experts do not think so as many persons approaching 70% sleep efficiency do not view this as an ongoing problem.

In the absence of more precise data on what constitutes a sleep problem, some analysts define sleep problems as too little sleep (5 or fewer hours a night), or too much sleep (9 or more hours a night). These two extremes are associated with higher mortality in adults (Gangwisch et al., 2008). An expert consensus panel reviewed research on sleep duration and health effects for older adults and determined that 7 to 8 hours of sleep was optimal (Hirshkowitz et al., 2015).

Sleep-Related Medical Disorders

Restless legs syndrome (RLS) is defined as intense discomfort in the legs during periods of inactivity, particularly at night. Movement alleviates the unpleasant symptoms but disrupts sleep, and RLS can recur when the legs are again at rest during sleep. About 10% of the population in the United States is afflicted with RLS, and most are over the age of 50 (Vorona, 2009). Patients are instructed to minimize caffeine and alcohol and to avoid antihistamines. Some are asked to take warm baths, to get massages, or to exercise. Medications, vitamins, and minerals may be helpful.

Obstructive sleep apnea syndrome is the repeated complete or near-complete occlusion of the upper airway during sleep. Often found in obese or older people, it is marked by cycles of loud snoring, obstruction, and gasping for breath. This is the most common sleep disorder and is age related, perhaps owing to loss of muscle tone that disrupts air flow, and peaks after age 65. It is considered to be a secondary cause of hypertension and is associated with heart problems, stroke, cognitive impairment, and dementia (Yaffe et al., 2011). Patients are often instructed to lose weight and to reduce or avoid alcohol. Keeping the airway open with continuous positive airway pressure (commonly referred to as CPAP) machines, using mouth guards, and undergoing surgery are possible interventions for obstructive sleep apnea.

There are a host of other sleep-related diseases and disorders to consider as well, such as gastroesophageal reflux disease (GERD), heart problems, stroke, dementia, depression, osteoporosis, and renal disease, to name a few. Inadequate sleep is associated with obesity (Jean-Louis et al., 2014). Insufficient sleep lowers the level of leptin, a hormone that tells the brain enough food has been consumed, and increases the level of ghrelin, which stimulates appetite.

Interventions

Identifying the cause of sleeplessness can be rather complicated, but it is necessary for identifying effective interventions. Potential causes of insomnia can be far ranging, as can interventions to alleviate the condition (Table 7.2). Most sleep specialists recommend the application of behavioral interventions for nonmedical sleep disorder problems rather than the long-term use of sleep medications.

Regarding exercise, older adults with moderate sleep complaints slept almost an hour longer and reduced by half the amount of time it took to fall asleep as a consequence of participating in a low-impact aerobics program (King et al., 1997). Even a sample of healthy older adult caregivers with no major sleep complaints saw improvements in sleep quality after completing a moderate-intensity exercise program (King et al., 2002).

Another effective exercise may be tai chi. Older adults with moderate sleep complaints improved self-rated sleep quality with a 6-month, low- to moderate-intensity tai chi program (Li et al., 2004). In another study, persons aged 59 to 86 with moderate

TABLE 7.2 CAUSES OF AND INTERVENTIONS FOR SLEEP DISORDERS

CAUSES		
Arthritis	Hyperactive thyroid	Sleep apnea
Restless legs syndrome	Anxiety	Too much caffeine
Noise, temperature, light	Inadequate sleep hygiene	Inactivity
INTERVENTIONS		
Restricting caffeine Managing daytime napping Avoiding heavy meals at night Cognitive/behavioral therapies	Keeping a regular bedtime schedule Avoiding reading and watching television in the bedroom Medical interventions Manage noise, temperature, light	Using relaxation techniques Limiting drinking, particularly alcohol, after dinner Monitoring medications More exercise

sleep complaints were randomized into a tai chi group or a health education class. A significantly higher percentage of the former group moved from the poor sleeping range into the good sleeping range compared with the latter group (Irwin et al., 2008).

Cognitive behavioral therapy (CBT) not only is effective for alleviating insomnia symptoms but also reduced healthcare-related costs by more than $200 on average (McCrae et al., 2014). In another study, CBT was slightly more effective than drug therapy in the short run, but follow-up assessments up to 14 months later indicated that *only* CBT led to sustained benefits (Morin et al., 1999; Sivertsen et al., 2006). In the long run, persons build up drug tolerance, the dosage must be raised, and the risks for memory impairment, hypertension, and more frequent accidents are increased. Even brief behavioral therapies have shown benefit.

Another sleep aid alternative is music. Sixty people aged 60 to 83 who had difficulty sleeping listened to music tapes before bedtime. Sleep improved over a 3-week period in terms of duration, efficiency, and perceived quality (Lai & Good, 2006).

Sleep hygiene is a major component of most sleep interventions. Attention to the environment is important in terms of such factors as modulating noise level, bright light, and room temperature, and avoiding use of the bed for television viewing or working. Bedtime reading with an iPad or smartphone—versus reading print—interfered with sleep onset, levels of melatonin, and REM sleep. Electronic devices reduce sleepiness at night and alertness in the morning (Chinoy et al., 2018).

Attaining a calm mental state is also important; relaxation techniques can be used to deal with mood issues or to avoid perseveration on anxiety-producing topics. Maintaining consistent bed and wake times is helpful, as is avoiding certain foods after 4:00 p.m., and limiting drinks after dinner. Finally, it is useful to identify any medical issues that may be in play, such as a medical problem or use of certain medications, and intervene as appropriate.

Although data on the United States are not available, the median amount of time spent on sleep-related issues during medical training in the United Kingdom was 5 minutes (Stores & Crawford, 1998). Not surprisingly, the typical treatment for chronic insomnia by physicians is to prescribe benzodiazepines, which have known side effects, rather than referral to CBT interventions (Montgomery, 2002).

Thus, a widespread approach to sleep problems, and one that is gaining even more popularity as a result of television advertising, is the use of sleeping pills. Sleeping pill prescriptions increased more than 60% over the past 15 years. The latest generation of sleep aids that reduce neural activity in brain neurotransmitters—products such as Ambien, Lunesta, and Sonata—have been advertised heavily in the United States and have led to substantially increased consumption of sleeping pills. In older patients, however, sedative medications are more than twice as likely to produce an adverse effect as they are to help improve quality of sleep, according to a meta-analysis of 24 randomized, controlled trials (Glass et al., 2005). Benzodiazepines like Valium and so-called Z-drugs such as Klonopin, Xanax, and Ativan are increasingly being used as sleep aids, accompanied by a higher risk of drowsiness, dizziness, and two and a half times the likelihood of hip fractures (Donnelly et al., 2017).

Over-the-counter sleep aids like Tylenol PM are antihistamines that may work for occasional sleeplessness, but should not be taken chronically. In older adults, they may have side effects like cognitive clouding, grogginess, dry mouth, constipation, and incomplete bladder emptying (Albert et al., 2017; Vitiello, 2018).

Many dietary supplements are reputed to act as sedatives, such as chamomile, tryptophan, exotic passion flower, and valerian extract, but their effectiveness is not supported by randomized, controlled research studies. The same holds true for the popular hormone melatonin, which is found in most health food stores and drugstores. There is little controlled research that supports its use as a sleeping aid, and prolonged use may be unsafe.

Sleep Resources

The *American Sleep Association* links people interested in sleep health and ***sleep disorders***, and is a complete source of sleep information communication (www.americansleepassociation.org).

The *National Sleep Foundation* posts research and lists sleep treatment centers (www.sleepfoundation.org).

The American College of Physicians recommends a CBT program for patients with insomnia, referred to as C.B.T.-I. This program is provided face-to-face or online. For more information, access www.med.upenn.edu/cbti.

SUMMARY

Health educators constitute an important profession that is necessary for promoting health. They must learn how—and be allowed—to collaborate with health providers who may not recognize their worth, and with patients/clients who may resist their guidance. Practical health research findings are reported in academic journals or popular media almost every day of the year, and it is a challenge for health educators, providers, and patients/clients to stay current. A collaboration among the three groups is essential.

Perhaps the most successful outcome of health education is smoking cessation. The number of smokers in the United States declined by two thirds since the mid-1960s, and the percentage of older adults who smoke is down to 8.8%. Alcohol use disorder is also quite low among older adults, estimated to be in the single digits, but unlike smoking cessation, this percentage is likely to increase because of the advent of the more booze-friendly boomers entering the ranks of those age 65+. Although not prevalent among older adults, the addictions of smoking and alcohol can have deadly consequences.

Medication usage is a different story, with almost 90% of older Americans taking at least one prescription medication during the past month (two thirds take three), and close to 50% not taking a medication properly. Unintentional injuries among older adults are on the rise in the United States, and the mortality rate for older adults is twice that of other age groups. The most common unintentional injury is from falls, and a significant percentage of older adults never regain their baseline mobility or independence following a fall. Motor vehicle and pedestrian safety issues also disproportionately affect older adults, but there are devices, programs, and policies that can significantly reduce injuries and fatalities.

Sexual activity and ***physical intimacy*** can unnecessarily decline in late life because of stigma, lack of opportunity, and poor policies, particularly in long-term care institutions. The Hebrew Home at Riverdale provides a role model for enlightened thinking and practice when it comes to sex and intimacy in a long-term care facility.

Almost 50% of older adults complain about sleep problems at least once a week. Sleep issues are associated with accidents, anxiety, depression, forgetfulness, slow healing, reduced cognitive acuity, hypertension, weight gain, and ... well, that should be enough to convince the reader of the importance of sleep efficiency. Cognitive behavioral interventions are effective, while long-term use of sleep medications is not. Over-the-counter supplements may be useful as placebos but have not established superiority to placebos in rigorous research endeavors.

REFERENCES

Only key references appear in the print edition. The full reference list can be accessed by visiting www.springerpub.com/courseconnect. See inside front cover and tear-out card for CourseConnect details.

Agimi, Y, Albert, S. M., Youk, A., Documet, P., & Steiner, C. (2017). Mandatory physician reporting of at risk drivers: The older driver example. *The Gerontologist*, *58*(3), 578–587. https://doi.org/10.1093/geront/gnw209

Albert, S. M., King, J., Boudreau, R., Prasad, T., Lin, C. J., & Newman, A. B. (2014). Primary prevention of falls: Effectiveness of a statewide program. *American Journal of Public Health*, *104*(5), e77–e84. https://doi.org/10.2105/AJPH.2013.301829

Fralick, M., Bartsch, E., Ritchie, C. S., & Sacks, C. A. (2020). Estimating the use of potentially inappropriate medications among older adults in the United States. *Journal of the American Geriatrics Society*, *68*(12), 2927–2930. https://doi.org/10.1111/jgs.16779

Han, B. H., Sherman, S. E., & Palamar, J. J. (2019). Prescription opioid misuse among middle-aged and older adults in the United States, 2015–2016. *Preventive Medicine*, *121*, 94–98. https://doi.org/10.1016/j.ypmed.2019.02.018

Humphreys, K., & Shover, C. L. (2023). Twenty-year trends in drug overdose fatalities among older adults in the US. *JAMA Psychiatry*, *80*(5), 518–520. https://doi.org/1001/jamapsychiatry.2022.5159

Kelly, J. F., Abry, A., Ferri, M., & Humphreys, K. (2020). Alcoholics Anonymous and 12-step facilitation treatments for alcohol use disorder: A distillation of a 2020 Cochrane review for clinicians and policy makers. *Alcohol and Alcoholism*, *55*(6), 641–651. https://doi.org/10.1093/alcalc/agaa050

Kiel, D. P., Magaziner, J., Zimmerman, S., Ball, L., Barton, B. A., Brown, K. M., Stone, J. P., Dewkett, D., & Birge, S. J. (2007). Efficacy of a hip protector to prevent hip fracture in nursing home residents. *Journal of the American Medical Association*, *298*, 413–422. https://doi.org/10.1001/jama.298.4.413

Parish, W. J., Mark, T. L., Weber, E. M., & Steinberg, D. G. (2022). Substance use disorders among medicare beneficiaries: Prevalence, mental and physical comorbidities, and treatment barriers. *American Journal of Preventive Medicine*, *63*(2), 225–232. https://doi.org/10.1016/j.amepre.2022.01.021

VanFrank, B. (2024). Adult smoking cessation—United States, 2022. *Morbidity and Mortality Weekly Report*, *73*(29), 633–641. https://doi.org/10.15585/mmwr.mm7329a1

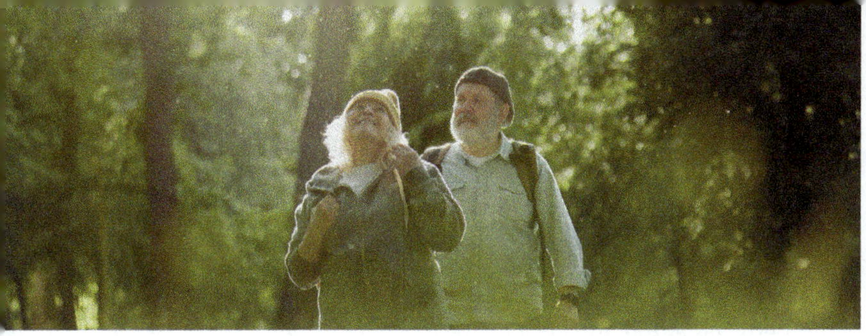

8

MENTAL HEALTH AND AGING

KEY TERMS

Alzheimer disease
anxiety disorder
brain games
chronic stress
cognitive behavioral therapy
cognitive reserve
cognitive stimulation
dementia
depression
emotional regulation
empowerment theory
ethical will
gerotranscendence
intergenerational support and programs
isolation and loneliness
life review
mental health
mental health parity
mental health resources
mental illness
online support
peer support
pet support and pet therapy
placebo effect
psychoneuroimmunology
relational management skills
religious or spiritual resources
self-transcendence
social networking
social support, social/emotional support
socioemotional selectivity
stress management

LEARNING OBJECTIVES

- Compare the *mental health* of older adults with that of younger and middle-aged adults.
- Define mental health and *mental illness*.
- Explain the relationship between aging and *emotional regulation*.
- Review the causes and consequences of *depression* in late life and explain why depression is not a normal part of the aging process.
- Examine the challenges of screening and diagnosing depression in older adults and the consequences of untreated or undertreated depression.
- Contrast the pharmacologic and nonpharmacologic treatments for depression.
- Describe the *life review* process and its impact on mental health.
- Apply the life review technique to an older adult.
- Explain the purpose of an *ethical will*.
- Define *Alzheimer disease (AD)* and *preclinical AD* and identify the stages of both.
- Contrast the pharmacologic and nonpharmacologic treatments for AD.
- Explain *cognitive stimulation* and its benefits and limitations.
- Analyze the validity of *brain games*.
- Summarize mental disorders that affect older adults.
- Review the history of ***mental health parity*** in insurance coverage.
- Define *chronic stress* and explain how it is measured and treated.
- Explain *psychoneuroimmunology*.
- Critically evaluate the impact of a *positive attitude*.
- Explain the downside of relentless positivity.
- Define the *placebo effect* and state your opinion about its ethical justification in medicine.
- Explain whether trying to look younger in old age is an ageist reaction to a natural process or an effective way to cope in a youth-oriented society.
- Identify mental health and creativity resources useful for older adults.
- Contrast social support and social network.
- Examine the impact of social and emotional support on health and longevity.
- Discuss whether there is more social isolation in America today than in generations past.
- Recognize the involvement of baby boomers and older adults in online ***social networking***.
- Discuss the advantages and disadvantages of *online support* and social networking.
- Review the influence of *pet support* on the mental health of older adults.
- Critically evaluate whether religious activity promotes physical health and extends longevity.
- Identify aging and spiritual resources.
- Discuss whether health professionals should concern themselves with the religious beliefs and practices of clients.
- Review the *peer support* movement and its implications for older adults.
- Explain ***empowerment theory***.
- Discuss the strengths and limitations of *peer support*.
- Cite examples of model *intergenerational support* programs.

MENTAL HEALTH

Mental health is a multifaceted concept and difficult to define. In addition to clinical diagnoses, such as major depression or generalized ***anxiety disorder*** (GAD), it may include indicators of morale, such as life satisfaction, ability to cope, positive functioning, emotional regulation, finding meaning and purpose in life, and so forth. ***Mental health resources*** are equally diverse.

If mental health is defined as life satisfaction, researchers consistently report that the vast majority (about 85%) of older adults are satisfied with their lives, and that older adults are at least as satisfied with their lives as middle-age and younger adults. On a scale of 1 to 5, older adults in the U.S. National Health and Retirement Study reported a mean of 3.92 in life satisfaction, with 4 indicating "very satisfied" (Hudomiet et al., 2021).

But a growing number of studies go beyond life satisfaction, and ***social support*** the contention that older adults are more than just satisfied with their lives, but may be better than younger adults at:

- regulating their emotions with age,
- emphasizing positive emotions,
- curtailing negative emotions, and
- using their ***relational management skills*** to negotiate effectively with others.

There may be a biological basis for older adults' ability in these four areas. In the aging brain of older adults—but not in younger adults—the amygdala showed decreased reactivity to negative information, along with maintained, or increasing, reactivity to positive information (Mather et al., 2004). There may also be changes with age in the orbitofrontal cortex, impairing anger recognition (Ruffman et al., 2006). Older adults appear to be less driven by emotional impulsivity and less likely to respond thoughtlessly to negative emotional stimuli (Jeste & Harris, 2010) or perceive stress and anxiety (Thomas et al., 2016), perhaps because their brain function has slowed down compared with younger persons.

Psychology, however, may play a larger role in a shift over time in the four areas listed. Older adults become more selective in socioemotional regulation. First, there is increasing awareness in the second half of life of the limited amount of time left to live. As one comes to recognize time as finite, the regulation of one's emotional state in the present becomes more important (Carstensen, 2006). Present-oriented goals regarding psychological well-being are prioritized over future-oriented goals (Lockenhoff & Carstensen, 2004). Two of these present-oriented goals are maximizing positive emotions in the present and managing interpersonal conflict.

One study in support of ***socioemotional selectivity*** involved 184 participants aged 18 to 94. They were each given an electronic pager, and when buzzed multiple times each day were repeatedly questioned about how they felt "at this moment" (Carstensen et al., 2000). In general, "periods of highly positive emotional experience were more likely to endure among older people and periods of highly negative emotional experience were less stable." Perhaps in this study, argued some critics, there were *age cohort differences*—differences due to people being born within different historical periods—rather than *maturation* or age changes over time. However, follow-up research showed that each age cohort—young, middle-age, and older adults—focused increasingly on positive emotions over a decade-long study (Carstensen et al., 2011).

Second, you cannot help but gain experience with age. Repeated experiences in dealing with stressful and challenging encounters can help older adults acquire more effectiveness in handling emotional situations and interpersonal confrontations. Although not everyone learns new behaviors from repeated experience, many are able to take advantage of this opportunity.

Experience with age may relate to *relationship management skills*. Older adults appear to be better at seeing multiple perspectives and acquiring an enhanced ability to compromise. Regulating one's emotions and managing relationships are two components of *emotional intelligence.*

The following list includes studies that support the idea that these two skills—***emotional regulation*** and relationship management—develop with age. The first nine studies focus on *regulating one's emotions* and emphasizing the positive, and the remaining six focus on *relationship management*:

1. When reminiscing, older adults are more likely to focus on positive emotions than younger adults (Kennedy et al., 2004; Pasupathi & Carstensen, 2003).
2. Older adults select people and situations that will maximize positive emotions and minimize negative ones (Mroczek & Spiro, 2005).
3. Older adults have more emotionally gratifying memories of past choices and other autobiographical information than younger adults (Mather & Carstensen, 2005).
4. When shown images on a computer screen, followed by a distraction task, older adults recall more positive and fewer negative images than younger and middle-age adults (Charles et al., 2003).
5. When shown a series of faces portraying positive, negative, and neutral emotions, eye-tracking technology shows that older subjects are more likely to focus on happy faces and younger subjects on fearful faces (Isaacowitz et al., 2006).
6. When examining facial expressions, older adults are less likely than younger adults to give a negative rating to people who may look dangerous (Ruffman et al., 2006).
7. A content analysis of the collected works of 10 well-known novelists, playwrights, and poets who lived within the past 500 years found that with increasing age, the authors used more positive affect words and fewer negative ones (Pennebaker, 2003).
8. A study of 3,000 participants who were interviewed repeatedly over a 23-year period revealed that later generations of family members reported fewer negative emotions over time (Charles et al., 2001).
9. A Gallup phone survey of 340,000 adults ages 18 to 85 reported that older adults experienced negative emotions, such as anger and stress, less frequently than younger adults. Enjoyment and happiness decreased gradually until age 50, then rose steadily for the next 25 years (Stone et al., 2010).
10. When reading stories about interpersonal conflict, older adults were better able to see the need for assessing multiple perspectives, compromise with others, and accept uncertainty in outcome (Grossman et al., 2010).
11. Adults peaked in their 40s and 50s, with little decline thereafter, when accurately assessing the moods of others through viewing photographs of strangers' eyes on a computer screen (Hartshorne & Germine, 2015).
12. Older adults tended to act less confrontationally when problems came up in their relationships. They regulated their reactions to problems better than did younger persons, argued less, and picked their battles more carefully (Birditt & Fingerman, 2005; Birditt et al., 2005).
13. Older adults were best at reinterpreting negative images in positive ways by using positive reappraisal, which is a coping mechanism that draws heavily on life experience and lessons learned (Cappeliez & O'Rourke, 2006; Shiota & Levenson, 2009).

14. In later life, when people become sensitized to sadness, it does not necessarily lead to a higher risk for depression, but instead to a greater intimacy in interpersonal relationships (Seider et al., 2011).
15. When asked to view a repugnant television clip that elicited negative feelings, and then engage in a memory exercise, older adults were better able to regulate their negative emotions without a subsequent decrease in memory performance relative to younger people (Scheibe & Blanchard-Fields, 2009).

Other studies have extended these early findings to show that older adults are more successful at regulating desires (Burr et al., 2021) and maintaining positive affect even with declines in brain regions involved in executive control (Lantrip & Huang, 2017). Despite the likelihood of physical and emotional losses accumulating in old age, the old, according to psychiatrist Gene Cohen, become connoisseurs of "deep pleasure and satisfaction, especially in relationships with family and significant others." Older adults appear to recognize greater complexity in interpersonal and romantic relationships (Shavit et al., 2023). One author concludes, "if you want to be happy, learn to think like an old person" (Leland, 2018).

Emotional regulation is a feature of ***gerotranscendence*** (Tornstam, 1989). Older people become less interested in the material and superfluous and more selective in their social engagement and ***spiritual resources***. Levenson et al. (2005), using the idea of ***self-transcendence***, report a greater openness to experience, more agreeableness, increasing spirituality, and a connectedness to past and future generations.

Erikson's theory (1950) of stages of psychosocial development describes a process whereby psychologically mature older adults have a greater need to contribute to the lives of others, referred to as *generativity*, as well as to seek a basic acceptance of one's life, labeled *ego integrity*. Erikson and others suggest that to achieve these goals, a life review, a systematic review of one's life, will be helpful (Haber, 2006).

MENTAL ILLNESS

According to estimates from the World Health Organization (2019), 10% to 15% of older adults meet diagnostic criteria for ***mental illness***. Prevalence roughly doubles for people near the end of life or with severe stages of disease. The most common mental illnesses in old age are major depression and GAD.

DEPRESSION AND ANXIETY

Major depression is defined as five or more of the following symptoms lasting for 2 weeks or longer: depressed mood, diminished interest or pleasure in most or all activities, significant weight loss or gain, insomnia (or hypersomnia), psychomotor slowing, fatigue or loss of energy, feelings of worthlessness or guilt, diminished ability to think or concentrate, and recurrent thoughts of death (not just fear of dying) or suicide severe enough to cause distress or impairment. The most likely causes of ***depression*** in later life are the loss of a spouse or other family support; chronic medical conditions, pain, and loss of functional independence; and difficulty adapting to changing circumstances within the home, family, or living situation.

The disease–depression relationship is reciprocal. Disease increases the risk of depression, but depression also increase the risk of some diseases. For example, diabetics have a 30% increased risk of incident depressed mood (Maraldi et al., 2007). But depression also increases the likelihood of heart disease, diabetes, obesity, and other physical problems (Vogelzangs et al., 2008) and also raises the risk of poor outcomes among people with disease (Zhang et al., 2023). Even mild depression can weaken the immune system in older persons if it goes on long enough (McGuire et al., 2002).

While depression is not more prevalent among older adults, the severity of this disease may be worse. Symptoms of depression are more likely to persist, and the likelihood of remission is lower compared to other age groups (Schaakxs et al., 2018).

QUESTION: Why do White men over age 85 have the highest suicide rate?

Depression also plays a significant role in *suicidal behaviors*, and older persons have the highest suicide rate of any age group. In 2022, older adults accounted for 21% of all suicide deaths, though they make up only 16.8% of the general population (Barnett & Curtin, 2024). This elevated suicide rate, however, is largely accounted for by White men aged 85 and older. In stark contrast to the U.S. population rate of 14.2 suicides per 100,000 in 2022, this group of older White men saw a rate of 58.1 per 100,000, a fourfold difference, and greater use of firearms.

Depression Screening

The U.S. Preventive Services Task Force (USPSTF) advises that physicians screen adults for depression in the clinical setting. The Task Force concluded that there was good evidence that screening improves the accurate identification of depressed patients in primary care settings, and that treatment of depressed adults identified in these settings decreased clinical morbidity.

The USPSTF did not find evidence to select one screening method over another and recommended that clinicians choose the method they prefer based on patient population and setting. Asking two simple questions may be more efficient than administrating a longer instrument: "Over the past 2 weeks have you (a) felt down, depressed, or hopeless; or (b) felt little interest or pleasure in doing things?" An affirmative response to either question indicates the need for more in-depth diagnostic tools.

Screening adults for depression should take place only when adequate diagnosis, treatment, and follow-up are in place, according to the USPSTF. Treatment and follow-up are based on the availability of *staff-assisted depression care supports*. This term refers to staff in the clinic who can assist the primary clinician by providing direct depression care, such as care support or coordination, case management, or mental health treatment.

The minimum level of staff-assisted support consists of a screening nurse who advises the physician of positive screening results and implements a protocol that facilitates referral to behavioral or medical treatment. Treatment may include antidepressants, ***cognitive behavioral therapy*** (CBT), other types of brief psychosocial counseling, or a combination of these interventions.

Depression Diagnosis

Depression in older adults often goes undetected until it is too late. Even with screening, referral and treatment are suboptimal. As reported in the 2012–2013 Medical Expenditures Panel Study, only 25.1% of older adults age 65+ received treatment after positive depression screening (Olfson et al., 2016).

Videotapes of 385 physician appointments with older patients revealed that more than half of the patients whose responses to survey questions suggested they were depressed never talked with their doctors about their emotional state (Tai-Seale et al., 2007). Even when the older patients let their physicians know about their mental health problems, the physician responses averaged 2 minutes long and were often ineffective.

A substantial proportion of depressed older patients, therefore, receive inadequate treatment from physicians in primary care settings (Alexopoulos et al., 2009). Yet, according to the Surgeon General's report (U.S. Department of Health and Human Services [DHHS], 1999), up to 37% of older adults in the primary care setting suffer from depressive symptoms. These percentages vary among surveys, and some of this discrepancy may have to do with the definition of *major depressive disorder* versus *depressive symptoms* of lesser scope or intensity.

Older adults are also less likely than younger adults to report some of their feelings—perhaps irritability, guilt, or worthlessness—which reduces the likelihood of a formal diagnosis of major depression.

Detection of depression is hampered not only by the underreporting of symptoms by older patients but also by biases on the part of physicians and family members. In one study, admittedly dated but interesting nonetheless, 75% of physicians thought that depression was understandable in older persons, that is, a normal facet of old age (Gallo et al., 1999). Family members may also view the signs and symptoms of depression as "normal aging," when in fact the persistence of depressive symptoms is not normal.

QUESTION: Given the emotional and physical losses that accumulate in late life, why is depression not considered a normal part of the aging process?

The diagnosis of depression is even more problematic because of cultural factors. African Americans are significantly less likely than Caucasians to have mental health–related office visits to a physician (Wu et al., 2012). Once there, African Americans are significantly less likely to receive a depression diagnosis from a healthcare provider than Caucasians because of greater stigma, shame, and denial, which prevent seeking professional help (Akincigil et al., 2012).

Diagnosis of depression in older adults has improved in the last few years in part because of better education of primary care physicians. Physicians have been alerted to the need to screen older adults for depression when staff is available for treatment and follow-up, through the recommendation of the USPSTF. Also, under the Affordable Care Act, depression screening became part of the free Welcome to Medicare visit for new beneficiaries and also part of free annual wellness visits thereafter.

Treatment for Depression

There are many modalities for the treatment of depression among older adults, including medication, CBT, other forms of counseling, exercise, life review, social support, and ***pet therapy***.

The effectiveness of medications for the treatment of depression is debatable. A minority of researchers claim they are no better than placebos and may be worse, as they may engender one or more of a wide range of potential side effects. Meta-analyses, however, conclude that they are effective for some, just not for everyone (Cipriani et al., 2018), and for more severe depression (Fournier et al., 2010).

The National Institute for Health and Clinical Excellence in Great Britain reported that antidepressants have low-to-moderate effectiveness, with about 50% of those on medications reporting significant improvement compared with 30% taking a placebo. And though there are a wide range of side effects reported—dizziness, low sex drive, headaches, insomnia, nausea, diarrhea, and so forth—they tend to diminish over time depending on the person and the type of medication. Older adults had more frequent and serious adverse medication reactions than younger adults did to the earlier generation of tricyclic antidepressants, but the subsequent generation of antidepressants, selective serotonin reuptake inhibitors (SSRIs), produced fewer side effects among older adults, superior to serotonin-norepinephrine reuptake inhibitors (SNRIs; Sobieraj et al., 2019).

The effectiveness of medication and CBT combined is better than either modality alone (Keller et al., 2000). CBT is designed to replace dysfunctional thoughts, emotions, and behaviors with more effective ones. It can be delivered one-on-one or in groups. The technique has been effective when applied to clinically depressed older adults (Peng et al., 2009; Pinquart et al., 2007), even when administered over the phone or video conferencing (Simon et al., 2004).

Other psychotherapy techniques have been effective with depressed older adults as well, including problem-solving social skills, interpersonal psychotherapy, psychodynamic therapy, reminiscence therapy, and so forth. Some argue that the skill of the provider and the quality of the relationship between the provider and the patient are more important factors than the choice of therapy. Lay delivery of psychotherapy after training has also shown promise (Dias et al., 2018; Seeley et al., 2017).

Another intervention for depression is mindfulness meditation. Primary care patients who completed an 8-week program lowered their depression scale scores by 50%, which was comparable to results with CBT (Reangsing et al., 2021; Sundquist et al., 2015). The advantage of meditation is that after an initial brief training, patients can practice on their own without additional cost.

Physical activity, aerobics, and weightlifting can also be effective treatments for depression, or reduce the risk of becoming depressed, among older adults (Blake et al., 2009; Singh et al., 2001; Strawbridge et al., 2002). The most common form of physical activity in these studies—walking—reveals that neither high-intensity exercise nor elaborate equipment is necessary for significant results.

Still, use of antidepressant medications has increased steadily, with about 13% of the American population using a medication over the prior 30 days (Brody & Gu, 2020). Analysts speculated that the stigma of depression has declined, while Americans' penchant for treating problems with pills has strengthened. Thanks in part to medication advertisements, which quadrupled over the first decade in this millennium, antidepressant prescriptions doubled during this time.

Collaborative care refers to comprehensive care for late-life depression provided in physician offices or primary care clinics. Following a diagnosis of depression, a trained nurse or psychologist serves as a "depression care manager," working with older patients to develop treatments and monitor progress. Referrals to psychiatrists or other providers are made when necessary. The effectiveness of collaborative care is more than 50% over usual care (Unutzer & Park, 2012). The extra cost involved in this treatment is likely to be offset by reduced visits to doctors and emergency departments, fewer hospitalizations, and decreased complications associated with depression-affected physical diseases.

Anxiety often accompanies depression but counts as a distinct mental illness in the absence of symptoms of depression. GAD in old age is common, with a prevalence similar to major depression (10%–20%). GAD symptoms include uncontrollable feelings of fear or apprehension, obsessive thoughts, reactions disproportionate to the fear, restlessness, trouble with memory and focus, insomnia, nightmares, and alterations of behavior related to fear, such as refusal to engage in routine activities or ritualistic behaviors. GAD often comes with recognition that this nervousness is excessive but out of control. It is often accompanied by disabling physical symptoms (e.g., heart racing, shortness of breath; https://www.ncoa.org/article/anxiety-and-older-adults-a-guide-to-getting-the-relief-you-need/). Antianxiety medications and psychotherapy may offer benefit.

Treatment with medications for anxiety disorders tends to be similar between older and younger patients. Benzodiazepines and other anxiety medications, however, are marginally effective in treating chronic anxiety in older patients. For anxiety associated with depression, an antidepressant may be effective; for mild dementia, a more structured environment may alleviate symptoms; for bereavement, CBT or an exercise program may be of benefit.

Life Review

The universe is made of stories, not of atoms.

—Muriel Rukeyser, poet

A ***life review*** refers to an autobiographical effort or a memoir (a collection of memories) that is preserved in print, audio, or video. The review is typically guided by a series of questions in specific life domains, such as work and family. Memories may be further stimulated through a review of the family photograph album or other memorabilia, a genealogy, musical selections from an earlier time, or a trek back to an important place in one's past.

A life review can be conducted by oneself, in a dyad (Box 8.1), or as part of a group process. It is more likely to be conducted by or with an older adult who is relatively content with their life and not seeking therapy, than it is to be used therapeutically with an older adult. Nonetheless, life reviews are believed to have therapeutic powers, and they are incorporated into a wide variety of counseling modalities (Haber, 2006).

BOX 8.1 ARE YOU SAVED?

Harry Moody reports a meeting with Rabbi Zalman Schachter. In talking about the search for meaning in old age, Schachter stressed "eldering," sharing the wisdom that comes with growing old. This is the work of reviewing one's life to leave a legacy. In a video interview (https://vimeo.com/502633735), the rabbi notes that leaving a legacy allows us to contribute to life after death: "The body will say this is enough, [but] I know life will go on" (Living Tao, 2021).

This idea contrasts sharply with the attitude of some older adults approached about participating in a life review: "My life is not interesting enough to take up that much of anyone's time." Despite this initial attitude, most of these older adults can be persuaded to participate. Here is a reaction to a reader of a life review:

> "... I thought my older adult was lonely, somewhat depressed and negative. She told me her family does not have time to visit often, and she has serious health problems. I felt sorry for her. By the end of the life review experience, I had quite a different impression. She shared great memories, smiled often, and seemed happier than when we started. We shared some great laughs together. She may be a bit lonely, but she is certainly not negative. In fact, she has had an amazing life. I'm glad I was given the opportunity to get to know her. I am thinking about the idea of writing older people's life stories for a living, but I can't believe you can get paid to do something that is this enjoyable!" (Haber, 2008)

The psychiatrist Robert Butler first extolled the benefits of the life review process to his colleagues and the public as early as 1961, as a way of incorporating reminiscence in older adults as part of a normal aging process. Dr. Butler described the life review as more comprehensive and systematic than spontaneous reminiscing, and perhaps more important in old age when there may be a need to put one's life in order and to come to an acceptance of present circumstances (Butler, 1995).

The review of positive and negative life experiences by older adults can enable them to overcome feelings of depression and despair (Watt & Cappeliez, 2000). A study of the life review process reported positive outcomes in terms of stronger life satisfaction, psychological well-being, and self-esteem, as well as reduced depression among older adults (Haight et al., 1998). Similar results have been obtained with depressed older adults in long-term care institutions (Hsu & Wang, 2009).

QUESTION: Find additional reading material on conducting a life review and then conduct a life review segment (for instance, the development of a hobby, early work career, courting, childhood holiday celebrations, or the impact of a historical event) with an older adult. What did you learn about aging that was most important to you?

An ***ethical will*** is another resource and can be a component of a life review or completed as a separate project. Unlike traditional wills that transfer worldly possessions, ethical wills bequeath values through heartfelt words. Though ethical wills were first described 3,000 years ago in the Hebrew Bible, they have become increasingly popular in contemporary America among Jews and non-Jews alike. Ethical wills document the essential lessons that one has learned in a lifetime or one's hopes and dreams for future generations. They can be as brief or as long as you like.

ALZHEIMER DISEASE

Dementia refers to progressive, degenerative brain dysfunction, and about two thirds of dementia is ***Alzheimer disease*** (AD). Other types of dementia include vascular dementia (about 15% to 20% of all dementias), and less common types such as alcohol-associated dementia, Lewy body dementia, frontotemporal degeneration, and so forth. There are also reversible conditions that mimic AD and other forms of dementia, such as hypothyroidism, depression, prescriptions that impair memory, and vitamin B_{12} deficiency. About 10% to 15% of people age 65+ meet criteria for probable or possible dementia, but diagnostic criteria continue to evolve as biomarkers of the disease process are identified, such as beta amyloid and tau imaged in the brain and now assessed in blood.

There is good news on the dementia front: While prevalence is increasing—due to the rapid rise in the number of older adults reaching ages 85 and above, when one is most susceptible to dementia—the incidence, or percentage of new cases, is declining (Derby et al., 2017). There has been a 20% decline in dementia incidence per decade, starting in 1977 (Satitabal et al., 2016). In the National Health and Aging Trends Survey, the prevalence of probable dementia declined from 11.9% in 2011 to 9.2% in 2019 and 8.2% in 2021 in people aged 72+ (Freedman & Cornman, 2024). Researchers can only speculate on the reasons but offer two: (a) better control of blood pressure, cholesterol levels, and other modifiable risk factors, and (b) higher levels of formal education and greater participation in informal education that stimulate neural reserves.

Given that AD is close to 70% of all types of dementia, how is it identified? AD consists of (a) *beta-amyloid plaques*, dense deposits around neurons that may block cell-to-cell signaling at synapses; and (b) *neurofibrillary tangles*, tau protein fibers twisted into a helix inside the neurons that keep nutrients from moving through the cells. These plaques and tangles appear to be impervious to lifestyle changes, though it is not uncommon for marketers of one product or another to suggest otherwise.

The main risk factor for AD is age, and if you live long enough, you likely will develop it. It is uncommon to have AD at age 65 or younger, but after age 65 the risk doubles every 5 years. At age 85 and above, about 50% of people will at some point have symptoms of AD. When autopsied, though, many of these people with tangles and plaques did *not* exhibit AD symptoms to family and friends prior to death, such as significant forgetfulness, difficulty with common tasks, becoming lost in familiar areas, poor judgment, and inappropriate behavior or emotions.

This may be due to ***cognitive reserve***, the brain's ability to develop and maintain extra neurons and recruit spared brain areas for cognitive tasks (Garibotto et al., 2008; Morbelli et al., 2013). Perhaps due to brain-stimulating educational and social activities, extra connections may develop to help compensate for dementia-related brain pathology.

For those with full-blown AD, it is a particularly cruel disease for women for two reasons: (a) The lifetime risk of developing demonstrable AD beginning at age 65 is one in six for women, but only one in 11 for men. This is due mostly to greater longevity in women, but other factors not yet understood may also play a factor. (b) Women are 2.5 times more likely than men to provide on-duty unpaid care 24 hours a day for a family member in the late stages of the disease.

Characteristics and Stages of Alzheimer Disease

In the *early* stage of AD, the most common symptom is diminished short-term memory. Word finding becomes difficult and may be accompanied by personality changes, emotional lability, and poor judgment.

In the *intermediate* stage, the ability to dress, bathe, toilet, and perform other activities of daily living becomes impaired.

In the *severe* stage, people are totally dependent on others, and the ability to recognize even close family members may be lost.

Drug Treatment

Short of a vaccine that could immunize the central nervous system against AD neurodegeneration, the next best thing is a drug that modifies the course of disease (as opposed to simply reducing symptom burden); that is, drugs that delay or slow disease progression. Early drug therapies, such as donepezil and memantine (Aricept and Namenda), had only limited effectiveness (Courtney et al., 2004; Howard et al., 2007; Lichtenberg, 2009; Schwartz & Woloshin, 2012). Despite only a short-term indication, some patients were on these antidementia drug for as long as a decade (Carter & Purvis, 2018). Not surprisingly, geriatricians, who are most knowledgeable about research findings pertaining to older adults, are least likely to prescribe a dementia drug, and neurologists and psychiatrists most likely to prescribe one (Koller et al., 2016). More than half of Medicare beneficiaries with diagnosed dementia are prescribed a dementia drug.

In a contentious decision, in 2023 the Food and Drug Administration (FDA) approved a new monoclonal antibody therapy for dementia: lecanemab (Leqembi). Another monoclonal antibody, aducanumab (Aduhelm), was approved earlier by FDA, but the manufacturer ultimately withdrew it from the market because of lower efficacy and high risk of adverse events. The drugs remove brain amyloid concentrations effectively, but their benefit on cognition and functional status is less clear. Other drugs promoting amyloid clearance, such as donanemab, have received FDA approval, and others are in the development pipeline.

Lecanemab showed modest benefit in delaying disease progression in people with mild cognitive impairment or early-stage AD. Over 18 months, disease progression (measured by the Clinical Dementia Rating Scale) was about 27% slower in the lecanemab group (van Dyck et al., 2022). However, the absolute difference in change was small and its clinical significance unclear. The drug requires infusions and is expensive. It is also associated with important adverse effects, such as brain edema (amyloid-related imaging abnormalities [ARIA]), which can be lethal. People carrying a particular genotype (*APOE e4*), which is common in AD, are at risk for this potentially severe adverse effect. The ideal candidate for this therapy is the patient with amyloid evident in brain imaging but with no or only mild cognitive impairment. Thus, prescribing the drug is complex because of the need for screening imaging, access to infusion technology, monitoring for brain edema, and financial assets. For these reasons, extensive uptake of the therapy is unlikely. The search for better pharmacotherapy continues.

It is also not uncommon for antipsychotic drugs to be used for controlling agitation and combative behavior in residents with dementia in nursing homes. It is estimated that about 20% of nursing home residents with AD in the United States receive an antipsychotic each year, despite only some 2% with conditions appropriate for such prescriptions. The drugs can leave residents in a stupor and increase falls. Some experts refer to antipsychotic medication use in the nursing home as a chemical restraint.

Pharmacologic therapies (including drugs for depression and anxiety) are not particularly effective for the management of psychiatric symptoms of dementia or for the reduction of disability. Nonetheless, they are prescribed because it is easier to medicate than to engage. A 2002 study by the Kaiser Foundation found that the staff in a typical nursing home spent a total of only 2 hours and 20 minutes per day with each resident and relied substantially on medications to manage residents. Perhaps the money spent on dementia medications could be redirected to better social support and more creative interventions, such as music therapy, aromatherapy, and pet therapy (Sink et al., 2005).

Finally, a study of more than 5,000 nursing home residents with advanced dementia (a terminal disease) reported that more than half of the residents continued to receive medications of questionable benefit, including medications to treat dementia and to lower cholesterol level, at a substantial financial cost (Tjia & Briesacher, 2015).

Nondrug Treatments

Arlene Astell, a researcher at the University of St. Andrews in Scotland, has had success with improving the mental health of dementia patients in institutional, community, and home settings by showing them familiar movies and photographs, or playing familiar musical selections. Based on the principles used in Montessori schools for children, a training program for older persons with early-stage dementia helps them to better perform simple, but meaningful, tasks (Camp & Skrajner, 2004).

A remarkable video went viral in 2012, showing Henry, a 94-year-old African American man suffering from dementia who resides in a Brooklyn, New York, nursing home. Henry, who rarely speaks, became revitalized when listening to an iPod loaded with his favorite music. The video is titled *Alive Inside* and is narrated by neurologist Oliver Sacks and social worker Dan Cohen, founder of a nonprofit organization called *Music and Memory* that has been implemented in 50 nursing homes in 15 states.

From being hunched over in his chair and incapable of answering questions beyond a "yes" or "no," Henry immediately lights up with the music, his eyes wide open, his face full of expression, and even engages in dialogue when asked what the music means to him: "It gives me the feeling of love, of romance. I figure right now the world needs to come into music, singing. You've got beautiful music here." He then mimics the song of his favorite artist Cab Calloway, scat singing a credible "I'll Be Home for Christmas."

Arts interventions have shown some promise. A small study by researchers at Johns Hopkins University reported that an active singing program with older residents with dementia in an assisted living facility led to cognitive improvements (Maguire et al., 2015). A program called *Meet Me at MoMA* (Museum of Modern Art) in New York City brings groups of patients and caregivers to selected artworks for observation and discussion. *TimeSlips* shows photographs to people with memory loss and then asks them to imagine what is going on—not to try to remember anything, but to make up a story (www.timeslips.org). Many participants in a Seattle senior center who engaged in this program talked very little to others, including relatives, prior to participation. But once they joined in, they became enthusiastic about making up a story, for example, of a photograph of a fit older man wearing a banana-yellow wet-suit vest who is water skiing.

Persons with dementia in the mild to moderate stages may benefit from ***cognitive stimulation***, such as social day programs that can provide cognitive-stimulating activities that take into account patient and family preferences. A review of 15 randomized controlled trials, mainly with persons with AD or vascular dementia, reported a consistent benefit from social activities on measures of psychological or behavioral function (Woods et al., 2012). Results for music therapy are mixed (Fusar-Poli et al., 2018).

Another resource is the *Dementia Café*, which first sprung up in the Netherlands and in Seattle in 2008 and later other American cities (to access a U.S. directory, access www.memorycafedirectory.com). The purpose of the cafes is to socialize and improve the spirits of those with early-stage dementia. The early years of dementia need not lead to the isolation of the patient and the caregiver. For those who are not mobile enough or do not live close enough to access a Dementia Café, there are virtual resources that are easy to navigate online by caregivers (www.dementiamentors.org).

A 4 year study of the MIND diet (Mediterranean-DASH Intervention for Neurodegenerative Delay) reported a 53% lowered risk of developing AD if followed strictly, and a 35% risk reduction if followed moderately well (Morris et al., 2015). The diet focused on vegetables, nuts, beans, whole grains, fish, poultry, olive oil, and wine.

Prevention of Alzheimer Disease

The 2024 *Lancet Standing Commission on Dementia Prevention, Intervention, and Care* added untreated vision loss and high low-density lipoprotein (LDL) cholesterol to its growing list of factors that increase risk of dementia. Other factors include low education, hearing loss, hypertension, smoking, obesity, depression, physical inactivity, diabetes, excessive alcohol consumption, traumatic brain injury, air pollution, and social isolation. Synthesizing evidence and applying attributable risk estimates, the authors argue that about 40% of dementia cases could be prevented by public health efforts and clinical interventions addressing these risk factors (Livingston et al., 2024). Thus, public health efforts can play a central role in reducing risk of dementia in late life. The American Academy of Neurology has similarly identified these factors as central to promoting brain health across the lifespan (Selwa et al., 2025).

Among these population health risks for dementia, the most closely investigated is education. An early study of an American order of nuns noted how educational attainment early in life was associated with lower risk of dementia in late life (Snowdon et al., 2000). Religious orders offer the advantage of relatively uniform backgrounds and fewer variations in lifestyle to confound associations.

The researchers found that lower linguistic ability in terms of ideas and sentence structure (Snowdon et al., 2000) and greater negative emotional content (Danner et al., 2001) in early-life writings had a strong association with dementia in later life and premature death. Also, higher participation in cognitively stimulating activities reduce the risk of AD (Wilson et al., 2002). The association between early-life education and cognitive performance in late life is well established, suggesting that education may offer neuroprotection through increased brain reserve.

The intensity and regularity of physical activity may also reduce dementia risk. Physical activities affect the blood flow to the brain and may help sustain mental faculties. Again, early studies have shown that people who report greater physical activity between the ages of 20 and 60 had a lower risk for vascular dementia in later life (Friedland et al., 2001; Wang et al., 2006).

Regarding AD, researchers are still seeking a biological explanation as to how increased mental or physical activity might impact the brain. One study reported that the person's AD status at death (i.e., the degree of plaques and tangles in the brain) did not correlate with a high versus low cognitive lifestyle score. However, an active cognitive lifestyle was associated with greater neuronal density and cortical thickness in the frontal lobe (Valenzuela et al., 2012). This *cognitive reserve* may help compensate for noticeable dementia-related brain pathology (Garibotto et al., 2008).

Brain Games

Warner Schaie, a leading researcher in the field of cognitive development, suggested that the "use it or lose it" principle applied not only to muscles but to the brain as well. He reported that by 80 years of age, virtually everybody has some decline in mental function, but how much you slip in your 60s and 70s depends in part on mental stimulation.

Some of our memory performance in old age depends on our expectations about the effects of aging. Older adults who were trained to perceive greater control over their cognitive functioning improved memory performance (Lachman & Andreoletti, 2006). By the same token, lower expectations, induced by ageism, can adversely affect performance.

Whether brain training in old age can enhance cognitive performance remains controversial. The question is challenging because of training effects. Older people will improve performance in computer games and puzzles over time, but this enhanced performance does not usually transfer to everyday activities. The most extensive study of cognitive training, the large, multisite ACTIVE study (Advanced Cognitive Training for Independent and Vital Elderly) showed a mixed picture of benefit (Rebok et al., 2014). ACTIVE provided 10 to 14 weeks of organized cognitive training in memory, reasoning, or speed-of-processing and compared cognitive performance and self-rated disability in participants relative to a control group. The interventions produced improvements in trained cognitive abilities, which persisted up to 10 years for reasoning and speed-of-processing training. Self-reports of disability were lower in participants receiving training. The authors conclude that "this is the first demonstration of long-term transfer of the training effects on cognitive abilities to daily function." However, they also note that the effects of cognitive training on daily function were small and that performance-based measures of disability did not show benefit. These findings challenge or at least qualify the claim of transfer of training skills.

The question is also challenging because of commercial interests. Nintendo came out with a video game in Japan called *Brain Training for Adults* in 2005; by March 2006, 3.3 million copies had been sold to eager consumers. By December 2022, the franchise had sold over 35.5 million copies worldwide. (https://vgsales.fandom.com/wiki/Brain_Age). In January 2007, a brain gym opened in Sarasota, Florida. Seniors attempting to prevent or delay the decline of cognitive function are joining these types of brain fitness centers, and engaging in *neurobics,* or exercises for the brain. These centers are like traditional fitness centers in that the member pays a monthly fee, has access to the club's mental exercise equipment, and can pay an additional fee for consultation with a personal cognition trainer.

Caution is appropriate. A review of 132 studies on ***brain games*** showed that improvement is not generalizable to the real world; that is, to everyday cognitive function (Simons et al., 2016). In 2016, Luminosity paid a $2 million fine to settle Federal Trade Commission charges about making unfounded claims of benefit. This has not stopped growth in the brain training market. Sales of brain game products in the United States increased from $2 million in 2005 to about $225 million in 2009 (Papp et al., 2009) and have grown to $2.8 billion in 2023 (https://dataintelo.com/report/global-brain-game-market).

OTHER MENTAL DISORDERS

Schizophrenia, characterized by delusions, hallucinations, paranoia, disorganized speech, catatonic behavior, and affective flattening, can extend into or first appear in later life. The prevalence of schizophrenia among older adults, however, is less than 0.5% (Cohen et al., 2015), about half the rate for the population aged 18 to 54. Pharmacologic treatment of schizophrenia in late life is challenging, as the first generation of antipsychotic medications had a high risk of persistent and disabling side effects. The second generation of antipsychotics, such as clozapine, risperidone, and others, may be somewhat more effective with older adults than the earlier neuroleptics.

Posttraumatic stress disorder (PTSD) is expected to increase in prevalence among older adults as Vietnam veterans reach old age. The percentage of community-dwelling (civilian, nonveteran) older adults with a diagnosis of PTSD over the past year ranges from less than 1% to 3% (Glaesmer et al., 2010).

Alcohol abuse, deliberate misuse of medication, and illicit drug abuse are considered mental health disorders. While deliberate misuse or illicit use of drugs rarely occurred among previous cohorts of older adults, affecting less than 0.1%, this is rapidly changing. The Substance Abuse and Mental Health Services Administration (SAMHSA) has documented the baby boomers' increasing addiction to, and misuse of, prescription drugs such as opioids for pain, or the more powerful oxycodone, as well as the use of illicit drugs like heroin (see Chapter 7).

Finally, there are *compulsive behaviors* that are being labeled as mental disorders and treated with the SSRI antidepressants. These behaviors include such activities as gambling addiction, kleptomania, shopping addiction, and social phobia. Some argue that these are legitimate mental disorders that should be treated medically. Others contend that these behaviors are everyday maladies that are escalated into medical problems by drug company marketing.

Since the advent of the SSRIs, such as Prozac, the threshold has been lowered for what constitutes an emotional disorder that requires medication. Prescriptions for this generation of antidepressants tripled during the 1990s, and sales for these types of drugs doubled between 2000 and 2005. Data from the National Ambulatory Medical

Care Survey show that prescriptions for antidepressants among older adults increased from 9.9% to 12.3% between 2003–2005 and 2010–2012 (Maust et al., 2017). An increasing percentage of SSRI drugs are directed toward compulsive behaviors.

MENTAL HEALTH AND INSURANCE COVERAGE

For many years, advocates have publicly and strongly objected to the unequal Medicare coverage of mental illness and physical illness. Beginning in 2008, parity in reimbursement for treatment of mental and physical health has made gains, as the Medicare copay (after meeting the Medicare Part B deductible) is 20% for both kinds of medical services (https://www.medicare.gov/coverage/mental-health-care-outpatient). Inpatient care still shows lack of parity: There is no cap on care in a medical hospital, but Medicare has a 190-day lifetime limit on inpatient psychiatric hospital care.

Disparities in Medicare reimbursement between physical and mental treatments increase the stigma surrounding mental illness in older adults (Unutzer et al., 2003). This stigma, along with other financial barriers, may be responsible for generally low rates of mental health services use in older adults. According to the 2019 National Health Interview Survey, the percentage of adults who receive counseling or therapy from a mental health professional in the past 12 months decreases with age, from 11.6% among those aged 18 to 44, to 9.1% among those aged 45 to 64, and to 5.7% among those aged 65 and over (Terlizzi & Norrris, 2021).

Lack of parity also fueled the misperception that mental illness cannot be treated as effectively as physical conditions in older adults. As noted by the Surgeon General's report on mental health (DHHS, 1999), 65% to 80% of depressed older adults improve with medication, psychotherapy, or a combination of both—a success rate higher than many current common medical treatments for nonpsychiatric illnesses.

CHRONIC STRESS

Chronic stress contributes to depression and anxiety disorders and interferes with memory processing. Several days of exposure to high levels of the stress hormone cortisol leads to memory and learning impairment. One study reported that stressful activity makes older adults more cautious in decision-making but has little effect on younger adults (Mather et al., 2009). The researchers suggested that the stress hormones that accumulate over the life cycle are likely to shrink the brain regions involved in decision-making, particularly with decisions involving risk.

Measurement of Chronic Stress

Perhaps the best-known stress measurement tool of the past half century is the *Social Readjustment Rating Scale* (SRRS; Holmes & Rahe, 1967). The SRRS ranked 43 life-change events according to a score derived from more than 5,000 interviews over two decades. Men and women of different socioeconomic status, age, and marital status were asked to assign numeric values higher or lower than an arbitrary score of 50 for marriage. Ten of the top 15 scores related to the family, with death of a spouse receiving the top score of 100. Surprisingly, the ratings of events were consistent across ethnicities (African Americans and Latinx) and countries (Europe and Japan).

Holmes and Rahe's classic study (1967) correlated the ratings of life-change events over a 12-month period with health risk. Thirty-seven percent of the participants who scored under 200 underwent an appreciable change of health, compared with 79% of those who scored over 300.

An interesting facet of the SRRS is its validity, despite its norm-based approach to life events. The instrument does not, for instance, determine whether the person's perception of a life event is stressful or not. For example, the death of a cantankerous and burdensome spouse may be met with relief by one person, whereas a codependent spouse may experience hysteria. Yet the SRRS treats both with a common stress value based on the population norm for loss of a spouse.

Over the past several decades, researchers have been looking for ways to make stress-measuring instruments more precise and powerful by weighing individual perceptions of stressful events. Lazarus and Folkman (1984) focused on daily hassles (e.g., weight gain, rising prices, losing things) and found stronger statistical associations with health outcomes than those obtained by merely counting life events. It is also clear during this time that the Holmes and Rahe scale was not as responsive to the later years as it could have been, because many of the life events included in the scale are unlikely to have occurred in late life. Age-specific scales are now available.

Perspectives on Stress

Stress can be viewed from three perspectives. The first is external, focusing on threatening stimuli from the environment. Measuring stress from this perspective may consist of counting stressful events like widowhood or calculating the impact of daily hassles, such as being stuck in traffic.

A second perspective on stress focuses on internal forces, such as our psychological response to stressors. Being stuck in traffic, for instance, can produce anger, anxiety, and frustration, or we can perceive the traffic delay as an opportunity to converse with our companions or listen to a few additional podcasts.

The fact that we do not all perceive events in the same way is illustrated by the well-known picture in Figure 8.1. Do you see a young woman or an old woman? Is it difficult to shift your perception between the two?

From the third perspective, stress is viewed as a transactional process, an interaction between forces in the environment and our perception. For example, because we are in a hurry, traffic triggers a stress response. Our anger and frustration then escalate our stress. In this transactional process, however, we can deliberately take a pause from our escalating stress level and choose to do a deep-breathing exercise. Thus, we can attempt neither to fight nor flee, but rather to flow.

Psychoneuroimmunology

Over the past three decades, researchers have found a number of physiologic linkages between the nervous system, mood, and the immune system, giving rise to the field of ***psychoneuroimmunology***. When the brain perceives a stressful event, for example, immunological changes result, such as a decline in the cells that fight tumors and viral infections.

Unfortunately for stress researchers, many other factors can also suppress immunity, such as lifestyle habits (alcohol consumption, smoking, nutritional habits, etc.) and the overall status of the immune system. This latter variable is particularly relevant for older adults, because the robustness of the immune system declines with age.

One landmark study, which examined the relationship between lifestyle stress and the immune system of older adults, compared 69 older caregivers of spouses with AD to a matched sample of older adults living in the community. During this 13-month

FIGURE 8.1 What do you see?

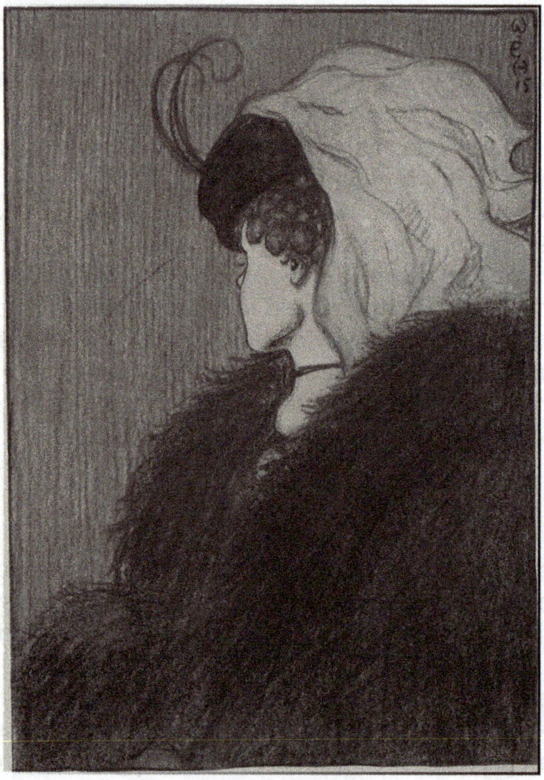

study, the chronic stress of caring for a family member with dementia led to the reduced function of the immune system of the older caregivers, which in turn led to more frequent respiratory tract infections compared to the matched sample in the community (Kiecolt-Glaser et al., 1991).

The brain's perception of mental stress may be a better predictor of future heart problems than physical stress recorded through conventional treadmill testing with heart function measured on an electrocardiogram. Persons who responded adversely to mental stress testing (which include reactions to engaging in public speaking or solving math problems on a deadline) were two to three times more likely to suffer a heart attack or progressive chest pain in the future (Jiang et al., 1996).

STRESS MANAGEMENT

Although many Americans report that stress has had some effect on their health, it is less likely to be reported by older adults (about one third) than younger adults (about half). Similarly, in response to the broader question of how much stress they feel in their daily lives, the American Board of Family Practice reported that older adults were less likely to report considerable stress (about half) than younger adults (almost two thirds). A large national study involving survey data confirmed these findings (Stone et al., 2017).

It is possible that older adults manage their stress better than younger adults, perhaps through more effective coping skills and other informal ***stress management*** techniques. One study reported that stress changes with age, and that older adults get better at managing stress over time (Almeida et al., 2002). More recent research suggests no greater impact of stressful events on older people compared to younger people (Crosswell et al., 2021).

It is also possible that older adults are less willing to report stress. They may find it more of a stigma than do younger adults and are reluctant to admit to it; or they may be less able to recognize it, either owing to lack of knowledge about what stress is or because the stress is masked by depression.

Regardless of age, many adults report a great deal of stress from time to time, and the great majority of them consciously take informal steps to control or reduce it. Only a few, however, try formal stress management techniques. The most popular stress management measures are the informal strategies of physical exercise, psychological denial, and avoidance.

Regarding exercise, a group of older adults with arthritis of the knee significantly lowered their depressive symptoms as a consequence of low-impact aerobic exercise. The subjects also reduced their disability and pain and increased their walking speed (Penninx et al., 2002). Another study used a variety of more formal stress management techniques (anger coping, muscle relaxation, deep breathing, etc.) and individualized them according to the needs and preferences of subjects with high blood pressure. The researchers reported that blood pressure level was reduced through stress management, in comparison with a control group (Linden et al., 2001). A systematic review found positive effects for exercise in reducing stress in older adults (Churchill et al., 2022).

The effects of *journal writing* or expressive writing may alleviate stressful experiences and reduce symptoms (Smyth et al., 1999). This randomized trial in patients with asthma or arthritis reported significantly greater symptomatic improvement (lung function and disease activity) in the journal-writing groups, compared with the control groups that wrote about emotionally neutral topics. It is possible that the participants' immune functions improved after they unburdened themselves, or that they learned ways to cope better with the current stresses in their life by reading their journaling efforts. Other controlled studies have demonstrated the short-term benefits of journal writing on patients with high blood pressure (McGuire et al., 2005) or fibromyalgia (Broderick et al., 2005). Meta-analyses confirm these findings (Guo, 2023).

Journal writing is a popular method for stress management and personal growth. For information on techniques and workshops, contact the Center for Journal Therapy at www.journaltherapy.com, or the Progoff Intensive Journal Program for Self-Development at www.intensivejournal.org.

A Positive Attitude

None are so old as those who have outlived enthusiasm.

—Henry David Thoreau

The Harvard Study of Adult Development was a 60-year longitudinal study of 824 persons from adolescence to late life, conducted for the purpose of learning about successful aging (Vaillant, 2002). In addition to looking at privileged men and women from Harvard University and from California, the study examined healthy aging among inner-city men (Vaillant & Western, 2001).

The psychiatrist George Vaillant, director of the study, concluded that good mental health with aging, regardless of background, involved a capacity for gratitude, forgiveness, and love; a desire to connect with people and replenish social networks; an interest in play and creativity; and a commitment to lifelong learning.

A longitudinal study of 23 years' duration reported that older adults with more positive self-perceptions of aging lived 7.5 years longer than those with less positive self-perceptions of aging (Levy et al., 2002). This advantage remained after controlling for a number of potentially confounding variables, such as whether participants were young-old or old-old, men or women, higher or lower income, lonely or not, or better or worse off in functional health. This finding appeared to be a more powerful predictor of longevity than blood pressure level, cholesterol level, smoking, or exercise.

From 1998 to 2007, the *Georgia Centenarian Study* followed a group of older people into very old age. The investigators concluded that mental health is more important to survival than the longevity of your parents or what you have eaten over a lifetime (Poon et al., 1992). Survivors over the age of 100 appear to be optimistic, to be passionately engaged in some activity, and to have the ability to adapt to repeated losses over time.

Positive affect also predicted subsequent functional independence and survival after a major health event among older Mexican Americans (Ostir et al., 2000) and among older Blacks and Whites (Ostir et al., 2002). Scheier et al. (1999) reported that optimism predicted a lower rate of rehospitalization after coronary artery bypass graft surgery. Optimism is good medicine (Rozanski et al., 2019) and not just good for rehabilitation.

Conversely, negative attitudes like anger, pessimism, and gloomy self-perceptions of aging can lead to a host of unpleasant consequences. A high level of anger is associated with subsequent heart disease (Chang et al., 2002; Williams et al., 2001) and stroke (Ostir et al., 2001; Williams et al., 2002). A 30-year follow-up study of 723 patients revealed that those with pessimistic personalities had a 19% increased risk of death (Maruta et al., 2000).

The protective effect of a *positive attitude* on physical health and mental performance may work in a variety of ways. Positive emotions can increase confidence in performance capacity, strengthen social support, stimulate motivation for self-care, and encourage more physical activities that lead to higher level mental and physical functioning (Cabrita et al., 2017; Penninx, 2000).

An Opposing View

Studies of patients with cancer have reported that a positive attitude and social support did *not* affect survival rates (Coyne et al., 2007; Ehrenreich, 2009; Stefanek et al., 2009). Perhaps a positive attitude is more important in the prevention process than after disease has come into play. Some argue, though, that even in the realm of prevention we cannot assume that a positive attitude is best.

Researchers surveyed adults age 60 and older and asked them to rate their physical and social expectations. Those who had *less* optimistic views of their future well-being had more positive scores on psychological well-being measures. The researchers concluded that those who were able to make more realistic, and even overly negative, estimates of their future health and wellness were more satisfied with themselves than those who were more positive (Cheng et al., 2009). Perhaps unrealistic expectations of the future, given the well-known physical changes with aging, will lead to disappointment and have a negative impact on psychological well-being. In short, having negative expectations of the future can have a positive impact on health.

Adding to the skepticism toward positive expectations, the well-known investigative journalist Barbara Ehrenreich (2009) wrote the book *Bright-Sided*, with the provocative subtitle: *How the Relentless Promotion of Positive Thinking Has Undermined America*. Her challenging thesis is that being positive is a strong American value and a virtue that is flaunted at the risk of being stigmatized. In her chapter on breast cancer, Ehrenreich related her personal experience with breast cancer to how she was bombarded with positive thinking after her diagnosis. She received pink ribbons, teddy bears, new terms such as *survivor* rather than *patient*, slogans such as "cancer is a gift and an opportunity," visualization techniques to defeat her cancer, and self-help books. The overriding theme was this message: "A positive attitude is essential for recovery."

Ehrenreich (2009) argued that the relentless positivity "requires the denial of understandable feelings of anger and fear, all of which must be buried under a cosmetic layer of cheer" (p. 41). She concluded the chapter with the following:

> What [breast cancer] gave me, if you want to call this a "gift," was a very personal, agonizing encounter with an ideological force in American culture that I had not been aware of before—one that encourages us to deny reality, submit cheerfully to misfortune, and blame ourselves for our fate. (p. 44)

If this doesn't provoke you to think more about the benefits and pitfalls of positive thinking, then read this book, with the author's message embedded in its title: *The Antidote: Happiness for People Who Can't Stand Positive Thinking* (Burkeman, 2012).

A more prosaic explanation for the association between optimism and health outcomes may be simply that optimistic people have more resources (and pessimistic people less), in health, social networks, and otherwise, which go unmeasured in observational studies or which may motivate people differently to respond to disease and care challenges.

QUESTION: Do you believe a positive attitude can extend longevity? Explain your answer. Then, argue the opposite.

THE PLACEBO EFFECT

The ***placebo effect*** is often referred to as the power of positive thinking. It is a positive expectation (in contrast to the *nocebo*, a negative expectation). *Placebo* is Latin for "I shall please," and refers to a dummy substance or treatment that is designed to look like the real thing. People may respond favorably to a sham substance or treatment if they do not know it is phony and if they think it is a credible attempt at helping them. For example, patients who believe they are taking painkillers—with doses that contain no medication—may release chemicals in their brain that relieve pain (Zubieta et al., 2005). People in the placebo arm of such clinical trials involving medications, perhaps as many as 15% to 20%, report improvements or side effects (Colloca & Barsky, 2020).

A survey of 1,200 practicing internists and rheumatologists in the United States reported that half of these physicians regularly prescribe placebos to patients. Placebos in this study, however, were not restricted to just inert substances (about 5% used saline or sugar pills), but also analgesics, vitamins, subtherapeutic medication doses, herbal supplements, antibiotics, and sedatives—drugs used for their effect on patients' psyches but not their bodies (Tilburt et al., 2008).

One interesting study reported that a higher price for a placebo created the impression of higher value: a $2.50 placebo worked better than one that cost 10 cents (Waber et al., 2008).

In a similar study, patients with Parkinson disease were told that they would receive an injection of a substance that was either expensive ($1,500) and known to be effective, or not expensive and unproven ($100)—but they would not know which they were getting. In fact, they were given identical injections of a plain saline solution. Those who were later told that they received the expensive injection improved twice as much on a test of physical ability, and brain imaging revealed increases in the neurotransmitter dopamine (Espay et al., 2015). However, the power of placebos may be exaggerated. In a review of 114 studies, only subjective reports, particularly ratings of pain, demonstrated a placebo effect (Hrobjartsson & Gotzsche, 2001).

QUESTION: Aside from research projects, is it ethical to give someone a placebo? Why do you believe that?

MENTAL HEALTH AND ACCEPTANCE OF AGING (*PROAGING*)

The Botox (botulinum toxin type A) craze came along in 2002 when the FDA approved use of this drug to smooth out aging faces. Small doses of the toxin are injected into the forehead, for example, every few months to temporarily paralyze the injected muscle. The drug is expensive, requires repeated application, may have adverse side effects, and can make one look more zombie-like than youthful, but that has not discouraged the generation that has already accepted hair transplants, breast augmentation, collagen injections, chemical peels, lip augmentation, and liposuction.

An interesting essay by Blair (2001) called "The Many Faces I See" talks about the *matryoshka* doll that comes from Russia: a wooden doll that is hollowed out, with a smaller version of the doll inside, which is also hollowed out with a smaller version inside, and so forth. Ms. Blair wrote about feeling like a matryoshka, with all her earlier *me's* inside and fitted into one another. The rest of the world may only see the wrinkled older woman on the outside, but she knew all the earlier selves still inside her. Instead of making her external face look younger, Ms. Blair accepted herself as a little girl, a young mother, a middle-aged woman, and an older woman—all rolled into one. Instead of ignoring the old lady with wrinkles and gray hair, she and society should admire the woman who not only knows what it is like to be an old person but also knows what it is like to be a child, a teenager, a parent, a worker, a mortgage holder, a grandparent, and a retiree.

An interesting video is *Let's Face It: Women Explore Their Aging Faces* (Bare Face Productions, 2003). About a dozen women from age 40 to their early 60s literally explore their faces in the mirror and then discuss their reaction to the effects of aging, comparing their looks to earlier times. These close friends are coming to terms with growing older, with several expressing their disappointment at their diminished beauty (evaluated in terms of societal values), but all of them attempting—with varying degrees of success—to be positive and affirming toward the aging process. A rare photographic record of aging is available for the four Brown sisters, who were photographed in the same position and location over 40 years (and counting; Nixon, 2014). (https://www.nytimes.com/interactive/2014/10/03/magazine/01-brown-sisters-forty-years.html).

I have heard strong arguments that mental health can improve with age if those who so choose change their looks to be more youthful in appearance. For instance, a more youthful appearance may help a person in their 50s land a job or attract a mate. Indeed, those age 55 and over accounted for 25% of all cosmetic procedures in 2013, according to the American Society of Plastic Surgeons. In 2023, people aged 55 to 69 were the biggest consumers of plastic surgery, representing more than half the people undergoing face and neck lifts, forehand lifts, cosmetic eyelid surgeries, and facial fat grafting (https://www.plasticsurgery.org/documents/news/statistics/2023/plastic-surgery-statistics-report-2023.pdf).

However, it may be wiser to make the opposite argument: Mental health can improve more with age if we accept the appearance of old age and all that goes with it. This argument would be greatly strengthened if there was more societal support of a new genre of older people images, where positive visions of older adults are portrayed more frequently in movies, television, theater, books, and popular lyrics. Instead, the title of one scholarly article says it all: "The Aging Woman in Popular Films: Underrepresented, Unattractive, Unfriendly, and Unintelligent" (Bazzini et al., 1997).

The same negative stereotype holds true for television. Older Americans are 17% of the population, but are severely underrepresented in television. This is true of primetime television characters, television advertising, game show contestants, and cartoon figures (Harwood, 2007). Not only are older adults underrepresented, but approximately 70% of older men and 80% of older women seen on television are portrayed disrespectfully, treated with little if any courtesy, and often perceived as negative ("Is 'Change in the Wind,'" 2009). This situation is changing, especially in growing recognition of middle-aged women, but television and movies remain overwhelmingly young.

Instead of William Shakespeare's description of old age as "second childishness and mere oblivion/*sans* teeth, *sans* eyes, *sans* taste, *sans* everything," the arts could discover and reinforce the image of old age as one that embodies not just physical diminution but also wisdom, joyfulness, spirituality, resiliency, and integrity—and even beauty.

Integrity versus despair is the challenge of the last stage of Erik Erikson's stages of psychosocial development (Erikson et al., 1987). One task of the older adult at this stage of existence is to reflect on their life, review experiences and accomplishments, and integrate these memories into a story that captures a meaningful, well-lived life. Botox will not accomplish this. Those who accept the aging process and find integrity rather than despair in late life may find it personally satisfying and also become role models for succeeding generations.

QUESTION: Is trying to look younger in old age an ageist reaction to a natural process, or an effective way to cope in a youth-oriented society? Explain your answer.

MENTAL HEALTH AND AGING RESOURCES

The Friendship Line in California is a 24-hour toll-free hotline (for a crisis) and warmline (for emotional support and well-being check-ins) for older adults (age 60 and older) and their caregivers. The call-in service is for people who are lonely, isolated, grieving, depressed, anxious, or suicidal. (https://www.ioaging.org/mental-illness/ioas-friendship-line-offers-support-for-seniors-experiencing-social-isolation/).

The National Alliance on Mental Illness provides information on mental illness and its treatment, including the publication *Mood Disorders, Depression and Manic Depression*. Referrals are also made to local support groups (www.nami.org).

For additional information on mental illness and mental health, visit the following two websites: the National Institute of Mental Health at www.nimh.nih.gov, which provides literature and other resources designed for older adults; and National Mental Health America at www.nmha.org, which provides information on advocacy, education, support groups, research, and service.

AARP offers the Reminiscence Program for facilitating life reviews; the Widowed Persons Service is a peer support program of trained volunteers who assist the newly widowed recover from their losses (https://wpsgr.org/).

Creativity and Aging Resources

Fostering creativity in older adults can also improve their mental health.

> There is some degree of creativity in every person, and the health practitioner's function is to assist the aged person to recognize and believe in his or her full potential. Products of creativity are less important than fostering a creative attitude. Curiosity, inquisitiveness, wonderment, puzzlement, and craving for understanding are creative attitudes. It is possible to help older persons to break free. (Ebersole & Hess, 1990)

To obtain information about the following creative-arts therapies or to identify certified therapists near your location, contact the following nonprofit organizations: the *American Music Therapy Association*, www.musictherapy.org; the *American Dance Therapy Association*, www.adta.org; the *American Art Therapy Association*, www.arttherapy.org; or the *National Association for Poetry Therapy*, www.poetrytherapy.org, and Senior Theatre (www.seniortheatre.com).

QUESTION: Theodore Roszak wrote, "Aging changes your consciousness more surely than any narcotic; it does so gradually and organically. It digests the experience of a lifetime and makes us different people—sometimes so different that we are amazed, embarrassed, or even ashamed at the person we once were." Do you think most older adults view their younger selves as someone completely different than who they are now? Why or why not?

Koch's (1977) *I Never Told Anybody: Teaching Poetry in Nursing Homes* describes how he taught poetry to nursing home residents and provides interesting samples of their work.

The *National Center for Creative Aging*, founded by Susan Perlstein in 2001, is a clearinghouse throughout the United States for information, research, and training on arts and aging. The mission of the center is to promote creative expression and healthy aging (www.creativeaging.org).

The *Center on Aging, Health & Humanities*, founded by the late Dr. Gene Cohen at George Washington University, has a focus on studying and promoting creativity (www.nursing.gwu.edu/center-aging-health-and-humanities).

The *Osher Lifelong Learning Institutes* promote lifelong learning and community service opportunities for retirement-aged adults (www.osherfoundation.org).

SOCIAL/EMOTIONAL SUPPORT

Social/emotional support can be defined as the perceived caring, esteem, and assistance that people receive from others. Support can come from spouses, family members, friends, neighbors, colleagues, health professionals, or pets. The literature is rife with elaborate taxonomies of support, but it can be reduced to four basic types:

1. *Emotional support* provides people with a sense of love, reassurance, and belonging. When people feel they are being listened to and valued, they develop a healthy sense of self-worth. Emotional support has a strong and consistent relationship with health status. Clearly, emotional support is the foundation of social support in general.
2. *Instrumental support* refers to the provision of tangible aid and services that directly assist people who are in need. Examples are financial help and household maintenance. Good instrumental support has been correlated with a decrease in psychosomatic and emotional distress, and with greater life satisfaction.

3. *Informational support* is the provision of advice, feedback, and suggestions to help a person address problems.
4. *Appraisal support* is help in keeping perspective, essential for effective coping skills.

Social networks are defined in terms of structural characteristics: the number of social linkages, the frequency of contacts, and so on. Although the characteristics of people's social networks do not necessarily reflect the quality of social support, they correlate with positive health outcomes.

There is a tendency, however, for social networks to shrink with age. Older people have more time for friendships and report more close friends than younger people, but they also lose friends over time to death and relocation. The quality of social relationships for older people may be better because older people are more selective and invest more carefully in time spent with others as part of greater socioemotional selectivity, as described earlier.

The popular stereotype that older adults become more socially isolated with age is not borne out by research. Although the size of one's social network declines with age, older age is positively associated with frequency of socializing with neighbors, religious participation, and volunteering (Cornwell et al., 2008). Major later life transitions, such as retirement and widowhood, may prompt greater social or emotional connectedness through other venues.

Social support appears to lower the risk of mortality in older adults (Eng et al., 2002; Obisesan & Gillum, 2009) and perhaps the risk of dementia as well. Social support is associated with many positive health behaviors, including less sedentary time, healthier diets, less alcohol consumption, greater adherence to medical care, and greater regularity in sleep. Social support is as important as fitness for reducing mortality (Glass et al., 1999). In the United States, older persons who were satisfied with the support available to them were twice as likely to report better health as those who were not satisfied (White et al., 2009). Social support may bolster cognition (Kelly et al., 2017).

Support can be helpful in trying times. It can lower the risk of late-life depressive symptoms (Isaac et al., 2009), reduce anxiety and depression in older cancer patients (Lien et al., 2009), improve self-rated health after a disaster such as a hurricane (Ruggiero et al., 2009), and encourage older women to exercise while recovering from a hip fracture (Casado et al., 2009). Social strain, in contrast, can discourage older adults with osteoarthritis from exercising (Cotter & Sherman, 2008).

Social and emotional support may affect the likelihood of a person becoming obese. One study reported that people with obese friends are significantly more likely to develop obesity themselves (Christakis & Fowler, 2007). Friendship, perhaps, may provide permission to overindulge in an unhealthy consumption of food. Also, social support from friends who are physically active can encourage physical activity among those who had been less active (Scarapicchia et al., 2017). These research findings could, however, foster blame on obese or inactive people and their choice of companionship, rather than place attention on the overall environmental challenge in the United States that fosters obesity and inactivity.

FAMILY, FRIENDS, PLACE OF WORSHIP, AND OTHERS

Large-scale epidemiologic studies have shown that membership in a social network of family, friends, church, and other support structures is correlated with lower mortality risk. In a classic study of 7,000 residents of Alameda County, California, residents who were married, had ample contact with extended family and friends, belonged to a church, and had other group affiliations were half as likely to die over the course of the 9-year study as those with less adequate social supports (Berkman, 1983).

Over the next decade, research findings on the relationship between social support or social networks and mortality were replicated by large-sample studies (Goodwin et al., 1987; House et al., 1988; Williams et al., 1992) that controlled for other factors possibly affecting mortality, such as lifestyle, socioeconomic status, age, race, and access to healthcare. It turned out that inadequate support by itself among older adults is comparable to smoking, poor diet, and inactivity as risk factors for mortality (Holt-Lunstad et al., 2010).

A spouse or supportive family member is important in helping people adopt or sustain good health habits. Using 8-year longitudinal data from the Health and Retirement Study, researchers found that when one spouse improved their health behavior, the other spouse was more likely to do so as well (Falba & Sindelar, 2008). These behaviors ranged from smoking, drinking, exercising, cholesterol screening, and obtaining a flu shot.

A study reported that lifestyle interventions targeted at men and women as couples, rather than as individuals, resulted in a greater reduction in cardiovascular risk factors like cigarette smoking, systolic blood pressure, and cholesterol level (Pyke et al., 1997). Targeting the couple may strengthen outcomes through the mutual reinforcement of lifestyle changes (Carr et al., 2019).

Community-dwelling older men and women were more likely to have obtained preventive care when they lived with their spouse than when they lived alone or with adult offspring. Specifically, those living with a spouse were more likely to obtain an influenza vaccination, cholesterol screening, colorectal cancer screening, routine physical checkup, and routine dental care (Lau & Kirby, 2009). Observers of a focus group reported that spousal support influenced dietary changes following a diagnosis of type 2 diabetes in middle-aged and older adults (Beverly et al., 2008).

An interesting study reported that the greater the marital strain over time, the steeper the decline in health for both men and women. When the researchers separated study participants into three age groups—ages 30, 50, and 70—only the oldest group showed negative health effects (Umberson et al., 2006). The researchers speculated there may be a cumulative effect over time among couples unhappy with their marriage, combined with age-related declines in immune function and a higher rate of health problems such as heart disease.

Isolation and loneliness are psychological states, not simply the absence of social contacts (Box 8.2). People can feel lonely regardless of the amount of social contact with other people. A review of 70 studies, with participants averaging 66 years of age, revealed that the *perception* of loneliness or isolation increased the risk for dying sooner by 29% (Holt-Lunstad et al., 2015). A study of loneliness in people over age 50 reported greatly increased risk of high blood pressure (Hawkley et al., 2006). Loneliness is a risk factor for cognitive decline and psychiatric illness (Solmi et al., 2020).

Adults over the age of 50 who reported chronic loneliness over a 4-year period reported more problems with daily living tasks, a greater number of depressive symptoms, and more visits to their physician (Gerst-Emerson & Jayawardhana, 2015).

The loss of a spouse or loved one can be quite severe, and in one study the risk of a heart attack in the week after a spouse's death is six times greater than normal (Mostofsky et al., 2012). The death provokes bereavement, which is accompanied by depression, anger, and anxiety, all of which can elevate heart rate and blood pressure and increase the risk of blood clotting. Persistent grief is now recognized as a psychiatric diagnosis.

Spouses as a source of support are increasingly unavailable with age, particularly among older women. Although 84% of males and 67% of females live with their

BOX 8.2 Bowling Alone?

In 1995, Robert Putnam published an article titled "Bowling Alone: America's Declining Social Capital," (Putnam, 1995), and then followed up subsequent criticism of his article with a book, *Bowling Alone: The Collapse and Revival of American Community* (Putnam, 2000). Putnam argued that both television and a generation that is less civically engaged than their parents has created more social isolation—to the detriment of themselves and society. His conclusion generated much discussion, including from those who argued that there has only been a change in type of social support (e.g., cyberspace, nontraditional small groups like book clubs and support groups, and prayer fellowship) in contemporary America, rather than the quantity or quality of social involvement.

The question of whether there is a trend toward less social support or to different types of social support in American society remains unanswered. Also unexamined are the qualitative differences between obtaining support online versus in person. However, Putnam's writing has emphasized the importance of monitoring social activity in America and stimulated discussion on what we should do to improve it.

spouses during late middle age, the percentages drop to 72% of males, but to less than half, 46%, of females at age 65 and over. Fortunately, older women living independently manage well psychologically and may fare even better than women living with a spouse, provided they have supportive relationships from other relatives and from friends (Michael et al., 2001).

QUESTION: **Do you think there is more social isolation in America today than in generations past, and on what do you base your assertion?**

Adult children can be a primary source of social support for older adults, though their support for parents often has to compete for time and energy with their own needs and those of their children. Because of the limitations of spousal and child support, friendships take on increasing importance in late life. In a study of 1,500 Australians age 70 and older, friends rather than children or other relatives were most important in lengthening survival (Giles et al., 2005). Qualitative interviews with 40 unmarried women ages 40 to 75 led to the recommendation that nurse practitioners who routinely prescribed exercise to improve the health of older adults may be more effective if they enlist the support of older friends and other older adult peers to join them (Dorgo et al., 2009).

The different types of relationships for researchers to consider will be greater among baby boomers than is the case with the present cohort of older adults. Among the boomers, for instance, the number of unmarried older people who *live together romantically* more than doubled in the decade from 2000 to 2010 (Lin & Brown, 2012). Among people aged 65 to 74, census data from 2023 show that 3.9% of men and 2.6% percent of women live with a partner, not a spouse (https://www.nytimes.com/2024/11/10/health/elderly-unmarried-couples-caregiving.html). Are these cohabitant friends comparable to spouses? They may not marry for practical reasons such as to protect their individual nest egg in order to pass it on to their children. Or they may not want to jeopardize a pension or Social Security payment earned through a former relationship. Or they may not want to be financially responsible for taking on the other person's medical debts. Or they may fear caregiving responsibilities when a partner's health declines. Does this affect the quality of the emotional support they give or receive?

Another category likely to need more analysis is *divorce*. Only 10% of people who got a divorce in 1990 were over 50, versus 25% in 2010. By 2019, over one third of divorces involved people over age 50 (Brown & Lin, 2022). Divorce and choosing to remain single have contributed to about one third of boomers being unmarried today versus just 20% at a comparable age in 1980.

Whether divorced, widowed, or never married, numerous *dating sites* for older adults have been launched, with names like ourtime.com, youngatheart.com, and silversingles.com. AARP partnered with HowAboutWe.com, a dating website (now merged with match.com), and offered a 50% discount to AARP members who joined. Filmmaker Steven Loring filmed a speed dating event at an Italian restaurant for 15 men and 15 women ages 70 to 90. When a segment about this event was aired on National Public Radio in 2015, the reactions ranged from "encouraging" to "sad."

ONLINE SUPPORT

People with medical conditions are forming ***online support*** groups (e.g., *PatientsLikeMe Inc.*; www.patientslikeme.com) to communicate about symptoms, medications, treatments, results, and other medical data with people with similar conditions. Online cancer information and support repositories allow patients find peer support and health providers through this service. Researchers often use the sites to recruit study participants.

There are internet sites that help people support each other on topics other than just health concerns. For example, *Meetup.com* (www.meetup.com) helps people set up face-to-face meetings anywhere in the country to discuss politics, the environment, caregiving, hobbies, and so forth.

Social media usage is dominated by the young—temporarily. In 2018, about 88% of young adults between the ages of 18 and 29 used some form of social media. Close to three quarters used *Snapchat* or *Instagram*, sites for sharing images and videos. But as older adults are being replaced by the boomers, social media usage is evening out among the age groups. In 2018, only 37% of those age 65+ used social media (though up from 26% in 2010), compared to 64% of those between the ages of 50 and 64. In 2021, three quarters of people aged 50 to 64, and nearly half of people age 65+, used social media regularly (Auxier &Anderson, 2021).

A gerontological concern about Facebook is that it is a source of ageism. The title of one research article is cogent: *Facebook as a Site for Negative Age Stereotype* (Levy et al., 2014). Young adults, mostly in their 20s, when commenting about older adults were critical 74% of the time, with 41% of their descriptions referring to physical deterioration and 27% to cognitive decline. More than one third advocated banning older adults from public activities, including driving cars. The negative comments cited in the article ranged from subtle to blatant, with an example of the latter being: "Anyone over age 69 should face a firing squad." The authors concluded that ageism is a common occurrence on Facebook.

PET SUPPORT

Between one third and one half of all households in the English-speaking world have pets, yet there has been limited research on the effects of animal companionship. Though meager and not rigorously conducted, research suggests that the positive effects of pet ownership on human health should be taken seriously (McNicholas et al., 2005).

Many of the studies have focused on older persons with a great need for companionship. For example, ***pet support*** among older women living in the community (Krause-Parello, 2008), older residents living in long-term care facilities (Banks & Banks, 2002), and hospital patients (Coakley & Mahoney, 2009) alleviated loneliness and increased energy level. The vast majority of these *pet intervention* studies, however, did not include control groups, and did not separate out the overall attention and novelty that typically accompanies pet support programs (Gee & Mueller, 2019; Obradović et al., 2020).

On a practice level, a survey of nursing homes in Ohio revealed widespread support for the health benefits of pets, but few had policies on health and safety concerns. Missing were important policy and procedural guidelines such as vaccinations, hand hygiene, biting prevention, temperament testing, and staff training (Stull et al., 2018).

In contrast to live animals is the idea of robotic dogs hatched by two researchers from the veterinary school at Purdue University. They pilot-tested robotic dogs with older adults in retirement homes and reported that there were positive psychological effects on the older residents. The researchers also noted that the older adults did not have to worry about remembering to feed them or about being fit enough to walk them (Eisenberg, 2002). The downside of this experiment might be its short-term emotional value and the less-than-ideal tactile sensation that the robot dog provides. Robot social companions represent a new and potentially important component of care for people with dementia (Guerra et al., 2022).

Pet Support Programs

Home for Life provides a sanctuary for pets if an older pet owner has to move into a nursing home or another residence that does not allow pets, or if the pet owner dies. The animal is guaranteed a home for life in this pet sanctuary. This program not only provides a safe and affordable residence for pets but can arrange for travel to the sanctuary (for contact information, visit www.homeforlife.org). *Pets for the Elderly Foundation* pays the fees to 58 animal shelters in 30 states for adults aged 60 and older to adopt a companion dog or cat from a participating shelter (www.petsfortheelderly.org).

The *Delta Society* and its national program, *Pet Partners*, brings volunteers and their trained pets (mostly dogs, followed in frequency by cats and, surprisingly, miniature horses) to nursing homes, hospitals, and schools (https://petpartners.org/). To observe the effects of one visiting dog, see Figure 8.2.

A creative aging charity in London, called Equal Arts, provides hens to 700 older adults residing in 20 long-term care facilities (https://www.equalarts.org.uk/our-work/henpower). In addition to children being attracted to the facilities to see the hens, the older residents gather outside to watch them. Most impressive of all, the hens love to be carried or to sit on laps and be hugged.

RELIGIOUS OR SPIRITUAL SUPPORT

Religious and spiritual activities are often not differentiated in research, though typical measures assess religious beliefs or practices (Atchley, 2009). When a distinction is made, *spiritual activity* is more varied in its manifestations and focused on the internal process, whereas *religious activity* is considered to be more institutional and doctrinal.

In the 1990s, there was widespread belief that religious or spiritual people not only live longer but also have stronger immune systems, are physically healthier, and are less depressed than those who are not (Koenig et al., 1997, 1999; Strawbridge et al., 1997).

FIGURE 8.2 Dog from a pet companion program visiting an older adult.

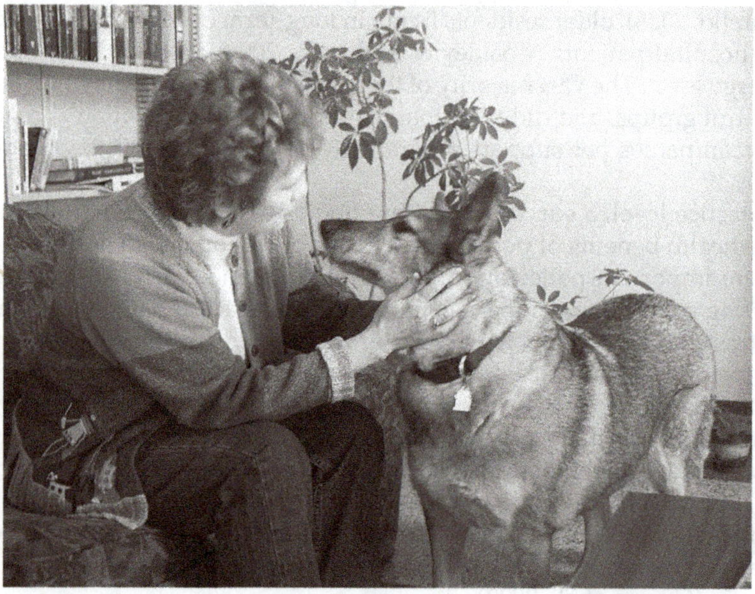

The relationship between religious activities and good health remained even when researchers controlled for potentially confounding variables, such as chronic illnesses, functional abilities, age, race, and other health and social factors. Explanations for the positive relationship between religion and health included the impact of religion on healthy lifestyles (e.g., less addiction to smoking and drinking); positive and supportive social relationships; positive ideologies and prayer, which lower harmful stress hormones; and more stable marriages.

One interesting study on the effect of religious involvement on longevity reported that Christians and Jews tended to die less frequently in the month before their own group's major religious holidays (Idler & Kasl, 1992). A study on prayer reported that people who engaged in private prayer before surgery for coronary heart disease were more optimistic about the outcome and then recovered more effectively than those who did not so engage (Ai et al., 2002). Conversely, sick patients who were pessimistic about their religious faith had a higher risk of mortality within 2 years (Pargament et al., 2001).

Harold Koenig, a physician and leading researcher on religion, spirituality, and medicine, reviewed 350 studies on the impact of religious involvement on physical health and reported that the majority of the studies support the finding that religious people are physically healthier and require fewer health services. Moreover, an additional 850 studies examined the relationship among religion, spirituality, and mental health, and about 70% of them reported that people experience better mental health and adapt more successfully to stress if they are religious (Koenig, 2000).

However, there is *no* compelling evidence of a relationship between religious or spiritual activity and health and longevity, according to two psychologists from Columbia University. The psychologists reviewed all 266 articles published during the year 2000 on religion and medicine and reported that only a few demonstrated the beneficial effects of religious involvement on health (Sloan & Bagiella, 2002).

One of the common mistakes made by the researchers in the studies they reviewed is the failure to control for multiple comparisons, commonly referred to in research as a fishing expedition. In other words, if you examine enough variables, you will find some of them significant on the basis of chance alone. When studies with multiple dependent variables are statistically corrected for—a standard practice in statistical analysis when examining multiple comparisons—the significance levels of these variables commonly disappear.

The psychologists also noted that most studies were correlational rather than causal, and that religious behavior can be the product of good health, rather than its cause; and, conversely, the lack of religious behavior can be the product of poor health, rather than its cause.

One particularly rigorous study, which supported the contention that the effect of religion on health was overblown, was a 14-year longitudinal analysis that carefully controlled for potentially confounding covariates. Over this length of time, religious activity no longer had predictive value in terms of physical health or psychological well-being (Atchley, 1998). A systematic review of randomized controlled trials involving religious and spiritual interventions found only small benefits for physical activity and promotion of health behaviors. Other outcomes, such as cardiac measures, did not show benefit (Gonçalves et al., 2017).

Nonetheless, many remain convinced of both the health and longevity benefits of religion. Regardless of your opinion (about the effects of religious belief), it is reasonable to endorse the idea that health professionals who work with older clients should be sensitive to their religious and spiritual needs and provide the time to listen to, and empathize with, their concerns.

Health professionals can strengthen the mental health of their clients by finding out whether they have an interest in, and access to, a pastor, rabbi, or religious study group. If the client is primarily home bound, the health professional can encourage the client to inquire about receiving visits from volunteers at the client's previously attended religious institution.

It should be noted that religious activity may not affect all older adults equally. It may, for instance, be especially important as a source of social support for Black older adults (Krause, 2008). Holding strong religious or spiritual beliefs appeared to protect older African Americans from contemplating or committing suicide (Cook et al., 2002). Involvement in religious activity correlated with greater self-esteem and personal control in a sample of older African Americans (Krause, 2008).

African American caregivers were found to be more likely than White caregivers to use religion as a means of coping and to receive greater consolation in the face of adversity (Ferraro & Koch, 1994). Finally, a national sample of 1,500 older adults, equally divided between Blacks and Whites, concluded that "older Black people are more likely than older White people to reap the health-related benefits of religion" (Krause, 2002).

Aging and Spirituality Resources

An academic journal in this field is the *Journal of Religion, Spirituality, & Aging*, published by Routledge, the academic branch of Taylor & Francis, Inc. "Spirituality" was added to the title in 2005.

A widely read book on spirituality was authored by Schachter-Shalomi, titled *From Age-ing to Sage-ing: A Profound New Vision on Growing Older* (1995). His message is that with age and experience can come wisdom and the opportunity to mentor the young.

Another spiritually oriented book is *Still Here: Embracing Aging, Changing and Dying* by Ram Dass (2000). Ram Dass, a well-known spiritual leader and former Harvard professor, suffered a crippling stroke while in the midst of writing this book. Yet this septuagenarian at the time managed to eloquently integrate this experience into the rest of his writing. As he notes in his book, "These days I'm the advance scout for the experiences of aging, and I've come ... to bring good news. The good news is that the spirit is more powerful than the vicissitudes of aging" (Dass, 2000, p. 204).

PEER SUPPORT

Growing older presents the challenge of coping with chronic conditions—either one's own or those of loved ones. A significant number of older adults are discovering the benefits of evidence-based *peer counseling programs* implemented by their fellow older adults (Dias et al., 2018), or *peer mentoring programs* (Seeley et al., 2017), which basically constitutes a name change by a few service organizations to avoid the perceived stigma of the term "counseling" held by some older adults. These free volunteer services may be vital to older adults who otherwise might not have access to evidence-based interventions with fees.

More ubiquitous are the ***peer support*** groups that unite older adults with common health concerns so that they can share ideas and feelings, exchange practical information, and benefit from knowing they are not alone. In short, older adults attempt to help their peers learn to live as fully as possible, despite the limitations that accrue with age.

A peer support group can be located online or in person for many chronic health conditions—AD caregiving, cancer, arthritis, heart disease, lung disease, stroke, hearing or visual impairment, and others. The groups have certain commonalties: most operate informally, meet regularly, and do not charge fees. Most distribute leadership responsibilities among their peer members, and many involve health professionals in educating members in an adjunct role.

Peer support groups, however, can differ widely in the way they operate. Most AD groups, for example, focus primarily on the emotional needs of caregiving members, though practical information is provided as well. Other support groups may emphasize education, whereas others focus on health advocacy in the legislative arena. Some groups meet in an institutional setting, such as a hospital, with strong professional leadership that differs markedly from groups that meet in a home or church and do not include professional involvement.

Research on support groups, whether focused on older adults or not, tends to be qualitative. The samples are small, and few utilize a control group. The results are almost always that groups reduce isolation, provide practical information, and empower participants. We know little about ineffective or damaging groups. Of several dozen support groups, the participants expressed how much they benefited from attending. One group, however, included a peer leader who made inappropriate comments regarding medical care and medications and expressed unusual ideas about what constitutes good coping practices. A rigorous comparison of peer-to-peer versus standard community services support showed increases in anxiety and greater risk of hospitalization in the peer-to-peer group, and no difference in other health domains (Jacobs et al., 2020; Schwei et al., 2021).

Still, the self-help group movement is a phenomenon to be reckoned with. As far back as 1979, there were an estimated 15 million participants in almost 500,000 groups, and growth has been steady since then. More than four decades ago, based on a probability sample of more than 3,000 households, self-help groups had already become the number one source of assistance to persons with mental health problems. More people in the United States participated in self-help groups at that time (5.8%) than sought help from mental health professionals (5.6%) or consulted with clergy or pastoral sources (5%; Mellinger & Balter, 1983).

Fitzhugh Mullan (1992), a physician and former director of the Bureau of Health Professions, suggested that newly diagnosed patients, "instead of simply going to that white-coated doctor and medical establishment (go) to people who have already 'been there' in some way ... people who have already had the condition, or who are coping with it." Self-help groups and institutionalized versions, such as community peer navigators, are now part of the landscape of American care.

QUESTION: Visit a peer support group and then describe your experience in neutral terms—respecting the anonymity of the participants—to an older adult. What is the older adult's opinion of the peer support group you visited, and what does it reveal about their attitude toward this type of support?

Age-Related Peer Support Groups

Peer support groups, at least theoretically, may be especially appropriate for aging persons with chronic impairment and their caregivers. Age-related peer support groups may provide support when younger family members are geographically distant and/or involved with their children. Declining birth rates after the baby boom generation mean that fewer children and grandchildren are available to serve as support persons. Job mobility, retirement relocation, and neighborhood growth and renewal result in the dispersion of family, friends, and neighbors. An increasing percentage of women—who constitute a majority of the caregivers in America—have entered the workforce over the past few decades and have reduced the amount of caregiving support available to assist older adults with health challenges.

Creative models, such as Share the Care, have emerged to build volunteer caregiving networks from family, friends, and neighbors to support older people without caregivers (https://sharethecare.org/). The organization provides tools and guidance to "transform and bond a group of people who may not know each other and want to help."

In response to shrinking family support systems, Haber embedded a peer support group component into programs focused on older adults and health promotion (Haber, 1983, 1984, 1986, 1989, 1992; Haber & Lacy, 1993). Some participants in these peer support groups continued to provide social support and practical assistance to each other for years afterwards the funded project and the participation of health professionals had terminated. One health promotion class, for instance, continued to meet a decade later as a monthly peer support group. A member of the group sent a letter that appears in Figure 8.3.

INTERGENERATIONAL SUPPORT

Generations often live far away from one another. Grandparents and grandchildren may be both geographically and emotionally separated from each other. If personal interactions occur infrequently, they can at least be memorable. There were several travel companies that specialize in intergenerational travel; for example, Road Scholar (www.roadscholar.org), formerly Elderhostel, a longstanding travel and educational program for older adults, began to offer intergenerational trips that focus on grandparents and grandchildren (parents allowed as well).

FIGURE 8.3 "Dear David" letter.

April 1

Dear David,

You might already know - but the outgrowth of your classes is a continuation of socialization among nearly 20 persons. The "Prime Timers" are going strong - we meet once a month.

We are never at a loss for agenda! April 24, we will meet at Kountz Memorial Church for Fred Aliano's famous spaghetti, and a relaxation tape to improve our mental health.

Everyone sends love and we miss you. From your friends....

Jackie Devaney, secretary for the day

Travel experts report that the best age for traveling with a grandchild is when the child is between 11 and 14 years old. A grandchild at that age is old enough not only to appreciate the trip, but to be responsible as well. The child is also not so old as to be set in their ways or to be totally into their own things.

Older adults can also be a tremendous source of support to children who are unrelated to them. The *Foster Grandparent Program* is a national program that trains volunteers aged 60 and over to serve 20 hours a week with children in hospitals, shelters, and special-care facilities. Low-income volunteers receive a small stipend (https://americorps.gov/serve/americorps-seniors/americorps-seniors-foster-grandparent-program).

Marc Freedman, founder and CEO of Encore.org (now CoGenerate) reported that the Foster Grandparent Program inspired him to write a book, *How to Live Forever: The Enduring Power of Connecting the Generations* (2018). The theme of his book is the importance of intergenerational connections for both young and old, and how older adults can go about strengthening these connections.

In Bend, Oregon, through the Central Oregon Council on Aging, a *TECH (Teenager Elder Computer Help)* program was born (www.councilonaging.org). High school students sign up to teach local senior citizens about Facebook, Skype, smartphones, taking and sending digital pictures, and other tech challenges.

For information and ideas about ***intergenerational support and programs*** and projects, contact the *Intergenerational Center* at Temple University, www.Templecil.org. The center has a toolkit for intergenerational program planners titled *Connecting Generations, Strengthening Communities* (see Figure 8.4).

To order a free copy of the *Intergenerational Projects Idea Book*, contact AARP Fulfillment, 601 E St. NW, Washington, DC 20049, and request stock #D15087.

SUMMARY

Ever notice how the topic of mental *health* invariably emphasizes mental *illness*? When it comes to aging, the content of many textbooks usually focuses on depression and dementia, with several other illnesses, such as anxiety, addiction, stress, isolation, suicide, and so forth. This chapter, by contrast, focuses on *mental health and aging*, not mental illness and aging. Did you know a life review, for instance, can enhance the mental health of an older adult? Also effective for mental health and aging are journaling, peer support mentoring, peer support groups, pet support, dementia cafes, intergenerational activities, and so forth.

FIGURE 8.4 Older adult assisting student with her reading comprehension.

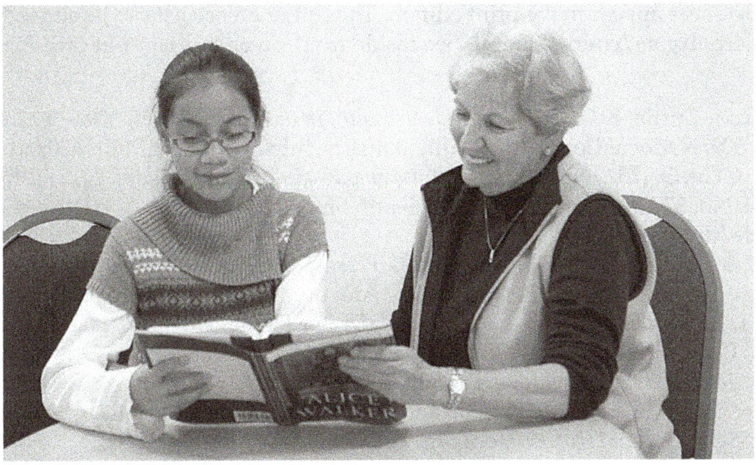

But the most impressive mental health and aging finding may be the increased likelihood of gaining wisdom with age. A lot depends, of course, on how you define wisdom, and some definitions are not advantageous to aging adults. But the most promising definition of wisdom, in my opinion, is our enhanced ability to regulate our emotions with age. It is not clear whether this phenomenon is explained better by a biological theory involving changes over time in our amygdala, or by a psychological theory that suggests, as future time shortens, we focus more effectively on positive feelings in the present and management of interpersonal relationships to support these feelings.

So back to the commonly addressed topics of depression and dementia: There is even good news on these fronts. Depression is not age related, as the popular stereotype suggests. It is much more strongly related to health issues, daily stressors, and negative life events. Each stage of the lifecycle presents its unique challenges, and most people are resilient at any age. There are also effective ways to treat depression if it is identified and adequate follow-up is implemented.

Regarding dementia, it is true that its prevalence keeps rising over the decades, but so do the number of older adults who reach the most vulnerable stage of the life cycle for dementia, age 85 and above. When you look at the incidence (new cases) of dementia, however, prevalence is declining, about a 3% decline per year since 1997. Perhaps this is due to greater educational attainment and increasing cognitive stimulation in our society over the past few decades, which builds up our neural reserves.

Forget the brain games, though. No need to spend money to stimulate your brain, just like there is no need to spend money to exercise your body. Instead, there are many free options such as interacting with friends or borrowing a book from the library. That book may inspire you to tackle a new hobby, learn a language, increase your knowledge, and expand your vocabulary. Good stuff for the brain!

SPRINGER PUBLISHING CONNECT™ | **A robust set of instructor resources designed to supplement this text is located at http://connect.springerpub.com/content/book/978-0-8261-8386-6. Qualifying instructors may request access by emailing textbook@springerpub.com.**

REFERENCES

Only key references appear in the print edition. The full reference list can be accessed by visiting www.springerpub.com/courseconnect. See inside front cover and tear-out card for CourseConnect details.

Barnett, M. F., & Curtin, S. C. (2024). *Suicide mortality in the United States, 2002–2022*. NCHS Data Brief, No. 509. National Center for Health Statistics. https://doi.org/10.15620/cdc/160504

Brody, D. J., & Gu, Q. (2020). *Antidepressant use among adults: United States, 2015–2018*. NCHS Data Brief, No. 377. National Center for Health Statistics. https://www.cdc.gov/nchs/data/databriefs/db377-H.pdf

Brown, S. L., & Lin, I. F. (2022). The graying of divorce: A half century of change. *The Journals of Gerontology: Series B*, *77*(9), 1710–1720. https://doi.org/10.1093/geronb/gbac057

Carstensen, L. L., Turan, B., Scheibe, S., Ram, N., Ersner-Hershfield, H., Samanez-Larkin, G. R., Brooks, K. P., & Nesselroade, J. R. (2011). Emotional experience improves with age. *Psychology and Aging*, *26*, 21–33. https://doi.org/10.1037/a0021285

Colloca, L., & Barsky, A. J. (2020). Placebo and nocebo effects. *The New England Journal of Medicine*, *382*(6), 554–561. https://doi.org/10.1056/NEJMra1907805

Freedman, V. A., & Cornman, J. C. (2024). Dementia prevalence, incidence and mortality trends among U.S. adults ages 72 and older, 2011–2021. *The Journals of Gerontology, Series A: Biological Sciences and Medical Sciences*, *79*(Supplement_1), S22–S31.

Kelly, M. E., Duff, H., Kelly, S., McHugh Power, J. E., Brennan, S., Lawlor, B. A., & Loughrey, D. G. (2017). The impact of social activities, social networks, social support and social relationships on the cognitive functioning of healthy older adults: A systematic review. *Systematic Reviews*, *6*, 1–18. https://doi.org/10.1186/s13643-017-0632-2

Livingston, G., Huntley, J., Liu, K. Y., Costafreda, S. G., Selbæk, G., Alladi, S., Ames, D., Banerjee, S., Burns, A., Brayne, C., Fox, N. C., Ferri, C. P., Gitlin, L. N., Howard, R., Kales, H. C., Kivimäki, M., Larson, E. B., Nakasujja, N., Rockwood, K., Samus, Q., … Mukadam, N. Dementia prevention, intervention, and care: 2024 Report of the Lancet Standing Commission. *The Lancet*, *404*(10452), 572–628.

Nixon, N. (2014, October 13). Forty portraits in forty years. *The New York Times*. https://www.nytimes.com/interactive/2014/10/03/magazine/01-brown-sisters-forty-years.html

Rebok, G. W., Ball, K., Guey, L. T., Jones, R. N., Kim, H.-Y., King, J. W., Marsiske, M., Morris, J. N., Tennstedt, S. L., Unverzagt, F. W., Willis, S. L., & ACTIVE Study Group. (2014, January 13). Ten-year effects of the ACTIVE cognitive training trial on cognition and everyday functioning in older adults. *Journal of the American Geriatrics Society*. *62*(1), 16–24. https://doi.org/10.1111/jgs.12607

Solmi, M., Veronese, N., Galvano, D., Favaro, A., Ostinelli, E. G., Noventa, V., Favaretto, E., Tudor, F., Finessi, M., Shin, J. I., Smith, L., Koyanagi, A., Cester, A., Bolzetta, F., Cotroneo, A., Maggi, S., Demurtas, J., De Leo, D., & Trabucchi, M. (2020). Factors associated with loneliness: An umbrella review of observational studies. *Journal of Affective Disorders*, *271*, 131–138. https://doi.org/10.1016/j.jad.2020.03.075

Terlizzi, E. P., & Norris, T. (2021, October). *Mental health treatment among adults: United States, 2020*. NCHS Data Brief, No. 419, pp. 1–8.

WHO. (2019). *Mental health of older adults*. https://www.who.int/news-room/fact-sheets/detail/mental-health-of-older-adults

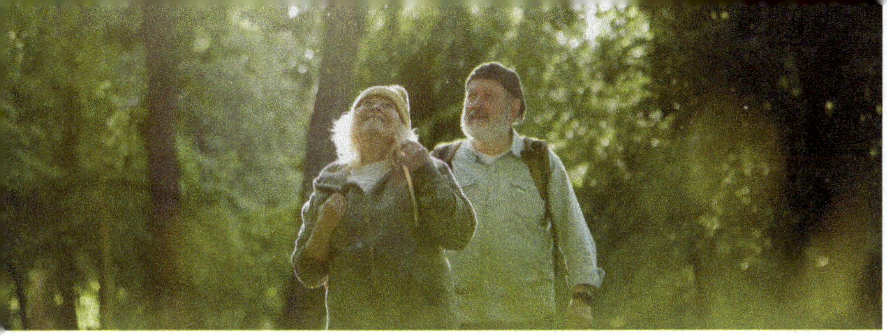

9

COMMUNITY HEALTH AND AGING

KEY TERMS

AARP
aging network
Area Agency on Aging
BenefitsCheckUp
boomers and entrepreneurship
chronic disease self-management programs
community volunteering
Emeritus Centers
Encore Careers
environmental advocacy
Experience Corps
Foster Grandparent Program
Gray Panthers
horticulture and community garden
lifelong learning institutes
long-term care ombudsman program
Mather Cafés
National Council on Aging, NCOA Center for Healthy Aging
National Senior Services Corps
Older Americans Act (OAA)
parish nurses
professional associations
Project Enhance
Red Hat Society
Retired Senior Volunteer Program
Road Scholar
senior center
Senior Companion Program
SeniorNet
Service Corps of Retired Executives
Shepherd's Centers of America
shopping mall–based educational programs
Strong for Life
worksite wellness

LEARNING OBJECTIVES

- Identify your local *Area Agency on Aging (AAA)* and describe what it does.
- Describe the *Older Americans Act (OAA)* and the *aging network*.
- Explain the need for *senior centers* to be responsive to baby boomers.
- Recognize the role that religious institutions play in providing health-promoting and educational services.
- Identify community resources for health promotion, such as universities, shopping malls, hospitals, and so forth.
- Review the history of *worksite wellness*.
- Examine the evolution of the *Road Scholar* program.
- Describe *lifelong learning institutes*.
- Describe a shopping mall–based health program.
- Analyze why boomers are becoming entrepreneurs disproportionate to other age groups.
- Identify and describe a computer education program for older adults.
- Identify the health benefits of gardening for older adults.
- Describe several model health promotion programs for older adults.
- Identify several *professional associations* that provide health-promoting services for older adults.
- Explain the importance of volunteering for contributing to the mental health of older adults and the improvement of society.
- Identify model volunteer programs that involve older adults.
- Describe the work of community health advocacy programs.
- Evaluate the value of the *BenefitsCheckUp* website.

COMMUNITY ORGANIZATIONS

Unless they live in rural settings, older persons are likely to have a wide array of community-based health-promoting programs, resources, and services available to them. Moreover, neither frailty nor disability automatically prevents older adults from gaining access to them. Programs and services for older adults are housed at religious institutions, senior centers, institutes of higher education, public service agencies, ***AARP*** chapters, hospitals, clinics, and other community sites, and they are often responsive to the health needs and limitations of older adults in their homes, in the community, or in long-term care alternatives. Increasingly, communities are developing their own networks and conduits for gaining access to services, as seen in the "age-friendly" movement, aging "villages," and organizations linking aging services providers to community organizations.

The Aging Network

In 1965, Congress passed the ***Older Americans Act (OAA)***. It was signed into law by President Lyndon Johnson and was one of the major pieces of legislation of the Great Society initiative, which also included Medicare and Medicaid. Over the subsequent decades, the OAA developed and expanded an infrastructure referred to as the aging network. The U.S. Administration on Community Living (ACL; formerly the Administration on Aging [AOA]) completed an update of OAA regulations in 2024 based on comments from all levels of the aging network. These include individual county-based Area Agency on Aging (AAA) and the statewide networks that link them, State Units on Aging that administer OAA funds (and typically are part of state governments), and the national USAging, which links AAAs across states. The 2024 final rule is available at https://acl.gov/sites/default/files/oam/2024/OAA_FinalRuleOverview2024.pdf.

The ***aging network*** serves older adults and helps them maintain their independence and well-being, covering everything from in-home personal care to senior centers, along with guardianship, caregiver support, transportation services, and home-delivered meals. While historically OAA provided free access to many services for anyone over the age of 60, without consideration of income level, over the years limitations on funds have led states to limit eligibility to low-income older adults.

The ***National Council on Aging (NCOA)*** reported that between 2011 and 2015 federal funding for the then AOA (now ACL) either did not increase or suffered as much as a 15% reduction. Even with an infusion of pandemic funding in 2020 to 2021, funding levels did not increase enough to meet growing needs (https://www.usaging.org//Files/AAA-Survey-Report-23-508.pdf). There is an equal push from the other side of the debate, however, to avoid the OAA being viewed as a welfare program, which might reduce its favorability rating among the majority of older adults.

What does the funding for the aging network provide for persons age 60 and over? Although the services vary by state, generally they consist of the following:

- *access assistance*—Outreach, information, referral, care management, and transportation;
- *nutrition programs*—Home-delivered meals, congregate nutrition sites, and nutrition education;
- *long-term care*—Home and personal care, adult day care, family caregiver support, and oversight of nursing home alternatives in some service areas;
- *health promotion*—Fall prevention and ***chronic disease self-management programs;*** and
- *protection*—***Long-term care ombudsman program***, older abuse and neglect protective services, and legal assistance.

Area Agencies on Aging

At the heart of these services, and the logical place for older persons and their caregivers to begin to locate relevant community health resources, is the local AAA. These 655 agencies cover the entire U.S. population and are responsible for planning, monitoring, and coordinating services at the local level, even though not all of the services are under the control of the AAA.

An effective AAA not only provides a wide range of services to older adults but is also aware of the aging programs and services sponsored by others, such as the local hospitals, universities and colleges, voluntary and faith-based programs, Road Scholar programs, AARP services and programs, senior centers, private case managers, home health agencies, and so forth.

As an example of the many services offered by AAA, consider the Allegheny County, Pennsylvania, agency, which covers the Pittsburgh region. It is part of the county's Department of Human Services. It "assists Allegheny County residents, 60 years of age and older, to live safe, healthy and, when possible, independent lives" (https://www.alleghenycounty.us/Services/Human-Services-DHS/DHS-Offices/Area-Agency-on-Aging). In 2021, the Allegheny County AAA served over 36,000 people through 71 contracted, community partner organizations. The range of services offered can be categorized according to who is served: (i) *all older adults and their loved ones* (health insurance counseling, protection from abuse and neglect, and opportunities for social participation and security (senior community centers, support for parenting grandparents, transportation, and assistance with obtaining additional services, such as subsidies for utilities and prescription medication, property tax and rent abatements, and supplemental nutrition assistance); (ii) *older adults who face challenges but want to remain in their homes* (adult foster care, nursing home alternatives, supportive services in the home, and personal assistance care); (iii) *older adults who need skilled care* (Ombudsman program); and (iv) people who provide care for older adults (caregiver support program). A factsheet summarizing the services shows the great breadth and complexity of delivering such services (https://www.alleghenycounty.us/files/assets/county/v/2/services/dhs/documents/publications/office-profiles/aaa.pdf).

Unfortunately, the 600+ AAAs across the U.S. do not have uniform names and can be difficult to locate in a telephone directory. USAging (formerly the *National Association of Area Agencies on Aging*, (https://www.usaging.org/) can provide current information on local AAAs. Information about USAging is available here: https://www.usaging.org//Files/USAging_Local%20Leaders%2023_508.pdf. The *Eldercare Locator* (https://eldercare.acl.gov/Public/Index.aspx) can provide current information on local caregiver services and resources, provided either by the local AAA or affiliated agencies.

Senior Community Centers

Older adults seek health information more actively than do younger adults. A major source of information for older adults is the neighborhood ***senior center***. In 2024, over 11,000 senior centers offered services to more than 1 million older adults daily (https://www.ncoa.org/article/get-the-facts-on-senior-centers/). More than half receive at least partial support through the OAA, and all of them provide some type of health-related program. The term "senior center" is increasingly giving way to the "older adult community center" (as they are now called in New York City), in keeping with a new focus on exercise, financial planning services, computer classes, immunization, organized travel, cafes, and a variety of other new functions.

At one end of the continuum, though, are senior centers that only provide a hot meal and bingo. At the other end are *multipurpose senior centers* that provide not only education and screening but also a variety of exercise and nutrition classes, self-help groups, social services, medical services, and referrals. About 75% of senior centers are multipurpose.

Some of the senior centers around the country are excellent places to go to access innovative, health-promoting activities. Two early innovators among senior centers include these Texas sites:

1. The *Geriatric Wellness Center of Collin County* offers a wide array of health programs, including health assessments, medical screenings and immunizations, health education, caregiving programs, and support groups. In addition, this senior center is unique in that it (a) identifies itself as a comprehensive wellness center to the community, (b) provides a leadership role for older adults on its board of directors, and (c) matches trained volunteers with older adults discharged from a medical center to provide short-term practical support. Contact Wellness Center for Older Adults of Collin County at www.wellnesscenteronline.org.

2. After a flood, the participants at the *Comal County Senior Citizens Center*, disassembled, hand-sanded, and reassembled into squares thousands of inch-long pieces of wood for the parquet tile floor. Retirees continue to make contributions to this senior center, including the operation of a thrift shop that provides considerable revenue for center activities. It also has an excellent fitness center. Contact the Comal County Senior Citizens Center, https://www.nbsenior.org/.

The ***Mather Cafés*** in Chicago sought a name, décor, and menu that removed the negative features of the "senior center." The café component was stylish, with an open kitchen and inventive foods and drinks that cater to (and are open to) all age groups. It was meant to be a neighborhood place, not a senior site. The programs, however, were designed for older adults, ranging from gentle yoga for those with arthritis to computers for shopping online and keeping up with grandchildren.

Religious Institutions

The church, synagogue, or mosque has the potential to be one of the most important sources of health-promoting programs in the community. Congregational members share values, beliefs, traditions, cultural bonds, and the trust and respect that these engender. Among minority groups, religious institutions may be the only community organizations deemed trustworthy of providing health information and social support (Wheldon et al., 2020). In addition, religious institutions are able to connect with hard-to-reach older adults, who may be isolated from other sources of healthcare.

Religious institutions are often called upon to provide a wide array of educational, counseling, and social support services for those persons who are least served by healthcare institutions: minorities and the poor. It would entail only a small additional step—collaboration with health professionals—for many of these institutions to be able to implement medical screenings and health education programs. Yet the immense potential contribution of religious institutions toward the health promotion of congregation members remains only partly tapped.

The site of most volunteer activity is a house of worship and its programs. In 2010, the U.S. Bureau of Labor Statistics (BLS) estimated that 25% of people age 55+ had volunteered in the previous year. People aged 65+ devoted a median of 96 hours annually, about 2 hours weekly. Nearly 10% of volunteers aged 65+ put in 500 or more hours annually, 10+ hours weekly. Adults aged 35 to 44, by contrast, contributed a median of 48 hours annually (Population Reference Bureau, 2011). In 2021, the proportion of those age 65+ who provided volunteer services was 22.1% (America's Health Rankings, 2025).

Health programs implemented at religious institutions have contributed to the health of congregation members in a variety of ways. These programs, for example, have improved mammography adherence (Sauaia et al., 2007), prostate cancer screening (Husaini et al., 2008), diabetes and hypertension screening (Boltri et al., 2008), short-term metabolic control (Samuel-Hodge et al., 2009), fruit and vegetable intake (Thorogood et al., 2007), and weight reduction (Quinn & McNabb, 2001). In a sample of 100+ churches serving the African American community, each church offered a mean of six different health programs (Woodard et al., 2020), Many religious institutions have broadened their mission to include mental health–promoting services. Surveys of self-help groups, for instance, reveal that churches and synagogues far exceed any other type of host community site.

Finally, there is the growing role of ***parish nurses*** who are members of a congregation and provide health services for members. They are either volunteers or part time and salaried, and engage in health screening, health counseling, grief support groups, and community referrals. Though most parish nurses report prior work experience in health settings, only about half of them hold at least a baccalaureate degree in nursing.

Many parish nurses focus on the relation between faith and health, and they and their congregational clients are disproportionately over the age of 55. Parish nurses can also provide services that are not accessible in much of the traditional healthcare system—community case management, community advocacy, and community health education (McGinnis & Zoske, 2008). They may become patient navigators or community health workers in Medicaid-funded programs to support diabetes management and mental health.

The ***Shepherd's Centers of America*** is a national association of interfaith organizations, typically housed in local neighborhood congregations, which offers older persons an array of educational courses, services, and resources with a wellness approach. Formed in Kansas City, Missouri, in 1972 by Dr. Elbert Cole, this organization originally consisted of six men who delivered hot meals to seven homebound women.

In 2015, the organization had 57 centers, with approximately 9,000 volunteers, 26,000 persons receiving educational services, and 35,000 receiving caregiving services. The centers provide health education, life enrichment and life review classes, caregiver seminars, bereavement support, exercise and nutrition classes, medical screenings, medication seminars, peer support groups, transportation services, respite care programs, advocacy, and other activities.

The empowerment philosophy of the Shepherd's Centers is embodied in the saying, "No one should do for older persons what they can do for themselves." The organization is now known as *Aging Forward* (https://aging-forward.org/).

Jewish Community Programs and Aging

American Jews aged 65 and older are overrepresented in the population of older Americans. The Jewish Population Survey in 2020 estimated that 30% of Jews were aged 65+ (Maurice and Marilyn Cohen Center for Modern Jewish Studies, Brandeis University, 2021), compared to about 17% of the population as a whole. This high percentage of older Jews is matched by an inadequate number of adult children caregivers. Jewish baby boomer adult children have in general an above-average educational level, which is associated with a lower fertility rate and greater geographical mobility in their careers—hence fewer accessible caregivers.

As a consequence, and drawing as well on scriptural and cultural traditions, the Jewish community has a strong legacy of supporting older adults through innovative and high-quality community and long-term care programs. Some examples follow.

The *Mitzvah Model*: Rabbi Dayle Friedman defines *mitzvah* as an act of kindness, and the Mitzvah Model expects all Jews, regardless of age, to perform them. Even impaired older adults can ask: "What can I contribute?" As Rabbi Friedman writes, "We are called to invite and facilitate elders' contributions so that they may not only experience meaning but also help to repair our broken world" (2008, p. 20).

An example of this is the *Hands and Hearts* program, which allows nursing home residents to reach out to newcomers and others in the community with handmade gifts. This program was created by the chaplain Sheila Segal and her colleagues at the Abramson Center for Jewish Life (formerly the Philadelphia Geriatric Center). Founded in 1959, it was also the first research center in the United States sponsored by a geriatric facility.

Lilmod: Elders as Students of Torah: *Lilmod* is the Hebrew word for learning and studying. Rabbi Friedman believes that aging is enriched by the study of the Torah, the Talmud, and other Jewish texts. The Torah is the five books of Moses, referred to by non-Jews as the Old Testament. The Talmud refers to the vast body of Jewish law and traditions. Older adults are not only students who study the Torah and the Talmud but teachers and mentors to the young as well. The enthusiasm for Jewish study among older people can be seen in the *Florence Melton Adult Mini-Schools*, located at 49 sites in 26 cities in the United States.

Rabbi Friedman notes that the *andragogical* approach to education (see Chapter 3) is practiced at these adult learning sites. Adult learners are encouraged to talk about their life experiences in order to build from the known to the unknown, to encourage personal reflection and sharing with others, and to set their own learning objectives and evaluation criteria.

L'Dor Vador: This Jewish term means "from generation to generation." Intergenerational activities, encounters, or messages between older adults and the young put L'Dor Vador into practice. One such example is the *ethical will*, first described in Genesis of the Hebrew Bible 3,000 years ago. Initially, these wills were transmitted orally, but over time they evolved into written, video, or audio recordings. Whatever form it takes, the ethical will fulfills a Jewish mandate: "You shall teach them diligently to your children" (Deuteronomy 6:7).

The purpose of an ethical will is to share values, lessons, hopes, dreams, loves, and the benefits of forgiveness with succeeding generations. The richest sharing of life occurs in the last stage, when an older adult is able to assimilate all of life's lessons over the life cycle, and the younger generation can contemplate on a full life and its lessons.

A related intergenerational activity frequently practiced in the Jewish community is the *life review*. By listening attentively and perhaps helping older adults to record their life stories, younger people can help these adults come to terms with their lives and teach succeeding generations about their roots.

DOROT: DOROT was established to enhance the lives of Jewish and other older adults in the greater New York metropolitan area. It fosters interactions between the generations, including volunteer opportunities for youth to serve and enhance the lives of older people. DOROT provides training and consultation, and has published a manual, *Friendly Visiting Plus: A Proven Method for Enhancing Connections Between Older Adults and the Community* (DOROT, www.dorotusa.org).

Innovative nursing home models, in which community care is linked to long-term care, include the *Hebrew Home, a* not-for-profit geriatric care centers that include strong research efforts. The Hebrew Home of Riverdale, New York, developed *Generation2Generation*, an intergenerational program that links groups of Jewish students and older residents. The students learn about Jewish attitudes on aging and how to improve understanding between generations. The Jewish Home and Aging Services in Detroit developed *the Art of Jewish Caregiving,* a program designed to educate caregivers and healthcare professionals about the diversity of the Jewish culture and traditions in order to enhance well-being at a critical time in a person's life. The *Jewish Eldercare of Rhode Island Outreach Program* offers in-service caregiving training for nursing home staff on Jewish observances, traditions, and dietary customs, and similar training to visitors to private residences. *Hebrew SeniorLife* in Boston includes a rehabilitation center, along with adult day healthcare, home healthcare, outpatient specialty clinics, and community-based health and wellness programs. It developed *NewBridge on the Charles*, a multigenerational campus that provides housing options for seniors amidst a K–8 school and an early childhood education program. The *Menorah Park Center for Senior Living* in Cleveland sponsored the *Chutzpah Mission*, which sent 10 residents, age 77 to 94, with their wheelchairs, oxygen tanks, and nebulizers, to Israel for educational and tourism purposes.

Spiritual Eldering refers to the movement to recognize the potential for aging with wisdom, or *sage-ing*. This movement was founded by Schachter-Shalomi (1995) and sprang from his book, *Age-ing to Sage-ing: A Profound New Vision on Growing Older*. *Sacred Aging*, conceived by Rabbi Richard Address, seeks to help older adults become a meaningful part of the congregation, community, and family. He has written on how to incorporate Jewish values into end-of-life decision-making, caregiving for aging parents, and developing programs and resources for older adults (Address, 2005). This includes new rituals for older adults who experience loss or personal growth occasioned by lifespan transitions, such as becoming a grandparent, reaching an unusually advanced age or wedding anniversary, entering retirement, moving into a retirement home, and completing a year of mourning.

Educational Programs

Road Scholar

Less than 9 months after *Elderhostel* renamed itself *Exploritas*, it was renamed ***Road Scholar***. The first name change was an attempt to rid itself of "elder" in the name and appeal more to younger persons, particularly the huge cohort of baby boomers in their 50s and 60s. In its 50 years, over 6 million people aged 50+ have participated in Road Scholar educational travel to over 100 countries (https://www.roadscholar.org/).

Many of the Road Scholar programs are quite innovative. An interesting example that took place at Texas A&M University at Galveston was a sea camp that focused on the coastal environment and endangered species. During the 5-day residential learning program, the students attended classes, took sailing trips, and did netting aboard the *Roamin' Empire*, a 48-foot research vessel. Another program was intergenerational, in which grandparents who wanted to share an experience with their grandchildren (ages 9 through 12) participated in on-the-water activities during 5 days in the summer and resided in dormitories on campus at night.

Road Scholar also provides aid to low-income adults who otherwise would not be able to afford travel. In addition, they provide scholarships for family caregivers who are in need of respite.

Educational Opportunities for Older Adults in Higher Education

Rosabeth Moss Kanter, a professor at the Harvard Business School, envisions a future where going to a university in your 50s or 60s is the norm, not the exception, in order to make a transition from the primary income-earning career to subsequent years of flexible service. No idea would be too idealistic for these older college students, from raising literacy rates to ending poverty to helping to reverse global warming.

Kanter envisions the development of these graduate programs at colleges and universities around the country, designed for older students who want to serve and solve problems. These students would be financially supported by foundations, employers, and governments through scholarships and tax breaks. Kanter refers to this opportunity as "even higher" education.

Let us begin with the more than 400 ***lifelong learning institutes*** affiliated with colleges and universities in the United States and Canada. Typically, older volunteers provide labor and leadership to these continuing-education programs (Manheimer, 2009). A related initiative is the *Osher Lifelong Learning Institutes* (OLLI), funded by the Bernard Osher Foundation. OLLI is "a national lifelong learning network for seasoned adults" and is integrated into the campuses of 125 institutions of higher education (https://www.osherfoundation.org/programs.html).

The National Center for Education Statistics has estimated that about 340,000 adults age 50 and over were enrolled in degree-granting public or private colleges in 2022 (https://nces.ed.gov/programs/digest/d23/tables/dt23_303.50.asp). This growth of older adult learners has inspired universities to adopt age-friendly core principles to encourage intergenerational interaction on college campuses as part of a broader diversity initiative. Age-friendly universities encourage older adult participation in all aspects of university life including taking courses, enrolling in degree programs, obtaining career preparation for the second half of life, and accessing the university's health, wellness, arts, and recreation programs. These efforts are typically spearheaded by a gerontology program on campus or a Center on Aging.

Emeritus Centers bring retired professors back to campus. These educational programs offer retired faculty members a chance to socialize, discuss topics with fellow academics, teach a course or give a lecture, advise a junior professor or student, or even pursue scholarly endeavors. At Emory University, for instance, there is a discussion group for emeriti that focuses on late-life issues, such as relations with adult children, long-term care, and managing care for a spouse.

Even though UCLA started the first emeritus center in 1969, the one launched at the University of Southern California (USC) in 1974 is considered to be particularly innovative and comprehensive. In 1993, USC began offering retired scholars research stipends of up to $2,000, and endowed an annual lecture that recognizes continuing achievements in scholarly publications. There is also an off-campus lecture program that allows emeriti to give lectures throughout southern California (USC Emeriti Center; https://emeriti.usc.edu/). USC's center also serves retired staff members as well as faculty.

In 2004, representatives of 40 universities attended the first meeting of the *Association of Retirement Organizations in Higher Education* (AROHE; www.arohe.org). The goal of this organization and its national conference is to encourage the continuing engagement of retired faculty and staff in the life of the university.

College-affiliated retirement communities have sprung up in about 60 college towns across the country, next to such institutes of higher education as Notre Dame, University of Florida, Stanford University, Pennsylvania State University, Oberlin College, Cornell University, Indiana University, Iowa State University, and the University of Michigan. In addition to socializing with former college classmates—though some choose to retire in communities affiliated with colleges that they did not attend—these retirees can attend classes at reduced rates or for free, and gain priority access to sporting or cultural events.

The *American Association of Community Colleges* is developing a nationwide program to retrain adults age 50 and older who want to find new work after traditional retirement age. The organization represents 1,200 community colleges and received a $3.2 million grant from the Atlantic Philanthropies to develop a program to retrain older adults at community colleges because these sites already provide relatively inexpensive classes within a nationwide infrastructure. In 2022, about 145,000 students attending 2-year community college were aged 50+.

A large number of older adults attend nondegree–granting programs at institutes of higher education. For instance, the *Fromm Institute* at the University of San Francisco (USF) is an educational program for retired persons taught by retired professors (https://www.fromminstitute.org/). The institute presents about 50 courses each year over three 8-week sessions. Program participants enjoy being in class with their peers and have the opportunity to interact intergenerationally with more traditional students on the USF campus. Other examples of nondegree programs, apart from the Osher network, include the *Plato Society* of Los Angeles (Office@theplatosociety.org) and *Renaissance Society* (renaissa@csus.edu). Contact nearby colleges and universities to find out if they offer similar educational programs.

In 2011, *massive open online courses* (MOOCs) took hold. This latest iteration of virtual education is often free, though they tend not to offer academic credit. About 10% of students are aged 60+. For older adults with transportation issues, this is a wonderful resource. But for those who want to build their social network or enjoy the camaraderie of in-class learning, contact one of the many lifelong learning institutes, such as the ones implemented by the Osher network, described earlier.

Educational Opportunities for Older Adults in Other Settings

Experience Corps (www.experiencecorps.org) is an AARP-AmeriCorps program that has placed over 2,000 mostly low-income older adults as tutors and mentors with 20,000 low-income children in urban public elementary schools and after-school programs in eight states and 23 metropolitan areas. Older adults who complete 25 hours of annual training, and serve 5 to 15 hours a week during the school year, receive a stipend ranging from $100 to $200 a month (Fried et al., 2004; Rebok et al., 2004; Tan et al., 2009). An important randomized trial compared Experience Corps participants to other older volunteers and showed benefit: less sedentary time and, for women, greater physical activity (Varma et al., 2016); increased generativity (Gruenewald et al., 2016); for men only, increases in hippocampal volume (Carlson et al., 2015); less intraindividual variation in cognitive performance but not in average cognitive scores (Brydges et al., 2021); and less referrals for discipline among children relative to comparison schools but no differences in reading or math performance (Rebok et al., 2019). This uneven pattern of benefit shows the challenges of intervening in late life but also suggests that volunteering is undervalued as a source of health promotion.

QUESTION: Can you locate a model health program in your community, oriented toward older adults, and describe it in sufficient detail to satisfy the curiosity of an interested older adult? Choose a program that is located at one of the following sites: hospital, senior center, AARP chapter, religious institution, retirement community, university, community college, AAA, or shopping mall.

Shortly before he died, Senator Ted Kennedy sponsored the *Serve America Act*, which became law in April 2009. One component of this legislation was *Encore Fellowships*, for persons age 55 and over who are willing to serve 1 year half-time, or 6 months full-time in areas of national need. CoGenerate (then Civic Ventures) launched the Encore Fellowships program to promote "encore careers," postretirement careers in the nonprofit sector (https://cogenerate.org/encore-fellowships/).

Shopping Mall–Based Programs

OASIS (Older Adult Service and Information System) originally provided ***shopping mall–based educational programs*** at May Company department stores in 43 cities in 25 states. It began in 1982 through its founder and president, Marylen Mann, in collaboration with Margie Wolcott May of the May department Stores. In 2020, Oasis programs were active in more than 250 communities through eight education centers and a national network of over 700 partners in 22 states (https://www.oasisnet.org/). The organization offers courses focused on mental and physical health, intellectual stimulation on a wide scope of subjects, and fun.

Computer Education

SeniorNet is an award-winning national program and the largest computer-training program for adults age 50 and older. The organization began in 1986 with 22 members, and now has educated over 2 million older adults at 130 learning centers in communities around the country.

SeniorNet (www.seniornet.org) provides training for teaching staff; offers hardware, software, and 150 course curricula; and shares strategies with community organizations for effective marketing to seniors. SeniorNet also provides online computer courses, discussion rooms for computer users, discounts on computer hardware and software, and newsletters.

WORKSITE WELLNESS AND ENCORE CAREERS

While ***worksite wellness*** programs are well-established, few focus on older workers (Haber & Wicht, 1987). A study of worksite wellness at PepsiCo by RAND and PepsiCo, over a 7-year period, revealed that health cost savings were largely attributable to the disease management savings among older workers (Caloyeras et al., 2014). In contrast, the lifestyle programs, like weight-loss programs, did not provide more savings than they cost to offer.

In general, corporate leaders continue to believe that wellness programs have both health benefits for their employees and financial benefits for their organizations. They are aware of studies reporting that participation in worksite wellness programs leads to fewer medical insurance and disability compensation claims and increased productivity. However, results from randomized clinical trials are less positive. A study of 33,000 workers reported that worksite wellness programs improved self-reported health, but did not improve clinical outcomes or healthcare utilization or spending (Song & Baicker, 2019).

In 2014, financial incentives to participate in worksite wellness programs kicked in through the Affordable Care Act (ACA). These incentives could be as much as 30% of the cost of the worker's insurance premium (50% if the program included a tobacco cessation program), and could be positive and reward based or punitive through increased insurance costs. Some employers, though, were going one step further and linking financial incentives to health goals (weight, blood pressure, etc.) that were not truly voluntary.

Architects of the ACA are revisiting the involuntary nature of employee participation in some of the worksite wellness programs that associated financial outcomes with employee health goals. They are also concerned about requiring employees to involuntarily provide health information to employers, which could be particularly discriminatory against older workers who would have to reveal sensitive health information.

One of the major shortcomings of worksite wellness programs has been the tendency for those who need these programs the least—the younger and healthier workers—to utilize them the most. This is due, in part, to the youth of staff members. At General Electric, Campbell Soup, and Johnson & Johnson, the average age of wellness staff members was less than 30. Unless trained or self-educated in the special needs, interests, and motivations of older employees, youth-oriented fitness center staff may not be effective.

An estimated three fourths of major employers offer *preretirement* programs that include a wellness component. Even more encouraging, many of these companies do not wait until employees reach their 60s, but reach out to employees in their 40s and 50s as well. At the other end of the spectrum, about 15% of companies with wellness programs permit retirees to participate. However, many retirees are excluded from worksite wellness programs for such reasons as space limitations, added staff costs, and possible legal liability.

Institutional Change in the Business World

Wellness in the workplace means more than just wellness programs. It means institutional change in order to be responsive to the needs of older workers. Only a minority of employers offer flexible work arrangements that appeal to the needs of older workers, even though a majority of older employees express interest in this option.

Why should employers accommodate the needs of the older worker? In contrast to the stereotype that older workers want to disengage from work, they are more satisfied with their jobs than younger workers, are more engaged in their work, have lower absenteeism, only marginally raise healthcare costs, and interact effectively with clients (Mori et al., 2024). Also, older adults of retirement age have the potential to be a financial bargain for their employers, as they may have retirement savings and not need or seek a full salary.

Some employers have received the message that older adults are desirable employees and should be pursued. Home Depot, for instance, offers "snowbird specials"—opportunities for older workers who live in Maine to do part-time summer work but also part-time winter work in Florida, where they are snowbirds (i.e., maintain a second residence or live for an extended period in a warmer climate during winter).

Fifty percent of registered nurses are expected to retire in the next 15 years, just as boomers will step up the demand for nursing services. Of the approximately 1 million registered nurses older than age 50 in 2023, as many as one third could retire in the next 10 to 15 years (Haddad et al., 2023). Hospitals and clinics are starting to find ways to reduce hours and change job responsibilities in order to take advantage of the experience and training of older nurses and extend their careers. Modifications in the work environment are also taking place. An increasing number of hospitals have now installed new patient beds that make it easier for older nurses to lift and move their patients.

Hospitals are getting more creative with recruiting older volunteers as well. They offer more flexible hours, free lunches or parking, and access to medical seminars. Older volunteers are given the opportunity to enjoy delivering positive results from hearing screenings to parents of newborns (while medical professionals deliver bad news). Older adults remain volunteers over a longer period of time than do young student volunteers. They also handle difficult situations in a calming manner, know how to offer emotional support to patients, and apply their maturity to often challenging tasks.

Religious institutions may be considering older leadership more. "***Boomers*** are the fastest-growing demographic at U.S. divinity schools, according to the Association of Theological Schools" (Newsome, 2011). This trend is partly due to the aging process and a growing interest in theology with age, and partly to the comfort among congregation members toward a religious leader who has experienced the challenges and losses of aging and who communicates more effectively on these issues.

The *AARP National Employer Team* is a program to link job seekers who are 50 and older with employers who are older-worker friendly. These employers may provide such benefits as flexible hours, seasonal months-off programs, tuition assistance, older adult wellness programs, allocation of pretax earnings toward eldercare needs, large-screen computer monitors with ergonomic chairs, discounts on medications, or programs that pay grandparents to supervise play activities at on-site daycare facilities. On occasion, AARP provides these companies with favorable publicity. Employers can pledge to promote a level playing field for older adults in opportunities for employment (https://www.aarp.org/forms/employer-pledge-form.html).

There are companies that exclusively match people over age 50 with age-friendly businesses. *RetirementJobs.com, Inc.* (www.retirementjobs.com) is one such company. Employee applicants pay for access to age-friendly employers, résumé editing, interviewing skills and other online workshops, job-seeking guides, self-employment and work-at-home opportunities, and other services. Businesses pay for job postings, for being designated an age-friendly company, and to gain access to employee applicants.

ReServe connects New York City retired professionals with opportunities in the workplace, particularly in service positions at nonprofit and public agencies. In its first 2 years of operation, ReServe placed 275 older adults with 110 nonprofit organizations. It launched a joint program with AARP and won a contract to place people with city agencies. ReServe envisions itself as a model for other cities in the future, but it is currently focused on the NYC area (www.reserveinc.org, *https://www.reserveinc.org/brochures*).

The federal government has recognized the potential of older adults to enhance the workplace. In addition to long-standing AmeriCorps programs such as Senior Companions, VISTA, Foster Grandparents, Seniors RSVP (https://americorps.gov/serve/americorps-seniors), the U.S. Environmental Protection Agency Senior Environmental Employment (SEE) Program seeks to employ older adults to remain active "using their matured skills in meaningful tasks that support a wide variety of environmental programs" (https://www.epa.gov/careers/senior-environmental-employment-see-program). This is a potentially valuable model for expanding the pool of older adults employed in the public sector.

The last word on institutional change in the business world will go to an expert on innovation at work. The late Peter Drucker, who died a few days short of his 96th birthday in 2005, remaining an innovative thinker and productive author on the topic of work until the year he died, declared: "The best way to predict the future of work is to create it." Which leads to . . .

Boomer Entrepreneurs

Capitalizing on experience and the networking skills accumulated over a career, boomers are jumping into the exciting and risky world of ***entrepreneurship***. Nancy Kessler of Mount Kisco, New York, for instance, following a layoff at age 58 from her career as a museum curator, launched Memoirs Plus, which helps older adults write their life stories (more content on life stories is in Chapter 8, Mental Health and Aging). She first took a class that helps women launch businesses, wrote a business plan, and did the necessary research on her start-up.

Marilyn Arnold retired from her position as a managing partner at a life insurance company and began Marilyn Arnold Designs in her mid-60s. This start-up custom designs and sews (her lifelong hobby) 18-by-18-inch pillows made from cherished clothing long since relegated to the back of a closet. She also stitches quilts assembled from beloved T-shirts and other garments. Everything she makes is from repurposed materials.

Before she retired, Ms. Arnold took up her sewing and quilting skills once again, and after regaining her skills and confidence, personally financed the $12,000 needed for equipment and supplies. After launching her business, she created a website, opened an online web storefront on Etsy, and began posting her designs on Pinterest.

John Goodenough at age 94 led a team in 2017 that invented a low-cost battery that could power the next generation of electric cars. This person ever-so-slightly increased the median age of 47 for innovators in science and technology, according to a 2016 study by the Information Technology and Innovation Foundation in Washington, DC.

According to the Kauffman Index of Entrepreneurial Activity, Americans between the ages of 55 and 64 have had a higher rate of entrepreneurial activity than those aged 20 to 34 for the past two decades (and all other age groups for the past decade). A survey by MetLife Foundation reported that 25 million people aged 44 to 70 expressed an interest in starting their own business or nonprofit organization within the next 5 to 10 years.

Many aging baby boomers have the disposable income, discretionary time, experience, and optimism to try new ventures—once the exclusive preserve of younger adults. However, a word of caution is in order. If your start-up costs are substantial and your retirement income is not, you need to find the right balance between risk and following your bliss. Is it wise to draw down on your savings and home equity to the point that if the new venture fails, you are in serious financial hardship?

On the other side of the risk/benefit ledger is the desire to work for oneself and create a meaningful business with social impact at a time of life when workers over age 50 have a hard time getting hired. If the financial risk is manageable, and the desire strong, then full steam ahead!

MODEL HEALTH PROMOTION PROGRAMS

The first directory of evidence-based health promotion programs was published in the 1980s by the AOA (now ACL) and distributed by the NCOA. Other directories were published by AARP and the U.S. Public Health Service's Office of Disease Prevention and Health Promotion. A few of the best-known, evidence-based health promotion and aging programs are briefly summarized next.

The National Council on Aging Center for Healthy Aging

The latest effort to list model health promotion programs is focused on evidence-based programs summarized by the NCOA's Center for Healthy Aging. To obtain more information, contact the ***NCOA Center for Healthy Aging*** (https://www.ncoa.org/page/contact-us/). This resource center provides healthy-aging materials such as manuals, toolkits, and links to other healthy-aging websites and conducts formal reviews of programs to assess their evidence base. Effective programs are eligible for funding using OAA Title III-D funds, which means that states can use their federal allocation of funds for providing services to older adults to deliver these health promotion programs. The NCOA Center also houses two ACL-funded national clearinghouses for fall prevention and chronic disease self-management programs (https://www.ncoa.org/evidence-based-programs/). The full set of approved evidence-based programs as of 2025 is shown in Table 9.1.

Some of the most well-known and extensively disseminated programs are described here. The author conducted research on two of the programs in Pennsylvania that received which allowed them to receive NCOA evidence-based certification (Healthy Steps for Older Adults, Healthy Steps in Motion).

Chronic Disease Self-Management Program

Kate Lorig and colleagues at the Stanford University School of Medicine have been evaluating community-based, peer-led, ***chronic disease self-management programs*** (CDSMPs) for many years, beginning with the Arthritis Self-Management Program. This initial limited program has evolved into a curriculum that is applicable to a wide array of chronic diseases and conditions.

Typically, each program involves about a dozen participants, led by peer leaders who have received 20 hours of training. The peer leaders, like the participants, are typically older and have chronic diseases themselves.

TABLE 9.1 EVIDENCE-BASED HEALTH PROMOTION PROGRAMS THAT MEET THE ADMINISTRATION FOR COMMUNITY LIVING CRITERIA FOR OLDER AMERICANS ACT TITLE IIID FUNDING

PROGRAM	LINK
A Matter of Balance	https://ncoa.org/article/evidence-based-program-a-matter-of-balance
Active Choices	https://ncoa.org/article/evidence-based-program-active-choices
Active Living Every Day	https://ncoa.org/article/evidence-based-program-active-living-every-day
AEA Arthritis Foundation Aquatic Program	https://ncoa.org/article/evidence-based-program-aea-arthritis-foundation-aquatic-program
AEA Arthritis Foundation Exercise Program	https://ncoa.org/article/evidence-based-program-aea-arthritis-foundation-exercise-program-land-based
Better Choices, Better Health (CDSMP) (Online)	https://ncoa.org/article/evidence-based-program-better-choices-better-health
Bingocize	https://ncoa.org/article/evidence-based-program-bingocize
BRI Care Consultation™	https://ncoa.org/article/evidence-based-program-bri-care-consultation
Cancer: Thriving & Surviving (In-Person)	https://ncoa.org/article/evidence-based-program-cancer-thriving-surviving-in-person
Cancer: Thriving & Surviving (Online)	https://ncoa.org/article/evidence-based-program-cancer-thriving-and-surviving-online-in-real-time
Cancer: Thriving & Surviving (Toolkit)	https://www.ncoa.org/article/evidence-based-program-cancer-thriving-surviving-mailed-tool-kit
Cáncer: Triunfando y Sobreviviendo (Cancer: Thriving & Surviving in Spanish) (In-Person)	https://www.ncoa.org/article/evidence-based-program-cancer-triunfando-y-sobreviviendo-cancer-thriving-surviving-in-spanish-in-person
Cáncer: Triunfando y Sobreviviendo (Cancer: Thriving & Surviving in Spanish) (Online)	https://www.ncoa.org/article/evidence-based-program-cancer-triunfando-y-sobreviviendo-cancer-thriving-surviving-in-spanish-online-synchronous
CAPABLE	https://ncoa.org/article/evidence-based-program-capable
Care Transitions Intervention	https://ncoa.org/article/evidence-based-program-care-transitions-intervention
CDC Diabetes Prevention Program (DPP)	https://ncoa.org/article/evidence-based-program-cdc-diabetes-prevention-program-dpp

(continued)

TABLE 9.1 EVIDENCE-BASED HEALTH PROMOTION PROGRAMS THAT MEET THE ADMINISTRATION FOR COMMUNITY LIVING CRITERIA FOR OLDER AMERICANS ACT TITLE IIID FUNDING (*CONTINUED*)

PROGRAM	LINK
Chronic Disease Self-Management Program (CDSMP) (Toolkit)	https://ncoa.org/article/evidence-based-program-chronic-disease-self-management-mailed-tool-kit-mailed-cdsmp
Chronic Disease Self-Management Program (CDSMP) (In-Person)	https://ncoa.org/article/evidence-based-program-chronic-disease-self-management-workshop-in-person
Chronic Disease Self-Management Program (CDSMP) (Online)	https://ncoa.org/article/evidence-based-program-chronic-disease-self-management-workshop-online-in-real-time
Chronic Pain Self-Management Program (CPSMP) (Toolkit)	https://ncoa.org/article/evidence-based-program-chronic-pain-self-management-mailed-tool-kit-mailed-cpsmp
Chronic Pain Self-Management Program (CPSMP) (Online, Synchronous)	https://ncoa.org/article/evidence-based-program-chronic-pain-self-management-program-cpsmp-online-synchronous
Chronic Pain Self-Management Program (CPSMP) (In-Person)	https://ncoa.org/article/evidence-based-program-chronic-pain-self-management-workshop-in-person
Diabetes Self-Management Program (DSMP) (In-Person)	https://ncoa.org/article/evidence-based-program-diabetes-self-management-program-in-person
Diabetes Self-Management Program (DSMP) (Toolkit)	https://ncoa.org/article/evidence-based-program-diabetes-self-management-mailed-tool-kit-with-or-without-telephone-scripts
Diabetes Self-Management Program (DSMP) (Virtual)	https://ncoa.org/article/evidence-based-program-diabetes-self-management-program-virtual-real-time
Eat Smart, Move More, Weigh Less	https://ncoa.org/article/evidence-based-program-eat-smart-move-more-weigh-less
Enhance Fitness	https://ncoa.org/article/evidence-based-program-enhancefitness
EnhanceWellness	https://ncoa.org/article/evidence-based-program-enhancewellness
FallScape	https://ncoa.org/article/evidence-based-program-fallscape
FallsTalk	https://ncoa.org/article/evidence-based-program-fallstalk
Fit and Strong!	https://ncoa.org/article/evidence-based-program-fit-strong

(*continued*)

TABLE 9.1 EVIDENCE-BASED HEALTH PROMOTION PROGRAMS THAT MEET THE ADMINISTRATION FOR COMMUNITY LIVING CRITERIA FOR OLDER AMERICANS ACT TITLE IIID FUNDING (*CONTINUED*)

PROGRAM	LINK
Florida BRITE Project (Brief Intervention & Treatment for Elders)	https://ncoa.org/article/evidence-based-program-florida-brite-project-brief-intervention-treatment-for-elders
Geri-Fit® Strength Training Workout for Older Adults	https://ncoa.org/article/evidence-based-program-geri-fit-strength-training-workout-for-older-adults
Health Coaches for Hypertension Control	https://ncoa.org/article/evidence-based-program-health-coaches-for-hypertension-control
HealthMatters Program	https://ncoa.org/article/evidence-based-program-healthmatters-program
Healthy IDEAS (Identifying Depression, Empowering Activities for Seniors)	https://ncoa.org/article/evidence-based-program-healthy-ideas
Healthy Moves for Aging Well	https://ncoa.org/article/evidence-based-program-healthy-moves-for-aging-well
Healthy Steps for Older Adults	https://ncoa.org/article/evidence-based-program-healthy-steps-for-older-adults
Healthy Steps in Motion	https://ncoa.org/article/evidence-based-program-healthy-steps-in-motion
Home Hazard Removal Program (HARP)	https://www.ncoa.org/article/evidence-based-program-home-hazard-removal-program-harp
HomeMeds	https://ncoa.org/article/evidence-based-program-homemeds
Manejo Personal de la Diabetes (DSMP in Spanish) (In-person)	https://www.ncoa.org/article/evidence-based-program-manejo-personal-de-la-diabetes-dsmp-in-spanish-in-person
Manejo Personal de la Diabetes (DSMP in Spanish) (Toolkit)	https://www.ncoa.org/article/evidence-based-program-manejo-personal-de-la-diabetes-mailed-tool-kit-mailed-dsmp-in-spanish
Manejo Personal de la Diabetes (DSMP in Spanish) (Online)	https://www.ncoa.org/article/manejo-personal-de-la-diabetes-dsmp-in-spanish-online-synchronous
Manejo Personal del Crónico (CPSMP in Spanish) (Online)	https://www.ncoa.org/article/evidence-based-program-manejo-personal-del-cronico-cpsmp-in-spanish-online-synchronous
Mind Over Matter: Healthy Bowels, Healthy Bladder (MOM)	https://ncoa.org/article/evidence-based-program-mind-over-matter-healthy-bowels-healthy-bladder-mom

(*continued*)

TABLE 9.1 EVIDENCE-BASED HEALTH PROMOTION PROGRAMS THAT MEET THE ADMINISTRATION FOR COMMUNITY LIVING CRITERIA FOR OLDER AMERICANS ACT TITLE IIID FUNDING (*CONTINUED*)

PROGRAM	LINK
On the Move	https://ncoa.org/article/evidence-based-program-on-the-move
Otago Exercise Program	https://ncoa.org/article/evidence-based-program-otago-exercise-program
PEARLS (Program to Encourage Active, Rewarding Lives for Seniors)	https://ncoa.org/article/evidence-based-program-pearls-program-to-encourage-active-rewarding-lives
Positive Self-Management (In-Person)	https://ncoa.org/article/evidence-based-program-positive-self-management-program-in-person
Positive Self-Management (Virtual)	https://ncoa.org/article/evidence-based-program-positive-self-management-program-virtual-real-time
Powerful Tools for Caregivers	https://ncoa.org/article/evidence-based-program-powerful-tools-for-caregivers
PREPARE For Your Care	https://ncoa.org/article/evidence-based-program-prepare-for-your-care
REACH Community (Resources for Enhancing Alzheimer's Caregivers Health in the Community)	https://ncoa.org/article/evidence-based-program-reach-community
REACH-TX	https://ncoa.org/article/evidence-based-program-reach-tx
Respecting Choices	https://ncoa.org/article/evidence-based-program-respecting-choices
¡Sí, Yo Puedo Controlar Mí Diabetes! (¡Sí, Yo Puedo!)	https://www.ncoa.org/article/evidence-based-program-si-yo-puedo-controlar-mi-diabetes-si-yo-puedo
SHARE (Support, Health, Activities, Resources, and Education) for Dementia	https://www.ncoa.org/article/evidence-based-program-share
Stay Active and Independent for Life (SAIL)	https://ncoa.org/article/evidence-based-program-stay-active-independent-for-life-the-sail-program
Stepping On	https://ncoa.org/article/evidence-based-program-stepping-on
Stress-Busting Program for Family Caregivers	https://ncoa.org/article/evidence-based-program-stress-busting-program-for-family-caregivers
Tai Chi for Arthritis and Falls Prevention	https://ncoa.org/article/evidence-based-program-tai-chi-for-arthritis-and-falls-prevention
Tai Chi Prime	https://ncoa.org/article/evidence-based-program-tai-chi-prime

(*continued*)

TABLE 9.1 EVIDENCE-BASED HEALTH PROMOTION PROGRAMS THAT MEET THE ADMINISTRATION FOR COMMUNITY LIVING CRITERIA FOR OLDER AMERICANS ACT TITLE IIID FUNDING (*CONTINUED*)

PROGRAM	LINK
Tai Ji Quan: Moving for Better Balance	https://ncoa.org/article/evidence-based-program-tai-ji-quan-moving-for-better-balance
TCARE® Support System (Tailored Caregiver Assessment and Referral®)	https://ncoa.org/article/evidence-based-program-tcare-support-system-tailored-caregiver-assessment-and-referral
Tomando Control de Su Salud (In-Person)	https://ncoa.org/article/evidence-based-program-tomando-control-de-su-salud-cdsmp-in-spanish-in-person
Tomando Control de Su Salud (Mailed Tool Kit Phone)	https://ncoa.org/article/evidence-based-program-tomando-control-de-su-salud-mailed-tool-kit-mailed-cdsmp-in-spanish
Tomando Control de Su Salud (Virtual)	https://ncoa.org/article/evidence-based-program-tomando-control-de-su-salud-cdsmp-in-spanish-online-synchronous
Walk With Ease (group program and self directed program)	https://ncoa.org/article/evidence-based-program-walk-with-ease
Wellness Initiative for Senior Education (WISE)	https://ncoa.org/article/evidence-based-program-wellness-initiative-for-senior-education-wise
Wellness Recovery Action Plan (WRAP®)	https://ncoa.org/article/evidence-based-program-wellness-recovery-action-plan
Workplace Chronic Disease Self-Management Program (wCDSMP) (In-Person)	https://ncoa.org/article/evidence-based-program-workplace-chronic-disease-self-management-workshop-wcdsmp-in-person
Workplace Chronic Disease Self-Management Program (wCDSMP) (Online, Synchronous)	https://ncoa.org/article/evidence-based-program-workplace-chronic-disease-self-management-workshop-virtual-real-time
YMCA Moving for Better Balance	https://ncoa.org/article/evidence-based-program-ymca-moving-for-better-balance

Source: National Council on Aging. Evidence-Based Programs. https://www.ncoa.org/evidence-based-programs/

The topics that are covered in the CDSMP are contained in the textbook, *Living a Healthy Life With Chronic Conditions,* 5th edition (Lorig et al., 2020). This content focuses on three main areas:

Medical management refers to the ability to communicate effectively with health professionals and bcome an educated consumer of medical resources.
Social management refers to maintaining valued roles while living with chronic disease.
Emotional management refers to regulating the emotional consequences of chronic conditions.

The CDSMP is taught by volunteer lay leaders who receive 20 hours of training. Upon completion of training, the course they facilitate typically consists of seven weekly sessions, each 2.5 hours in length, with 10 to 15 participants. The location can be a senior center, a church, a retirement community, a hospital, or another site that will not charge for space.

The theoretical basis of the program has been to promote a sense of personal efficacy, or confidence, among participants (Bandura, 1997) by using such techniques as guided mastery of skills, peer modeling, reinterpretation of symptoms, social persuasion through group support, and individual self-management guidance.

The evaluation of the CDSMP program (Lorig et al., 2001) concluded that graduates reported reduced emergency department and outpatient visits; decreased health distress, fatigue, and limitations in role function; and greater energy and self-confidence.

With the help of the ACL Evidence-Based Disease Prevention Grants Program, the NCOA's Center for Healthy Aging, and the nationwide network of AAA, the CDSMP has gone nationwide. This CDSMP effort was further enhanced by a 3-year, 2012 to 2015, $10 million grant sponsored through the ACA. By 2024, over 400,000 older adults have participated in CDSMP (National Council on Aging, 2024). Grantees are charged with the responsibility of finding new partners (e.g., state agencies, YMCAs, employers, unions, retiree organizations, Veterans Affairs) and new funding sources, and have been successful with accomplishing this. In the national evaluation (unfortunately not a randomized trial), CDSMP led to improvements in social/role activities, depression, and communication with physicians as well as improvements in physical activity and lower utilization of the emergency department and hospital (Ory et al., 2013).

There is also an online version of the CDSMP, with funding from Atlantic Philanthropies, to help people with arthritis, asthma, diabetes, lung and heart disease, stroke, and other chronic conditions.

Enhance Fitness, Enhance Wellness

Senior Services of Seattle/King County began ***Project Enhance*** (formerly the Senior Wellness Project) in 1997 at the North Shore Senior Center in Bothell, Washington. It is a research-based health promotion program that included a component of chronic care self-management that was modeled after CDSMP. The program also includes health and functional assessments; individual and group counseling; exercise programs; a personal health action plan with the support of a nurse, social worker, and volunteer health mentor; and support groups. The Project Enhance Resource Portal can be accessed by contacting projectenhance@soundgenerations.org.

A randomized controlled study of chronically ill seniors who attended this program reported a reduction in number of hospital stays and average lengths of stay, a reduction in use of psychotropic medications, and better functioning in activities of daily living (Leveille et al., 1998).

Enhance Fitness began as a partnership among a university, an AAA, local and national foundations, health departments, senior centers, primary care providers, older volunteers, and older participants. Versions of this model program are being replicated at senior wellness sites around the country (80+ sites in the United States) and globally to test its effectiveness in a variety of communities in an assortment of sites, all serving diverse clienteles. One study of this program demonstrated higher levels of physical activity and lower levels of depression among its participants (Dobkin, 2002).

The program has been divided into two components: Enhance Fitness and Enhance Wellness. *Enhance Fitness* is an exercise program that focuses on stretching, flexibility, balance, low-impact aerobics, and strength training. Certified instructors have undergone special training in fitness for older adults. Classes last an hour, involve 10 to 25 people, and participants can track their progress through a series of functional evaluations. Participants who completed 6 months of Enhance Fitness improved significantly in a variety of physical and social functioning measures, and also reported reduced levels of pain and depression. There was also a reduction in healthcare costs (Ackerman et al., 2003).

Enhance Wellness focuses on mental health, with an emphasis on lessening symptoms of depression and other mood problems, developing a sense of greater self-reliance, and lowering the need for drugs that affect thinking or emotions. Enhance Wellness typically consists of a nurse and social worker working with a participant. An analysis of the effectiveness of the program found that it reduced depression when measured 1 year after the program was completed, and improved exercise readiness, physical activity levels, and self-reported health (Phelan et al., 2002). The programs have been replicated in almost every state, with over 80,000 participants.

Strong for Life

The ***Strong for Life*** program is a home-based exercise program for disabled and nondisabled older adults. It focuses on strength and balance, and provides an exercise video, a trainer's manual, and a user's guide. The program was designed by physical therapists for home use by older adults, and relies on elastic resistive bands for strengthening muscles. The exercise program led to a high rate of exercise adherence among older participants, as well as increased lower extremity strength, improvements in tandem gait, and a reduction in physical disability (Jette et al., 1999).

QUESTION: **Which one of the model health promotion programs summarized in this chapter is of most interest to you? Find out more information about this program (or a similar health and aging program), and describe it in sufficient detail to adequately inform a health professional.**

A BROADER VIEW OF HEALTH PROMOTION ACTIVITY

A Model Health Program in China

A self-led tai chi class observed in China as far back as 1978 provides a good example of a community-based health promotion program. Tai chi is a mindful sequence of physical movements derived from the ancient Chinese martial arts. These movements attempt to increase energy, improve balance, and enhance mental and spiritual health. The participants, over half of whom were older adults, had maximum accessibility to this program—they had only to exit their front doors. There were no fees to be paid and no professionals to depend on. Figure 9.1 shows one group of people practicing tai chi (Haber, 1979).

Since that time, several studies have reported that tai chi is beneficial for older adults with balance problems (Wolf et al., 1996; Wolfson et al., 1996), and it is now being taught at many senior centers and other community sites throughout the United States. Meta-analyses and randomized controlled trials support the effectiveness of tai chi (Yang et al., 2021).

FIGURE 9.1 Tai chi in China.

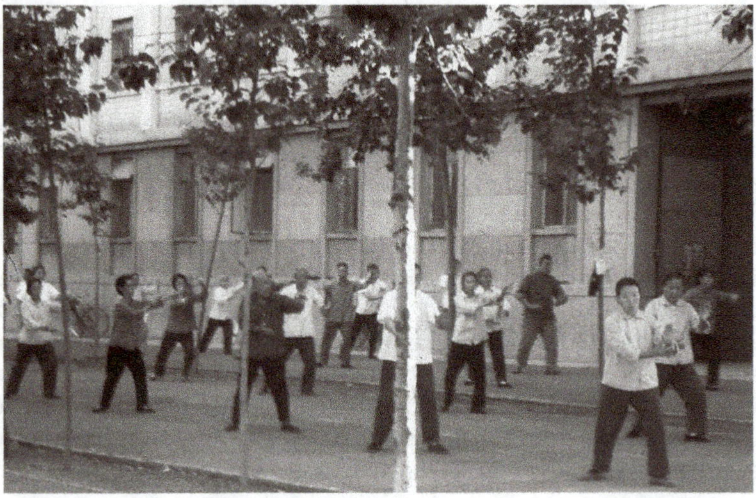

Horticulture and Community Gardening

How can you go wrong listening to Michael Pollan, the Knight Professor of Journalism at the University of California, Berkeley, one of *Time* magazine's 100 most influential people in the world, and the author of several popular books on food? In his book *Food Rules,* Pollan (2011) recommends that you plant a vegetable garden if you have the space, a window box if you do not. In addition to communing with nature, your garden produces the freshest, most nutritious produce possible. He also notes the side benefits: being outside, getting exercise, and saving money (a $70 dollar investment yields $600 worth of food, according to Pollan). Also, ***horticulture*** is age-friendly.

On March 20, 2009, a hopeful gardener began to plant in her backyard. Not just any backyard, but the South Lawn of the White House. And not just any gardener, but the First Lady at the time Michelle Obama who had come up with yet another project to foster one of her goals, improving the health of Americans. She had lots of questions, besides whether she would be allowed to do this on the White House grounds. \Was the soil fertile enough? Was the sunlight sufficient? Was her gardening inexperience too much of a barrier? Did she have enough time?

Ms. Obama had more on her mind than eating fresh vegetables. She wanted to send a message about the food we eat and the lives we live. Her first plan of action was to recruit 23 fifth graders from a local elementary school to help plant the lettuce, peas, spinach, broccoli, kale, and collard greens. After three successful crops, Ms. Obama wrote about her experience in *American Grown: The Story of the White House Kitchen Garden and Gardens Across America* (Obama, 2012). Her goal in writing this book was to inspire families, schools, and communities to try their hands at gardening and "enjoy all the gifts of health, discovery, and connection a garden can bring" (p. 19).

If space is limited, there are still options. If viable soil is inaccessible, plant in raised beds or on a sunny windowsill, patio, or balcony. You do not get the exercise of using hoes and shovels or tilling the ground, but you do get the fruits and vegetables.

If expertise is not available, read a book or go to a garden show in your community and learn from master gardeners. You will have to learn about what is best to plant in your area, when to plant, what amounts of sun and water are needed, soil management and plant nutrients, how to control weeds, what to watch out for—pests, birds, rabbits, deer, soil erosion, the least toxic approach to pest control—and many other interesting and challenging topics.

Mrs. Obama said her first crop cost $200 for soil, seeds, seedlings, and soil nutrients, and produced 740 lbs of produce—not a bad financial payoff. Whereas fresh food is generally more expensive than convenience food (thanks to misdirected government subsidies), this is not so when you grow your own.

Your produce can also make thoughtful gifts and strengthen your emotional connections to others. You may also work with others on an individual garden or on a ***community garden***. What makes this project gerontological in nature is that many community gardens are intergenerational, involving local youth and older adults. There are about 30,000 community gardens in the United States and Canada, reclaiming empty or neglected land and changing it into crops.

Many examples of community gardens are provided by Michelle Obama in her book. The most ambitious one is in Seattle, Washington, where there are 76 gardens on 23 acres with 4,700 gardeners, about a third of whom donate their harvest to food banks and feeding centers. In 2010, 21,000 lbs of fresh produce were given away. There is an *American Community Garden Association* (www.communitygarden.org), which informs you about existing community gardens in your area or how to start your own.

Gardening is good for the health of older adults. A review of 22 studies on gardening by either community-dwelling or institutionalized older adults revealed that this activity improved physical strength, flexibility, cognitive ability, socialization, and overall quality of life (Wang & Macmillan, 2013). The researchers noted that the studies took place in both urban and rural communities as either individual or group activities. National data also support the benefit of gardening (Veldheer et al., 2023).

Another review of 17 studies reported that watering plants, or sitting or strolling in a garden can help soothe the anxiety of dementia patients in nursing homes (Whear et al., 2014). Yet another example of the benefits of ***horticulture*** with older adults is a study in a nursing home that reported that horticulture therapy increased interpersonal intimacy among older residents and improved psychological well-being (Jueng et al., 2023; Yao & Chen, 2017).

PROFESSIONAL ASSOCIATIONS SUPPORTING HEALTH PROMOTION IN OLD AGE

Health promotion and health education programs are sponsored by many disease-specific ***professional associations***. The *Arthritis Foundation*, for example, offers several health education programs, among them self-help and peer support programs, including the Arthritis Self-Help Course, PACE Exercise, arthritis clubs, and aquatic programs. All programs are taught by trained volunteer instructors, many of whom cope with arthritis themselves.

It is believed that everyone over the age of 60 has some degree of osteoarthritis, and about 40% to 60% of older Americans recognize some of its symptoms. Osteoarthritis, the most common form of arthritis, is the gradual wearing away of tissue around the joints of the hands, feet, knees, hips, neck, or back. Arthritic pain may vary from mild to severe, and it may come and go. Arthritis cannot be prevented or cured, but the function of arthritic joints can be improved and the pain often can be alleviated.

More than 100 local chapters of the Arthritis Foundation offer a 6-week course that provides information on medications, exercise, nutrition, relaxation techniques, coping skills, and the practical concerns of daily living. Practical information can range from the identification of places to purchase Velcro-modified clothing, to the location of aquatic exercise programs.

Many of the Arthritis Foundation programs were developed and evaluated at the Stanford Arthritis Center over many years and are offered around the country. Participants are typically asked to pay a small fee for courses and instructional materials. Besides health education programs, local arthritis chapters distribute free booklets on arthritis as well as information about most arthritis medications. For additional information, contact the Arthritis Foundation (www.arthritis.org).

Many other professional associations also offer health education programs and materials. If you cannot locate a state or local chapter of a specific professional association, contact one of the following national headquarters for information on local educational opportunities and support groups, as well as for resource materials:

Alzheimer's Association (24-hour toll-free telephone link to access information about local chapters and community resources, free catalogue of educational publications, and research program): www.alz.org
American Cancer Society (education and support programs, workshops, transportation programs, publications, and financial aid): www.cancer.org
American Diabetes Association (local chapters for support and referrals, and outreach programs for minority communities): www.diabetes.org
American Heart Association (cookbooks, guides on treatment and prevention, and research funding program): www.americanheart.org
American Lung Association (education, advocacy, and research on asthma, emphysema, tuberculosis, and lung cancer: www.lung.org
National Stroke Association (survivors, caregivers, family, and medical professionals): www.stroke.org
American Parkinson's Disease Association (local chapters, educational materials, referrals, and research): www.apdaparkinson.org
Better Hearing Institute (information on medical, surgical, and rehabilitation options): www.betterhearing.org
National Association for Continence (advocacy, education, and support): www.nafc.org
National Association on Mental Illness (support groups, education, advocacy, and research): www.nami.org
National Council on Alcoholism and Drug Dependence (advocacy, information, and referrals): www.ncadd.org
National Council on Problem Gambling (guides to counselors, support groups, and treatment facilities): www.ncpgambling.org
National Osteoporosis Foundation (research, education, and advocacy): www.nof.org

QUESTION: Visit the website of one of the professional associations listed in this section. What is the most innovative or interesting component of the program that involves older adults that you can find? Please describe it and explain why you chose it.

COMMUNITY VOLUNTEERING

The United States finds itself with two parallel phenomena that invite convergence. On the one hand, the country has vast unmet community service needs; on the other hand, the United States draws only partially on the large and growing productive potential of older people.

—Caro and Morris (2001)

Although many analysts see the rapidly growing older adult population in the United States in terms of being a financial burden on future generations, others see a vast, untapped social resource for improving the health and well-being of older adults and society itself. An AARP survey reported that 50% of Americans age 50 to 75 were planning to incorporate community service into later life (Freedman, 2002). The Bureau of Labor Statistics of the U.S. Department of Labor, however, reported that in that same year the volunteer rate for people age 65 and older was less than half of that (22.7%).

If the potential tidal wave of ***community volunteering*** could be unleashed, there would likely be greater fulfillment in, and purpose to, the latter part of the life cycle. A meta-analysis of 37 independent studies reported that the sense of well-being among older volunteers was consistently enhanced as a consequence of their volunteer efforts (Wheeler et al., 1998). The authors also noted that while this mental health phenomenon was taking place, significant experience and energy were being directed toward the service needs of society's more vulnerable groups. Research continues to support the many benefits of volunteering (Kim et al., 2021) and suggests that the effect is not due to the greater likelihood of healthier people volunteering.

About a century ago, many services in America—education, law enforcement, firefighting, hospital care, social service—relied upon volunteers. Over time, however, community services began to be dominated by paid personnel, with the more affluent obtaining services privately if desired and the less affluent relying exclusively on publicly funded services. In addition, volunteering in the public sector became less attractive and peripheral to the main work of paid staff. Volunteer responsibilities were not only becoming marginal to the mission of public organizations, but when volunteers were utilized, they were often lacking in training, supervision, and recognition.

Marc Freedman, president of Civic Ventures, described the volunteer opportunities available to most older adults as "incapable of capturing the imagination of a new generation of older Americans." In his book *Prime Time: How Baby Boomers Will Revolutionize Retirement and Transform America,* Freedman (1999) argues that we need to "learn how to tap the time, talent, and civic potential of the group that is our country's only increasing natural resource." To accomplish this goal, volunteers need to be adequately trained and offered ongoing support, including stipends (Morrow-Howell et al., 2009). Persons of low socioeconomic status report the most benefit from their volunteer experience when stipends are provided to cover costs. Linda Fried, one of the developers of Experience Corps (discussed previously), has made the case for volunteering in old age as an unprecedented resource gifted to the world through our current expansion of longevity and healthy aging (https://www.youtube.com/watch?v=GNLucqxn-7w). Volunteer opportunities must be tailored to older people's interest and capacities, but the source of attrition among older volunteers is more likely to be underchallenging tasks that do not take advantage of the range of skills older people bring to the table (Kaur et al., 2022).

Encore Careers, at www.encore.org, is a follow-up initiative by Marc Freedman to help older adults transition out of their work careers and into jobs or volunteer opportunities in the nonprofit and public sectors. Encore careers are those that are extended into personally fulfilling public service opportunities, sometimes providing modest income. Freedman (2007) provides many examples in his book *Encore: Finding Work That Matters in the Second Half of Life.* Encore careers have a positive impact on society's greatest problems.

A surprisingly large number of baby boomers and older adults ages 44 to 70 are interested in an encore career, according to a 2008 MetLife Foundation/Civic Ventures Encore Career Survey (www.metlife.com). An encore career focuses on personal meaning, often with social impact. Retirees move into jobs or volunteer opportunities in such fields as education (30%), healthcare (23%), government (16%), and nonprofit organizations that serve a public good (9%). Almost 10% of the age 44 to 70 population surveyed were already engaged in encore careers, and almost half of the remaining surveyed (45%) were interested. In a 2014 survey, about 4.5 million people aged 50 to 70 had started encore careers (Encore.org, 2014).

Encore, in cooperation with AARP, has encouraged older adults to join the *Peace Corps*. Established in 1961 under the initiative of a baby boomer role model, President John F. Kennedy, the Peace Corps over time has been reaching out more to older adults. Beginning with Lillian Carter, former President Carter's mother, who volunteered in India at the age of 68, those age 50 and older now constitute 7% of Peace Corps volunteers. In 2015, the oldest volunteer was age 80; the oldest ever in the Peace Corps was 86. Older Americans can serve a traditional 2-year period or take part in shorter (3 months to 1 year) assignments.

Regardless of one's impact on the community, the volunteer experience seems to be consistently beneficial to one's mental health (Morrow-Howell et al., 2003). The beneficial effect of volunteering may be particularly timely during widowhood. People who have experienced spousal loss report a greater likelihood of volunteering a few years after the death of their spouse. The volunteer experience then appears to be protective against depressive symptoms, while enhancing one's confidence in oneself (Kim et al., 2021; Li, 2007).

Another study reported that volunteer opportunities produce mental health benefits in nursing homes. These were not volunteer opportunities to help nursing home residents, but volunteer opportunities performed *by* nursing home residents. Residents from five long-term care facilities were given the opportunity to tutor students in English as a second language. The treatment participants improved their psychological well-being in comparison with nursing home control groups (Yuen et al., 2008).

FEDERAL VOLUNTEERISM

The following federally funded programs provide training, supervision, and recognition for older adult volunteer activity. Program evaluations, though limited, show that these programs enhance the lives of the persons they serve as well as the mental health of older volunteers (Morrow-Howell et al., 2003; Tan et al., 2016).

The ***National Senior Services Corps*** (now known as AmeriCorps Seniors) was established in 1973 and is the principal vehicle for federal volunteerism for Americans age 55 and older (www.seniorcorps.org.). Every year, over 143,000 AmeriCorps Senior volunteers take on service opportunities offered by community partners (https://www.federalregister.gov/documents/2024/08/30/2024-19348/americorps-seniors-regulation-updates). These older Americans, most of whom are low income, participate in the corps and receive a small stipend for their effort. Volunteers serve primarily through one of the following three programs:

1. The ***Retired Senior Volunteer Program*** (RSVP), which matches the personal interests and skills of older Americans age 55 and over with opportunities to solve problems in their local communities.
2. The ***Foster Grandparent Program,*** which trains low-income adults age 60 and over to serve 20 hours a week helping children with special needs (e.g., a seriously ill child with cancer).
3. The ***Senior Companion Program,*** which trains low-income adults age 60 and over to support peers who are frail and disabled (e.g., a stroke victim who is confined to a wheelchair and suffering from depression), to help them remain as independent as possible. In 2011, 13,600 older volunteers in 220 programs served 61,000 clients.

Other federal volunteer opportunities include the ***Service Corps of Retired Executives*** (SCORE), which operates in conjunction with the Small Business Administration (www.score.org). Since 1964, SCORE has helped retired executives and business owners counsel younger entrepreneurs who are launching America's small businesses. There are nearly 400 SCORE chapters. The 2024 report from SCORE notes that its volunteers have helped more than 17 million entrepreneurs. Its 10,000 volunteers provide volunteer services throughout the United States.

OLD AGE VOLUNTEER ADVOCACY

AARP

More than 70 years ago, the founder of ***AARP***, Ethel Percy Andrus, said that the way to lead a life with purpose and meaning was "to serve, and not to be served." This tradition can be found among the large number of AARP's 38 million members who volunteer annually. In 2023, 50,000 AARP volunteers provided nearly 8 million hours of service (AARP, 2023).

Three of the most popular AARP community volunteer programs are the following:

1. AARP's *55 Alive Driver Safety Program* is implemented by volunteers who are trained to provide driver education. This program helps older adults drive safely, and can significantly lower their automobile insurance rates. It has been offered to older adults for over 30 years, producing several million graduates.
2. AARP's *Tax-Aide* provides free tax counseling and preparation service for middle- and low-income taxpayers age 60 and older. Volunteer tax counselors are trained and certified by the Internal Revenue Service. The Tax-Aide program assists more than 2 million people each year and is staffed by more than 30,000 AARP volunteers.
3. AARP's *Senior Community Service Employment Program* (SCSEP) is implemented in conjunction with the Department of Labor. This program trains and transitions low-income older people into paid employment. Since its inception, over half a million people have found employment through the program.

Founded in 1958, AARP (formerly the American Association of Retired Persons) eventually became an organization with less than half of its members *retired*. Given universal recognition of its name, though, a compromise was struck and rather than giving up entirely on its name, it shifted to its acronym AARP. Any way you call it, its influence is great. The bimonthly *AARP The Magazine* has 38 million readers and is mailed free to households with AARP members, the largest circulation of any magazine in the United States. Every older person is eligible for AARP membership and receives an invitation when they turn 50.

> **QUESTION:** Describe a volunteering experience you have had. Were you trained, supervised, and recognized? Was it a satisfying experience? How could your experience have been improved? If you have never done volunteer work, become a volunteer and report on your experience.

Gray Panthers

The best-known role model for community health advocacy in aging was Maggie Kuhn (1905–1995), founder of the ***Gray Panthers***, an intergenerational advocacy group. Figure 9.2 shows her in 1978, literally on a slow boat to China (as part of a gerontology

FIGURE 9.2 Maggie Kuhn, founder of the Gray Panthers advocacy group.

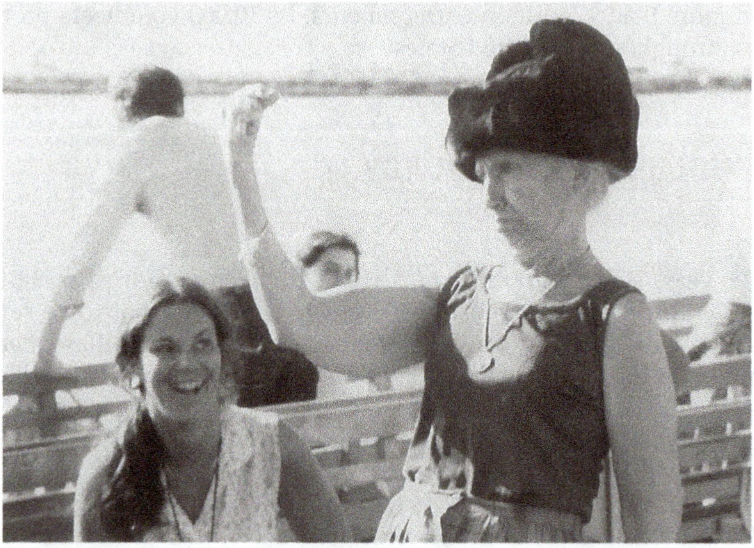

study tour), at a time when Chinese relations with the Soviet Union were very strained. Ever the feisty one, Maggie thought posing in a Russian hat might amuse her Chinese guides. The expressions on the faces of the guides, however, were inscrutable.

To find out about the advocacy issues and activities that the Gray Panthers are currently involved in, you need to contact individual chapters. A Google search revealed websites for chapters in New York City, San Francisco, and Albuquerque. A national website is no longer available.

To purchase or rent an excellent creative video on Maggie Kuhn's life, called *Maggie Growls*, e-mail orders@wmm.com, or visit the website at www.wmm.com. There is also an interesting written review of this video (see Bradley & Todd, 2005).

Environmental Advocacy

Environmental advocacy is a strong interest among many older adults, perhaps as part of their (increasingly unlikely) quest to leave Planet Earth in as good a condition as when they were born into it. Unfortunately, several environmental advocacy organizations listed in a prior edition of this book are no longer active. Perhaps that is the nature of advocacy groups. They come and they go.

One that still seems to have survived, though it has moved and changed leadership, is *Great Old Broads for Wilderness*, founded in 1989 by Susan Tixier of Escalante, Utah. She was concerned about motorized vehicles in designated wilderness areas and rampant grazing and mining scarring the Utah landscape. She organized an annual hike (the Broadwalk), published a newspaper (the *Broadside*), and organized a variety of environmental advocacy efforts. Susan also declared that women members younger than 45 would have to be called "Great Old Broads-in-Training." Later on, Great Old Bros (men) were declared welcome as well.

In 2003, the organization moved to Durango, Colorado, and is currently under the leadership of Shelley Silbert. The organization proclaims 40 chapters—called Broadbands, in 16 states, with about 8,000 members. For more information, contact https://www.greatoldbroads.org/find-a-broadband/.

An online group of older adults who aspire to create a green legacy is called *Gray Is Green* (https://grayisgreen.org). The group produces periodic newsletters, includes a speaker's bureau, engages in advocacy, provides fact sheets, and serves as a central clearinghouse for ideas and communication among older adults passionate about the environment.

Retirees in Service to the Environment (RISE) is an environmental education and leadership training program for adults over age 60. This program was created at Cornell University's College of Human Ecology; citra-rise.human.cornell.edu.

Granny Peace Brigade and the Raging Grannies

In an article from *The New York Times* (Hartocollis, 2006, p. A21), there was a summary of a trial of 18 women between the ages of 59 and 91. Some of the women used canes, one was legally blind, and one used a walker. They called themselves the *Granny Peace Brigade*, and they had been arrested for blocking the entrance to a military recruitment center in New York City's Times Square when they *tried to enlist*. They claimed they wanted to join the armed forces and spare the lives of younger soldiers in Iraq.

The judge, sensing a public relations disaster, found grounds to claim that the frail older women had been wrongly arrested, and that they had left room for people to enter the recruitment center. When the trial was over, the Granny Peace Brigade sang the song "God Help America," composed by a member of a sister group called the *Raging Grannies* in Tucson, Arizona—a group that has inspired several videos and films.

On a related note, when Occupy Wall Street was active in the fall of 2011, Frances Goldin decided to join in, holding a sign that stated: *"I'm 87 and mad as hell."* She also decided to get arrested because she was fed up with the growing gap between rich and poor, and wanted to call attention to the issue. The police refused to cooperate.

Seems to me older adults can play a unique role on the front lines of protest movements.

QUESTION: If you were to start up an advocacy group in retirement, what would you focus on and how would you go about it? What would be the advantages and disadvantages of recruiting older adults into this advocacy group?

Long-Term Care Ombudsman Program

Long-term care (LTC) ombudsmen can be paid or volunteer advocates for residents of nursing homes, board and care homes, assisted living facilities, and similar adult care facilities. In 2022, state LTC ombudsman programs were responsible for the care of 3 million residents in approximately 76,000 LTC facilities (U.S. Government Accountability Office, 2024). Begun in 1972 as a demonstration program and continued under the federal OAA, every state is required to have an ombudsman program that addresses resident complaints and advocates for improvements in the LTC system. Ombudsmen are often the only recourse for LTC residents who face improper treatment. The most frequent complaints in board and care, assisted living, and other residential care communities include discharge or eviction, medications, food services, physical abuse, and staffing. The most frequent nursing facility complaints include discharge or eviction, response to requests for assistance, physical abuse, unattended symptoms, and medications (Administration on Community Living, 2024).

BenefitsCheckUp

BenefitsCheckUp was launched nationally in June 2001 by the NCOA. It is the first national website for older adults and service providers to identify federal and state program benefits available to older adults. The site includes information on more than 2,500 public benefit programs and has 40,000 local entry contacts. Seniors may be eligible for Supplemental Security Income, food stamps, utility bills assistance, home weatherization, vocational rehabilitation, in-home services, caregiving support services, legal services, nutrition programs, training and education opportunities, and so forth.

In 2003, BenefitsCheckUpRx was launched, a national website to allow older adults to determine which of 250+ programs can help them save money on their prescriptions. Since 2001, 9.9 million people have used BenefitsCheckUp (https://benefitscheckup.org/page/about-us). Users receive a printed report that tells them which programs they may likely qualify for and where to enroll. What may have taken the older consumer days or weeks to ascertain, BenefitsCheckUp can do in minutes. In 2015, the organization reported having helped more than 4 million people find over $15 billion worth of benefits. To access this service, go to the website www.benefitscheckup.org.

Red Hat Society

The ***Red Hat Society*** is an advocacy group, but it is like no other (https://redhatsociety.com/). This group advocates for fun and a sense of humor. In 1997, Sue Ellen Cooper gave a friend a crimson fedora and a copy of Jenny Joseph's poem "Warning," which encourages old women to wear purple with a red hat that doesn't match. In some mysterious way, this led to a loose-knit social movement of 41,000 Red Hat chapters in more than 30 countries, with 1.5 million members. The chapters are for women age 50 and over who are willing to organize social functions and attend them in a red hat and a purple outfit. Many local chapters have adopted memorable names, like "Red Hot Mamas" and "RedNReady." The primary rule for each chapter is that the women who organize social events must attend them dressed in "full regalia."

SUMMARY

AAAs cover the entire U.S. population and are designed to be the focal point for identifying aging services, resources, and activities in one's local community. Although they may be a good starting point for identifying what is going on in one's community, no single agency or organization can address all the needs of older people or administer the full spectrum of aging services. This chapter covered more than 45 age-related resources, many of which already exist in an older adult's community (though much less so in most rural communities), and only scratches the surface of the aging services network.

What to do about this challenge of locating aging resources? Plenty of legwork will be required. Certainly you'll want to visit your local senior center(s); the religious institutions engaged in community outreach; universities and community colleges especially if they house a gerontology program; professional medical associations that focus on age-related diseases; hospitals that host age-related support groups and educational activities; the local AARP office—for starters.

The good news is that even if you never uncover all the aging services and resources available in your community, you will discover exciting and useful activities you did not know existed and meet compassionate staff persons who gravitate toward older adults out of respect and love. Many of these staff persons and volunteers are older adults themselves. And as far as older adults who seek services from these organizations or attend activities, you will meet engaged and enthusiastic people who defy old-age stereotypes.

It is a good time to be old, or to look forward to being old.

SPRINGER PUBLISHING CONNECT™ **A robust set of instructor resources designed to supplement this text is located at http://connect.springerpub.com/content/book/978-0-8261-8386-6. Qualifying instructors may request access by emailing textbook@springerpub.com.**

REFERENCES

Only key references appear in the print edition. The full reference list can be accessed by visiting www.springerpub.com/courseconnect. See inside front cover and tear-out card for CourseConnect details.

Encore.org. (2014). *Encore careers: The persistence of purpose.* https://cogenerate.org/wp-content/uploads/2022/10/2014EncoreResearchOverview.pdf

Gruenewald, T. L., Tanner, E. K., Fried, L. P., Carlson, M. C., Xue, Q. L., Parisi, J. M., Rebok, G. W., Yarnell, L. M., & Seeman, T. E. (2016). The Baltimore Experience Corps Trial: Enhancing generativity via intergenerational activity engagement in later life. *The Journals of Gerontology. Series B, Psychological Sciences and Social Sciences, 71,* 661–670. https://doi.org/10.1093/geronb/gbv005

Kim, E. S., Whillans, A. V., Lee, M. T., Chen, Y., & VanderWeele, T. J. (2021). Volunteering and subsequent health and well-being in older adults: An outcome-wide longitudinal approach. *American Journal of Preventive Medicine, 59,* 176–186. https://doi.org/10.1016/j.amepre.2020.03.004

Lorig, K., Holman, H. R., Sobel, D., Laurent, D., González, V., & Minor, M. (2020). *Living a healthy life with chronic conditions* (5th ed.). Bull.

Morrow-Howell, N., Hong, S. I., & Tang, F. (2009). Who benefits from volunteering? *The Gerontologist, 49,* 91–102. https://doi.org/10.1093/geront/gnp007

Ory, M. G., Ahn, S., Jiang, L., Lorig, K., Ritter, P., Laurent, D. D., Whitelaw, N., & Smith, M. L. (2013). National study of chronic disease self-management: Six-month outcome findings. *Journal of Aging and Health, 25,* 1258–1274. https://doi.org/10.1177/0898264313502531

Tan, E. J., Georges, A., Gabbard, S. M., Pratt, D. J., Nerino, A., Roberts, A. S., Wrightsman, S. M., & Hyde, M. (2016). The 2013–2014 Senior Corps study: Foster grandparents and senior companions. *Public Policy & Aging Report, 26*(3), 88–95. https://doi.org/10.1093/ppar/prw016

Varma, V. R., Tan, E. J., Gross, A. L., Harris, G., Romani, W., Fried, L. P., Rebok, G. W., & Carlson, M. C. (2016). Effect of community volunteering on physical activity: A randomized controlled trial. *American Journal of Preventive Medicine, 50,* 106–110. https://doi.org/10.1016/j.amepre.2015.06.015

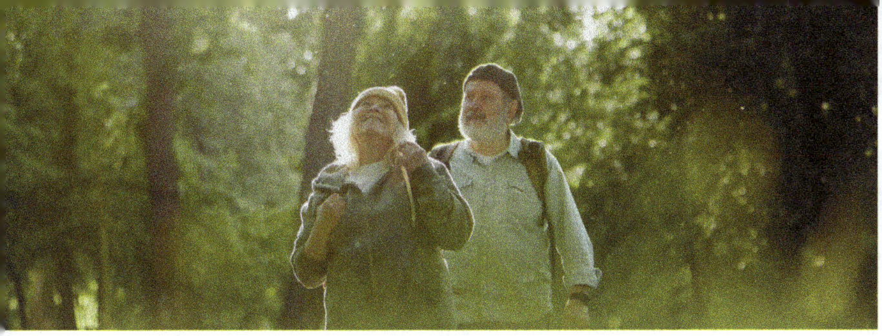

10

LONG-TERM CARE AND END-OF-LIFE CARE

KEY TERMS

activities of daily living (ADLs) and instrumental activities of daily living (IADLs)
adult foster homes (AFHs)
advance directive: living will, durable power of attorney for healthcare, and POLST
Amazing Village
assisted living facilities
Buchwald phenomenon
certified-aging-in-place (CAP) program
continuing care retirement communities
death doulas
Death with Dignity Act
Eden Alternative
elder cohousing
euthanasia
foreign-based home care
granny flats
green burials
Green Houses
guided care
hospice
informal versus formal caregiving
long-term care
long-term care alternatives
long-term care insurance: private versus public
memory care facilities
naturally occurring retirement communities (NORCs)
niche retirement communities
nursing homes and culture change
palliative care
Programs of All-Inclusive Care for the Elderly (PACE)
respite care
shared housing for older adults
smart homes and telehealth
virtual villages
voluntarily stopping eating and drinking

LEARNING OBJECTIVES

- Define *long-term care (LTC).*
- Distinguish between informal and formal caregiving.
- Distinguish between *activities of daily livings (ADLs)* and *instrumental activities of daily living (IADLs).*
- Examine the burdens and rewards of caregiving.
- Compare traditional nursing home care with culture change in LTC.
- Examine the variety of LTC alternatives.
- Describe *Green Houses* and analyze their potential for future success.
- Review home modifications and home care alternatives.
- Analyze LTC insurance, public and private.
- Describe the options for caring for people with dementia.
- Examine advance directive options.
- Describe the growth of the *hospice* movement and discuss the barriers and opportunities for further growth.
- Define and compare *palliative care* and hospice care.
- Examine alternative explanations for the *Buchwald phenomenon* and their impact on hospice use.
- Describe the *Death with Dignity Act* and offer your opinion of it.
- Analyze the ethics and legality of *voluntarily stopping eating and drinking.*
- Define *euthanasia.*
- Describe the role of the *death doula.*
- Describe and offer your opinion on *green burials* and cemeteries.

Most older Americans express a clear preference for spending their last years at home, surrounded by the people they love.

—*William Thomas*

LONG-TERM CARE

Long-term care **(LTC)** is part of the final chapter in most older people's lives. It refers to personal care and assistance with household tasks on an ongoing basis owing to disability or illness that limits the ability of the person to function independently. About half of Americans who turn 65 will need LTC, with one in seven requiring care for more than 5 years. A 2015 projection suggests that one in six will spend at least $100,000 for LTC (Office of the Assistant Secretary for Planning and Evaluation, 2015).

Perhaps the ideal goal for quality LTC in this country was articulated best by William Thomas, the founder of the Eden Alternative and the Green House (to be reviewed later). He stated that we should seek home- or community-based LTC developed on a cornerstone of love (Thomas, 1996).

Skilled Nursing Facilities

The reality of LTC today, however, is not based on love, but on institutional care based on control over resident routines and endless safety regulations. As noted by R. A. Kane (2001) about two decades ago, but still applicable today, the "bulk of LTC public dollars go where older people do not want to go." LTC supports (including skilled nursing facilities) account for approximately 1.3% of the gross domestic product, and government programs (primarily Medicaid) cover about 75% of the total (Centers for Medicare & Medicaid Services [CMS], 2021).

Since Kane made these comments, there has been a steady decline in the percentage of residents receiving nursing home care, but not necessarily toward noninstitutional care and certainly not to care based on love in the home and community.

Some argue that the for-profit philosophy and practice in LTC has not been ideal. Of the 15,300 skilled nursing facilities in the United States, with some 1.6 million licensed beds, about 70% are owned by for-profit operators (National Center for Health Statistics [NCHS], 2020a). For-profit homes tend to be less focused on quality of care than non-profit homes and more concerned about keeping costs down and profits up (Harrington et al., 2012; Ronald et al., 2016), though nonprofits have also been faulted (Chidambaram et al., 2024). In 2020, 1.3 million Americans lived in skilled nursing facilities; 82% were people aged 65+ (National Center for Health Statistics, 2020b).

Regarding profits, one study reported that for-profit nursing homes appear to be incentivized to maximize the profits associated with therapeutic services, even among the sickest of their residents. Moreover, the sickest residents receive such services as late as the last week of their lives and sometimes even on the day of their death (Temkin-Greener et al., 2019).

Conversely, one study reported that nonprofit nursing homes deliver higher quality care than for-profit nursing homes, and if all nursing homes in the United States were converted to nonprofit homes, residents would receive 500,000 more hours annually of nursing care (Comondore et al., 2009). For-profit institutions are less likely to meet mandated staff requirements (Blanco et al., 2024).

Staff–resident ratios are not all that is wrong with nursing homes. The for-profit philosophy leads one to cut costs where possible. One egregious example of where this can lead—by no means typical but nonetheless instructive—occurred in the Evergreen Gridley Health Care Center in Northern California. This institution spent $1.91 per day to feed residents (extraordinarily cheap even by 2002 standards), which was about $1 a day less than California spent on food for inmates in state medical prisons at that time. This was also about $2 a day less than the U.S. Department of Agriculture cited as the minimum necessary for a nutritious diet for older adults (Schmitt, 2002).

Treatment of dementia in nursing homes is also not ideal. According to Dr. Patrick Conway, chief medical officer for the CMS, almost 40% of nursing home residents with signs of dementia were receiving antipsychotic drugs at some point in 2010, even though there was no diagnosis of psychosis. The inappropriate use of this medication was primarily for the purpose of calming agitated behavior, but as a consequence it also increased the risk of significant mental and physical health problems as well as death. Overuse of antipsychotic medications for managing dementia behaviors is still a concern, despite its status as a quality benchmark in Nursing Home Compare, the rating system used by the CMS to determine eligibility for reimbursement (https://www.medicare.gov/care-compare). Only 13% of skilled nursing homes have dedicated memory care units (NCHS, 2020b).

Nursing home quality is assessed through a number of metrics, including the star rating system of Nursing Home Compare and newer value-based payment programs. These are still evolving. The star rating system is based on inspections, staffing, and quality measures, which, for long-term stay residents, include the proportion of residents whose mobility has declined; whose need for help in personal care has increased; who have pressure ulcers, in-dwelling catheters, incontinence, or injurious falls; who are receiving antipsychotic medicine; and as well the number of hospitalizations and emergency department visits per 1,000 resident days (CMS, 2025).

Nursing Home Compare is a tool for consumer appraisal of quality and is designed to help families find skilled nursing facilities nearby. But the best way to determine nursing home quality is to personally visit and engage a sharp eye, not to mention nose and ear, toward the environment. Short of that, two sites can help with the selection process. In addition to *Nursing Home Compare* (https://www.medicare.gov/care-compare), there is also ProPublica's *Nursing Home Inspect* (https://projects.propublica.org/nursing-homes/), which allows consumers to examine inspection reports and citations.

There are many good nursing homes in the United States, staffed by dedicated and competent people who alleviate the institutional and bureaucratic feel of these facilities. Yet remaining in one's own home is the ideal way to get LTC, according to most surveys of Americans. The problem is that adequate in-home assistance is hard to obtain and even harder to afford. We will, therefore, summarize a variety of LTC options, most of which are innovative, attractive, and promising, though some represent only slight improvement over the traditional nursing home. In some cases, however, such as a need for 24-hour care or lack of alternatives or designation in hospital discharge as "unsafe to go home," skilled nursing facilities may be the only choice.

INFORMAL CAREGIVING

There are only four kinds of people in the world—those who have been caregivers, those who currently are caregivers, those who will be caregivers, and those who will need caregivers.

—*Rosalynn Carter, former First Lady of the United States*

We could add that people will likely occupy more than one of these roles in their lifetime. Informal caregivers are family and friends who support their loved ones facing chronic illness or disability. They, not paid caregivers, are the primary source of help to the frail elderly. The Family Caregiver Alliance reported that if informal caregivers had to be replaced by paid services, it would more than triple the amount we spend on home healthcare and nursing home care combined. AARP estimated that family caregivers provided 36 billion hours of unpaid care worth $600 billion in 2021. Caregivers, or more properly speaking, "care partners," also pay more than $7,200 annually in out-of-pocket costs for caregiving supports (AARP Public Policy Institute, 2023).

Ascertaining precisely how many informal caregivers there are in America is a daunting proposition. On the one hand, the U.S. Bureau of Labor Statistics (BLS, 2023) will include a grandchild as a caregiver if they made as few as two 20-minute visits to a grandparent over the past 3 months. On the other hand, many caregivers provide substantial help with household chores, like laundry, preparing meals, and shopping for groceries, but do not view themselves as caregivers and are undetected.

Given these limitations, the best estimate is that approximately 40 million Americans over the age of 15 provide unpaid care to someone over age 65 because of a condition related to aging. According to the BLS, male and female care partners contribute about equal amounts of caregiving support, but longitudinal studies suggest a female preponderance of care labor.

Care recipients need assistance with daily functioning. The most commonly used measure for the functional assistance needed by care recipients is termed ***activities of daily living (ADLs)***. This measure summarizes a person's ability to perform basic personal care tasks such as eating, bathing, dressing, toileting, getting in or out of a bed or chair, and indoor mobility (the latter being the most common ADL limitation for older adults).

Instrumental activities of daily living (IADLs) summarize a person's ability to perform more complex, multidimensional activities in the environment, such as home management, money management, meal preparation, getting to places outside the home, making a phone call, laundry, and light grocery shopping (the latter being the most common IADL problem). These limitations typically precede limitations associated with ADLs. On average, caregivers help with 1.7 of the 6 ADLs, and 4.4 of 7 IADLs (AARP & the National Alliance for Caregiving, 2020).

Care recipients at home vary widely in the amount of assistance they need, from help with one or two IADLs to four or more ADLs. This need for assistance is lower than what we see in skilled nursing residents, who require assistance in almost all ADLs. (Indeed, need for at least partial assistance with one or more ADLs nearly all the time is a criterion for "nursing facility clinically eligible," which state Medicaid offices use to determine eligibility for personal assistance care in homes.) The greater the ADL need, the greater the caregiver strain, so most informal caregivers experience some amount of stress. ***Informal caregiving*** for an older adult often has a negative impact on health, personal freedom, employment, privacy, finances, and social relationships for the caregiver (Bom et al., 2019; Hooyman & Kiyak, 2011).

Yet even the onerous task of unpaid caregiving has its intimate and positive qualities. Two separate studies of older caregivers reported about 70% had positive feelings toward at least one aspect of caregiving for an older adult (Cohen et al., 2002; Wolff et al., 2007). Some of the positive aspects included companionship, fulfillment, enjoyment, and the personal satisfaction of meeting an obligation.

One group of researchers went so far as to report that under some circumstances, caregiving behaviors are associated with *decreased* mortality risk among those caregivers (Brown et al., 2009). The lead researcher, Stephanie Brown, speculated that helping a person you love may relieve some of the harmful stress effects of seeing that person suffer. Other research supports this benefit (Leggett et al., 2020; O'Reilly et al., 2015), but any mortality benefit likely reflects the greater physical vitality of people able to take on caregiving responsibilities rather than a benefit of caregiving itself. On the whole, negative effects outweigh positive gains, a robust finding from 30 years of caregiving research (Schulz et al., 2020).

There is a national trend toward increasing the amount of LTC provided in the home, rather than in the nursing home. At the state level, this has been manifested in *Medicaid-managed LTC* programs that shift the care of frail elders from nursing homes to homes. In addition, Congress allocated $4 billion in funds ($3 billion from the Affordable Care Act [ACA]) through a program called *Money Follows the Person*, which gives states Medicaid dollars to help this transition.

Also at the federal level, Medicare regulations in 2010 mandated that every nursing home resident is asked quarterly: "Do you want to talk to someone about the possibility of returning to the community?" If the resident responds yes at any time, contact with an outside agency is mandated, along with a discussion of how this might be put into operation. Obviously, the transition out of a nursing home is not always possible.

Yet some progress has been made. At the turn of this century, 73% of Medicaid dollars went to institutional care versus home or community services. By 2010, that percentage declined to 55%. In 2022, the majority of U.S. spending on long-term services and supports (LTSS) went to home and community-based services (HCBS). Spending on HCBS was $284 billion and the remaining $131 billion was spent on institutional LTSS, such as nursing facility care (Chidambaram, & Burns, 2024). This represents success in rebalancing the LTSS portfolio.

Some of the decline in nursing home occupancy has been due to the expansion of ***assisted living facilities*** (ALFs). Although the cost is lower and the regulations less burdensome, these facilities are still institutions. However, many cover the full spectrum of housing options for people in need of support or who anticipate such need. Such campuses include independent apartments, ALFs, and skilled nursing facilities. This should be contrasted with Section 8 Senior housing, subsidized apartments that provide little or no services.

For those who want information on informal caregiving, there is a website created by *AARP's Caregiver Resource Center* and can be accessed through www.aarp.org/home-family/caregiving. Other resources are www.eldercare.gov, and www.caregiver.org.

Informal Caregiving for Dementia

Owing to the protracted and difficult period of decline with Alzheimer disease and related dementias, older adults are at greater risk for abuse by caregivers, and caregivers in turn are at greater risk for depression and anxiety as well as injury. Despite the greater risk, about 75% of cognitively impaired older adults are cared for in a home setting, with limited outside support. AARP estimates that approximately 11 million family members and other unpaid caregivers provided an estimated 18.4 billion hours of care to people with Alzheimer or other dementias in 2023 (Alzheimer's Disease Facts and Figures, 2024). The number of men caring for loved ones with Alzheimer or dementia has increased, changing the tone of local support group meetings.

Caregivers for persons with dementia can benefit from cognitive behavioral therapies (CBTs), which help caregivers identify, plan, and increase positive activities for the patient, and can improve the mood and reduce depressive symptoms of Alzheimer caregivers as well as care recipients. These therapies are incorporated into a variety of venues, including caregiver education and social support, and can lead to reduced caregiver burden, depression, and dysphoria (Lee et al., 2007; Mittelman et al., 2004). This support option can be effectively provided over the internet as well (Marziali & Garcia, 2011). Caregiver support, in turn, can lead to the delay of institutionalization of older persons by almost a year (Andren & Elmstahl, 2008).

FORMAL CAREGIVING

Although older people overwhelmingly want to remain in their homes, the availability of family members continues to decline because of smaller family size, greater mobility among adult children, a higher percentage of single-parent families among adult children, and rising employment rates among women.

Formal caregiving refers to paid caregiving in the home or in the institutional setting. In the *home setting*, competent care workers are not easy to find or retain. Part of the problem was that in 1974, Congress decided to exempt paid domestic workers who provided services in the home from wage and overtime protections. The intent of the law was to exempt the babysitter or neighbor who provided the occasional support, but the law also included professional home care aides. This *companionship exemption* was finally reversed more than 40 years later. In 2015 the

U.S. Department of Labor applied federal overtime and minimum wage laws affecting nearly 2 million home care workers provided they worked 20% or more of their time in care services.

Home healthcare workers earn about $19/hour, and aides providing personal assistance earn only $14/hour in American cities (estimates from Chicago, 2024), leading many to work multiple shifts and rely on public benefits like Medicaid and food stamps. Nationally, 3.7 million home health aides or personal assistants earn an average of $16/hour (BLS, 2024a). About a quarter of home care workers live below the federal poverty line; more than half rely on public assistance (American Public Health Association [APHA], 2020). The projection by the BLS that by 2030 about 13 million older adults will need daily assistance to live outside a nursing home was woefully undermatched by the projected number of formal caregivers available to them. A conservative estimate suggests a need for 1.3 million additional home healthcare workers (U.S. Administration on Community Living, 2024).

Lifting the companionship benefit to increase wages and benefits and providing a time-and-a-half premium when working more than 40 hours a week, can make a small dent in reducing the shortage of workers and unmet demand. But it will not be enough. Paid caregivers in the home need considerably more compensation to make a decent living. Not surprisingly, paid homecare workers include groups traditionally underpaid: women (87%) and immigrants (42% of home health aides and 27% of personal care aides; BLS, 2024b).

Another problem with formal caregiving is the lack of background checks at many healthcare agencies (Lindquist et al., 2012) that family members and older adults rely on. A survey of 180 agencies in seven states revealed that some of the agencies even resorted to recruiting random strangers from Craigslist.

Overall, only 55% of the agencies did a federal background check on their employees, only 33% did a drug test (particularly problematic given that many older adults have pain medication, including narcotics, in the home), and only 33% administered a test for caregiver skill competency, including cardiopulmonary resuscitation (CPR) certification, lifting and transfer skills, behavioral management, cognitive support, or help with ADLs. Only 30% of agencies sent supervisors to a home to check on caregivers, with some not checking with the care recipient at all, and most relying on asking the caregiver over the telephone about how things are going. The National Background Check Program, established by the ACA, developed a nationwide system for conducting comprehensive background checks (CMS, 2024).

What about converting informal family caregivers into formal paid caregivers? One study reported that when states allowed spouses to become paid personal care providers, there were fewer nursing home admissions compared with the use of nonfamily paid caregivers (Newcomer et al., 2012). The fear, of course, is that paying for unpaid family care would increase public costs. If it resulted in fewer nursing home admissions, though, this could be a cost-effective alternative for the state.

In the *institutional setting*, formal caregiving relies primarily on certified nursing assistants (CNAs) who are underpaid (average hourly wage $18 in 2024), overworked, undertrained, insufficiently respected, and typically without opportunity for career advancement in their facility. Not surprisingly, turnover rate is estimated at greater than 100% annually, meaning that people start and stop more than one position each year (Gandhi et al., 2021).

Moreover, most nursing homes are not only understaffed but they have had even fewer caregiving staff than they had reported to the government for years. Thanks to the ACA, daily nursing home payroll records were required to be collected and made public. Kaiser Health News conducted a survey in 2018 and found that 70% of the 14,000 nursing homes included in the survey (of 15,600 overall) had lower staffing ratios than they had previously reported (Rau, 2018).

One advantage that nursing homes have over less regulated ALFs (to be described more fully later), despite the greater popularity of the latter, is the required CNA certification of nursing home staff. The federal government sets a minimum level of training for CNAs and requires a state agency to certify them. Moreover, the federal government requires that CNAs be backed up by 24-hour nursing supervision. ALFs, in contrast, do not have to (and rarely do) hire CNAs, and do not have 24/7 nursing supervision on the premises.

One improvement of formal caregiving in the nursing home would be for CNAs and their supervising nurses to consistently work with residents in the same unit, with no rotation. Consistent or permanent assignment to units (or neighborhoods) is correlated with a higher quality of life for nursing home residents (Jurkowski, 2013). This consistency leads to a clearer understanding of resident preferences and habits, fewer behavioral difficulties among residents, and greater compassion for residents among staff members. However, greater flexibility in assignments may also offer advantages to CNAs and residents (Roberts et al., 2015).

NURSING HOMES AND CULTURE CHANGE

Nursing homes are institutions licensed by the state to offer room, board, 24-hour nursing care, and therapy in a medical setting. Because of detailed federal regulations covering every aspect of nursing home care and the requirement to care for residents who are too frail for any alternatives to nursing home care, they are expensive, averaging about $82,000 per resident per year nationwide (and $92,000 for a private room; U.S. Administration on Community Living, 2020).

Thus, despite the growth of the frail older adult population in America, the number of residents in nursing homes—about 1.4 million (or 3% of the older adult population)—is stagnant despite the increasing number of older adults in the United States. Occupancy rate has declined, from 87% in 2011 to 82% in 2018 to 77% in 2024 (Kaiser Family Foundation, 2024), along with state Medicaid dollars that have shifted from nursing homes to ALFs. Thus, less expensive and less regulated options like ALFs are growing.

Even though the industry has made a concerted effort to change the term nursing "home" to nursing "facility," the nursing home term still prevails. Yet no one thinks a nursing home is a home. The needs of a large number of residents must be met, and this is done as most institutions must do it, through numerous bureaucratic rules and regulations.

Large-scale food service, for instance, is not organized to meet individual preferences for food or how it is prepared, much less when and where residents might want to eat it. There are also rules for bathing, waking, sleeping, and even the choice, or lack of, for a roommate. There are long corridors, medication carts, nursing stations, and large dining rooms in nursing homes. Incorporating resident preferences into daily care is a major challenge but also an important initiative in skilled nursing facilities.

Staff is not family; instead, they are underpaid and underappreciated workers. They take care of bodily and basic medical needs, and they tend to do it short-staffed in most nursing homes. Activities are scheduled and initiated by staff and traditional in content. Many residents have few or no visitors from outside. What about this description reminds you of *home*?

While institutions are not homes, nursing facilities do have a mechanism for reconciling complaints among residents, their families, and staff. The Older Americans Act mandates that every state have a *long-term care ombudsman program* to help families and older adults navigate the bureaucracy of LTC, mediate conflicts, and advocate for residents and family members fighting for better care.

The ombudsman program is universally recognized as an important monitor of nursing home life, but there are problems with the program. The recommended caseload by the federal government, for instance, is that each ombudsman is responsible for 2,000 nursing home residents. The national average per ombudsman, however, is more than 2,500 residents. There is also a recommendation that each nursing home be visited four times a year, but this too is generally not met.

Ombudsman positions are funded jointly by the state and federal governments and each program develops a system for recruiting volunteers to help compensate for the shortfall in funding to meet the recommended standards for oversight. In 2010, there were 1,167 full-time equivalent paid staff nationwide in ombudsman offices, and 8,813 trained volunteers, or eight times the number of volunteers versus paid staff. Yet substantially more trained volunteers are needed in most, if not all, states. The federal Administration on Community Living monitors ombudsman activity at a national level and county area agencies on aging at a local level.

More important than resolving complaints, though, is improving the general culture of the nursing home, to approach what Dr. William Thomas calls "long-term care based on a cornerstone of love." ***Culture change***, or *person-centered care*, in LTC is focused on choice, self-determination, dignity, respect, purposeful living, and community. Even attempts to ensure that residents are not involved in activity, a quality assurance issue, can result in a violation of personal preferences, in this case the wish not to participate (Stone et al., 2009). Even well intentioned regulations do not always encourage a feeling of shared humanity, community, and love.

Nonetheless, as far back as 2007, the Commonwealth Fund's National Survey of Nursing Homes reported that almost one third of nursing homes engaged in some type of culture change to approach these goals. Currently, more than 80% are engaged in culture change (Miller et. al., 2018). A complete effort at culture change would include:

- action to create a more homelike environment;
- individual rooms or resident choice to have a roommate;
- a more personalized dining experience;
- implementation of resident choices, when possible, in all other aspects of living;
- empowerment and recognition of staff;
- efforts to build personal relationships among residents, among staff, and between residents and staff; and
- ongoing assessments and improvement of overall quality of life for residents and staff.

The *Pioneer Network* (www.pioneernetwork.net, www.residentcenteredcare.org, and www.planetree.org) began in 1997 to advocate for more *person-directed care*; that is, LTC models that emphasize flexibility, self-determination, and community. The network sponsors workshops and conferences to promote caring and loving communities, regardless of the type of long-term housing in which it is located.

There are specific state government initiatives that could foster culture change or improve quality of life in nursing homes. These initiatives cost money when funding for LTC is in short supply. Nonetheless, here are a few such ideas:

- Mandate increased wages and benefits and better training for nursing home aides to improve quality of care and reduce exceptionally high turnover rates.
- Provide financial awards to exemplary LTC settings.

- Give stiff fines to owners of LTC settings that consistently perform poorly.
- Respect residents' preferences when it comes to eating, bathing, waking, and going to bed.
- Eliminate forced roommates.
- Establish state LTC clearinghouses for information and support.

In the absence of culture change, traditional nursing home residents are viewed as sick and dependent, which fosters learned helplessness and induced disability. For example, wheelchair dependency may be encouraged to serve the needs of staff members, who must transport residents down long hallways and are pressed for time. Dressing, feeding, bathing, and toileting are routinized and sped up for aides needing to stay on schedule. A staff member is more likely to rely on incontinence briefs than to take the time to develop individualized toileting routines.

Most Americans state that the idea of being placed in a nursing home is unacceptable. This discontent has triggered a nationwide movement toward LTC alternatives (Rahman & Schnelle, 2008).

LONG-TERM CARE ALTERNATIVES

By 2026, when the leading edge of boomers will turn 80, there will likely be a rapid growth in ***long-term care alternatives***. This innovation will be inspired by the educational attainment of boomers and their formal and informal caregivers, a history of activism (e.g., Vietnam War protests and civil rights), and a desire for supportive housing that is not institutionalized, bureaucratized, or medicalized in late life.

It seems likely that frail boomers later in life will want to be surrounded by caring people and with the opportunity for purposeful activities, regardless of their circumstances. Some of the LTC alternatives to meet these needs have yet to be created, but many are already in development. Several innovative LTC alternatives will be summarized next.

Assisted Living Facilities

I debated whether to even include ALFs in this section on LTC *alternatives*. First, there are now almost as many residents in ALFs as there are in nursing homes—making ALFs more mainstream than alternative. Second, the innovations created by its founder have been mostly co-opted into an institutional, profit-oriented venture. Nonetheless, it is instructive to examine the beginning of the ALF movement.

When Keren Brown Wilson built the first ALF in 1983 in a state (Oregon) that would soon be known for several LTC innovations, the goal was to replace the traditional nursing home with a home that would allow freedom and autonomy irrespective of the physical or mental impairment. The first ALF was built in Portland and called Park Place. Its 112 units filled up quickly.

Why? The rules were different. Care providers were entering a resident's apartment (which could be locked!) and catered to the wishes of the older adult: when they got up and went to bed, when and what they ate, when and how they bathed, and whether to keep a pet or drink alcohol. If the person was demented, then the family or designate helped negotiate the risks and choices that were acceptable.

While the nursing home industry was up in arms over these innovations, the popularity of Park Place was undeniable. Wilson expanded her company, Assisted Living Concepts, from the three facilities she founded, to providing development and management services to more than 200 ALFs in 18 states. By 2018, the number of people nationwide in ALFs almost equaled the number of residents in nursing homes.

But something affecting quality happened along the way. In 2000, Wilson stepped down as CEO and sold all of her shares of Assisted Living Concepts (Gawande, 2014). The ALF industry had changed in ways in which she did not approve. Instead of building small facilities in small towns, the profits were to be made in larger facilities in larger cities. And, equally discouragingly, many ALFs did not accept low-income elders.

The industry moved on without her. It is still the fastest growing alternative to a nursing home because there is no federal oversight with its daunting and costly regulations. ALF owners save money and aggravation, even in the 85% of states that require state oversight as well as the 60% that require licensing. The state regulations are much less onerous than the federal requirements for nursing homes.

The challenge for ALFs is that while they tend to be smaller institutions with fewer regulations than nursing homes, they are still institutional in appearance and bureaucratic in function. In many states, they are primarily private pay and not affordable for a great many people.

Also, as the average age of an ALF resident continues to rise, approaching that of nursing home residents, the policies for transferring residents to nursing homes when healthcare needs become overly burdensome for an ALF are typically unclear.

ALFs provide room, board, 24-hour supervision, housekeeping, meal preparation, and assistance with ADLs. But as noted earlier, they do not require a nurse on the premises 24 hours a day, do not require certified nursing aides, and do not have the expertise and resources to deal with the most medically challenging residents. The decision to relocate residents late in life, when they are most frail, can lead to confrontations among residents, family, and ALF administrators.

For more information about ALFs, contact the National Center for Assisted Living, www.ncal.org. In 2015, the Assisted Living Federation of America (www.alfa.org) became Argentum (Latin for silver; i.e., the silver generation). Perhaps this association for ALF operators decided that a euphemism might enhance its image.

Green Houses

For people who are frail, William Thomas, MD, has created the Green House (www.thegreenhouseproject.org), an innovative LTC home that avoids the problems of institutionalization and the restrictions of the medical model. Dr. Thomas's philosophy on older adults and how to care for them is summarized in his interesting book (2004), *What Are Old People For?*

Green Houses can be licensed as nursing homes, assisted facilities, or ***adult foster homes (AFHs)***, and can be a large home, part of an apartment building, or something else. They are homes and not just "homelike," no matter how they look on the outside or if they are licensed, and certainly are not facilities.

The first ones were constructed in Tupelo, Mississippi, in 2003 and were 6,400 square feet in area—obviously bigger than the average home, but otherwise a home in appearance. Each resident's room is individual, not shared, and is designed to look like a bedroom, with a hidden ceiling lift if needed, locked individual medicine cabinet to avoid the need for institutional medical carts circulating from room to room, and often a couch that can be a pull-out for a guest to stay over.

About 10 to 12 people live in a Green House, though this (and much of what follows) varies depending on the model adopted. Individual autonomy is emphasized, catering to a resident's desire for waking, eating, bathing, and sleeping. This applies to residents with dementia as well.

The care workers are the Green House *shabazzim* (singular, *shabazz*; Thomas's preferred term derived from the mythical Persian royal falcon that protected the king in ancient times, with the primary job responsibility to protect, nurture, and sustain people). They are paid more (about 40% more) than aides in traditional settings and are better trained (an additional 120 hours) than traditional nursing home staff.

These extra salary costs are offset by employee satisfaction, which reduces staff turnover and associated recurrent training expenses. The annual turnover rate was less than 10% in the first Green Houses in Tupelo. Every one of the early Green Houses was fully staffed during the first 3 years of its existence, with never a day understaffed. Moreover, not one staff person left during those first few years.

Shabazzim are trained in a variety of skills and are the managers of the Green House. They are at the top of the totem pole of responsibility, rather than at the bottom, as is typically the case in nursing homes. Shabazzim are trained in the culinary arts and safe food handling, purchasing food and managing a budget, providing CPR and first aid, communication and problem-solving, scheduling, housekeeping, and dementia care.

There is a *central hearth* where cooking and socializing are done. The shabazzim encourage shared meal preparation and eating. Residents have the option to eat in a group or alone, with a personal menu and pleasant surroundings—referred to as a *convivium*. A local cookbook is assembled to cater to the tastes of people born in a particular region. Shabazzim can eat with residents and participate in activities with them, along with family and friends.

There is a surrounding garden for contemplative walks and for growing vegetables and flowers. In each individual room, windows can be opened to view the garden outside or the door opened to view the hearth inside or closed for privacy. With the square or rectangular structure of the modest-sized building, both the garden and the central hearth are within 30 feet. Strategically placed furniture helps residents "cruise" to central areas and contributes to gains in resident mobility.

Green Houses promote autonomy. Residents get up, eat, and go to bed when they want. They may decide on which foods to eat, which can even include pizza, wine, or ice cream. Induction cooking in the kitchen prevents residents from burning themselves when they are helping the shabazzim cook. Stoves have shutoff valves, with pot trappers to prevent hot pots from burning residents. A safety gate around the kitchen can be used when necessary.

People in the first 10 Green Houses were selected from nursing homes in an attempt to represent a typical nursing home population. Of the first 40 residents selected, 12 had advanced dementia. Green House residents had an array of physical and cognitive limitations and medical challenges associated with the average nursing home resident.

The desired, or model, staff-to-resident ratio in a Green House is 1:5; the nurse-to-resident ratio is 1:20 (based on nearby residences); and one administrator (and one assistant) is available for every 12 houses or 1:120 people. Financial realities alter these ratios for most Green Houses.

Decision-making lies with shabazzim and residents, unless there are safety or budget issues that cannot be handled at that level. Shabazzim coordinate replacements for themselves if they are sick, either through a substitute pool or through other staff working overtime (which is managed within the allowable budget).

Studies reported that wheelchair use in Green Houses declined, and strength of residents increased. One 2-year longitudinal study compared Green House residents to residents at a traditional nursing home with the same owner (Kane et al., 2007). The Green House residents reported a higher quality of life, better emotional well-being, and a lower incidence of decline in late-loss ADLs. More research into Green Houses and culture change in LTC is needed (Rahman & Schnelle, 2008).

Thomas notes that "the conventional long-term care facility has struggled with, but never satisfactorily resolved, its split personality. As Mr. Hyde, it poses as a home. In its propaganda, the long-term care facility tells its staff members that 'this is the resident's home; we just work here.' Meanwhile, Dr. Jekyll maintains, with full professional authority, that the facility is actually a 'healthcare services workplace' (Shapiro, 2005). In the skilled nursing facility, routines are organized around the needs of the institution, not its residents.

The Robert Wood Johnson Foundation provided a $10 million grant (between 2006 and 2010) to establish Green Houses around the United States, and to allow other LTC owners and administrators to replicate them through training support and up to $125,000 in predevelopment loans. The latest count had the Green House concept spread to 260 homes operating in 32 states. To receive a free copy of the *Green House Project Guide Book* or the 8-hour orientation workshops, contact The Green House Project, 849 International Drive, Linthicum, MD 21090.

Virtual Villages

Naturally occurring retirement communities (NORCs) preceded ***virtual villages*** and were created by federal grants initiated by the United Jewish Communities in 1985. An initial $10 million grant by the Administration on Aging went toward 29 communities in neighborhoods that were primarily older adult (50% or more age 50 and older). The goal was to help older adults "age in place."

These federally supported NORCs inspired the idea of virtual villages a few years later. The villages, however, rely on individual and family fees and charitable foundations to support lower income residents rather than on federal grants. Virtual villages are nonprofit, dues-paying, membership communities to help older residents stay in their own homes for as long as possible. These communities are often not self-sufficient from dues and depend on local donors to subsidize the services they provide for low-income residents within their virtual village boundaries.

Services in virtual villages are prescreened, and hourly rates are low because of the expected volume of work offered to providers. The services typically include some combination of home maintenance, home repairs, yard work, home healthcare, check-in or companion services, transportation, social and educational programs, grocery shopping, quick-response medical support, and so forth. Sometimes these villages organize an exchange of donated volunteer hours among residents that can also be accumulated in volunteer credit hours that are formally recorded.

The virtual village idea began with the Beacon Hill Village in Boston in 2001. Several friends and neighbors developed a plan to help each other stay in their homes. They used a nonprofit organization to screen and organize programs and services to help accomplish the goal of aging in place. At Beacon Hill Village, residents are charged an annual membership fee of $600 for an individual and $850 for a couple, with discounts for those in financial need (Thomas & Blanchard, 2009).

Two decades later, the Beacon Hill Village model had spread to other parts of the country, with more than 300 at last count, but the number is rising rapidly. These supportive communities have the virtue of allowing older residents to remain in the same environs with long-standing neighbors and friends, as well as sustaining a more natural intergenerational neighborhood. Residents are less dependent on their grown children, who are often dispersed around the country and have their own families to support.

For more information, visit the original virtual village site at www.beaconhillvillage.org. Also, there is a *Village to Village Network* (www.vtvnetwork.org) that provides information on how to start a village and how to network with other villages, and information about workshops and a national conference.

Niche Retirement Communities

Niche retirement communities refer to specialized retirement housing organized around a hobby, culture, religion, or some other belief, activity, or interest that the older residents share in common.

For instance, there are *university-based retirement communities* (UBRCs) that offer retirees the opportunity to attend nearby campus activities, like athletic events, lectures by nationally recognized speakers, art exhibits, plays, and the like. Occasionally, the university resource can come to the retirement facility. At a retirement community named Kendal, near Oberlin College in Ohio, the school sends string quartets to perform at the retirement facility.

Typically, there is an opportunity for the older residents in a UBRC to sit in on certain classes at the university without being tested or graded. At Lasell Village on the campus of Lasell College in Newton, Massachusetts, the 210 older residents are required to participate in 450 hours of education a year (9 hours a week), and cultural and fitness activities count.

There are about 60 UBRCs, with more in the planning stage or in development. About half of the residents of the typical UBRC are alumni or former faculty and staff; the other half are interested in this type of living arrangement even without a former affiliation.

The UBRCs are a win–win–win situation. The older adults gain an educational and culturally enriched lifestyle, the college students gain an intergenerational component to their educational experience, and the university can receive assets from the estates of grateful older residents who appreciated their retirement years at a nearby retirement facility. The Osher program links older adults to colleges and universities, with college-level classes taught by faculty or retirees.

There are *artistically oriented* niche retirement communities. The Burbank Senior Artist Colony in Burbank, California, for instance, attracts persons interested in painting, writing, or other artistic endeavors in their retirement years. This 141-unit community has a 40-seat performance theater, artist studios, art display galleries, and classrooms.

For an interesting fictional version of this type of niche retirement community, see the 2013 movie *Quartet*, about retired musicians living in creative splendor and angst in a retirement home.

Hippie communes are not niche retirement communities, but if they last long enough, they become intergenerational communities. The Farm in Summertown, Tennessee (www.thefarmcommunity.com), has survived since 1971 by adapting to the needs of succeeding generations. Aging hippies needed to work and support children, so the residents created a midwifery school; raised, consumed, and sold organic vegetables and fruits; and engaged in environmental businesses. The older generation teaches the younger generation on this commune in a community-oriented school that caters to students as individuals with unique needs.

The Farm was founded by Stephen Gaskin, self-proclaimed Cultural Engineer, Shade Tree Mechanic, and Hippy Priest, who remained a leader in the community until he died in 2014 at age 79.

There is an *intergenerational retirement haven* called NewBridge on the Charles, in Dedham, Massachusetts. A K–8 Jewish day school is on the premises. Older adults help children with reading challenges, and some of the computer-oriented children teach the retirees their computer skills.

Astronomy lovers can select Chiefland Astronomy Village in Chiefland, Florida, where the skies are not affected by light pollution as much as other locations. Also, nearly every home has a built-in telescope.

Nalcrest, a *letter carriers' retirement community*, about 70 miles east of Tampa, prohibits dogs that bite, a former occupational hazard.

Fox Hills Club in Bethesda, Maryland, is a *wellness retirement community* that offers gyms, spas, health-conscious restaurants, an organic herb garden, outdoor walking trails, and onsite personal trainers and physical therapists.

The Ridge at Chukker Creek in Aiken, South Carolina, attracts *retired equestrians* with horse pastures, horseback trails, and community-shared barns to house the horses.

There are *retirement communities for lesbian, gay, bisexual, and transgender (LGBT) older adults* in California, Minneapolis, Chicago, Pennsylvania, New York, Florida, and elsewhere. The one in Philadelphia, the John C. Anderson apartments, is situated in the affectionately nicknamed Gayborhood.

Smart Homes and Telehealth

The preferred LTC alternative for most people is to stay in their homes with the assistance of people and technology. The key to both of these caregiving resources is availability and affordability. The availability and affordability of care workers in the home setting is a great challenge. Regarding technology, we are making rapid progress with availability and slower progress with affordability.

Smart homes are residences equipped with technology designed to enhance older residents' safety and independence, and to monitor their health status in their homes. If a person with dementia wanders from the home, a global positioning system (GPS) device placed on a shoe can detect their location. If a person falls, sensors in the floor alert emergency medical staff. If a person remains in bed and does not perform a daily activity like opening a refrigerator, someone is also electronically alerted.

Telehealth refers to transmitted health information from the home to a health specialist. For example, an older person's vital signs and urinalysis can be transmitted electronically from the person's home to a physician's office, ambulatory care setting, or other medical location. Proteus Digital Health manufactures a pill that passes through you and transmits medical data to a physician.

The future may be more amazing, as Google is working on a pill composed of nanoparticles that it hopes will one day detect malignant cells. It has also unveiled a smart contact lens for diabetics that is still in the experimental stage. It takes a glucose reading from the tears that wash over your eye when you blink and transmits the data to a nearby device. You can monitor glucose, blood pressure, and heart rate all through simple wearable devices.

The Oregon Center for Aging and Technology (OCAT) at Oregon Health & Science University tests technology in more than 350 homes, apartments, and retirement communities. The goal is to find out how to keep aging adults in their homes safely. Motion sensors are installed throughout a home to alert outsiders if help is needed. Opening a pillbox and taking the proper medication is also electronically transmitted.

With another experiment, OCAT raised other questions: Can Celia the Robot, who has a video screen for a head and can be operated remotely by a faraway family member, reduce the isolation and improve the mental health of the older adult? Or is it too intrusive? Or weird?

A Thai company called Dinsow 2 developed an impressive robot that acts as a personal healthcare assistant. It can serve medicine and food; pick up and carry items, avoiding obstacles in the way; and transmit blood pressure and heart rate to a physician's office. An older user can also say "Dinsow, come here," and then touch a menu on the robot's head in order to automatically call a family member, doctor, or another contact.

Paro, the robotic seal, has fur, big eyes, and responds to voice commands. This companion robot was developed at the Japanese National Institute of Advanced Industrial Science and Technology. AgeLab at the Massachusetts Institute of Technology (MIT) is testing it to see whether it can help calm older adults with dementia. Many simpler and less expensive robot companions are now available, including robot pets.

The Mayo Clinic Robert and Arlene Kogod Center on Aging sponsors a laboratory called HAIL (Healthy Aging and Independent Living). The researchers asked the following set of questions: Will older participants take their blood pressure, communicate through a tablet computer with video messaging to a health coach, and then follow suggestions on how to improve blood pressure? Would it be intrusive to wear a Band-Aid–sized cardiac sensor on the chest that transmits real-time information about heart health to a caregiving team?

As the evidence accumulates regarding the effectiveness of ***smart homes*** and ***telehealth***, the bottom line will be, well, the bottom line. Will these gerotechnologies save money? Will the cost of widespread implementation be offset by reduced institutionalization, hospitalization, emergency department visits, and other medical costs? In addition, ethical issues such as privacy and confidentiality must be addressed.

One final note. Consider the movie, *Robot & Frank*. The protagonist starts to have memory problems, and his children purchase a robot for him, similar to Dinsow 2. Frank, initially resistant to this robot companion, forms an unusual bond with him. He finds the robot useful for picking locks and casing a home to burgle. *Robot & Frank* won the Alfred P. Sloan Foundation prize at the 2012 Sundance Film Festival, an award for films that explore themes of science and technology.

The Eden Alternative

The basic premise of the ***Eden Alternative*** is that nursing homes should treat residents as people who need attentive care in a homelike setting. To accomplish this goal, nursing homes need to consider the involvement of pets, plants, children (Figure 10.1), and other amenities that make life worth living. Regarding dogs, cats, and other pets, they live permanently (rather than just visiting) with residents in LTC facilities through some Eden Alternative programs. This enhances bonding.

Plants are distributed throughout the home, with individual resident responsibility to care for them. Also, the Eden Alternative makes extra effort to recruit students from nearby schools and sponsor intergenerational activities.

The Eden Alternative was initiated by Dr. William Thomas in 1991 when he was medical director at a nursing home in New York. Since then, more than 300 nursing homes have been registered in this movement (in the United States, Canada, Europe, and Australia). Studies that support the benefits of the program—reductions in mortality, urinary tract infections, respiratory infections, staff turnover, resident depression, and medication costs—are reported in Thomas's book *The Eden Alternative* (1994).

An Eden Alternative Train-the-Trainer program was launched in 1996. The 3-day program demonstrates how to create a LTC environment that supports residents emotionally and spiritually as well as physically. To find out about the training, or the location of Eden Alternative sites in your state, go to www.edenalternative.com. Currently, approximately 350 sites have been certified in Eden principles.

QUESTION: What are three reasons that a nursing home administrator might offer resistance to the idea of converting the home into an Eden Alternative? How would you address these barriers and help change the mind of this administrator?

FIGURE 10.1 Visiting a resident in a nursing home (1984).

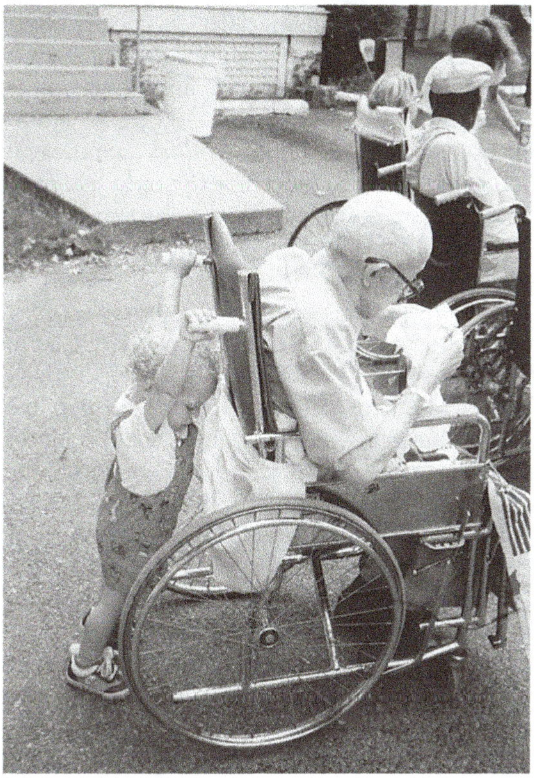

A radical remake of the nursing home industry along the lines of the Eden Alternative, however, has been slow and difficult. Over the past decades, only about 2% of U.S. nursing homes have adopted major components of the Eden Alternative. Even when they do, most institutions remain pretty much an institution, no matter how much you "Edenize" it.

Which is why William Thomas has mostly moved on from the Eden Alternative to create the Green House Project, previously described.

Elder Cohousing

If you are in your 50s or 60s, you may have had a conversation with friends centered around the following question: Wouldn't it be neat if several of us who share similar values could get together in retirement and live out our remaining days together in a supportive community? The details vary, of course. Some boomers discuss buying homes near each other. Others discuss building or taking over an apartment building, or acquiring a large home and dividing it up, and figuring out ways to live together and share expenses.

A housing concept, called *cohousing*, is based on adults figuring out how to live interdependently as housemates or neighbors. Cohousing refers to privately owned homes that are socially and architecturally innovative with resident input, in a caring, noninstitutional environment.

The concept was imported from Denmark in the early 1990s, and the number of cohousing communities in the United States has grown to more than 100. There are cohousing organizations (e.g., www.cohousingpartners.com) that provide ideas on shared visions and values; strategies for architectural innovation, such as designs to enhance the sense of community that allow both common areas and privacy; and approaches to shared management and decision-making.

The cohousing concept has been extended to ***elder cohousing*** (see www.seniorliving.org/cohousing), which is designed to help older people live more communally in late life, where common interests are emphasized (e.g., hiking, gardening), while other activities are no longer relevant (e.g., child care). Eligible residents are over a certain age, typically beginning at age 55 or older.

One example of a cohousing project began in 2002 and called itself the *Glacier Circle Community* (https://www.cohousing.org/directory/glacier-circle-community-association/). About two dozen people in their 70s and 80s, mostly friends from a Unitarian Universalist Church in Davis, California, hired lawyers and architects to help them create a small cooperative-style housing community of seniors. The members of the community participated in facilitation training at the local university in order to enhance their communication skills with each other in the planning of their vision.

They came up with a plan for eight townhomes, ranging in size from 1,000 to 1,400 square feet and designed for energy efficiency with skylights and sun tubes. There is a common garden that includes fruit trees, vegetables, and flowering plants, and a common house with an affordable second-floor apartment that is offered to an individual or couple in exchange for help with cooking and maintenance as the residents age in place. For additional information, contact Glacier Circle Senior Community, https://www.cohousing.org/directory/glacier-circle-community-association/.

Elderspirit is also one of the first senior cohousing communities, founded by former nuns who left their order over philosophical differences. They wanted to build their own community dedicated to personal growth, mutual support, and the deepening of spirit in later life. This model project has now grown to 29 homes of mixed-income housing for persons at least 55 years of age who share the values of spiritual growth and emotional support. The development is built along a scenic trail within easy walking distance of shops and downtown Abingdon, Virginia. For more information, contact Elderspirit, https://elderspirit.org/.

Programs of All-Inclusive Care

The ***Programs of All-Inclusive Care for the Elderly (PACE)*** started off as a demonstration project in the early 1970s in a small community in the Chinatown and North Beach neighborhoods of San Francisco, California. Developers of the program conceived of a model of care based on keeping an older adult at home with the aid of an adult day-care center and an interdisciplinary team consisting of physicians, nurse practitioners, nurses, social workers, physical and occupational therapists, dietitians, and recreational therapists, among others. This model was already popular in the United Kingdom.

The name of the original demonstration project in California was (and is) On Lok, Cantonese for "peaceful, happy abode." The PACE model quickly expanded in the 1970s and 1980s, reaching 180 programs in 33 states serving about 79,000 enrollees in 2024. In the past few decades, however, the growth has been replaced by stagnation. Some of the concerns are the financial risk to healthcare organizations and recruitment. Specifically, there is a reluctance among older adults to take on a new set of primary care providers to replace their existing ones, and to receive some of their services in the adult day-care center rather than at home (Casiano, 2015).

The adult day-care center is at the heart of the PACE program. It includes a healthcare clinic open during weekday business hours that provides occupational and physical therapy services beyond what traditional Medicare or Medicaid would provide, and various other healthcare providers and resources. The PACE participant is encouraged to attend at least monthly and, on average, attends 2.5 days a week, with some spending 5 days a week if they live with a family member who works.

The PACE program requires Medicare and Medicaid dual eligibility and integrates all existing public and private insurances and LTC funding sources. The program targets those who are eligible for nursing home care but still live in the community. By combining Medicare dollars, state Medicaid funds, foundation grants, and individual resources, a more comprehensive range of services can be provided. Services and resources are mostly targeted toward the home (e.g., grab bars and ramps) or provided at the adult day-care centers.

The upside to the PACE program is that more individualized care may be provided at lower cost (Wieland et al., 2000). Evaluations have shown that PACE can achieve a substantial reduction in the use of institutional care (Arku et al., 2022).

Outcome studies have reported that PACE improves functional status and overall health, and reduces resident death rate (Hansen, 2008). A chief concern is that some persons who are *not* eligible for nursing home care *are* deemed eligible for the PACE program and included in the evaluations that suggest, perhaps unrealistically, that cost savings in general are achieved.

In 2015, the PACE Innovation Act was signed into law to develop pilot projects to reach more populations and to experiment with older adults who do not yet meet the nursing home level of care standard. In addition, the PACE program reached out to private equity firms, including a for-profit business in Colorado that invested $196 million in a PACE program. Some argue that appealing to venture capital firms in Silicon Valley will revitalize the PACE programs and is the way to go in the future, while others are concerned that private mercenaries will skimp on services in order to maximize profits.

For more information about PACE, contact the National PACE Association, www.npaonline.org.

QUESTION: Why is LTC more of a health promotion issue than a medical care issue? If you believe otherwise, support your position.

ADDITIONAL LONG-TERM CARE ALTERNATIVES

Granny Flats

The name comes from sharing your home with granny via structural renovations that allow for privacy and nearby assistance when needed. ***Granny flats***, also known as accessory dwelling units, Elder Cottage Housing Opportunity (ECHO) housing, or mother-in-law suites, can be a modified interior part of a dwelling or add-on to the main dwelling. This allows an older adult to have a separate yet supportive unit to live in, and to be close to family members when support is needed. The main challenge to granny flats centers around zoning regulations that attempt to avoid excessive population density in a community; that is, permitting "duplexes" where single-family homes exist.

AARP developed a ***certified-aging-in-place (CAP) program*** whereby a trained specialist can design a granny flat or other housing structure to help an older adult stay safe in their own home as independently as possible. This program trains people to identify and implement home modifications to circumvent barriers that impede independence. After completing the training program, CAP specialists need to successfully complete 12 continuing education units every 3 years.

Adult Foster Homes

AFHs are privately owned homes located in residential neighborhoods that are converted into care homes to serve a small number of older (and sometimes younger disabled) adults with ongoing care needs. The number of residents allowed in an AFH varies by state, with one to five residents allowed in Oregon. Costs are usually far lower than nursing home care, and resident autonomy is far greater, with the added benefit of being in a home environment. AFHs are licensed and regulated in most states that have them.

Although popular with many older adults who wish to live in a home rather than a facility, there are challenges. For instance, quality can vary significantly among homeowners. Some are extraordinarily dedicated to their residents, while others do not maintain a clean and organized setting. In addition, it is the homeowner, not the resident, who decides whether smoking, alcohol, or pets will be allowed.

An additional challenge is that it is not always clear when, or if, the resident needs to be transferred to a nursing home because of the increased physical or mental decline of a resident. Finally, a small number of residents can lead to a stronger sense of community, or there may be one unpleasant resident who cannot be avoided in such a small setting.

Continuing Care Retirement Communities

People typically enter ***continuing care retirement communities (CCRCs)*** through independent retirement housing. If they decline in health, they transfer to an attached or nearby ALF or nursing home. The advantage is that if one spouse declines faster than the other, they can still be on the same campus. CCRCs are very much profit oriented: Most have large entrance fees with monthly costs, though some have just monthly costs. None, however, take Medicaid or low-income adults.

A recent challenge for CCRCs occurred when a resident in an independent apartment relocated into an attached ALF. Immediately thereafter, she was denied access to a bingo game in the independent facility where she used to live. The management claimed they were worried about liability, but the reality was that management, and some residents, did not want intermingling among those with vastly different physical or mental capabilities. This reminder of one's physically diminishing future can prove upsetting to some healthier residents and in this instance the bingo-playing residents continued an exclusive game on their own.

The shunned resident's lawsuit against the CCRC, however, was successful—but it had an unsatisfying outcome. The CCRC-sponsored bingo game was disbanded, but then individual residents continued an informal bingo game on their own that did not allow the resident from the ALF to participate.

Respite Care

Respite care allows temporary relief for caregivers so an older adult can remain in their home. *Adult day-care* sites are one type of respite program. They generally operate during normal business hours, 5 days a week, to provide respite for a working family caregiver or someone who just needs a break. The *social model* provides a safe and socially supportive environment for the older adult during the day; the *medical model* provides supervision of medications and limited nursing care and therapies. An expanded medical model is used by the PACE program.

There are other respite options as well, such as bringing in a home health aide on a temporary basis or bringing the older adult to a nursing home or ALF for a temporary stay.

One of the most innovative respite programs is *Elderserve at Night*, at the Hebrew Home at Riverdale in the Bronx, New York. Many people with dementia engage in "sundowning," whereby an older adult becomes agitated, confused, and prone to wandering late in the day or at night. There is a basic incompatibility when a person with dementia becomes more active at night, just when the caregiver needs to sleep. Thus, Elderserve at Night reversed the more typical adult day-care program for older adults with dementia and became an adult night-care program. Another innovative respite care program is the *Circles of Caring Adult Day Health Program*, www.circlesofcaring.org.

Memory Care Facilities

Memory care facilities (MCFs) can be located in separate facilities, but much more often they are units within a nursing home or an ALF. Persons with dementia in an MCF are kept within the perimeters of a secure setting to prevent wandering into unsafe areas.

In states where MCFs are accredited (like Oregon), the staff—both direct care and management—must meet minimum training requirements for caring for persons with dementia. There may also be requirements regarding floor plans, exit doors, secure outdoor areas, room temperature, noise levels, no-glare lighting, and individualized activity plans that are designed to stimulate residents with dementia.

In states that do not have dementia-related regulations added to existing regulations, facilities or units in facilities can declare themselves as dementia focused, even if there is no dementia training provided to staff and no adaptations are made to their facility.

Rather than a unit or even a separate facility for memory care, what about an entire village? Located in the Netherlands, there is a self-contained village, referred to as ***Amazing Village***, where people with dementia can shop, cook, get their hair done, and live together safely without the typical restraints of conventional dementia care.

Closed to the outside world with gates and security fences, inside it has restaurants, cafes, a supermarket, gardens, a pedestrian boulevard, and other aspects of village life. Residents with dementia are encouraged to shop in a grocery store, to cook and houseclean as able, and to walk or wander within the village. Caretakers wear street clothes and are available around the village to help guide residents when needed. Institutional characteristics are avoided throughout the village.

Other villages for persons with dementia have since been launched. In France, the layout of the village mirrors the design of surrounding small French towns. In Ireland, a village called Carebright is modeled after the Amazing Village in the Netherlands, but it is more compatible with Irish rural living and includes a farm, an orchard, and the employment of a community gardener. The first dementia village in the United States is Glenner Town Square in San Diego. It consists of two dozen buildings, several store fronts, a post office, a barber, a movie theater, a diner, and so forth. Its motif has a 1950s time frame.

These artificial villages raise ethical issues, such as whether deception is appropriate and whether care staff should participate in supporting such deception. Yet when the dementia villages are opened to outsiders, as some in Europe are, people find themselves welcome and enjoy participating in these artificial worlds. This may suggest room for inclusiveness and truly dementia-friendly societies rather than support for separate artificial villages.

Shared Older Adult Housing

Shared housing for older adults typically allows a widowed or divorced older adult to take advantage of a home that was once an appropriate size for their needs and is now too large, so they rent out space to other older adults. *The Golden Girls*, a 1980s sitcom, depicted the charms and challenges of shared housing for older adults.

For those who participate in shared housing, there is a written house agreement that includes rules about where to keep items in the refrigerator and how to share kitchen appliances, how to divide house cleaning duties, what is an appropriate noise level for day or nighttime, guidelines on visitors, and so forth.

For the newly divorced or widowed person, this allows for enlightened companionship, perhaps from someone sharing the same type of loss. Also important is the financial benefit from sharing costs.

Guided Care ("Hospital at Home")

This type of medical care keeps frail older adults in their homes and reduces costs by delaying or avoiding hospital or nursing home care. It is based on a specially trained registered nurse in a primary care practice working in partnership with two to five physicians in order to provide high-quality care for 50 to 60 chronically ill patients with particularly heavy healthcare use based on prior insurance claims.

The model includes assessing the patient and primary caregiver at home, providing an action plan, promoting patient self-management, monitoring conditions monthly, coordinating the effort of all healthcare providers, smoothing transitions between sites of care (particularly in and out of hospitals), educating and supporting family caregivers, and facilitating access to community resources (Leff & Novak, 2011).

The program has had extensive evaluation in randomized controlled trials. At 20 months, ***guided care*** patients experienced 21% fewer hospital readmissions, 16% fewer skilled nursing home days, 30% fewer home healthcare episodes, and only 4% more emergency department visits compared with a control group (Boult et al., 2011). Guided care reduced home healthcare episodes, suggesting the value of proactive, accessible care in heading off more extensive medical encounters (Boult et al., 2013). In addition, all participants, ranging from older adults to family caregivers, physicians, and nurses, reported improved quality of care. Guided care has been expanded and is being evaluated through the ACA.

A similar intervention program, with home-based primary care and an equivalent frail older adult population (i.e., focusing on the most costly Medicare beneficiaries), saved Medicare an average of $8,477 for patients receiving guided care (De Jonge et al., 2014). Reduction in costs is obtained mostly by savings in care at the end of life (Stanhope et al., 2018).

Foreign-Based Home Care

Foreign-based home care is an option for newly retired boomers. Americans have been heading down to Mexico or another location in Central or South America, where they rent an apartment, receive three meals a day, laundry and cleaning service, and 24-hour home healthcare from an attentive staff person at a fraction of what it would cost in the United States. An estimated 60,000 American retirees live in Mexico under these conditions. The downside to this home care solution is that you live in a foreign country far from family, and there is little government regulation to protect the consumer.

LONG-TERM CARE INSURANCE: PRIVATE VERSUS PUBLIC

Private long-term care insurance plays a minor role in financing home care and other LTC alternatives. Although estimates vary, in 2024 about 2% of Americans have invested in LTC insurance (Congressional Research Service, 2023). Although this type of insurance can provide peace of mind in times of need, it is expensive, premiums increase as the beneficiary ages, and contract benefits and exclusions are not easy to decipher. Private LTC insurance has not caught on as a successful LTC option.

There are numerous limitations in coverage under private LTC insurance, along with many other pitfalls. In California, in 2005, nearly one in every four LTC insurance claims were denied, many for technical and questionable reasons (5%–10% in 2022; National Association of Insurance Commissioners, https://content.naic.org/mcas_data_dashboard.htm). Moreover, many policyholders found the policy details to be confusing and not what they expected. This prompted an investigation in Congress by the House Committee on Energy and Commerce, which called for federal oversight of the industry rather than relying on lax state regulations (Duhigg, 2007).

LTC insurance rates rose by 15% between 2015 and 2020, according to the American Association for Long-Term Care Insurance (https://www.aaltci.org/long-term-care-insurance/learning-center/ltcfacts-2020.php#2020total). Plus new policies were being written with even more restrictions to limit insurers' risks. The greater cost and limitations were based on greater unpredictability of claimants' growing life expectancies and uncertainty over the prevalence and duration of Alzheimer and other forms of dementia.

Exacerbating these problems were extraordinary declines in interest rates after the 2008 recession, which limited the insurers' ability to generate financial returns on their income that were sufficient to pay claims. Despite double-digit rate hikes and additional restrictions, many of the major insurance companies decided to drop out of providing LTC insurance altogether, including Prudential, MetLife, and Unum.

The reduction in companies providing LTC insurance took place despite the fact that they collected premiums without having to pay out benefits for a significant minority of clients. More than 25% of those who bought LTC policies at age 65 let them lapse because of financial difficulties and other challenges (Friedberg et al., 2023). The insurance company pocketed what was previously paid, while the policy became defunct for the buyer. It seems to make more sense to build up a retirement savings account than to spend money on expensive LTC premiums. The latter are constantly going up in cost along with greater restrictions on what is covered; and, to make matters worse, there is the possibility the policy will lapse and money already paid will be forfeited. An even better idea than individual savings is for the nation's policy wonks to figure out how to incorporate LTC insurance into Medicare.

Public long-term care insurance was proposed by Senator Ted Kennedy and his senate colleagues shortly before he died. The *Community Living Assistance Services and Supports (CLASS) Act*, part of the ACA, would have created a premium-funded public insurance program. Working-age adults would become eligible for a cash benefit after paying into the program for 5 years.

The obvious problem with the CLASS Act was that it was voluntary. This was done for political reasons, but financially it was unfeasible. A voluntary LTC benefit is not that appealing to healthier and younger clients, and insurance only works with a large pool of contributors—many of whom are not at immediate risk of needing the benefit. As the CLASS Act was a stand-alone provision of the ACA, it was quickly terminated before it was even launched.

For those of us who support public LTC insurance, it has become clear that the only solution is for it to be an essential part of Medicare, an entitlement program that all Medicare beneficiaries are required to join. However, public LTC insurance is not likely to become a reality in the near future, given the Republican Party's opposition to expanding federally coordinated health services.

END-OF-LIFE CARE

Advance Directives

The Patient Self-Determination Act of 1990 was enacted to reduce the chance that a life would be shortened or prolonged against the wishes of that person. Part of this Act is to inform patients upon admission to a hospital that a ***living will***, a document that states one's wishes regarding end-of-life care, can be completed to make sure that one's preferences are respected. There is also a ***durable power of attorney for healthcare***, a document that designates an alternative decision-maker, family member or not, who becomes an advocate in the event that the person becomes incapacitated.

The need for at least one such document (both would be preferable) is still not sufficiently recognized. In 2016, 37% of American adults and 45.6% of adults age 65+ had an ***advance directive*** (Yaday et al., 2017).

Originally part of the ACA, this end-of-life legislation was derailed for a few years by opposition political leaders who referred to this educational planning resource as "death panels." Most sane people, though, understood the need for advance care planning conversations, and Medicare's coverage of this discussion now enhances the likelihood of it taking place. The Palliative Care and Hospice Education and Training Act, introduced in 2022, provides end-of-life training for physicians, nurse practitioners, physician assistants, and social workers, all of whom are eligible for reimbursement (Congress.gov, 2021–2022).

Too often a completed advance directive, particularly a living will, is not helpful. It may not be accessed in a timely manner, or the document is too general and provides insufficient guidance in a complex end-of-life situation. In one family's case, a living will, completed before undergoing heart surgery, stated clearly that if heart surgery were unsuccessful, there should not be a second effort. While recovering from heart surgery, however, the patient developed a leak in the surgical repair that could be rectified with a second surgery. The family agreed to it unanimously while the patient lay unconscious, and the patient lived several more years with independence.

The living will may not provide sufficient guidance to family members. Even with such guidance, inadequate communication between the dying person and the person with a durable power of attorney may negate end-of-life planning. The power of attorney is authorized to make medical decisions on an individual's behalf when incapacitated, but the power of attorney must understand the individual's reasoning to make informed decisions consistent with the individual's wishes.

Often, the advance directive is signed by an older adult who has no idea what really happens in a potential end-of-life event. To counteract this ignorance, older persons who view a video, rather than hearing a verbal description, are much more likely not only to more effectively communicate their wishes, but to choose comfort care over unnecessarily aggressive treatment (Houlihan et al., 2022; Volandes et al., 2008).

These types of videos show what is involved with CPR, what it is like to be on a ventilator, and what it is like to be in an intensive care unit hooked up to multiple tubes. The patient choices are (a) life-prolonging care, (b) limited medical care, or (c) comfort care.

Choosing the most aggressive, life-prolonging treatment has been the norm in our healthcare system; life must be preserved regardless of how hopeless or torturous the process. This continues to be the preferred choice for some people. However, this choice is less likely after viewing a video on end-of-life care options.

Ninety percent of older patients admitted to a skilled nursing facility who viewed an end-of-life video preferred to forego aggressive interventions and to die at home. Among those who did not see the video, 75% accepted the idea of aggressive intervention in a hospital (Volandes et al., 2012). The video did not attempt to scare patients with alarming images, and more than 95% who saw it would recommend it to other patients.

In another study, 75 seriously ill patients viewed a video about CPR and intubation. Afterward, 72% did not want intubation and 64% did not want CPR to be administered (El-Jawahri et al., 2015). The video also inspired most viewers to communicate directly with family members and their physician. Similar interventions confirm benefit for informed decision-making at the end of life (Nouri et al., 2022).

Most advance directives, however, take a back seat to emergency medical personnel, who operate under standing orders to attempt resuscitation. To prevent this lack of choice, one needs to complete a ***POLST*** form, which stands for *physician orders for life-sustaining treatment*. Oregon was the first state to use the POLST in the mid-1990s, and all states have adopted variants of the form. This document is voluntarily co-signed by a patient with high risk of dying and either a physician, physician's assistant, or nurse practitioner. It has two advantages over the better known living will.

First, a POLST addresses potentially unwanted emergency medical care by directing medical personnel on which actions to take, or not to take, in the event of a medical emergency. The directive is electronically accessed quickly by emergency personnel or a physician through an online statewide database. The digital version is available around the clock.

Second, the three choices about medical intervention are made clear. A person can choose to have CPR or full treatment; choose not to attempt resuscitation (do not resuscitate [DNR]) and allow natural death; or choose limited intervention that includes comfort care, and may or may not include IV fluids, antibiotics, and/or transfer to a hospital. Other issues are also addressed, such as the circumstances under which artificially administered nutrition is acceptable.

The need for an advance directive or POLST was revealed in one study in which 1,200 seriously ill Medicare beneficiaries were interviewed at five U.S. teaching hospitals. Among this sample, 40% requested a preference for treatment focused on extending life, and 60% expressed a preference for comfort care. However, while 86% of the patients who wanted aggressive treatment received care consistent with their preferences, only 41% who preferred comfort care received care consistent with their preferences (Teno et al., 2002). New efforts seek to document patient-provider conversations about preferences for care at the end of life (Glass et al., 2021).

Hospice Support

The philosopher (and humorist) Woody Allen once said, "I don't mind dying. I just don't want to be there when it happens." This sentiment may be shared by many Americans. For those who *are* willing to be there, those who want an open acknowledgment of the experience surrounded by family, friends, and compassionate caregivers, there is *hospice*.

The physician Cicely Saunders wrote about her experiences launching St. Christopher's Hospice, near London, established in 1967 (Saunders, 1977). The St. Christopher's Hospice prototype was an independent institution that provided inpatient care for dying patients. The first American hospice, Connecticut Hospice in New Haven, was founded a few years later in 1974 and was modeled after the London exemplar.

Hospice programs have since expanded their service sites, providing not only care in a hospice inpatient unit (now serving only a small percentage of hospice patients) but also in private homes, nursing homes, ALFs, and other settings. Hospice has evolved into a type of care, rather than the site of care.

Hospice's distinguishing characteristic is an emphasis on psychosocial and spiritual support over aggressive medical procedures, by which hospice attempts to improve the mental health and quality of life of clients, even as their physical bodies deteriorate.

The growth of the hospice movement in the United States has been tremendous. Between 1990 and 2010, the number of hospice programs in America increased from 1,800 to 5,000 and the number of terminally ill persons served from 210,000 to 1.6 million. In 2024, the United States has 5,200 hospice agencies that serve 1.8 million people annually (Levins, 2024). During the first decade of this century, Medicare dollars spent on hospice increased from $2 billion to more than $12 billion. The percentage of all deaths in the United States under the care of hospice increased to nearly half in 2024 (Hospice Facts and Figures, 2024). The growth of hospice care has been consistent and unrelenting.

The Centers for Disease Control and Prevention looked at the deaths of people over age 65 and noted encouraging trends. The proportion of older adults who died in a hospital dropped from 49% in 1989 to 33% in 2021, and the proportion who died at home increased from 15% to 39% during that same time period (Lei et al., 2021). Deaths in nursing homes are on the rise as well. While that may not be considered ideal for some, a death in a nursing home is likely to be more humane than in a hospital, where an unnecessary end-of-life aggressive procedure is more likely to occur.

One of the more startling statistics is that although 10% of older people in hospice visited an emergency department in their final month, 56% of those who were not enrolled in hospice visited the emergency department (Smith et al., 2012). Research looking at the last week of life sets the difference at 69.6 emergency department visits/1,000 beneficiary-days for nonhospice patients versus 7.6 for hospice beneficiaries, a ninefold difference (Obermeyer et al., 2016). Why is this important for people at the end of life and their families?

- Emergency personnel are unfamiliar with patient histories, goals, and preferences.
- Emergency departments are places to fix problems, some of which are not able to be fixed, rather than provide comfort.
- Emergency departments are frightening places, often followed by intensive care or care in the hospital, rather than care at home, where most people prefer to be.
- Emergency care is expensive, and one of the biggest contributors to why 25% of Medicare expenditures happen in the final 6 months of life (Nicholas et al., 2024).

An overlooked benefit of hospice care is bereavement support. Spouses of patients who receive hospice care for 3 or more days reported reduced depression symptoms compared with surviving spouses of patients who did not receive hospice care (Ornstein et al., 2015). The differences were even more pronounced a year after a spouse's death.

Although saving money is not the purpose of hospice care, it does. Hospice patients compared with nonhospice patients had significantly fewer hospitalizations and invasive procedures and were five times less likely to die in a hospital or nursing home (Obermayer et al., 2014). On average, patient cost was about $8,700 less per person in hospice care than for those not in hospice care.

One component of hospice care that can stand improvement is length of service. The majority of hospice patients die within 2 or 3 weeks of enrollment and, in 2009, 34% were in hospice fewer than 7 days. This means that hospice, despite its growing usage, is lagging behind in acceptance in a timely manner. Hospice is being thought of by too many as a very last resort. Ira Byock, director of palliative care medicine at the Dartmouth–Hitchcock Medical Center, quips: "This is brink-of-death care rather than end-of-life care."

There are several barriers to why more people do not receive more time in hospice care, or hospice care at all. First, many physicians are still reluctant to refer patients to hospice, seeing it as an admission of defeat. Many family members also see it in the same negative way. Second, most insurance companies, including Medicare, require that the physician certify that the patient has fewer than 6 months to live. The problem is that only late-stage cancer tends to be that predictable. Emphysema, congestive heart failure, Parkinson disease, dementia, and other conditions are not as predictable.

Consequently, the ACA funded several pilot programs that eliminated the need to predict 6 months to live or less, or to choose between comfort care and curative care. The programs involve 15,000 Medicare patients with terminal illness to *receive both hospice care and medical treatments* like chemotherapy or hospitalization. This allows for a continuation of medical personnel involvement rather than a shift to hospice personnel. It also removes the stigma of impending death, which has discouraged some from opting for the "hospice death sentence."

Third, older minority adults are less likely to use hospice services owing to fewer minority staff and volunteers, less trust of the healthcare system, and cultural beliefs that discourage the use of hospice care (Haber, 1999). In 2009, 44% of White decedents received hospice services in the last 30 days of life, versus 34% of Blacks and 31% of other minorities. Conversely, 26% of White decedents used intensive or critical care units in the last 30 days of life, versus 32% of Blacks and 33% of other minorities.

A major difficulty facing hospice clients and their families in the future may be the lack of a sufficient number of caregivers for people who choose to stay at home. Eighty percent of hospice clients are age 65 or over, and 83% are living in a private residence. Their spouses and increasingly their adult children are elderly themselves and physically unable to bear the exhausting burden of supporting the terminally ill in conjunction with hospice support (which plays a supplementary, not a primary, role). It is problematic whether sufficient numbers of volunteers and paid staff will be found to help meet the additional social support needs of the family of the terminally ill elderly who desire to remain at home with hospice support.

Inadequate social support not only prevents some older adults from participating in hospice at home; it may also characterize the situation of those who die in a hospital setting. Dying in a hospital largely means dying by oneself. According to one hospital study that used video cameras taped to patient doorways, seriously ill hospital patients were spending 75% of their day alone (Sulmasy & Rahn, 2001).

While the federal government publishes consumer data on the quality of care offered by hospitals, nursing homes, and home health agencies, it provides no such information about hospices. As the industry becomes more for-profit versus nonprofit (70% for-profit in 2024, and rising), research suggests nonprofit hospices are more likely to provide quality care (Soltoff et al., 2024). Another study reported that nonprofit hospices are more likely to partner with

QUESTION: Do you think it is likely that in 15 years more than two thirds of Americans will die with hospice support? What would it take for this to happen?

oncology centers, train their own staff better, and not disenroll patients prior to death (Aldridge et al., 2014).

Related to hospice care is ***palliative care***, which is designed for the purpose of alleviating pain from serious illness. Unlike hospice, palliative care is targeted toward all patients, not just those in terminal care situations. Palliative care programs are rapidly increasing in number. In 2015, 67% of hospitals with 50 or more beds had palliative care programs, up from 53% in 2008 and just 15% in 2001. In 2022, over 80% of hospitals had palliative care teams in place (Center to Advance Palliative Care, 2022). Why are palliative care programs increasing? Because there is greater recognition of the value of these programs, along with medical boards recognizing palliative care as an official subspecialty for the first time in 2008.

Why are palliative care programs important? One study of patients with metastasized lung cancer reported that those getting palliative care from the start of their diagnosis reported less depression, pain, nausea, mobility, worry, and other problems (Temel et al., 2010, 2017). Moreover, even though substantially fewer of the palliative care patients opted for aggressive chemotherapy, they lived almost 3 months longer than the group getting standard care.

One challenge for the future of palliative care is for a greater percentage of hospitals to meet national staffing recommendations. Almost two thirds of hospitals did not have a funded or unfunded physician, registered nurse, social worker, and chaplain all participating on the palliative care team (Spetz et al., 2016).

The Art Buchwald Phenomenon

Many people are scared off by hospice because they feel it is a death sentence. To be eligible, patients must be certified by two doctors as having 6 months or less to live. Yet there are two mitigating factors that make hospice less of a death sentence. First, hospice patients in one study lived an average of 29 days longer than comparable nonhospice patients (Connor et al., 2007). This may be due less to the social/emotional support provided by hospice care and more to the lethal nature of aggressive treatment for the terminally ill.

Second, many terminally ill diagnoses are not very predictable, certainly much less so than the gold standard of predictability—late-stage cancer. In fact, 17% of the 1.3 million hospice patients in 2006 were *discharged*, a rate that was mostly stable through 2020 (Medicare Payment Advisory Commission, 2022). One of those hospice patients was Art Buchwald, the Pulitzer Prize–winning newspaper humor columnist who in his prime was published in more than 550 newspapers. After 5 months in hospice, Buchwald left hospice care in 2006 and eventually died the following year, at the age of 81.

After kidney and vascular problems forced physicians to amputate one of his legs, Buchwald decided to refuse dialysis and entered hospice. Expecting to die in a few weeks, Buchwald, to the amazement of himself, his physicians, family, and friends, saw his kidneys start to work again. After leaving hospice, he wrote about his 5-month experience in a book titled *Too Soon to Say Goodbye* (2006). Once back in the community, he began to make the rounds of appearances necessary to support the sales of his book.

Although this is an unusual case, to say the least, publicizing it may reduce the stigma of hospice as a death sentence (but, on the negative side, strengthen our culture's denial of death). As Buchwald noted in his book, hospice provides as much comfort and support as possible and, if one should die, allows the person to die with dignity.

An entire team, consisting of volunteers, physician, nurse, social worker, therapist, spiritual advisor, and bereavement coordinator for the survivors, is dedicated to the goals of comfort, support, and dignity. Pain management is central, with families given access to opioids and instruction in their use. Until Americans change their attitudes toward dying and death, perhaps publicizing the ***Buchwald phenomenon*** can make the hospice option more palatable.

Hospice Resources

Since 1983, Medicare has covered hospice care provided by Medicare-approved agencies or facilities for terminally ill older persons who elect it in lieu of standard hospital treatment. Most private health insurance plans and state Medicaid programs also pay for hospice care.

For more information on hospice, including where to locate the one closest to you, contact the *National Hospice and Palliative Care Organization* (https://www.nhpco.org/), now renamed the *National Alliance for Care at Home* or contact the *Hospice Foundation of America*, (www.hospicefoundation.org).

DEATH WITH DIGNITY

In October 1997, after 3 years of legal challenges, the state of Oregon legalized physician-assisted death through the ***Death with Dignity Act***. In 2006, the U.S. Supreme Court rejected an effort by the Bush Administration to prevent Oregon and other states from creating Death with Dignity laws. In November 2008, voters in the state of Washington passed the second statewide Death with Dignity Act.

In 2009, Montana became the third state to approve right-to-die legislation, followed by Vermont. In 2016, a right-to-die bill passed in California in a special legislative session and was approved by the governor; however, in 2018, it was overturned by a California judge. In Massachusetts, voters narrowly rejected (51% to 49%) the Death with Dignity Act after opponents of the legislation outspent supporters by four to one. As of 2024, California, Colorado, Washington DC, Hawaii, Maine, Montana, New Jersey, New Mexico, Oregon, Vermont, and Washington have approved Right to Assisted Death legislation, and more states, undoubtedly, will follow. All states allow patients to decline treatment, but only these allow physicians to prescribe lethal drugs.

The Oregon Department of Human Services espouses that the term *physician-assisted suicide* is incompatible with the Death with Dignity Act and will use only the terms *physician-aid-in-dying* or *physician-assisted death*. Physician-assisted death legislation includes a rigorous process for determining which patients are eligible as well as waiting periods and independent confirmation of cognitive and psychiatric status. The preferred term now is *medical assistance in dying* or MAID.

The Oregon statute, which has been pretty much followed by subsequent states, mandates that an adult resident (age 18 or older) with a terminal illness (prognosis of less than 6 months to live) makes two separate requests 15 days or more apart, orally and in writing, with the written request signed by two witnesses—at least one of whom is not related to the patient; and that two physicians affirm that the patient has no more than 6 months to live and does not suffer from any mental disorder, including depression, that might impair judgment. The prescription, usually a lethal dose of barbiturates, cannot be administered by a physician and must be self-administered. (There are a few more requirements, but you get the point—it cannot be done on a whim.)

During the first 15 years of Oregon's law, 596 Oregonians availed themselves of it—about 40 persons per year, or 0.2% of dying Oregon patients, nearly all of whom were on hospice care. Among terminally ill persons who requested a prescription for lethal medication, less than half actually ended up using the medication. Regardless of whether they followed through, Oregon residents who requested assistance with death spent more time communicating about the issue through discussions with nurses, social workers, and physicians.

According to participating nurses and social workers, the primary reason patients make such a request is to be able to control the circumstances of death if they so choose, not to end their lives because they are depressed, lack social support, or fear being a financial drain on family members (Ganzini et al., 2002). In a later study of 56 Oregonians who requested physician-assisted death, few rated pain as a primary motivation. The primary reasons were a desire to be in control, remain autonomous, and die at home (Ganzini et al., 2009). Additional studies reported other frequently held motivations, such as the inability to enjoy activities or loss of dignity, both of which are more frequent motivators than inadequate pain control. A review of the total number of people requesting physician-hastened death in Oregon through 2024 (approximately 2,500 cases) showed increasing health insurance coverage from federal entities, shorter times of consultation with health care professionals, and continuing low rates of psychiatric referral (Regnard et al., 2024).

Although a good death is subject to interpretation, few would define it as being hooked up to machines in a hospital under the control of medical personnel and subjected to futile, painful, and extremely costly attempts to extend life. The Death with Dignity Act allows patients to place limits on their emotional and physical pain and be in control of the decision-making process.

About 80% of those who have died through the Death with Dignity Act were cancer patients (approximately 75%), and the diagnosis with the next highest percentage was amyotrophic lateral sclerosis (ALS, also known as Lou Gehrig's disease). This latter disease, due to muscle wasting, makes it difficult to comply with one component of the law, to self-administer the lethal dose of barbiturates. Dr. Richard Wesley, a retired pulmonologist and critical care physician with ALS, said he would find a way to meet this requirement even though he had lost the use of his limbs. He added: "I don't know if I'll use the medication to end my life, but I do know that it is my life, it is my death, and it should be my choice" (as cited in Hafner, 2012).

One final thought on palliative care, as it relates to physician-assisted death. A leading advocate of palliative care is a palliative care physician named Ira Byock. He argues that assisted death is immoral and unnecessary with adequate palliative and hospice care. Yet he admits that these options are not adequate. He believes that the hospice industry should employ more nurses to adequately serve their patients, and that too few clinicians are trained in palliative care.

So is it immoral? The ethicists will debate this. But pain and depression are common in the last year of life. The last months of life include a host of unwelcome symptoms, including breathlessness, anorexia, confusion, severe fatigue, loss of mobility, and incontinence (Singer et al., 2015). Perhaps the medical profession's increasing ability to prolong life exceeds its ability to extend comfort.

Other End-of-Life Options

Voluntarily stopping eating and drinking, also referred to as VSED, sounds like the simplest way to end life, but sometimes it is not. VSED is legal, based on the principles of patient autonomy and decision-making capacity. There are no government regulations surrounding it, and no terminal illness is required. It is difficult for some to accomplish it, though, with the hard part stopping fluids and suffering from dehydration. Just a few sips of liquid prolong the dying process.

The dying process through VSED typically takes about 7 to 14 days. One study of 102 hospice nurses who oversaw patients engaged in VSED reported that most patients died a peaceful death with little suffering (Ganzini et al., 2003; Mensger et al., 2024; Quill et al., 2018). Only 20% of the patients were deemed to have a poor quality of death or resumed eating or drinking.

Death doulas are sometimes referred to as transitional coaches. They are similar to midwife doulas who assist with the birthing process, except they support dying persons (but do not facilitate dying). They offer support to a dying person by being there, helping with physical and emotional care, and providing aroma therapy, guided visualization, and/or touch if desired. If in a home setting, household chores and other needed activities are provided.

A similar service is available at some hospitals. The *No One Dies Alone* (NODA) program began at Peace Health in Eugene, Oregon, in 2001 and is now a nationwide volunteer-centered program (see also, *No One Should Die Alone*, https://nosdaf.com/). NODA programs serve patients who are dying in a hospital and have no family or friends for support, or perhaps family members live out of state and their time for providing support at a hospital is limited.

A NODA companion sits by the bedside for typically 2- or 3-hour shifts and, along with other volunteers, a round-the-clock vigil takes place until the death of the patient. The companion can read to the person, use aroma therapy, play soft music, and offer physical comfort that is unskilled but unavailable from busy bedside nurses.

We can anticipate increasing acceptability of psychedelic drugs as an addition to palliative care. Use of the drugs may reduce anxiety and perhaps ease the transition to death.

Euthanasia is a deliberate action to end life in order to relieve suffering. It differs from Death with Dignity in that the physician takes an active role in administering the ending of a life. It is illegal in most countries, but was legalized in the Netherlands in 2002; Belgium, Germany, Spain, and Luxembourg followed suit. Other European countries, including Portugal, France, and Ireland, are debating whether to allow it. Involuntary euthanasia refers to termination of a life when the person is unable to provide consent owing to dementia, lack of consciousness, or other factors.

Euthanasia is always controversial but even more so when countries permit it for persons who cannot provide consent, for persons who are not terminally ill but may be suffering from a psychiatric illness, or for those who are suffering and unwilling to tolerate loss of independence, physical deterioration, and loneliness.

NURSING HOMES AND DEATH

The number of deaths in nursing homes is in the hundreds of thousands each year. Yet it is typically shrouded in secrecy. In one nursing home, the deceased was wheeled out when no one was looking. There was no recognition of the event, except when the name label near the door was removed. The reason for the secrecy was a belief by administrators that death was depressing and should be hidden.

However, attitudes toward death in the nursing home are evolving. Some nursing homes hold monthly memorial services to recognize residents who died. The new belief is that it is important to acknowledge the passing and to show the remaining residents that their lives mattered. This is a good time to highlight the interests, accomplishments, personality quirks, character traits, and family of the deceased. Perhaps a brief and selective life review by family members and friends could be presented orally or in succinct written form. It would also be a good time for music, poetry, laughter, and shared memories.

It may also be a time to recognize the needs of staff members who were closest to the deceased. Some can be given an opportunity to say a few words on behalf of the deceased at a memorial service, and some might deserve a paid day off to reflect on their feelings. All staff should receive training on how to cope with death.

Perhaps this evolution has been fostered by the presence of hospice or by the culture change movement in LTC. Both movements recognize that older adults have a lot of experience with, and ability to deal with, death. Older residents can help inform us of new rituals they would appreciate surrounding death in LTC. All can find comfort and support in sharing this experience and bringing the community together.

GREEN BURIALS AND GREEN CEMETERIES

Eco-friendly ***green burials*** and *green cemeteries* have been popular in Britain for years, with over 200 natural burial sites. But they are just starting to catch on in the United States, especially in three states: California, New York, and Washington. The first green cemetery in the United States, though, was established in 1998 in Westminster, South Carolina, and is called the Ramsey Creek Preserve. For additional information, read *The Green Burial Guidebook* (Fournier, 2018).

The green burial movement consists of biodegradable coffins costing as little as $100 or only wrapping the body in a shroud. In 2019, the state legislature of Washington went one step further and was considering the (most likely) first bill in the world (Johnson, 2019) to legalize above-ground composting of remains, or what the bill called recomposition. The body is wrapped in organic materials, with no coffin, embalming chemicals, fossil fuels for cremation, or expensive cemetery plot. When bathed in a stream of air warmed by microbes and periodically turned, the bodies essentially become soil in 30 days. You choose: environmentally sound, individual choice, or creepy?

The U.S. funeral industry, which generates an estimated $20 billion in revenue annually, is against both green burials and green cemeteries. Many others also find the idea unacceptable, relying on the comfort provided by funeral services, floral displays, vaults, and traditional burials and grave sites. But as Harris (2007) notes in his book *Grave Matters*, each year in the United States, 800,000 gallons of formaldehyde are injected into embalmed bodies. Formaldehyde is a carcinogen that eventually leaches into the environment. Also, there is enough metal buried with coffins and vault linings to rebuild the Golden Gate Bridge each year.

Cremations are considerably less expensive and use far fewer resources than traditional burials. The more orthodox advocates of the Green Movement argue, however, that they too involve hazardous emissions such as carbon monoxide and volatized mercury from dental fillings. There is also the cost of power to produce temperatures (about 1,800°F) to incinerate a human body. As an alternative, there are eco-friendly, flameless cremations known as *alkaline hydrolysis*, which use heat, lye, and water and have a light carbon footprint.

AARP reported that more than half of the boomers in the United States, about 38 million adults, can be classified as *green boomers*. These ecologically minded boomers are buying organic foods and goods produced locally (to reduce gasoline usage and air pollution), financially supporting green companies and nonprofit environmental groups, buying energy-efficient appliances, purchasing electric or gas–electric hybrid cars, using solar-powered water heaters, recycling, and monitoring their thermostat settings at home and water consumption in the yard. Eventually, some of these boomers will also join the ranks of those who opt for green burials and green cemeteries.

SUMMARY

In the 1970s, LTC in the United States basically consisted of families struggling on their own at home or relocating loved ones into a nursing home. There was little to no support for caregivers of frail elders in the home. And nursing home care was in dire need of reform.

Since that time, an increasing number of resources have been generated for caregivers, and in nursing homes, there was not just major regulatory reform but also culture change promulgated on a nationwide basis.

Moreover, alternatives to nursing home care in the United States have proliferated and now include Green Houses, ALFs, AFHs, virtual villages, elder cohousing, granny flats, CCRCs, MCFs, dementia cafes, and dementia villages. No one can deny the creativity and practicality of the LTC options that are now available.

There is no less creativity and practicality in the end-of-life movement in the United States. Hospice had not even come to America in 1971. Palliative care was not even a thing, except on occasion when it was done informally by an individual healthcare provider. There were no advance directives such as the living will, durable power of attorney for health, or POLST. Death with Dignity would have gotten you arrested in 1971. And you didn't die in nursing homes, you merely disappeared, without acknowledgment. Once dead, the funeral industry had a monopoly on profits, provided a scarcity of options, and successfully prevented green burial and green cemetery alternatives.

Births were celebrated while dying was often torturous, with aggressive medical care the only option. We are now much more responsive to the needs and wishes of persons in the last stages of the life cycle: frailty and dying. Although no one looks forward to the decline in the last two phases of life, we can at least celebrate the efforts that have been made during this juncture to make life more meaningful and humane.

REFERENCES

Only key references appear in the print edition. The full reference list can be accessed by visiting www.springerpub.com/courseconnect. See inside front cover and tear-out card for CourseConnect details.

AARP & the National Alliance for Caregiving. (2020). *Caregiving in the U.S.* https://www.aarp.org/content/dam/aarp/ppi/2020/05/full-report-caregiving-in-the-united-states.doi.10.26419-2Fppi.00103.001.pdf

AARP Public Policy Institute. (2023). *Valuing the invaluable.* https://www.aarp.org/politics-society/advocacy/info-2023/jenkins-family-caregivers.html#:~:text=AARP's%20recently%20updated%20%E2%80%9CValuing%20the,for%20transportation%20and%20other%20needs

APHA. (2020). *Supporting and sustaining the home care workforce to meet the growing need for long-term care.* https://www.apha.org/policies-and-advocacy/public-health-policy-statements/policy-database/2021/01/13/supporting-and-sustaining-the-home-care-workforce

Boult, C., Leff, B., Boyd, C. M., Wolff, J. L., Marsteller, J. A., Frick, K. D., Wegener, S., Reider, L., Frey, K., Mroz, T. M., Karm, L., & Scharfstein, D. O. (2013). A matched-pair cluster-randomized trial of guided care for high-risk older patients. *Journal of General Internal Medicine, 28*, 612–621. https://link.springer.com/article/10.1007/s11606-012-2287-y

Gandhi, A., Yu, H., & Grabowski, D. C. (2021). High nursing staff turnover in nursing homes offers important quality information. *Health Affairs, 40*(3), 384–391. https://doi.org/10.1377/hlthaff.2020.00957

Glass, D. P., Wang, S. E., Minardi, P. M., & Kanter, M. H. (2021). Concordance of end-of-life care with end-of-life wishes in an integrated health care system. *JAMA Network Open*, *4*(4), e213053. https://doi.org/10.1001/jamanetworkopen.2021.3053

Leggett, A. N., Sonnega, A. J., Lohman, M. C. (2020). Till death do us part: Intersecting health and spousal Dementia caregiving on caregiver mortality. *Journal of Aging & Health*. *32*(7–8), 871–879. https://doi.org/10.1177/0898264319860975

Mensger, M., Jiao, Y., Jansky, M., Banse, C., Nauck, F., Nothacker, M., & Stanze, H. (2024). Voluntarily stopping eating and drinking (VSED): A systematic mixed-methods review focusing on the carers' experiences, *Health Policy*, *150*, 105174. https://doi.org/10.1016/j.healthpol.2024.105174

Miller, S. C., Schwartz, M. L., Lima, J. C., Shield, R. R., Tyler, D. A., Berridge, C. W., Gozalo, P. L., Lepore, M. J., & Clark, M. A. (2018). The prevalence of culture change practice in U.S. nursing homes: Findings from a 2016/2017 nationwide survey. *Medical Care*, *56*(12), 985–993. https://doi.org/10.1097/MLR.0000000000000993

Schulz, R., Beach, S. R., Czaja, S. J., Martire, L. M., & Monin, J. K. (2020). Family caregiving for older adults. *Annual Review Psychology*, *71*, 635–659. https://doi.org/10.1146/annurev-psych-010419-050754

Smith, A. K., McCarthy, E., Weber, E., Cenzer, I. S., Boscardin, J., Fisher, J., & Covinsky, K. (2012). Half of older Americans seen in emergency departments in last month of life: Most admitted to hospital, and many die there. *Health Affairs*, *31*, 1277–1285. https://doi.org/10.1377/hlthaff.2011.0922

Temel, J. S., Greer, J. A., El-Jawahri, A., Pirl, W. F., Park, E. R., Jackson, V. A., Back, A. L., Kamdar, M., Jacobsen, J., Chittenden, E. H., Rinaldi, S. P., Gallagher, E. R., Eusebio, J. R., Li, Z., Muzikansky, A., & Ryan, D. P. (2017) Effects of early palliative care in patients with lung and GI cancer: A randomized clinical trial. *Journal of Clinical Oncology*, *35*(8), 834–841. https://doi.org/10.1200/JCO.2016.70.5046

U.S. Administration on Community Living. (2024). *Strengthening the direct care workforce*. Direct Care Strategies Center. https://acl.gov/programs/direct-care-workforce

U.S. Bureau of Labor Statistics. (2023a). *Unpaid elder care in the U.S.* https://www.bls.gov/news.release/pdf/elcare.pdf

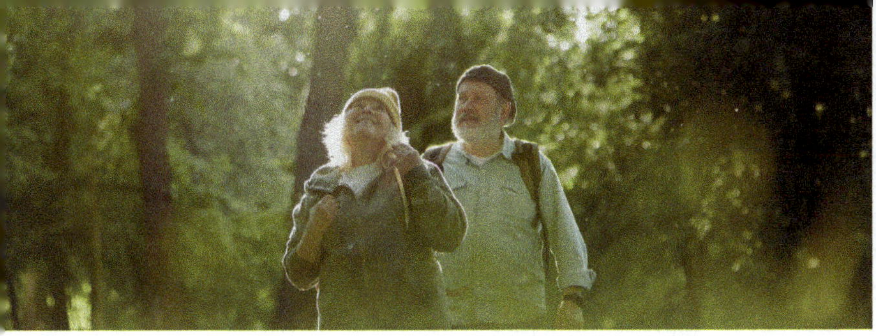

11

PUBLIC HEALTH POLICY AND AGING

KEY TERMS

- Affordable Care Act (ACA)
- age discrimination at work
- comparative effectiveness
- competition
- generic
- geriatric medicine
- geriatric research
- income security
- junk food tax
- managed care
- Medicare
- Medicare Part D
- Oregon as a model state
- patented versus generic drugs
- public health
- rationing
- Social Security
- student loan debt
- Surgeon General's reports

LEARNING OBJECTIVES

- Describe the role of *public health* in the United States, and how healthy aging can be strengthened through it.
- Critically evaluate the policy of implementing junk food and drink taxes.
- Cite the most influential *Surgeon General's reports.*
- State and support your opinion on the role of government in health promotion.
- Evaluate the future of *Social Security* and *Medicare.*
- Critically analyze the *Patient Protection and Affordable Care Act (ACA).*
- Assess the necessity of *rationing.*
- Analyze the role *competition* plays in the U.S. healthcare system.
- Critically evaluate the need for a single-payer, managed healthcare system.
- Critically evaluate *Medicare Part D* and medication expense in the United States.
- Differentiate between patented and generic drugs.
- Identify and summarize several important public health policy issues.
- Assess the future of *geriatric medicine* and *geriatric research.*
- Examine the importance of *comparative effectiveness.*
- Assess the likelihood of winning an age-discrimination-at-work suit.
- Argue the case whether *Oregon* does or does not deserve to be held up as a model state for health promotion.

Politics can be a strife of interests masquerading as a contest of principles.

—*Ambrose Bierce*

Americans live 30 to 40 years longer than they did a century ago; this progress is mostly due to triumphs in ***public health***, including improvements in sanitation, water and air quality, hygiene, immunization, and health education. Public health differs from medicine in that it focuses on preventing disease and promoting health in whole populations rather than treating disease and injury in a single patient.

Most Americans today have much less awareness of public healthcare in this country than they do about medical care. The best-known aspects of public health relate to the goals of maintaining safe water, attaining a clean environment, ensuring food safety, and controlling communicable diseases. But these public health roles come to the attention of the public only when there is a threat to water, food safety, the environment, or an outbreak of a drug-resistant infection.

Even less well known is the role that public health plays in gathering health information, conducting screenings and immunizations, providing health education, and conducting health interventions. These types of activities reflect public health's concern with a broad range of health factors that influence the quality of life of individuals, families, groups, and communities.

The public's lack of awareness of these endeavors is probably due to the fact that relatively little funding (minuscule in comparison to what we spend on medical care) is targeted to support public health activities. Even less is allocated to public health gerontology. Public health has largely ignored aging adults, despite the steady increase in the average age of the American population. One early report that is still relevant concluded with the following:

> The new challenge for public health is to develop a focus on healthy aging. ... Inadequate resources and attention are focused on health promotion and prevention of disease or secondary disability for older adults—the very population that experiences the highest rates of chronic disease and disability. (Palombo et al., 2003, pp. 1–2)

FUNDING PUBLIC HEALTH

One way to create a budget for health promotion for both the young and old is to craft federal legislation that mandates a small ***junk food tax***—candy bars, cookies, cakes, pastries, ice cream, soda, corn chips, tortilla chips, potato chips, ... you get the idea. Tax high-fat, high-sugar, or high-salt junk foods, which constitute over 20% of Americans' calories.

Jacobson and Brownell (2000) estimated that a national tax of 1 cent per 12-ounce soft drink would generate about $1.5 billion annually, and 1 cent per pound of candy, chips, and other snack foods would raise more than $100 million annually. A later analysis reported that a 1-cent-per-ounce tax on sugar-sweetened beverages would generate $14.9 billion in the first year alone (Chaufan et al., 2009).

This is not a strategy without controversy. The main argument against junk food taxes is that the government should not pry into people's personal business. Opponents of the nanny state prefer that we tackle obesity and inactivity with common sense and self-discipline rather than expecting government to do it for us.

Civil liberty concerns are raised as well. Wellness advocate Donald Ardell asked, "Don't we have a right to choose what we eat? Should we also tax those who do not exercise enough? What about those with no sense of humor? Now there's a group to sock with a big tax hit!" (D. Ardelll, personal communication, D. Haber). Those opposed to junk food taxes ask: If government gets more involved with promoting individual health, will it interfere with individual freedom and personal responsibility (Callahan, 2000)?

Those in favor of junk food taxes respond that there are long-time precedents for this. Of the main risk factors that enter our mouths, two are already regulated and taxed—tobacco and alcohol, first implemented by President George Washington and continued over two centuries;, while three, for the most part, are not—sugar, salt, and fat. Proponents argue that if government gets more involved with improving nutrition and exercise (and reducing obesity), the health outcomes will enhance the quality of life of individuals, as well as the financial and humanitarian interests of society. These differing opinions and values are difficult to reconcile and have become more complex with the advent of the new class of GLP-1 drugs (e.g., Wegovy, Ozempic) that offer effective but expensive weight loss.

Philosophical concerns aside, there are "sin" taxes that work. For example, cigarette taxes reduced smoking and were followed by a reduction in lung cancer rates. It may be unreasonable to assume, however, that taxes will also reduce the consumption of junk foods. Food consumption habits are probably shaped more by advertising dollars than by junk food taxes. Unlike tobacco products, there are no regulations to curb food product advertising.

There is little doubt, however, that junk foods are unhealthy and costly to our healthcare system—with an estimate of $147 billion in annual medical expenditures for diet-related diseases (Finkelstein et al., 2009). And it is advertising that fuels this medical bill. McDonald's and Coca-Cola's marketing budgets each reach more than $1 billion annually. Many additional billions of advertising dollars encourage the consumption of high-fat, high-sugar, and high-salt products. In contrast to this spending spree, the National Cancer Institute spent $1 million to promote its 5-a-Day (fruits and vegetables) campaign.

Sugar Taxes

More than two dozen cities in the United States levy taxes on some nutritionally deficient foods, especially sugary drinks, which constitute about 7% of all calories consumed, according to *Consumer Reports* (2017, October issue, p. 49). A 1-cent-per-ounce tax on sugar levied by Berkeley, California, in 2015 led to a 10% reduction in sugary drinks. National studies confirm decreases in sugar consumption, with population-wide health benefits, linked to imposition of taxes (White et al., 2023). The World Health Organization has endorsed taxes as an effective way to reduce the burden of obesity-related disease (https://iris.who.int/bitstream/handle/10665/260253/WHO-NMH-PND-16.5Rev.1-eng.pdf).

The rate of obesity in Mexico rose to 20.3% in 2016 from 7% in 1980, according to the Institute for Health Metrics and Evaluation at the University of Washington. Consequently, a 1-peso-per-liter tax on soda was implemented. This led to a 6% decrease in overall sales, and a 12% reduction among the most obese Mexicans—lower-income citizens. Chile also achieved a reduction in sugar-sweetened beverage sales through the implementation of taxes. This South American country then went two steps further by (a) requiring drinks with high-sugar content to include warning labels on their packaging and (b) prohibiting advertising aimed at children under age 14.

France not only instituted a soda tax but in 2017 banned restaurants from offering free refills of sodas and other sugary drinks. One Frenchman complained that restaurants might next be required to put weight scales by their front doors to discourage excess consumption.

The international outlier is China. In a few decades, China has gone from a nation plagued with food shortages to soaring obesity levels: from 20% of adults who were obese in 1991 to 42% in 2018. Thanks to Coca-Cola and other Western allies who have built thriving businesses in China, public health initiatives by the Chinese government promote exercise exclusively and do not mention sugar-sweetened beverages. Coca-Cola tried similar tactics in the United States, promoting the message that exercise, not diet, is the solution to the nation's obesity crisis. After mounting domestic scientific and public criticism, though, the food and beverage industries terminated this deceptive strategy in the United States, and shifted it abroad where sales were soaring and government oversight was more pliant (Jacobs, 2019).

A potential advantage of taxing sugar and junk foods with high salt and fat content (so-called sin taxes) is to apply the extra revenue toward health-promoting initiatives. Unfortunately, a significant percentage of junk food and cigarette tax revenues in the United States was spent on nonhealth activities. To combat this tendency, when the city of Philadelphia was struggling to pass legislation for a 1.5-cents-per-ounce soda tax in 2017, city officials promised that its millions in projected revenue would go toward funding prekidergarten programs (4,000 new prekindergarten slots in 2019, and another 1,000 in 2020). This promise led to increased public support and the passage of the legislation.

Another challenge is that raising taxes on junk food, particularly sugary products, at the state, county, or city level—no matter how modest—can provoke the food and drink industries to fight back. When the state of Washington, for example, imposed a 2-cent tax on soft drinks, the food and beverage industry spent $16 million on the referendum that repealed it. Moreover, in 2017 and 2018, thanks to overwhelming industry influence, California, Arizona, and Michigan passed laws to bar municipalities in their states from adopting soda taxes.

It may make more sense, therefore, to implement junk food or sugar taxes at the federal level, rather than at a lower level of government, but this won't be a picnic to accomplish either. When a sugar tax was proposed as part of the ***Affordable Care Act (ACA)***, the food and drink industry spent $58 million and blocked it.

It also makes sense, as was the case in Philadelphia, to link sugar or junk food taxes to the support of popular community programs, rather than emphasizing the goal of reducing the consumption of unhealthy food. Thus, it is important to not allow raised revenue to be used for nonhealth purposes, as was the case with the financial settlement the government made with the tobacco industry.

QUESTION: Examine the pros and cons of the idea to tax sugar or junk foods. What is *your* opinion of this idea, and why?

SURGEON GENERAL'S REPORTS ON HEALTH

Money is not the only tool for promoting health. Timely education based on rigorous research that is widely and effectively disseminated is important too. And the ***Surgeon General's reports*** on health have been doing that periodically for over a half century.

Despite the bizarre military term—"Surgeon General"—the person who assumes this role is neither a surgeon nor a general; they hold the top leadership position on public health in the federal government. With rare exception the person occupying this position has been anonymous. Would the anonymity recede if the position was shifted to the president's cabinet? Probably not, as the general public is not aware of these leaders either (except when they commit egregious ethical lapses or criminal behavior).

This does not mean that the periodic Surgeon General's reports suffer the same anonymous fate. The impact of some of these reports has been profound, beginning more than a half century ago. A few examples should suffice.

The *Surgeon General's report on tobacco* (Bayne-Jones et al., 1964) summarized the research into the health hazards of tobacco use, and most analysts believe it was the major stimulus in the subsequent 50% reduction in tobacco use that took place over the next three decades.

The *Surgeon General's report on health promotion and disease prevention* (U.S. Public Health Service Office of Disease Prevention and Health Promotion, 1979) became one of the most widely cited documents on the role that risk factors play in morbidity, mortality, and medical costs. This report helped launch the *Healthy People 1980* initiative, and five (so far) subsequent decade-long initiatives: *Healthy People 1990, 2000, 2010, 2020, and 2030.*

The *Surgeon General's report on physical activity and health* (U.S. Department of Health and Human Services [DHHS], 1996) did an excellent job of summarizing the research into the importance of moderate-intensity physical activity or exercise, the value of accumulating physical activity or exercise over the course of a day, the importance of resistance training along with aerobic exercise, and the utility of establishing an exercise habit of 30 minutes a day, most days of the week. These recommendations helped to change fitness practices.

The *Surgeon General's report on mental health* (DHHS, 1999) reported on the surprising prevalence of depressive and anxiety symptoms among the population, including older adults, and the inability of health professionals to identify and treat this problem. It also highlighted the reimbursement discrepancy between mental health and physical health problems, which was finally corrected a decade later.

The Surgeon General's report on bone health and osteoporosis (DHHS, 2004) warned that by 2020, half of all American citizens older than 50 will be at risk for fracture if no immediate action is taken. Scientific progress in the prevention, assessment, and treatment of osteoporosis to alleviate this serious health problem is ongoing.

The *Surgeon General's report on the health consequences of involuntary exposure to tobacco smoke* (Office on Smoking and Health, 2006) reported that there is no risk-free level of exposure to secondhand smoke. Nearly half of all nonsmoking Americans are still regularly exposed to secondhand smoke, which increases their risk of developing heart disease and lung cancer by about 25%. This report further spurred state restrictions on tobacco usage in public places.

More recent Surgeon General's reports have tackled related public health challenges. These include promoting breastfeeding (2011), reducing suicide (2012), preventing skin cancer (2014), developing walkable communities (2015), reducing addiction and substance abuse (2016, 2018), supporting maternal health (2020), confronting health misinformation (2021), addressing burnout in the health workforce (2022), reducing loneliness (2023), and tackling firearm violence (2024). The full set of reports provides a good history of public health efforts in the United States (https://www.ncbi.nlm.nih.gov/books/NBK45031/).

QUESTION: **Access one of the Surgeon General's reports. What do you find to be the most interesting or important age-related idea in this report, and why do you believe that?**

An Opposing Point of View (Sort of)

Fire the Surgeon General! Get government off our backs! If the government is going to be involved in health promotion at all, let it focus on the social, environmental, and particularly the economic contexts in which health behaviors are shaped. Improve living conditions, and health behaviors will follow suit. Give people freedom and self-responsibility instead of creating a backlash against health-promoting initiatives through government meddling.

What will the Surgeon General and big government do next? Should it encourage downhill skiers to take a safer 30-minute walk instead? Should it add to the stigmatization of overweight Americans by singling them out for ineffective interventions? Should it encourage insurance plans to be punitive toward smokers? If so, should it add overweight people, sedentary people, and, oh yes, those pesky downhill skiers to the list of scofflaws?

If this argument and these questions appeal to you, read Daniel Callahan's (2000) *Promoting Healthy Behavior: How Much Freedom? Whose Responsibility*? After reading

Callahan's book, read *Food Politics* (Nestle, 2002) and *Fast Food Nation* (Schlosser, 2001). Another set of questions should come to mind: Is it fair that the food and drink industries spend billions of dollars a year advertising high-fat, high-sugar, and high-salt products that influence our eating behaviors, while the federal government spends only a few million dollars on nutrition education? Or, as once stated by Kelly Brownell, the former dean of the Stanford School of Public Policy at Duke University and an internationally recognized leader on nutrition and obesity: "The entire federal budget for nutrition education is equal to one fifth of the advertising costs for Altoids mints."

QUESTION: Do you support a strong government role in promoting the health of an aging society? Explain why and state the advantages and disadvantages of such a strong government approach.

Is it fair that diet-related diseases resulted in $147 billion in annual medical expenditures in 2008 (Finkelstein et al., 2009)? This comes to just over 9% of all medical expenditures in that year. For Medicare beneficiaries, normal-weight persons averaged $4,700 a year in medical costs, whereas obese persons averaged $6,400. Sedentary behaviors may cost society a similar amount. Are we willing to ignore research on increased physical activity and exercise that show a significant effect on disease protection, improved functionality, and lower medical costs? Are we causing public health harm if we do so little to dislodge Americans from changing unhealthy behaviors?

And was it *un*fair that the federal government played such an important role (or meddled, depending on your point of view) in reducing the number of Americans who smoked cigarettes by two thirds? Clearly, this is no longer an opposing view and may indicate that government must play a major role in promoting the health of Americans, with appropriate community partnerships and communication. Three landmark pieces of legislation support this statement.

SOCIAL SECURITY

Few can argue that inadequate income is irrelevant to health. In the United States, its poorest citizens not only live their later years in worse health, but live, on average, more than 5 years less than affluent persons.

It is important, therefore, in a chapter on public health policy and aging, to examine the future of ***Social Security***. Social Security is indisputably one of the most successful pieces of legislation ever created, with a need to support the income of a population whose life expectancy at birth was 78.4 years in 2023 (Murphy et al., 2024).

The future of Social Security depends on its solvency. The good news is that compared to Medicare, fixing Social Security is a walk in the park. Yes, the percentage of people over age 65 has grown, from 6% of the population in 1935 to 18% in 2024. And, yes, the number of Social Security beneficiaries is expected to rise from 57 million in 2012 to 90 million in 2033. And yes, once again, the number of workers contributing to Social Security has decreased, from approximately four workers per beneficiary in the 1960s, to 2.9 workers in 2012, and the number of contributing workers is expected to decline further, to 2.1 workers per beneficiary in 2036.

But fixing Social Security is not that complicated (though it is exceptionally difficult, politically). Here are five ways, with the last one alone solving somewhere around 80% of the problem, though this percentage declines with each year we procrastinate.

1. Raise the retirement age.
2. Reduce the amount of money Social Security pays out to the highest earners.
3. Change the cost-of-living adjustment formula.
4. Increase the payroll tax rate for Social Security.
5. Remove the payroll tax cap from Social Security ($168,600 in 2024)—the simplest, easiest, and most politically palatable component.

The last option is politically feasible because the vast majority of wage earners are unaffected, and the lowest wage earners with the greatest need continue to be helped as much as before. But as previously noted, every year of delay makes the problem becomes more daunting. The last option would have solved 100% of the problem if enacted in 2010.

What about *privatizing Social Security*? There is nothing social and nothing secure about this strategy. If you became eligible for a privatized Social Security system just before the stock market crashed in 2008, you were ______ (insert your own dismal word here). Moreover, the cost of converting to a privatized plan is in the trillions, and where would we get this funding?

More than two thirds of respondents in their 20s and 30s in a 2011 Wells Fargo survey said they were not confident in the stock market as a place to invest for retirement, which is a likely destination for funds in a privatized Social Security alternative. In addition, pension plans outside Social Security are rapidly disappearing, with less than 10% of workers now having a pension plan in the work setting. Most everyone else relies on a 401(k)-type plan that, like privatized Social Security, is dependent on the performance of your investment, referred to as a *defined-contribution plan*.

In contrast to this is the greater predictability of a *defined-benefit plan* similar to Social Security, which is based on years of earning history. A defined-benefit plan pays out an annuity for the rest of the person's life, so you do not bear the risk of outliving your pension. When employees have a choice at work, they overwhelmingly opt for a defined-benefit plan. This choice at work, though, is rapidly disappearing.

In summary, to think that privatized Social Security is a good idea, you need to ignore the increased personal financial risk, not to mention the huge societal start-up costs that must come from somewhere.

What if we do nothing? In fiscal year 2018, Social Security expenditures ($991 billion) exceeded revenues ($912 billion) for the first time. At this rate, our reserves (the result of the accumulation of more money coming in over the years than going out) runs out in 2034, and we will only have enough revenue to pay out 79% of promised benefits beginning in 2035. Although bad, this is not the dire circumstance that many young adults have been led to believe; that is, only 31% expect any income at all from Social Security during their retirement years! Among people between the ages of 18 and 24, only 11% expect Social Security to still be around when they retire.

If we fix the problem, the last half of the 21st century is clear sailing. The percentage of the population that is older is expected to go down, and the percentage of the population contributing to Social Security should go up. A healthier older population can also be expected to work to later ages and perhaps delay receiving benefits.

MEDICARE

In 2022, 94% of older people not living in nursing homes were ***Medicare*** enrollees (Administration on Community Living, 2024). Medicare's Part A coverage, like Social Security, is an entitlement paid through deductions to wages over the lifespan. It covers hospitalization but also hospital discharge-related home healthcare and durable medical equipment, hospice care, care for younger people with special diseases (e.g., end-stage renal disease, motor neuron disease), and low-income younger people with chronic conditions eligible for Medicaid. It does not cover long-term care expenses, such as nursing home care, dementia respite services, and in-home and community-based services designed to support people with disabilities. Medicare special needs plans and low income subsidy programs extend Medicare accessibility to low-income beneficiaries, as Medicare requires beneficiaries to pay part of the cost of care. In fact, older adults cover about half of their health spending with other sources, including Medicare Part B (outpatient care) and Part D (prescription coverage) programs (ACL, 2024)

Medicare Advantage Plans combine these programs to varying degrees and function more like health maintenance organizations. In 2024, more than half of Medicare enrollees (approximately 54% or 32.8 million people) took advantage of these plans. As the Kaiser Foundation notes, Medicare Advantage plans go beyond traditional Medicare by providing coverage for allied health services (dental, vision, and hearing services) and limit out-of-pocket expenses (Freed et al., 2024). The downside is limited provider networks and stricter cost management (e.g., *prior authorization* for many procedures). Evidence suggests healthier older people are more likely to use Medicare Advantage programs.

Medicare is only one component of healthcare insurance in old age. Almost half of older adults (46%) had some type of private health insurance, 6% had military-based health insurance, 7% were covered by Medicaid, and 1% had no coverage (ACL, 2024). Medicare alone is insufficient for covering medical services, let alone long-term care needs. The latter are the province of Medicaid, state and county programs, family caregiving, and private insurance.

Medicare is widely and enthusiastically popular, and justifiably so. There were about 67.8 million people with Medicare coverage in 2024, 89.4% of which were age 65 or over (https://data.cms.gov/summary-statistics-on-beneficiary-enrollment/medicare-and-medicaid-reports/medicare-monthly-enrollment). Without Medicare, many of these beneficiaries would not be able to afford healthcare.

Even with universal Medicare coverage, older adults face increases in medical debt and medical-related bankruptcies. In 2022, 22% of adults aged 65 and older had unpaid debt related to medical or dental care (Cottrill et al., 2024). In some cases, this can mean bankruptcy due to medical expenses. As one study notes, "Older Americans are increasingly likely to file consumer bankruptcy, and their representation among those in bankruptcy has never been higher" (Thorne et al., 2018). Drawing on court bankruptcy records, between 1991 and 2016 filing for bankruptcy increased threefold among people age 65 to 74 (from 1.2 to 3.6 per 1000) and 10-fold (0.3-1.3 per 1,000) for people age 75+. In this period, the proportion of people age 65+ among people filing for bankruptcy increased from 2.1% to 12.2%.

Without Medicare, medical debt and bankruptcy would be much higher. Unfortunately, Medicare is far from being a self-sustaining program. More than half the amount spent on Medicare was *not* funded through payroll taxes, but by federal income taxes on all Americans or carried over into the future as debt. Yet another concern is the increasingly expensive new technologies, treatments, and medications that may or may not result in lowered costs. Hepatitis C drugs are a best case scenario: They are effective and may lower overall medical costs in the long run, and the immediate costs are declining significantly. Having noted all these benefits, it is still a drug that is hugely expensive for both insurance companies and for the out-of-pocket expenses borne by beneficiaries. There are also new medications and treatments that do not have all the benefits of hepatitis C drugs and cost several hundred thousand dollars while providing only a few months of additional life.

Complicating the financial future even more is the Medicare prescription drug program, Medicare Part D, that was passed in 2006. It included a cynical, self-serving, and costly-to-taxpayers effort by lobbyists and legislators to make it illegal for the government to negotiate prices with the drug companies. This policy continues to inflate costs despite a Kaiser Family Foundation survey that found that 87% of Americans want Medicare to have the authority to negotiate greater discounts with pharmaceutical companies. The policy debate continues, with the first progress on insulin and selected drugs only in 2024.

The bottom line is that the percentage of our spending on healthcare is double that of what most European countries spend, and we do not get longer life expectancy or health expectancy. Part of the problem is that we have more than a 2-to-1 ratio of specialists to primary care physicians (PCPs), whereas in other countries the ratio is 1-to-1. Consequently, nearly 40% of primary care services are provided by specialists in the United States owing to the well-documented shortage of PCPs and willingness of specialists to take on this role.

Specialists not only get paid more, but they also use more expensive interventions. One such intervention is the MRI scanner. The United States has 4.2 times more MRI scanners than Canada, and our utilization of them has been astonishing (as explained under "Rationing"). This is one of many reasons why Medicare is such a costly program.

Escalating costs did not stop Congress from adding much-needed new coverages in 2019. First, Congress eliminated the cap on therapy coverage, including physical therapy, speech therapy, and occupational therapy. Second, Medicare coverage tiptoed into the domain of long-term care in the home (though limited to selected Medicare Advantage and special needs plans). The goal of these two new initiatives is to avoid excess hospitalization and premature nursing home care, and thereby save money while providing more services. Studies are in progress to determine their cost-effectiveness.

MEDICAID DUAL ELIGIBLES

Medicaid is the U.S. health insurance safety net for Americans with low incomes. It provides health coverage for 7.2 million older adults who are also enrolled in Medicare. It also covers 4.8 million younger people with disabilities, who may also enrol in Medicare. These "dual eligibles" include more than 15% of all Medicaid enrollees (Medicaid, n.d.).

Importantly, unlike Medicare, Medicaid covers long-term care and allied health services. These include skilled nursing care beyond Medicare's 100-day limit, eyeglasses, and hearing aids. Coverage for services provided by both programs is shared by the programs. However, since Medicaid is partly funded by states, and since states vary in the generosity of their Medicaid coverage, Medicaid enrolless can have very different access to health services depending on residence.

Chapter 10 describes long-term care programs covered by Medicaid.

THE AGING SERVICES NETWORK

Evidence-based health promotion programs for older adults are funded through Older Americans Act (OAA) funding, which is overseen by the federal ACL, which "was created around the fundamental principle that older adults and people of all ages with disabilities should be able to live where they choose, with the people they choose, and with the ability to participate fully in their communities" (https://acl.gov/). ACL differs from other federal aging entities in that its funding goes to networks of community-based organizations, mainly state and county units on aging, who administer health promotion programs and long-term care funding.

For example, since 1987 Title III-D of the OAA has provided funding to states and territories to support programs that promote health and well-being among older adults. A condition of receiving such funding is evidence of program efficacy. Programs need to be tested and rigorously evaluated. Since 2003, the ACL has developed a detailed review process, now administered by the National Council on Aging (NCOA; https://acl.gov/programs/health-wellness/disease-prevention). Some of the well-established evidence programs have been launched nationally and have reached millions of older adults. Key programs involve falls prevention, chronic disease self-management, nutrition, and behavioral health.

THE FUTURE OF HEALTHCARE IN THE UNITED STATES

Here are four general principles relevant to health promotion among older adults:

Principle 1: *Universal healthcare coverage*. Americans need to have access to heat during cold winters, food when hungry and broke, shelter from the elements, and healthcare—all of which are rights, not privileges. The ACA, still a political hotcake in the United States after more than a decade, was a step in the right direction when it comes to healthcare, reducing the proportion of Americans without access to healthcare to less than 10%.

Principle 2: *Affordable healthcare*. Private enterprise works well in many domains of life, but not healthcare. Every other industrialized country manages its care and its costs through single-payer systems, and they are all considerably less expensive than the United States model and are associated with higher life expectancies and health expectancies.

Principle 3: *Rational allocation*. Healthcare needs to be *rationed* intelligently. Every healthcare system in the world rations healthcare, so it might as well be explicitly stated through *ration*-al discussion. Before the ACA, the major way healthcare was rationed was quite heartless—to deny health insurance to 50 million Americans, except under dire circumstances in an emergency department. And those with preexisting medical conditions? They were denied healthcare insurance (unless saved by a covered spouse), or went broke attempting to purchase unaffordable insurance.

Principle 4: *Health promotion and disease prevention supported by community initiatives*. Every American needs to be literate in health promotion but should also have the opportunity to adopt health protective behaviors through supportive age-friendly communities.

The ACA made progress on these four principles, but the future will be filled with trade-offs. For example, will the United States continue to maximize healthcare innovation (a worthy enterprise), or perhaps reallocate some of these resources toward caring for low-income citizens like the French and British healthcare systems? Irrespective of the priorities of the future, all industrialized countries with the exception of the United States practice universal healthcare coverage that requires all citizens to buy health insurance, and utilizes their governmental bulk purchasing power to manage the costs of medical care, particularly medications. Japan and other countries have begun to extend this principle to long-term care insurance as well.

RATIONING

Healthcare costs without limits inspire reckless spending. For example, $100,000+ medical procedures were being done on patients who had 6 weeks left to live (Singer, 2009). If this type of care is desired, then the patient needs to assume the cost. When there were 62 million CT (computed tomography, or three-dimensional images from x-rays) scans in 2008 for a nation of only 300 million people, there needed to be sensible guidelines for utilization. Other countries allowed many fewer scans and still had better health and life expectancy results.

Perhaps we also need to limit the number of specialists we train, and give incentives to encourage more medical students into primary care. There were twice the number of specialists and twice the rate of use of medical technologies in New York City than in Albany, New York, and—you guessed it—Medicare spent twice as much treating each patient in New York City as in Albany. Yet the overall medical outcomes were the same.

We have allowed unlimited EKGs (electrocardiograms) in this country. For healthy people with no symptoms of heart disease, the EKG is more likely to lead to unnecessary medications or surgeries than it is to identify early disease. Excessive EKGs also drive up the number of unnecessary CT scans. We also do annual blood work for many people who feel well. This is expensive and will more likely lead to unnecessary and costly follow-ups than identify undiagnosed disease.

Evidence-based medicine suggests we offer medical screenings too frequently (e.g., Pap smears every year or two), too soon in the life cycle (e.g., mammograms in one's 40s) or too late in the life cycle (e.g., colonoscopies in one's 80s and beyond), and too routinely (e.g., prostate-specific antigen tests, now no longer recommended). ***Rationing*** on the basis of scientific evidence makes sense in a country with runaway medical costs.

Rationing does not mean that you cannot acquire the medical care that you want regardless of cost, if you can afford to pay for it on your own. If you want proton beam treatment, an expensive therapy for prostate cancer, fine; pay for it. Proton beam therapy requires a particle accelerator in a football-field-sized building, and costs Medicare $50,000 to $100,000. This therapy does not cure more people or reduce side effects; in fact, the side effects may be greater (Leonhardt, 2009).

And it is definitely not the cheapest alternative. A targeted form of radiation, for instance, is half the cost. Surgery to remove the prostate gland is even less, and watchful waiting costs only a few thousand dollars in follow-up doctor visits and tests. There are no studies to show that the high-technology treatment does better at keeping men healthy or keeping them alive longer. In fact, most of these men will die of something other than prostate cancer. Yet which option grew most rapidly? You guessed it. Proton radiation therapy usage rose 10-fold from 2002 to 2006, resulting in several billion dollars spent in a medically unjustified fashion.

Because these treatments are so profitable for the provider, it did not seem to matter that the nine existing proton beam centers were underutilized, and there were 20 more in the planning or construction stages (Emanuel & Pearson, 2012).

In 2008, Medicare paid for 480,000 injections for Avastin to treat macular degeneration, at a cost of only $20 million. It also paid for fewer injections (337,000) of Lucentis at a cost of $537 million. The National Eye Institute sponsored a 2-year clinical trial (2011–2012) with results that reported the cheaper Avastin was just as effective as Lucentis at preventing vision loss. There were no significant differences in mortality or morbidity rates. No one benefits—other than the drug maker—from Medicare's inability to limit more expensive, but not more effective, drugs.

When it comes to paying for huge amounts of care for small amounts of benefit, surveys of Americans consistently demonstrate *approval* of this inefficient policy. Two thirds do not support cost–benefit analyses for healthcare decision-making. Americans focus on themselves as the patient when asked questions regarding rationing, rather than as the person who is paying for inefficient additional medical costs for someone else.

Consequently, one quarter of all Medicare expenditures are spent during the last year of life (I should caution that only a portion of spending in the last year of life is wasteful spending), costing more than six times what is spent on other Medicare beneficiaries. Should we place a value on how much we are willing to spend to prolong an older person's life, or should there be no control at all on costs?

A simple (simplistic?) way to ration healthcare, one that is popular with Republican conservatives, is to implement vouchers at the individual level and/or block grants at the state level. Under a voucher system, each beneficiary gets a flat amount of money to spend each year on health coverage. If care exceeds that level, the cost is borne out of pocket. Under a block grant approach, states get a fixed amount of money from the federal government for a state's Medicaid program. If the state exceeds the amount given to it by the federal government, the states have a choice: Make up the difference, cut benefits, or scale back on who is eligible.

There is a more thoughtful approach to rationing: What specific benefits need to be reduced or increased to maximize healthy behaviors, to reduce unhealthy behaviors, to curb less vital but costly services, or to increase services that may be cost-effective in the long run? These thoughtful and difficult decisions tend not to be made with a voucher or block grant approach.

We have reached a point in the United States at which more than 50% of all the healthcare spending is now government spending (Medicare, Medicaid, and Veterans Affairs). If we cannot control these taxpayer-supported costs, it will crowd out funds for infrastructure maintenance, such as repair of roads and bridges. It will crowd out support for public school education. It will crowd out funds for public safety. And it will crowd out funds for medical research.

The key question is whether age should be used as a criterion for allocating health dollars. For example, should we limit healthcare access for people aged 80 or older, as Callahan (2008) argued? Would this apply to all people over age 80, or just those with severe medical conditions likely to die in some defined interval? Callahan realized the difficulty of establishing such an age criterion. Many 80+ individuals do well with complex surgeries and can have many more productive years. Many are still active, even working; and many are adding new entries to their autobiographies. Callahan suggested that people at these late ages have had a full life and are not entitled to excess medical care. But even accepting the first claim, it remains difficult to define "excess" medical care. Perhaps the best solution to this ethical challenge is a medical breakthrough that would reduce time spent with chronic conditions and remove the need for protracted periods of long-term care. This is the promise of geroscience and "senolytic" therapies that improve "healthspan" by slowing the rate of aging. But we are not there yet.

COMPETITION

Although ***competition*** in many commercial markets in the United States drives costs down, in healthcare it appears to drive costs up. Competition means additional costs for maximizing profits, for advertising among competing private plans, for exorbitant executive salaries, and for individual practitioners who need to hire staff to decipher the rules among multiple plans. None of these expenditures inspire improvements in healthcare quality.

The physician Benjamin Brewer reported that he had 301 different private insurance plans to deal with. He wrote in an online column for *The Wall Street Journal* that he had to employ two full-time staff members for billing, and two secretaries who spent half their time collecting insurance information. "I suspect," Dr. Brewer wrote, "I could go from four people in the paper chase to only one with a single-payer system" (Brewer, 2006).

Moreover, private insurers compete for healthier and less costly Medicare enrollees, thereby leaving more of the frail and costly beneficiaries for traditional Medicare to take care of. This policy leads to more profit for private insurers, which goes back into higher administrative costs rather than improved quality of care. Traditional Medicare spends less than 3% on administrative expenses, whereas large private insurers spend about 15% to 20%.

Individual for-profit companies are also less effective than a single payer at negotiating lower rates from hospitals, doctors, and pharmaceutical companies. Of course, even a single-payer system can fall victim to powerful lobbyists, as noted previously with Medicare Part D. The creation of this piece of legislation came with a ban on government negotiation of medication prices.

QUESTION: Are you against a market-driven, fee-for-service, profit-oriented healthcare system? Consider that markets, profit, competition, and other elements of capitalism have proved their worth over the years in contributing to quality products at affordable costs. Are there elements of capitalism that can be helpful in encouraging quality healthcare in America? Explain your answer.

Competitive care raises costs in the healthcare industry. It also makes it extremely difficult for the health consumer to figure out which healthcare plan among competing plans is the best one to suit their upcoming needs. It may sound good politically to give consumers "choice." But even if consumers were given educational assistance in making this choice, they would have to be clairvoyant to know which healthcare plan, with its unique set of benefits and costs, will best meet their medical needs for the coming year.

Managed Care

The U.S. Department of Veterans Affairs is a single-payer, managed-care system with an integrated delivery system, salaried physicians, and medical information that is coordinated and tracked electronically. Each physician has access to a detailed electronic record of every patient visit, test, medication, and procedure. It allows patients to access their electronic medical records as well, and encourages their interest and involvement in their own healthcare.

Kaiser Permanente has a similar coordinated system. This integrated managed healthcare consortium with its 10 million members is based in Oakland, California. For more than 70 years, it has adopted or developed cost-saving technologies and policies without sacrificing quality care.

Internationally, there are a variety of ***managed care*** practices that appear to be effective in each industrialized country, perhaps none more so than France. Their Ministry of Health, for example, determines budgets, regulates the number of hospital beds and equipment that needs to be purchased, establishes how many medical students are to be trained, and sets prices for procedures and drugs. How does their extensive managed care affect quality of care? A panel of experts compared the quality of healthcare among eight industrialized countries: Canada, Britain, Singapore, Germany, Switzerland, Australia, United States, and France. France came out on top (Carroll & Frakt, 2017).

MEDICATION

Medicare Part D

On January 1, 2006, ***Medicare Part D***, a medication reimbursement program, was launched. Unsuccessful with an attempt to privatize Social Security, Part D was a step for the Bush administration toward privatizing Medicare. A major component of this legislation was the inclusion of a mandated middleman, private insurers, to cover the cost of medications. These private insurers offer different premiums and copayments, and cover different drugs.

Beneficiaries need to figure out which private plan among many in their geographical area is best for them. One study reported that older adults were "very confident" that they had chosen the right prescription drug plan that minimized total annual cost, when in fact they had not (Hanoch et al., 2009).

QUESTION: There will likely continue to be quite a lot of ongoing change in our healthcare system. Where will we be 20 years from now? Will there be a single-payer universal healthcare system? What else might or might not happen by then? Why do you believe that?

Comparing the different plans is a complicated process. In 2006, investigators from the nonpartisan Government Accountability Office (GAO) placed 900 telephone calls to 10 of the largest companies offering drug coverage to Medicare beneficiaries. Insurers failed to provide complete and accurate cost information more than 70% of the time. Staff at the same insurance company gave different answers to the same question. Even when GAO investigators were able to correctly identify the least costly plan, the insurance representatives provided a quote that was less than the actual cost to the beneficiary. The GAO investigators found that some of the private insurers referred callers to a toll-free government telephone number, 800-MEDICARE (633-4227). The Medicare office, according to the GAO investigators, was able to give accurate answers to consumer questions only 61% of the time. Has the situation gotten any better in the past 20 years? Probably. But it is still a complicated process.

Complexity is only part of the problem; cost is an issue, too. Medicare Part D does not allow the federal government to negotiate lower prices directly from drug manufacturers. This has not been the case with another government agency, the U.S. Department of Veterans Affairs, which pays nearly 50% less for drugs overall than Medicare. As a consequence, immediately after Medicare Part D was passed, drug prices rose sharply by 3.4%—three times the rate of inflation at that point in time. Prices rose even more during the first quarter after the Medicare prescription drug benefit went into effect, by 3.9%, which was almost four times the rate of inflation for that quarter.

Prices did start to go down a couple of years later, but, according to analysts, not as a consequence of competition in the private sector. Instead, a number of lower cost ***generic*** drugs that had been released into the open market were having an effect. Nonetheless, in comparison with five countries—Australia, Canada, Germany, New Zealand, and the United Kingdom—Americans were more likely to fail to fill a prescription medicine, or to take it regularly, because of its cost (Monaghan, 2006).

An added benefit to the pharmaceutical industry that was negotiated by lobbyists was the transfer of 6.5 million dual-eligible, low-income elderly and younger disabled poor from the lower paying Medicaid program to the higher paying Medicare Part D program. It is estimated that pharmaceutical companies received an additional 30% for comparable prescription drugs than they did through Medicaid, with which it was possible to negotiate, and achieve, deeply discounted drug prices. This led to a $2 billion annual windfall from this transfer—paid for by the American taxpayer.

Much of the formulation for Medicare and Medicaid public policy was created by lobbyists, rather than by the efforts of nonpartisan analysts. A congressional aide who helped write Medicare Part D, John McManus, formed his own lobbying firm the year after its passage and received $620,000 from drug companies and trade associations. Thomas Scully, the chief administrator of Medicare, was a hospital industry lobbyist *before* being appointed, and a lobbyist for the drug companies *after* he left government upon the passage of Part D. He was given a special ethics waiver to make this quick transition.

A leader on Capitol Hill in the creation of Part D, Representative Billy Tauzin, left Congress once Part D was passed to become the well-paid president (with a pay package estimated to be over $2 million a year) of a powerful drug industry lobby, the Pharmaceutical Research and Manufacturers of America.

Drug companies lobbied intensely in the development of this legislation. The healthcare industry spent $325 million to influence Congress, with drug companies leading the way with $87 million. Families USA, the major voice for healthcare consumers, spent $40,000. AARP attempted to influence the legislation in favor of the healthcare consumer, but it had a divided loyalty. After Part D was passed, AARP and its partner, the United Healthcare Insurance Company, quickly became the number one insurance provider of medications through Part D.

QUESTION: If we become more responsive to the healthcare needs of older adults, we will probably provide better healthcare for people of all ages in America. What do you think is the logic behind this belief?

The lobbying efforts paid off not only for insurers and drug companies but also for current Medicare consumers. They went from no help with medication costs to help. Consequently, 68% reported that they were better off than they were before they had Part D coverage. Researchers from a RAND Corporation study reported that the poor and disabled were the major beneficiaries, with lower out-of-pocket spending for prescription medications and an increase in the number of prescriptions filled.

While most agree that Medicare Part D has been good for beneficiaries, basic changes to the law are needed—especially giving Medicare the authority to negotiate drug prices and making it less complex so that the average consumer (or even the superbright one) can calculate which plan is best for them. Medicare even includes a counseling program to help guide consumers to optimal plans. Did I mention I prefer a single-payer, managed-care system?

Patented Versus Generic Drugs

A cheaper generic drug can come on the market only after a patent expires on a drug that has the same active ingredients. ***Generic drugs*** usually cost 60% to 90% less than brand-name versions, and the prices fall more as each new competitive generic drug enters the market. Unfortunately, drug companies producing brand-name medicines are able to pay generic drug makers to delay the marketing of less expensive generic products. These anticompetitive *pay-for-delay* settlements keep generic drugs off the market at the expense of American consumers.

And here comes more bad news. Generic drug costs started to go up in 2014 for no apparent reason. The cost of many generic drugs had increased so much during that year that prices for many common generic drugs in the United States have surpassed those of their brand-name equivalents in other developed countries—by a lot. One extreme example was Lannett, which raised the price of generic digoxin by nearly 1,000%!

With the federal government hog-tied by lobbyists, states are showing initiative. A law in Maine allowed residents to mail-order prescription drugs from licensed pharmacies in Canada, Britain, Australia, and New Zealand. These pharmacies have a comparable safety record to the United States and offer drugs that are jaw-droppingly less expensive. These practices continue to be challenged in court.

According to Angell (2004), in her book *The Truth About the Drug Companies: How They Deceive Us and What to Do About It,* few new drugs contained active ingredients that would make them better than drugs already on the market to treat the same condition. Of the 78 new drugs that the Food and Drug Administration (FDA) approved in 2002, for instance, only seven were truly innovative, and not one of those came from the major American pharmaceutical companies.

Rather than the $800 million on average that the drug companies claim it costs to bring out a new drug, these "me-too" drugs are likely to cost a small fraction of that amount. Nexium, for instance, was a me-too ***patented*** drug that took the place of Prilosec, which went generic and was reduced in price. Nexium was heavily advertised as something new and improved, and this expensive drug was promoted through such modalities as television and print advertising, and through "education" for—or marketing to—physicians ("academic detailing"). Spending on marketing and administration constitutes about 30% of pharmaceutical costs.

Effective lobbying is what allows drugs like Nexium to continue to be compared to placebos during clinical trials, rather than being compared to existing drugs on the market. If a new medication had to be superior to an existing drug, many could not be successfully navigated through clinical trials to gain FDA approval.

AND, BRIEFLY, OTHER PUBLIC HEALTH AND AGING POLICY CONCERNS

Leaning once again toward the side of a strong federal or state government role in promoting the health of an aging society, here are my *Top Ten* public health policy and aging ideas:

1. *Tobacco.* Now that tobacco is regulated by the FDA through the Family Smoking Prevention and Tobacco Control Act, it is important that the FDA set new standards to reduce the nicotine content of cigarettes and to regulate chemicals in cigarette smoke. Smoking in all public places should be banned throughout the United States. Federal and state taxes on tobacco products should continue to increase. E-cigarettes should be regulated to make sure they are safe, out of the hands of minors, and not a gateway drug to tobacco products.
2. *Alcohol and Cannabis.* Remove federal penalties on the latter and treat both the same. Raise federal excise taxes on both and use revenue to promote responsible usage. Establish guidelines for acceptable THC levels in the blood for driving.
3. *Physical Activity and Exercise.* For the benefit of future cohorts of older adults, require daily physical education classes in elementary through high school, and provide exercise options so that children can engage in the physical modality they

enjoy. Give recognition—perhaps through certification as a *heart-friendly location*—to shopping malls that promote walking and stairway use, communities that promote the use of bicycle and walking paths, and worksites that promote exercise for sedentary employees. Require commercial building codes to include safe, attractive, and accessible stairways (i.e., build stairwells in the centrally located sites where most elevators are now situated, pipe music into them, and hang attractive artwork on the walls). Recognize and reward transportation planners who shift their focus from cars to bike paths and sidewalks.

4. *Nutrition.* For the benefit of future cohorts of older adults, pass an amendment to the National School Lunch Act that mandates nutritional standards for all food and drinks sold on school premises, including cafeterias and vending machines, and at school-related events. Prohibit the marketing of junk foods directed at children. Add a 1-cent tax on high-fat, high-sugar, and high-salt junk foods, and use the resources for health-promoting initiatives. Require all restaurant menu boards and menus to state the caloric content of foods and drinks in a noticeable way. Set limits on the amount of salt allowed in processed foods and restaurant meals. Change nutrition labels so that sugar is included in the percentage of the daily value that they represent, and, most significantly, *apply the percentage to the specific product* (e.g., "this product is 40% sugar"), and not just to the daily intake for the day. Limit the sugar content of certain products such as breakfast cereals or else relabel them (e.g., "breakfast candy"). Shift federal agriculture subsidies from grain farmers to fruit and vegetable growers. Develop statewide policies to expand and support farmers markets that sell locally grown organic food.
5. *Geriatric Medicine, Nursing, and Allied Health.* There was an initial burst of enthusiasm in the 1970s when geriatric training programs were established, and again in 1988 when the first examination in ***geriatric medicine*** was administered. Thereafter, many physicians who were grandfathered in for a period of time, and who needed to take the examination to remain qualified, opted not to do so, and the number of physicians specializing in geriatrics began to decrease—from 8,800 board-certified geriatricians in the United States to 6,950 in 2018 (with only 3,590 full-time practitioners). Currently, the United States has only 7,100 board-certified geriatricians and only 8,220 practicing geriatricians. Since 30% of older adults would benefit from geriatrician-managed care, this workforce is clearly inadequate for meeting the demands of geriatric care (https://www.americangeriatrics.org/geriatrics-profession/about-geriatrics/geriatrics-workforce-numbers). A mere 250 geriatric fellowships are available annually and some go unfilled. The benefits of geriatric training and comprehensive geriatric assessment are clear. For example, one study reported that geriatricians were more efficient than other physicians in managing hospitalized older patients, with shorter lengths of stay and lower costs per admission (Sorbero et al., 2012).

   The best way to increase the supply of geriatricians is to provide better reimbursement for "high-touch" medicine versus "high-tech" procedures, and to elevate the income of geriatricians, who have been consistently ranked as one of the lowest-paid medical specialties. In the short term, something similar to the proposed *Geriatricians Loan Forgiveness Act* would also help. This Act, if passed, would forgive $35,000 of educational debt incurred by medical students for each year of advanced training to obtain a certificate of added qualifications in geriatric medicine or geriatric psychiatry. More standardized geriatric training across all medical specialties would be helpful as well.

   Equally challenging is the nursing shortage in our healthcare system—a deficiency that directly affects the quality of geriatric care, given the importance of nursing to the field of geriatrics. To provide more nurses trained in geriatrics to hospitals, clinics, and nursing homes, there is a need for higher pay for faculty with geriatric training in schools of nursing.

The same shortages plague geriatric physical and occupational therapy, pharmacy, dentistry, audiology and speech therapy, paramedicine, and related fields. Obstacles to training, certification, and reimbursement should be eased too.

6. *Geriatric Research.* The problem of meager funding for geriatric training spills over into the ***geriatric research*** arena as well. There is a need for increased funding for geriatric research to evaluate the effectiveness of preventing, delaying, or treating geriatric syndromes. There is also a need for health-promoting counseling and other behavior-changing strategies focused on helping older adults with such goals as remaining active and managing medication use judiciously. An innovative research initiative would be to evaluate whether older adults can become effective public health advocates, particularly in the areas of environmental protection and strengthening elementary school education.

   When health behavior change strategies are supported by research, incorporate these health strategies into Medicare—and encourage state legislatures and private healthcare plans to mandate reimbursement for them as well.

   In 2019, the National Institutes of Health implemented a new policy that required grant applicants to explain how they intend to include people of all ages, or provide justification for any age group left out. But what justifications are they accepting? Many research studies bar participants with multiple disorders or who are taking multiple medications (i.e., mostly older adults) or state an upper age limit of 75 or 80 for eligibility. When is it justified to exclude some or all older adults on the basis of eliminating confounding variables?

7. ***Comparative Effectiveness.*** Comparative effectiveness began as an important research consideration in the ACA. This term refers to research that provides unbiased information to make the best medical choices for a given patient. Congress, through the ACA, set aside a down payment of $1.1 billion to improve medical decisions that affect patients, a disproportionate number of whom are older. Despite the persuasive logic of such a program, lobbyists of all stripes are seeking to discontinue this program to determine best medical practices, as these decisions may negatively affect the practices and products they represent. Comparative effectiveness decisions need to be shielded from lobbyists.

   Destructive lobbying has been effective in the past. In December 2002, a rigorous research trial, costing $130 million and involving 42,000 patients over 8 years, produced what appeared to be solid evidence that generic diuretic pills for high blood pressure cost only pennies a day and were more effective and safer than newer drugs that were 20 times more expensive. However, pharmaceutical giants making big money on patented hypertension drugs managed to suppress the purchase of the inexpensive diuretics over the following 6 years. Their strategy consisted of heavy marketing of patented drugs, highlighting the limitations of their generic competitor's research results (no studies are flawless), and paying pharmaceutical representatives to convince physicians that the studies were fatally flawed. Only after some of the patents expired on the expensive hypertension drugs did the pharmaceutical companies relent (Pollack, 2008).

   A more general example of the need to evaluate effectiveness and cost-effectiveness is provided by the Dartmouth Atlas study of Medicare beneficiaries. There are large regional differences in spending and utilization that do not improve quality of care (Sutherland et al., 2009). In high-spending areas, Medicare patients are seen by physicians more often, are admitted to hospitals more frequently, and are the recipients of more screening tests of unproven benefit than in low-spending areas. Patient outcomes are not improved in the high-spending areas, and older adults do not feel they are being denied necessary care in the low-spending areas.

8. ***Age Discrimination at Work.*** Discrimination of any type (e.g., on the basis of gender, race, religion, age) is bad for worker health. There are eight types of discrimination prohibited by law, and redress involving age discrimination has the lowest success rate—14%—when it comes to charges filed with the Equal Employment Opportunity Commission.

   In a 5-to-4 ruling in 2009 (*Gross vs. FBL Financial Services*), the Supreme Court shifted the burden of proof in cases of age discrimination at work. Previously, if a worker could show that age was *one* of the factors in a layoff or other adverse employment decision, the *employer* was required to show it had acted for a legitimate reason and not on the basis of age bias. Now, the *worker* must bear the more difficult burden of proving that age was the *deciding factor*. Congress needs to act once again to pass a bill, the *Protecting Older Workers Against Discrimination Act*, to reverse the 2009 Supreme Court decision that has guided the lower courts to apply this onerous standard of proof to deny thousands of age-discrimination claims.

   Adults age 55 and older constituted 12% of the total workforce in 1990, but make up 25% of the U.S. workforce in 2024, according to the U.S. Bureau of Labor Statistics. An AARP survey in 2018 noted that 61% of workers over age 45 reported that they had seen or experienced age discrimination in the workplace. Strategies such as advocacy and education, therefore, are not likely to be sufficient for protecting the older worker. Legal action is important to prevent employers from forcing workers to retire simply because of age, rather than because of reduced ability and desire. This is an injustice that is not good for the mental health of older adults and can limit potential contributions of older workers to society. Moreover, the burden of proof for older workers who claim age discrimination should be the same as for workers who claim discrimination on the basis of gender or race.

9. ***Income Security.*** Low income and poor health are strongly correlated, and both depend on a solvent Social Security system. Eliminate the maximum amount of earnings that can be subjected to the Social Security payroll tax, and include state and local government workers who are now exempted from Social Security payments. This will go a long way toward making Social Security solvent and preserving a safety net for low-income elders. Social Security needs to live up to its name and be secure. Conversely, privatization of Social Security not only entails huge start-up costs, but would also make Social Security payments less predictable in the future.

   Require employees to opt out of their retirement program rather than requiring them to opt into it; currently less than half of eligible workers in organizations that offer 401(k) plans actually enroll in them. Eliminate the option of, or place restrictions on, lump-sum removal of retirement benefits when one is changing jobs or at any time prior to an age that makes one eligible for Social Security benefits.

   So-called registered or certified financial advisors for older adults, who now may obtain this title through minimal educational effort, should be required to pass a universal accreditation standard for financial advisors working with older Americans.

10. ***Student Loan Debt.*** This is not a misprint; it is a tip of the hat to my young students who struggle with debt. Most do not know that this is also an intergenerational problem that has to be resolved. The total outstanding older adult loan debt grew in 2005 to $18 billion in 2013, or 4% of households headed by people ages 65

to 75, up from less than $3 billion, and 1% of older households. This debt and percentage will continue to soar if nothing is done. Twenty percent of these loans were cosigned for children going to college, 80% for one's own education. Modify the current failed student loan system with the following: (a) give low-income students a 5-year grace period; (b) allow loans at excessive interest rates (compared to the current interest rates) to be refinanced; (c) limit loan payments to 10% of the current income level; and (d) levy fines on for-profit educational institutions that market heavily in place of an adequate budget for classes, teachers, and material, or have low student graduation rates.

OREGON: A MODEL STATE FOR HEALTH PROMOTION LEGISLATION

Here are 16 legislative examples from ***Oregon as a model state*** that show how policy can promote health in old age.

1967—A bill designated Oregon's beaches as public highways, resulting in the creation of many coastal state parks for recreational and meditative purposes, and granting public access to its residents to the entire coastline.

1971—The "Bottle Bill" required that deposits collected on beverage containers when sold in Oregon be refunded when containers are returned empty. Many other states followed suit to encourage recycling, reduce litter, extend landfill capacity, and decrease the incidence of glass lacerations.

1973—Oregon decriminalized simple possession of marijuana, from a jail sentence to a fine, which was followed by several other states in order to reduce the arrests of young people and to better use the limited resources of law enforcement. Legalization came 42 years later.

1973—An Oregon bill required every city and county to prepare a comprehensive land use planning program to comply with statewide goals. Farmers prevented suburban sprawl and private developers from infringing on the finite valley's agricultural industry. A number of states later developed similar statutes for growth management.

1981—Oregon was the first state to acquire a Medicaid waiver to create foster care homes and assisted living facilities as alternatives to nursing homes. Oregon continued to rank first per capita in nursing home alternatives.

1990—The Physician Orders for Life-Sustaining Treatment (POLST) was developed in Oregon. It is accessible in emergencies and continues to be adopted by other states.

1994—The Oregon Health Plan implemented a novel system of allocating scarce Medicaid funds to cover more poor residents. It prioritizes medical services through an independent commission that receives public input. It is more popular in good financial years than bad ones.

1994—Death with Dignity in Oregon was the first state legislation to legalize physician-assisted dying. The basic requirements in the legislation are being replicated in a growing number of states.

1998—Oregon was the first state to institute a medical marijuana registry, along with its Medical Marijuana Act, to coordinate the medical use of marijuana.

1998—Oregon became the first state in the nation to require all elections be conducted by mail. Expanding voting access can be thought of as a community mental health issue.

2006—Oregon became a national model for significantly reducing methamphetamine abuse by requiring key ingredients to become prescription drugs, expanding drug treatment, and reducing doctor shopping.

2009—Oregon became the first state to make POLST electronically accessible in emergency situations.

2011—Oregon made one more failed attempt at single-payer health insurance. Yes, it failed, and yes, Oregon was *not* the first state to propose a single-payer system. But it is the most persistent advocate for a single-payer system, with 2011 being its latest, and likely not last, attempt.

2015—Legalization of recreational marijuana. It remains to be seen how health promoting this is, but almost all agree that the war on drugs, and this drug in particular, has been a failure.

2015—With the New Motor Voter legislation, Oregon encourages voting by reducing the burden of voter registration. Interaction with the Department of Motor Vehicles results in a ballot being mailed to the resident for elections, unless the resident opts out.

2017—Oregon phases-in its pioneer state-run retirement plan. All private employers without a retirement plan (which included over 50% of the Oregon workforce) must register for the program. Employees can opt out of a 5% default retirement option (or change the rate). Employers are not required to make a contribution.

SUMMARY

Even the most enduring public policy and aging-related legislation, such as Social Security—about 90 years old and definitely geriatric—requires constant refinement in order to be responsive to changing needs. Another major piece of legislation, Medicare, is both age-related and aging over more than a half century, and requires constant attention if it is to survive and prosper in the coming years.

Related to Medicare is the ACA, which could be a bold step toward Medicare for All or some other legislation that implements universal access to healthcare and extends both life expectancy and health expectancy. Or the ACA could be repealed and replaced by something as bad as what we had before it was implemented. In case we forget, pre-ACA was marked by 50 million Americans without health insurance, denial of coverage for preexisting conditions, and runaway healthcare costs.

Many age-related public policies and legislation are in need of nurturing, change, or elimination. Our nation's stance toward geriatric medicine and geriatric research is lukewarm at best. Age discrimination in the workplace is alive and, unfortunately, robust. Medical bankruptcies are increasing among older adults. And even student loan debts impact on older adults who cosigned them.

On the bright side, long-term care policies have become more flexible and are encouraging interesting alternatives. Death and dying issues are being addressed, and more humane legislation is proliferating. And, to circle back to the beginning of this summary, we have had two pieces of major legislation, Social Security and Medicare, that have improved the lives of millions of Americans and have lasted more than a half century.

REFERENCES

Only key references appear in the print edition. The full reference list can be accessed by visiting www.springerpub.com/courseconnect. See inside front cover and tear-out card for CourseConnect details.

Administration on Community Living. (2024). *2023 profile of older Americans*. https://acl.gov/sites/default/files/Profile%20of%20OA/ACL_ProfileOlderAmericans2023_508.pdf

Callahan, D. (2008). *Setting limits*. Georgetown University Press.

Cottrill, A. Neuman, T., Lopes, L., & Hamel, L. (2024). *What are the consequences of health care debt among older adults?* Kaiser Family Foundation. https://www.kff.org/medicare/issue-brief/what-are-the-consequences-of-health-care-debt-among-older-adults

Freed, M., Biniek, J. F., Damico, A., & Neuman, T. (2024). *Medicare Advantage in 2024: Enrollment update and key trends*. Kaiser Family Foundation. https://www.kff.org/medicare/issue-brief/medicare-advantage-in-2024-enrollment-update-and-key-trends

Murphy, S. L., Kochanek, K. D., Xu, J., & Arias, E. (2024). *Mortality in the United States, 2023*. NCHS Data Brief, No. 521.

Thorne, D., Foohey, P., Lawless, R. M., & Porter, K. M. (2018). *Graying of U.S. bankruptcy: Fallout from life in a risk society*. Indiana Legal Studies Research Paper No. 406. http://doi.org/10.2139/ssrn.3226574

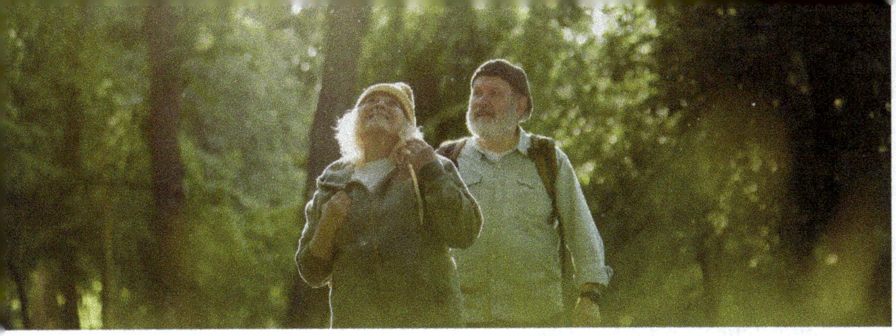

12

DIVERSITY AND AGING

KEY TERMS

acculturation
African American older adults
aging and the international cinema
Asian and Pacific Islander older adults
Chinese older adults
crossover phenomenon
culture
cultural competence
dependency ratio
ethnogeriatrics
global aging
Hispanic [Latinx] older adults
Japanese older adults
legalized gay marriage
lesbian, gay, bisexual, transgender, queer, and others
minority, racial, ethnic, or disadvantaged groups
Native American older adults
sex and gender differences
rural aging

LEARNING OBJECTIVES

- Analyze the role *culture* plays in health communication and health policy.
- Analyze the relationship between diversity and discrimination.
- Define culture, *cultural competence,* and *ethnogeriatrics.*
- Discuss the distinctions among the terms minority, race, ethnicity, and disadvantaged.
- Describe the health status of *African American, Hispanic American, Asian American,* and *Native American/Alaskan Natives older adults* in the United States.
- Discuss the reasons there may be a *crossover phenomenon.*
- Describe the differences between sex and gender.
- Examine how LGBTQ+ baby boomers may change aging institutions.
- Describe the process involved with the legalization of gay marriage.
- Describe the challenges facing rural older adults.
- Examine *global aging* and contrast old age in developed and developing countries.
- Examine the problems of *Chinese* and *Japanese older adults* and their caregiving family members.
- Discuss the role that the international cinema can play in improving the understanding of aging and old age.
- Compare aging men and women in the United States.
- Evaluate the recommendation that there should be demographic categories for the young old, the middle old, and the old old.
- Discuss the chronological age marker that you believe best delineates old age.

Diversity is not about how we differ. Diversity is about embracing one another's uniqueness.

—*Ola Joseph*

CULTURE AND PUBLIC HEALTH POLICY

Culture has been defined as our entire nonbiological inheritance. Among those who believe that cultural differences among older adults are at least as important as socioeconomic differences are the academicians who refer to themselves as ethnogeriatricians. The field of ***ethnogeriatrics*** focuses on the ability to provide healthcare in ways that are acceptable to older adults to ensure they are congruent with those persons' cultural backgrounds and expectations.

One study concluded that when the ***cultural competence*** of the healthcare organization is compatible with clients' perception of cultural need, cultural congruence leads to better treatment outcomes (Costantino et al., 2009). Specifically, when older Latinx clients received mental health services from culturally competent clinicians, depression, anxiety, and suicidal thoughts declined. To achieve cultural congruence or consonance may require modification of intervention programs and modes of delivery (Falgas-Bague et al., 2021).

One topic of particular interest to ethnogeriatricians is the degree to which the ***acculturation*** of the older person—the internalization of mainstream cultural values, beliefs, language, and skills—affects healthcare and health behavior. In other words, to what extent does identification with one's ethnic category affect one's belief in allopathic medicine and the efficacy of scientific treatments; one's ability to work with a healthcare provider of a different cultural background; one's need for dependence on family for decision-making in healthcare; one's belief in control, or lack of, over health outcomes; and one's willingness to negotiate with a complex medical bureaucracy?

Communication between persons with different cultural identification can be problematic. Some people prefer a slower pace of conversation in a healthcare setting, whereas others prefer a fast-paced conversation and expect to be interrupted. Some patients prefer close physical proximity when communicating, whereas others prefer to be at arm's length. Some cultures prefer eye contact, whereas others may consider this disrespectful. Some cultures value stoicism or mask their emotions with laughter or a smile, whereas others encourage open expression of pain, sorrow, and joy. The etiquette of touch, hand gestures, and finger pointing is highly variable across cultures. There is also a diversity of attitudes toward the subjects of death and dying, ranging from a preference for direct communication to the belief that these topics are inappropriate for discussion.

Communication is also hampered by the lack of appropriate foreign-language access in medical clinics and healthcare settings around the country, as cited in the Institute of Medicine's (IOM) report on unequal medical treatment. This situation is particularly burdensome for Latinx older adults, because 40% do not speak English.

Without widespread training in cultural competency, access to good healthcare is hampered. Practitioners remain ignorant of traditional medicine being practiced by patients, attitudinal barriers to allopathic medicine, ethnic diets, and health beliefs and practices that differ from the mainstream (Haber, 2005). State licensing boards are taking steps to reduce healthcare disparities and to make sure that healthcare professionals are more responsive to cultural and language differences among their patients.

MINORITY, RACE, ETHNIC, AND DISADVANTAGED GROUPS

Minority groups refer to subgroups within a population that are subject to discrimination, usually on the basis of race or ethnicity. The National Institutes of Health's (NIH) National Institute of Minority Health and Health Disparities recognizes the link between minority populations and health disparities:

> A health disparity is a health difference that adversely affects disadvantaged populations in comparison to a reference population, based on one or more health outcomes. All populations with health disparities are socially disadvantaged due in part to being subject to racist or discriminatory acts and are underserved in health care. (https://www.nimhd.nih.gov/resources/understanding-health-disparities/minority-health-and-health-disparities-definitions.html)

In the setting of a quickly growing diverse older population (***African American, Asian, Native American, Pacific Islander, Hispanic [Latinx] older adults),*** clinical services and aging policies will increasingly need to address these health disparities. Between 2022 and 2050, the non-Latinx White population is projected to decline from 75% to 60% (U.S. Census Bureau, 2023).

Racial and ethnic groups have definitional problems as well. ***Racial groups*** are categories based on parentage and physical appearance. Typically, skin color, hair texture, and face shape are its determinants. Yet race is increasingly problematic because of widespread intermingling, travel, and genetic diversity. It is a fluid construct, more the product of the human mind than nature. Nonetheless, the term continues to be used, and data continue to be collected.

Ethnic groups include those who share a cultural heritage, ancestry, history, homeland, religion, ritual, diet, appearance, and so forth—in other words, a hodgepodge of characteristics that do not all remain distinct among groups. Despite its vagueness, this term continues to be used, sometimes in combination, such as identifying one's racial/ethnic category.

The U.S. Census Bureau struggles with these categorizations as well. People of Middle Eastern descent, for instance, were considered White by federal census officials, whereas people from India, once classified as White, were placed into the Asian category. Latinx people are now considered an ethnic group, not a race. The situation was even more confusing in the 1960s, when the U.S. Census Bureau did not even count Latinx people separately, Asian Indians were classified as White, and many in the general population did not consider the Irish, Italians, and Eastern European Jews to be White.

Multiracial identification is also problematic. The 2010 census form allowed Americans to select more than one racial or ethnic category. However, when the Pew Research Center surveyed those who identified as multiracial, 29% at one time had identified themselves as single race. Conversely, 61% of the people whom Pew defined as multiracial identified themselves as just one race. Nearly 7 million Americans took the opportunity to identify themselves as a blend of two or more races. This category of multiracial, available for the first time in 2000, was selected by 2.4% of the country's population. In the 2010 census, this increased to 3%—though President Barack Obama stated at that time he was not one of the census participants who chose this category.

Though most biologists and anthropologists now deny the legitimacy of creating distinct racial and ethnic categories, the reality for older adults in America is quite different. The categories are in widespread use, and large amounts of data are collected by way of these categories and are useful in policy-making.

Another term to use with diverse populations is ***disadvantaged groups***. Older people disadvantaged by income and education do not engage in medical screenings in a timely manner and seek treatment later in the course of their disease. They are less likely to follow a treatment plan, more likely to cut back or discontinue medication because of cost, and have higher disease severity, disability, and mortality (Fuller-Thompson et al., 2009; Link & McKinlay, 2009).

As an example, type 2 diabetes patients who are disadvantaged by education and income are more likely to have problems reading prescription bottles, educational brochures, and nutrition labels. Consequently, they have more difficulty with blood sugar control and experience more diabetes-related complications than persons with higher income and literacy levels (Schillinger et al., 2002).

Environment can also be a disadvantage. Low-income older adults are worried about the safety of walking in their neighborhood, with less access to safe parks and recreational facilities. They have less access to fresh fruits and vegetables, which are often too costly when available.

DISPARITIES IN HEALTH AND HEALTHCARE

The IOM, an independent research institution that advises Congress, reported in March 2002 on the first comprehensive examination of racial disparities in healthcare among people who have health insurance. Previous studies reported on the lack of access to healthcare by racial/ethnic groups, as well as on how their lifestyles contribute to poor health. This study tackled the delicate issue of prejudice in healthcare.

The report reviewed more than 100 studies conducted over a decade and concluded that racial disparities contributed to higher death rates among minorities. It cited that minorities were less likely to be given appropriate medications for heart disease; less likely to be offered bypass surgery, angioplasty, kidney dialysis, or transplants; less likely to receive the most sophisticated treatment for HIV infection; and more likely to have lower limbs amputated as a result of diabetes (Stolberg, 2002). Some of these differences are longstanding. For example, the risk of leg amputation from complications of diabetes and peripheral artery disease is highest in the southeastern United States, areas with the highest proportion of slave labor some 150 years ago (https://features.propublica.org/diabetes-amputations/black-american-amputation-epidemic/). Why these disparities persist is less clear, but reasons include disproportionately fewer physicians of color serving the population, the limited resources of medically underserved communities, and bias based on low expectations of compliance with follow-up care.

DISTRIBUTION OF RACE/ETHNICITY GROUPS AGED 65+ IN THE UNITED STATES

According to the U.S. Administration on Community Living (2024), in 2023 25% of people 65 and older were members of racial or ethnic minority groups. Using U.S. Census racial categories, 9% were African American, 5% Asian American, 0.6% American Indian and Alaska Native, and 0.1% Native Hawaiian/Pacific Islander). Less than 1% identified as members of two or more races. People indicating Latinx origin (who can indicate any race) represented 9% of the older population.

This distribution should be distinguished from the proportion of people age 65+ within ethnic or racial groups. Within racial and ethnic minority populations, 11% were 65 and older compared to 22% of non-Latinx Whites, with 13% of African Americans, 14% of Asians, 11% of Native Hawaiian and Other Pacific Islanders, 14% of American Indian and Alaska Natives, 8% of Latinxs, and 6% of people indicating two or more races.

As a global measure of health status, self-rated poor or fair health (as opposed to good, very good, or excellent) indicates important disparities among older people by race and ethnicity. In 2019, about 40.3% of African Americans age 65+ and 35.5% of Latinx older adults rated their health as fair or poor in contrast to about 20% among White and Asian older adults (National Health Interview Survey, 2021).

African American Older Adults

Differences by race and ethnicity reflect a combination of differences in risk (based largely on socioeconomic factors), access to medical resources, and effective treatment. A review of cancer incidence shows the effect of this mix of disparities. While African Americans have a slightly lower incidence of any cancer than Whites, their mortality from cancer is higher, suggesting important differences in access and high quality treatment and follow-up. Differences tracked in the Surveillance, Epidemiology, and End Results (SEER) program from the NIH National Cancer Institute are shown in Table 12.1. The African American experience is similar to Native Americans. Asian/Pacific Islanders; Latinx populations do better on this measure of disease burden.

Treatment differences are almost certainly responsible for some of these differences. For example, African Americans are 27% less likely to get stroke-preventing medicines

TABLE 12.1 CANCER INCIDENCE AND DEATH RATES (PER 100,000) BY RACE/ETHNICITY

RACE/ETHNICITY	RATE OF NEW CASES	U.S. MORTALITY RATE
All Races	440.5	146.0
Hispanic	351.0	106.8
NH American Indian/Alaska Native	425.5	159.7
NH Asian/Pacific Islander	304.1	93.0
NH Black	452.1	168.6
NH White	471.8	151.3

Source: SEER 22, 2017–2021, Age-Adjusted Rate per 100,000/year. NH, non-Hispanic. https://seer.cancer.gov/statistics-network/

for atrial fibrillation, even in analyses controlling for socioeconomic differences (Essien et al., 2018). They are more likely to die after major surgery than White patients, controlling for patient characteristics such as severity of illness (Lucas et al., 2006). African American hospital patients have higher mortality than non-Blacks after abdominal aneurysm repair owing to their receiving care in lower quality hospitals that have fewer resources (Osborne et al., 2009).

Physicians who treat Black patients tend to have less clinical training and less access to important clinical resources (Bach et al., 2004). In yet another study, Black patients were found to be more likely than Whites to have a less experienced surgeon, and more likely to have complications from surgery to remove blockages from the carotid arteries (Halm et al., 2009).

Nursing homes remain relatively segregated, roughly mirroring the residential segregation within metropolitan areas. As a result, Blacks are much more likely than Whites to be located in nursing homes that have serious deficiencies, lower staffing ratios, and greater financial vulnerability (Smith et al., 2007). They are less likely to have access to and take advantage of hospice services,

QUESTION: **Black older adults appear to have the greatest amount of homogeneity among the four minority categories recognized by the U.S. Census Bureau. Is that an advantage or disadvantage when it comes to community advocacy? Why?**

On the bright side, for reasons not clearly understood, there is evidence of a ***crossover phenomenon*** for minorities relative to Whites. For example, once Blacks reach age 85, the remaining life expectancy for Blacks and Hispanics is higher than that of Whites, suggesting selection effects, in which minorities reaching very old age represent a genetically favored group that has survived high risk of earlier mortality. Some doubt, however, has been thrown on this finding based on errors in birth certificates.

Interestingly, caregiving appears to be less of a mental health burden on Black grandmothers who are raising grandchildren in their households compared with White grandmothers. A study of 867 grandmothers reported that Black grandmothers are more likely to embrace the prospect of raising grandchildren and consider this an important role in holding kin networks together (Pruchno & McKenney, 2002). In addition, older

African Americans may be better able than Whites to cope with the death of a spouse (Elwert & Christakis, 2006). This may be due in part to family connections, as older Black adults are much more likely to live with relatives, or it may be a consequence of having deeper ties to religious life and more emotional support from fellow church members.

Hispanic American Older Adults

Hispanic Americans (*Latinx* is the preferred term in some areas recently became the largest minority group in the United States. They are not homogeneous, in that they include Mexican Americans (49%); Cuban Americans (15%); Puerto Ricans (12%); and people from Central America, South America, and Spain (25%). Although the Hispanic populations share the Spanish language, there is much diversity in their dialects, their ability to speak English, and length of time spent in the United States.

Latinx in general have high rates of heart disease, diabetes, and cancer. This tends to be exacerbated by poor eating habits, smoking, lack of exercise, and excessive alcohol use. This vulnerability is enhanced by a language barrier that is experienced by many Latinx (Johnson-Kozlow et al., 2009), especially those with a lower acculturation level (Janz et al., 2009).

Latinx benefit from eating a higher proportion of traditional foods that are rich in fiber and complex carbohydrates, such as chickpeas, fava beans, pinto beans, plantains, cassavas, sweet potatoes, mangoes, guavas, papayas, and corn tortillas. Even in Mexico, however, the traditional diet of fresh foods is vanishing and is being replaced by imported fast foods, home-grown junk foods, and soft drinks.

Barriers to participation in community health promotion programs among primarily Spanish-speaking Latinx older adults include the following:

- Many Latinx older adults are unfamiliar with senior centers, whereas others who visit the centers find the programs to be culturally insensitive.
- Latinx physicians, followed by Spanish-speaking or bilingual health professionals, are preferred but are in short supply. The belief in folk medicine and divine healing power can often result in the postponement of timely doctor visits.
- Lack of experience with the American healthcare system, compounded by financial limitations and lack of transportation, constitute a major barrier to timely healthcare services.
- The most credible source of health information for Latinx older adults is Spanish-language television and radio—40% of Latinx elderly speak Spanish only—followed by the extended family, churches, community groups, and Latinx social clubs and organizations.

Health education programs need to involve the extended family, in both program development and implementation. Program presenters need to be sensitized to the spiritual beliefs and folk medicine of Latinx older adults and, when possible, to focus on ideas from both folk and Western medicine. The role of the *curandero*, a traditional healer who provides physical, psychological, social, and spiritual support for the Latinx family (not just the individual), should also be understood and incorporated into health education programs. Curanderos believe that morbidity and mortality are associated with strong emotional states, such as *biles* (rage) and *susto* (fright).

Latinx women who care for older relatives with dementia delay nursing home placement relative to White caregivers (Mausbach et al., 2004). The delay probably reflects cultural values that emphasize the importance of family and the expectation that family members will care for each other. Participants in the study also report greater benefit from, or more positive aspects of, caregiving. Latinx women who were more acculturated to U.S. society, however, are more likely to institutionalize their relatives.

Asian American and Native Hawaiian/Pacific Islander Older Adults

Asian Americans and Native Hawaiians/Pacific Islanders encompass at least 16 ethnic and cultural groups, many of which have little in common in terms of language, culture, religion, and immigration history. The largest group of older Asian Americans is Chinese (30%), followed by Japanese (24%), Filipino (24%), Korean (8%), Asian Indian (5%), and other backgrounds (Vietnamese, Cambodian, Laotian, Hmong, Thai, Pakistani, and Indonesian). The largest group of Pacific Island Americans is the Hawaiians and Samoans, followed by Polynesians, Micronesians, and Melanesians. Many other smaller islands could be included as well.

It is difficult to generalize within this diverse group. The poverty rates for older Japanese, Filipino, and Asian Indian Americans are low, whereas the poverty rates for older Southeast Asians are very high, reaching 47% among the Hmong older adults. Within this diverse group is the highest proportion of people with less than a ninth-grade education, but also the highest proportion of those with a bachelor's degree or more.

Interestingly, the prevalence of diabetes in this diverse ethnic group is more than double that of Whites, and this prevalence holds up regardless of body weight. The higher prevalence applies to native Hawaiians, who suffer from high rates of obesity, as well as to the Japanese, who have a relatively low body weight (Maskarinec et al., 2009).

Among Southeast Asian Americans, less than 5% of the population is age 65 or over because the refugee experience limited the number of older adults who could immigrate, and some still have not reached age 65 since their arrival. The percentage of Japanese older adults is expected to grow due to current limits on the immigration of younger persons from Japan.

After the Japanese attack on Pearl Harbor in 1941, 110,000 Japanese Americans living in the Western states were incarcerated. It is believed that many of these now-elderly Japanese Americans tried to suppress their Japanese ancestry, often teaching their children to do the same. This is one example of the dramatic differences in the life experiences of older adults among the various Asian American and Pacific Islander ethnic groups.

Asian and Pacific Islander cultures traditionally emphasize the importance of family bonds and the unquestioned authority of elder family members. The extent to which younger family members abide by these traditional values and beliefs, however, is varied. In fact, among Southeast Asian Americans, the traditional family roles are often reversed. More than 85% of older adults live with younger family members, the latter providing almost all of their economic and social support. This transfer of authority to the younger generation is one example of the difficulties that these older adults have had in adapting to American culture.

The proportion of middle-aged Americans providing caregiving support varies by race and ethnicity. According to the National Alliance for Caregiving and AARP's *Caregiving in the U.S.* survey (2015), Latinx (non-White, non-African American) have the highest proportion of family caregivers (21%), followed by African Americans (20.3%), Asian Americans (19.7%), and Whites (16.9%). Asian Americans and other minority groups are more likely to provide caregiving support than Whites.

Yet the erosion of family caregiving support over the past decades has been revealed in other ways. Vietnamese older adults, for example, are now being placed in nursing homes in America, something that was not condoned 20 years ago.

An interesting alternative that has begun to emerge in the Asian American community is *ethnically oriented assisted living facilities*—sprouting up across America, from Seattle to the Lower East Side of Manhattan—that cater to older Asian immigrants (Kershaw, 2003). These facilities provide ethnic foods, like miso soup, soba noodles, and dark-roasted teas, which are staples of the older Japanese American diet; and traditional games such as mahjong and rummikub. Even among Asians who were brought up to believe that they have a duty to take care of their aging parents in their homes, assisted living facilities that provide ethnic support for older residents are becoming an increasingly attractive option.

QUESTION: **Vietnamese older adults are now being placed in nursing homes in America, something that was not condoned 20 years ago. From the perspective of Vietnamese adult children caregivers, do you think this trend is a positive or negative contribution to their lives? Why do you believe that?**

Native Americans/Alaskan Natives Older Adults

Native Americans/Alaskan Natives are defined by the Bureau of the Census as American Indians, Eskimos, and Aleuts. As members of 562 federally recognized tribes (and about 100 nonrecognized tribes), they are exceptionally diverse both culturally and linguistically.

A study by the National Indian Council on Aging found that at age 45, reservation-dwelling Native Americans/Alaskan Natives had the health characteristics of the average American at age 65. Urban-dwelling Native Americans demonstrated these elderly characteristics at age 55.

Because many do not live long enough to develop them, Native Americans/Alaskan Natives have less heart disease and cancer than the general population, but have more pneumonia, influenza, diabetes, accidents, chronic liver diseases, septicemia, gallbladder disease, and hypertension (Butler et al., 1998). Since 1955, the Indian Health Service has focused its resources on treating infectious and acute diseases that occur in infancy through young adulthood, with few resources available for managing the chronic diseases of aging.

There is widespread poverty among Native Americans/Alaskan Natives, and as recently as 1984, 25% of them lived in households without plumbing. ***Native American/Alaskan Native older adults*** have a work history of high levels of unemployment and low-wage jobs, with 65% having worked as semiskilled workers, unskilled workers, or farm workers. Only about 22% graduated from high school, and 12% have no formal education at all.

SEX DIFFERENCES

Sex in survey research refers to biological attributes, male or female. ***Gender*** refers to the psychological and cultural aspects of being male, female, or self-identified in another way. This section focuses on sex differences.

As the population ages, it becomes decidedly more female. Life expectancy at birth in 2022 for a male born in the United States was 74.8 years, and that of a female was 80.2 years (Kochanek et al., 2022), a decline from previous years because of the COVID pandemic and increases in "deaths of despair" (deaths from opioid overdose, substance abuse, firearm violence, and suicide).

Though women are more likely to reach older ages, the prevalence of disability is consistently higher among women than among men. More than half of women age 70 and older report difficulty with mobility, such as walking across a room or climbing stairs, compared with 36% of men. Women age 70 and older are more than twice as likely as men (57% vs. 28%) to have difficulty with routine strength activities.

In addition, older women have higher rates of illness, physician visits, prescription drug use, acute illnesses, and chronic conditions. Among the chronic conditions that both women and men can acquire, osteoporosis is the most unfair to women, who represent 80% of those with the condition. Men, however, are more likely to encounter life-threatening acute conditions and to require hospitalization (Hooyman & Kiyak, 2011). Thus, Medicare, with its emphasis on hospital coverage and its weaknesses in providing long-term care, favors men.

Older women are more likely to be unpaid caregivers. Older wives are more likely to care for their spouses than are older husbands. Among adult children who care for their elderly parents, about 75% are daughters. And about two thirds of grandparents raising grandchildren are women.

The greater responsibility for caregiving is due primarily to cultural expectations. Society expects women to leave the workforce when family obligations beckon. The current cohort of older women has been considered the primary caregivers for family members, whereas men have been considered the primary breadwinners.

Unpaid caregiving responsibilities and lower wages for women are complicated by widowhood. Because women generally marry men older than themselves, live longer, and infrequently remarry in their 50s and older, it follows that more than three times as many women age 65 and over are widowed in contrast to men. Consequently, it is not surprising that women are more likely to experience economic insecurity in old age than are men.

According to the 2022 Profile of Older Americans, men age 65+ had a median income of $37,430 compared to $24,630 for women. The poverty rate of older women was 11.2% versus 9.0% for men. The average monthly Social Security benefit was 25% smaller for women than for men. As noted by the late Tish Sommers, founder of the Older Women's League, "Motherhood and apple pie may be sacred, but neither guarantees economic security in old age." This economic disparity, however, will diminish in the future if the higher percentage of women graduating from an institute of higher education results in the lessening of the wage disparity between the sexes.

Despite some of the disadvantages that accrue to women, older women are more health conscious and more resilient. They are more likely than men to have a regular physician, almost three times more likely to have seen a physician in the past year, and more likely to seek immediate medical care if they are sick or in pain (Shelton, 2000). They are also more likely to eat a healthful diet and to take a supplementary vitamin pill. In addition, older women have more frequent social contacts and more intimate relationships compared with older men.

Perhaps some combination of these factors contributes to greater resiliency and a lower likelihood of committing suicide. Between the ages of 65 and 69, male suicides outnumber female suicides by four to one; by age 85, this ratio increases to 12 to one.

It seems ironic that for many years clinical research trials sponsored by the NIH focused almost exclusively on male subjects, though men in general demonstrated little interest in their own health. This practice of excluding women from clinical trials was ended in 1991 by Dr. Bernadine Healy, the first woman to head the NIH. Also in 1991, Dr. Healy created the Office on Women's Health in the Department of Health and Human Services. There has been no interest on the part of male leadership to create a counterpart office. While women's health centers are commonplace in the community, men's health centers are a rarity.

A final note on the sex and age issue: Not only do differences between men and women increase with age, but aging women themselves are becoming more diverse. An article in the *Journal of the American Medical Association* reported that there is now no medical reason for excluding women in the sixth decade of life from attempting pregnancy on the basis of age alone (Paulson et al., 2002). No group is more diverse than women in their 60s, some of whom are new mothers, some of whom are grandmothers, and some of whom have never mothered.

QUESTION: Women live longer, are better connected socially, and commit suicide less often in late life. In contrast, they appear to have more health and financial burdens. Who is better off in America, older women or older men? Why?

LGBTQ+ AGING

LGBTQ+ is the commonly used acronym for ***lesbian, gay, bisexual, transgender, queer, and others.*** This topic does not appear in many gerontology textbooks (including, unfortunately, the first four editions of this book) or research articles in gerontology journals. This is beginning to change because the baby boomers started to become the gerontology boomers in 2011 and will become more visible in the gerontology field regarding LGBTQ+ issues (Haber, 2009).

It was not until 1973 that homosexuality as a pathological disorder was removed by the American Psychiatric Association from the *Diagnostic and Statistical Manual of Mental Disorders (DSM).* This was followed by a similar reversal by the American Psychological Association in 1974 and the beginning of a strong LGBTQ+ pride movement. In the scientific community, being gay was finally declared normal. One can argue, though, that these events in the early 1970s came too late for many adults who are of the silent generation (born between 1927 and 1945). Subsequent lifestyle and attitude changes, as well as advocacy efforts, would prove to be more difficult for them to embrace.

Now, as a cohort fast becoming gerontology boomers—the leading edge of the boomers reached age 65 in 2011—they are likely to be very different than the prior cohort of older adults in their willingness to advocate for more supportive age-related programs, organizations, agencies, and services. If the boomers are more likely to assert their rights as older LGBTQ+ Americans, it will be essential that healthcare professionals in the gerontology field become aware of practices and policies in community organizations and service agencies that affect the quality of their life.

Lesbians and Gay Men

A Gallup poll reported that 7.6% of Americans identify as lesbians or gay men (https://news.gallup.com/poll/611864/lgbtq-identification.aspx). Thanks to the aging of the large cohort of baby boomers and generation X (born 1965–1980), the number of older LGBTQ+ Americans will double by 2029 (Jackson et al., 2008). The 2024 Gallup poll estimates 2.3% of baby boomers and 4.5% of generation X identify as gay.

Today's older gays grew up in an environment where in they were vilified as sinful and considered undeserving of constitutional protection. They were "viewed as perverted by society, evil by the church, sick by the medical and psychiatric professions, and criminal by the police" (Reid, 1995, p. 217). Many of today's older lesbians and gay men have internalized these negative cultural attitudes and beliefs (Orel, 2004). The oppression and disempowerment that older lesbians and gay men have endured has unquestionably affected their mental health and, for many, their physical health as well.

A survey of 2,560 LGBTQ+ adults aged 50 to 95 across the United States revealed greater rates of disability, depression, and loneliness, and increased likeliness to smoke and binge-drink compared with heterosexuals of similar ages (Fredriksen-Goldsen et al., 2012). A survey of California gay and bisexual men between the ages of 50 and 70 reported higher rates of hypertension, diabetes, physical disability, and psychological distress than similarly aged heterosexual men (Wallace et al., 2011).

Another major concern for gay and lesbian older adults is the lower probability of support from significant others who live with them. Singlehood in late life is correlated with a variety of negative physical and mental health outcomes (Blank et al., 2009). A study by Anderson (2008) of gay older adults reported that they were twice as likely as nongay older adults to live alone in the latter part of the life cycle, four times less likely to have children to help them, and half as likely to have a significant other or close relative to call on for help.

The tragic decimation from AIDS in the 1980s and 1990s inspired several positive trends, such as a growing number of long-term monogamous relationships, the mass community outreach that took place during the mid-1980s, a wide spectrum of community services that humanized the face of a deadly epidemic, and acceptance and integration into one's neighborhood (Knauer, 2009).

Caitlyn Jenner

What a difference a year can make, especially if that year was 2015. The Supreme Court ***legalized gay marriage*** (to be discussed shortly) in 2015 (*Obergefell v. Hodges*), and that same year Bruce Jenner, winner of the men's decathlon in the 1976 Olympic Games, transgendered into Caitlyn Jenner. This latter phenomenon was significant for two reasons, one gerontological.

Research shows that gender identity has a basis in the brain (Kranz et al., 2014), and one's preferred gender can be mismatched with one's anatomy. The stress from this mismatch, referred to as *gender dysphoria*, can be alleviated by sexual reassignment. But given issues of harassment, discrimination and violence, and mental health impacts, it is also strongly associated with increased risk for premature death (Dhejne et al., 2011).

From a public health policy perspective, it should be noted that 41% of transgender and gender nonconforming individuals attempt suicide at some point in their lifetime (Friedman, 2015). Thus, there is an urgent need for better psychiatric care that begins as soon as gender dysphoria is recognized and does not cease if the person has chosen sexual reassignment.

Of particular gerontological interest is the fact that the 65-year-old (when she revealed her sexuality) Caitlyn Jenner did not come out as an *older* woman. Despite the fact that she was the oldest woman ever shown on the cover of *Vanity Fair* (and the photographer, Annie Leibowitz, was also age 65), her appearance was altered to look like a 35-year-old sexpot. So not only were all aspects of maleness removed from the magazine cover, so were all aspects of age.

Christine Jorgensen in 1952 became the first widely publicized person to have undergone sex reassignment surgery, in this case, male to female, creating a worldwide sensation. But it was not until Caitlyn Jenner's groundbreaking effort and courage to publicize her transition in 2015 did transgender people begin to rapidly gain acceptance in American society. Perhaps we should give a pass to that magazine cover, but underlying her message of acceptance for transgender people was a sad message of nonacceptance of aging.

LGBTQ+ Discrimination

More than a third of LGBTQ+ youth have been victimized by an immediate family member or by their peers at school. By the time they reach old age, the likelihood of victimization at home, in school, at work, or in the community by acquaintances or strangers, is very high. The fear and stress of expecting discrimination or experiencing actual discrimination can lead to low self-esteem, depression, involvement with risky sexual partners, alcohol abuse, drug abuse, and other types of victimization (Balsam & D'Augelli, 2006).

Access to programs and services is hampered by sexual orientation, including entrée into senior centers, meal programs, food stamps, domestic-violence shelters, counseling programs, and medical care. A study conducted by the U.S. Department of Health and Human Services reported that LGBTQ+ seniors are only 20% as likely to access needed services.

A survey of federally funded Area Agencies on Aging revealed that half of the senior centers would not welcome gay men and lesbians if their sexual orientation were known, and 72% of LGBTQ+ older adults reported that they were tentative about using such services, with only 19% participating in a senior center (Knauer, 2009). The Equal Rights Center investigated senior housing facilities in 10 states and found that 50% of the time the facilities were more likely to discriminate against research testers posing as same-sex spouses, than as opposite sex couples (Span, 2018). For the same-sex spouses, there were more burdensome application requirements, higher prices quoted, and fewer rental units offered.

Gelo (2008) reported that only 25% of gay older adults are completely open about their sexual orientation to healthcare workers. The average medical school allocates less than half a day within the 4-year curriculum to LGBTQ+ issues (Bonvicini & Perlin, 2003). Even LGBTQ+ boomers are highly skeptical and fearful of the medical profession caring for them in an unbiased manner (MetLife Mature Market Institute, 2006). LGBTQ+ discrimination is *slowly* declining—with a strong emphasis on the word "slowly."

Legalization of Gay Marriage and Its Consequences

On May 9, 2012, President Barack Obama became the first sitting president to endorse the legalization of same-sex marriage. Then came the Supreme Court decision in June 2015 that legalized gay marriage nationwide. And while considerable prejudice and discrimination remain, along with a need for more and better agency service and staff training programs, this one act unleashed many legal rights for the LGBTQ+ community.

These rights include eligibility for Social Security spousal benefits, as well as for 401(k) and other pension plans, health insurance, and inheritances associated with one's spouse. There is also Medicaid protection for the assets and homes of same-sex marriage partners; eligibility for the Family and Medical Leave Act, which guarantees 12 weeks of unpaid leave to employees to care for family; hospital visitation rights; filing of joint tax returns; and every other marital right previously denied to the LGBTQ+ community.

LGBTQ+ Community Programs

Services and Advocacy for Gay Elders (SAGE) is a model community program in New York City and now national clearinghouse. It links LGBTQ+ seniors in the five New York boroughs to innovative clinical and social services, including professional social workers for crisis intervention and ongoing assistance. Other services provided by SAGE include support groups, programs targeted at HIV/AIDS patients, volunteers who provide a wide range of assistance to older LGBTQ+ adults, a friendly visitor program, and training and workshops. A SAGE educational initiative encourages self-reflection and an examination of culture and society for the purpose of creating a more meaningful aging experience. The curriculum covers fears of aging, changing self-definitions, sexuality and aging, losses and gains with aging, religion and spirituality, physical and mental health, and community building. An online resource lists LGBTQ+-friendly housing options. Check out the National Resource Center on LGBTQ+ Aging, www.lgbtagingcenter.org.

Many of SAGE's programs are being replicated by community programs throughout the United States. SAGE also encourages local advocacy through professional conferences and workshops conducted nationwide. One of the goals of SAGE is to increase practitioner sensitivity and to provide information on how agencies and organizations can create policies and practices that support LGBTQ+ older adults. SAGE released a guide called *Inclusive Services for LGBT Older Adults: A Practical Guide to Creating Welcoming Agencies.*

The American Society on Aging (ASA) sponsors the LGBT Aging Issues Network (LAIN). This network's goal is to raise awareness about the concerns of LGBTQ+ older adults and the unique barriers they encounter in gaining access to housing, healthcare, long-term care, and other needed services. It provides online information on brief news items, a variety of informational sources, and timely announcements at www.asaging.org/lain.

Gerontologists of all stripes—educators, researchers, and practitioners—need to be sensitive to the needs and aspirations of the coming cohort of LGBTQ+ boomers.

RURAL AGING

While the overall percentage of people living in rural areas is declining compared to urban and suburban populations, the percentage of older adults is increasing (***rural aging***). About 17.5% of the rural population was 65 years and older compared to 13.8% in urban areas in 2012 to 2016 (Smith & Trevelyan, 2018). Living in a rural area increases the probability of living in poverty; income levels for older rural families are about one third lower than those for older urban families. Food stamps are disproportionately obtained by rural families, with 31% of rural grade-schoolers getting a free or reduced-price lunch versus 25% of urban grade-schoolers.

Rural living is associated with a higher ratio of convenience stores stocked with less variety and fewer healthy foods than supermarkets; substandard and dilapidated housing; a larger number of health problems; greater likelihood of living in a community without a doctor, nurse, or medical facility; inadequate caregiving support complicated by the migration of children to cities in search of work; challenging transportation issues due to longer distances to drive to needed services; lack of public transportation and poor roads; and greater likelihood of having an attitude of distrust toward the healthcare system or to have been instilled with an attitude of independence and self-reliance and a reluctance to demand needed health services (Health Resources and Services Administration [HRSA], 2002; National Rural Health Association (NRHA) blog, June 7th, 2019).

According to a 2017 Centers for Disease Control and Prevention report on potentially preventable deaths, rural Americans are far more disadvantaged than their urban counterparts. This holds true for heart disease, diabetes, stroke, cancer, respiratory diseases, and unintentional injuries.

Nurses, social workers, physicians, and other health professionals are in short supply in rural settings. This is due in part to health policies, such as lower reimbursement rates for health providers in rural settings (based on a formula where operating costs are assumed to be less), but also to the lack of community and healthcare resources in many rural locations. Health professionals are concerned about locating in rural areas that may lack quality public schools, cultural opportunities, job opportunities for a spouse, and sophisticated hospital equipment. Consequently, there are 10 physicians per 10,000 people in rural areas, compared to 31 per 10,000 in urban areas, according to a 2015 report by the NRHA.

Older adults who live in rural areas receive fewer services per home healthcare visit, and have poorer health outcomes than their city-dwelling older adult counterparts (Schlenker et al., 2002). These findings may represent accommodation of rural home health providers to rural realities, such as the lower availability of certain healthcare personnel like physical therapists or longer travel distances.

On a variety of measures, rural populations are in poorer health and at higher risk for poor health due to harmful health behaviors. Adults living in rural areas are more likely to smoke and have limited activity levels owing to chronic conditions (HRSA, 2002), have a higher rate of self-reported depression, and have a more negative self-appraisal of health (Thorson, 2000) than their counterparts in urban areas. To top it off, obesity rates are greater in rural areas, along with diabetes, cardiovascular disease, and arthritis (Lundeen et al., 2018). Disability, however, is comparable (Smith & Trevelyan, 2018).

Rural Resources

The *Rural Health Information Hub* makes referrals to federal and state agencies, provides publications, and serves as a clearinghouse for rural information. It provides a repository of rural information on more than 225 different federal health programs and additional private programs. The website includes searchable databases, congressional bill tracking, and quarterly newsletters. Contact the Rural Health Information Hub, www.raconline.org.

Inquiries can also be directed to the Office of Rural Health Policy, HRSA, 5600 Fishers Lane, Rockville, Maryland 20857; https://www.hrsa.gov/rural-health.

The *National Rural Health Resource Center* is a nonprofit organization that provides technical assistance, information, tools, and resources for the improvement of rural healthcare. Contact the National Rural Health Resource Center, Duluth, MN 55802; www.ruralcenter.org.

QUESTION: If you were launching a health promotion program for older adults, what are some of the details you would need to consider that are unique to a rural setting?

GLOBAL AGING

The average age of the world's population is increasing at an unprecedented rate. Between 2009 and 2040, the percentage of older adults will double from 7% to 14% of the total world population, according to the U.S. Census Bureau. Although *developed countries*, those with the most economic development, have the largest proportions of

FIGURE 12.1 Population aged 60 or over: World and developing regions, 1950–2050.

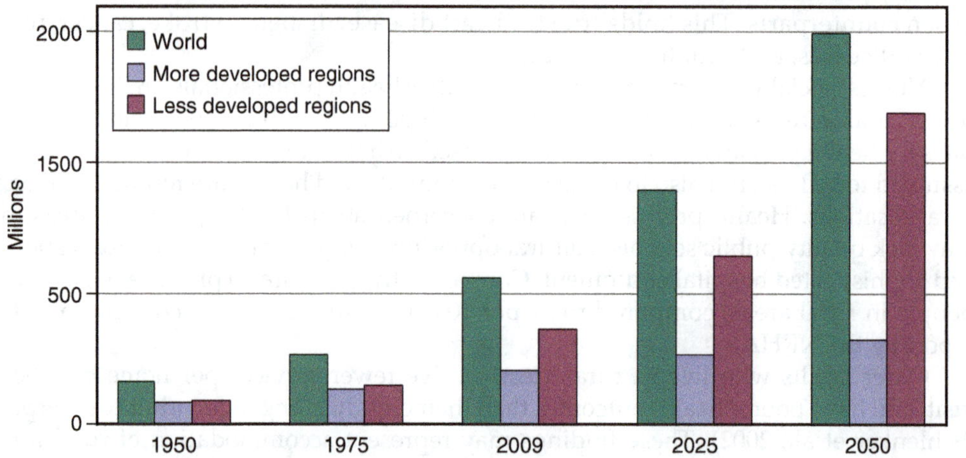

Source: United Nations. *World population aging, 1950–2050*. Author.

older people—of the 25 countries with the oldest populations, 23 are found in Europe—*developing nations* have the most rapidly growing senior cohorts.

Figure 12.1 highlights this differential growth. In 1950, there were 205 million people worldwide age 60 and over, which tripled to 606 million people between 1950 and 2000. It is projected to increase to almost 2 billion people worldwide by 2050; in other words, more than tripling again.

However, in developing countries, the growth rate is quite a bit faster during this century, reaching 15 times the population it was in 1950 compared to the projected population in 2050, versus only a fourfold increase during that century for developed countries.

The major source of diversity in ***global aging*** is whether a country is economically developed or not. In addition to the greater growth in older adults among developing countries, there is a much lower standard of living. This translates into almost a 20-year difference in life expectancy between India, a developing country, and Sweden, a developed country.

The increase in the percentage of older adults in developing countries presents additional challenges for the future. Demographers note that developed countries were rich before they got old, but less developed countries are getting old before they have a chance to get rich. While there is a rise in the number of countries with old-age disability or survivors programs, it is not keeping pace with the growing number of older adults in developing countries.

Thus, these developing countries may have to rely even more heavily on a less prosperous informal network of family and community to support their burgeoning older adult population.

China's Older Adults

Let us look at one rapidly developing country, and that is China. China has the world's largest older adult population with 201 million adults aged 60 and above in 2015, which is projected to increase to 479 million in 2050 (Wu et al., 2018). Owing to a significant decline in both fertility and adult mortality rates, persons age 65 and over constitute 11.4% of the Chinese population, and that percentage is projected to rise to 34% by 2050.

But as the number of older Chinese increased, the number of caregiving children was declining dramatically as a result of the *One-Child Policy*—a policy that limited married couples in urban areas to one child. This policy was implemented in 1979 to slow the rapid growth rate and the rising poverty level at that time.

However, for most ***Chinese older adults***, social security means relying on extended family. Seventy percent of Chinese older adults are supported by their families, and only 16% rely on the government's troubled pension system. Yet China's traditional extended family is dispersing more rapidly than ever before, and grown children are now leaving their elder parents to fend for themselves.

In 2013, China eased its one-child policy because there were too few adult children to provide caregiving assistance to their older adults. Married couples that included one parent who was an only child could have a second baby. However, because of the rising cost of child-rearing combined with rising expectations of a higher standard of living, only about half of eligible couples opted for a second child. In 2015, the policy was expanded: All married couples were allowed to have two children.

Another law instituted that same year also had trouble taking hold, perhaps because it was vague and a bit bizarre for the Chinese culture to accept. Adult children are required to visit their elder parents on a regular basis or risk being sued by the parent and fined by the government. The law, however, does not specify how often they must visit or what the penalty might be. A vague threat of detention, whatever that might mean, is also part of the law.

This law, called *Protection of the Rights and Interests of Elderly People*, was created in part because a survey found that 12% of young respondents had not visited their parents in years, and more than one third saw them just once a year. *Filial piety*, respect for older adults and ancestors in Confucian philosophy, which is arguably the most hallowed of traditional virtues in Chinese society, has now been converted from a moral obligation into a legal obligation.

About half of the 185 million people age 60 and older live far apart from their children, and most have needed to migrate to urban areas for employment. Owing to travel expense and work schedules, it will be difficult to enforce extra visits home, which for many young working adults only occurs during the Lunar New Year holiday.

Yet another public policy change is set to be launched in rural China, called *Mutual Assistance Eldercare*. With dwindling adult child caregiving support and a weak or nonexistent formal eldercare system in rural areas, the government is encouraging rural older adults to help those who are even older. The challenge with this policy is to have somebody in their 60s caring for somebody in their 90s, when there are medical and physical challenges, not to mention limited training. Like other initiatives, it does not seem adequate for the job.

Neither the villages nor the government can afford institutional care for every frail rural elder, but the problem of impoverished frail older adults in China is too big to ignore. Between 2016 and 2018, for instance, 200 nursing homes were built in China. This number was wholly inadequate, but even these few homes were finding it difficult to attract enough staff to take the low-paying jobs, and the work was deemed too unattractive by most young Chinese adults. And, unlike America, there were few immigrants to help out.

Another initiative that related to health insurance was passed in 2016, and launched the following year. Almost 6 million rural families that were impoverished by illness-related expenses qualified for lower copayments in 2017. In addition, 30,000 urban-based doctors were sent to perform medical duties in poverty-stricken areas. These types of healthcare initiatives will need greater resources in the future to deal with a growing population of rural older adults with increasing medical and long-term care needs.

Japan's Older Adults

Japan, a developed country, has a different set of healthcare challenges for their older adults. In 2016, Japanese women were the longest-lived in the world, with a life expectancy of 86.8 years. Japanese men were sixth in the world with a life expectancy of 80.5 years. There were 68,000 centenarians in Japan in 2017, an increase of almost 60,000 over the prior two decades. Japanese demographers predict that *more* than half of Japanese babies born in 2018 will live to be 100!

In the meantime, with 28% of the population over the age of 65 in 2018, and the time-honored tradition of adult children living with and caring for ***Japanese older adults*** weakening, two trends occurred: (a) The number of Japanese seniors living alone or with just their spouse doubled over the prior decade; and (b) the cost of government assistance to the elderly increased more than 70% over the prior decade, amounting to 12% of Japan's annual gross domestic product.

Smaller families, combined with adult children seeking jobs in cities, lead to lack of space, desire, and financial ability to care for parents in urban settings. Although many retirees are drawing pensions, fewer and fewer working-age people are paying into them. Consequently, premiums are expected to rise in Japan at the same time that older adult benefits are to be curbed.

There is also a shrinking pool of caregivers that is only beginning to get worse. In 2018, Japan suffered the largest natural population decline ever recorded. There was a record low birth rate that year, and the highest post-World War II death rate.

When asked: "How much of a problem is the growing number of older people in your country?" Japan topped the list, with 87% agreeing it is a major problem. China was third, with 67%, and the United States was near the bottom with 26% (2013 Pew Research Center Global Attitudes Project Survey).

Japanese policymakers have responded with a series of important initiatives, including universal mandatory long-term care insurance, a national structured geriatric assessment tool that assigns level of care needs and generates care plans delivered by local municipalities, and innovative community-based lay-led social and volunteering programs. Japan leads the world in social assistance robots to support dementia caregivers. People with dementia can attend (and even work in) the "Restaurant of Mistaken Orders," which allows people with and without dementias to mix.

Older Adults in the United States

Developed countries face the challenge of an aging population with substantial healthcare and long-term care needs. As the number of working-age persons relative to each older adult shrinks, we are learning about the magnitude of the economic strain that this dependency produces. The ***dependency ratio*** is the ratio between those not in the labor force (the dependent part of the population, mostly under age 15 and over age 65) and those in the labor force (the productive part).

QUESTION: What are the lessons that developed and developing countries can offer each other when it comes to both the role of older adults in society and the care of these older adults?

This changing ratio has the potential to incite conflict over funding for increasing pensions and healthcare for older adults, versus a country's need to support public schools and unemployment benefits for younger adults.

Yet while the United States has been getting older, the dependency ratio has been offset substantially by the absorption of many young immigrants. The ratio between those who are economically dependent and those who are economically productive in the United States is declining more slowly than in countries that are aging without much immigration. This has slowed down the reduction in overall workers contributing to Social Security and Medicare.

This trend delays the inevitable crisis in the United States, but does not prevent it, especially with pressure to limit immigration. As the dependency ratio inevitably increases, along with the huge baby boomer cohort reaching their 80s and older—prime decades for needing assistance—the shortage of home health aides and personal care assistants in long-term care settings will become ever more acute.

To find out more about international policy and research into aging, a free biannual e-mail newsletter, *AARP International*, can be obtained by contacting AARP's Office of International Affairs at www.aarpinternational.org. The World Bank is also a valuable resource, including its unlocking healthy longevity initiative (https://www.worldbank.org/en/topic/health/publication/unlocking-power-healthy-longevity).

Aging and the International Cinema

The June 2006 issue of *The Gerontologist* reviewed an English film called *Ladies in Lavender* (2004), about an older woman who converted a potentially foolish love experience into one of self-knowledge and inner peace. The journal also reviewed *Autumn Spring* (2003), a Czech film about an older husband full of mischief and an older wife ready to disengage from life and how they reconcile.

Another international film reviewed in the October 2012 issue of *The Gerontologist,* the Iranian film *A Separation,* tackled several themes, including the challenge of middle-aged caregiving for an increasingly frail parent. *Amour,* which won the Palme d'Or in 2012, the highest prize awarded at the Cannes Film Festival, was about an octogenarian couple facing their mortality.

Since then, it has become commonplace for gerontological films to gain international recognition. Too many, in fact, to summarize here (though I include an abbreviated and "dated"—I like to think of them as classics—list of films in Box 12.1). I encourage you to take advantage of these cinematic opportunities to learn about cross-cultural aging.

THE DIVERSITY OF AGING

Because this is a book about aging, but mostly about being old, it is perhaps tardy to define the term at the very end of this book. But there is a reason for this. I am uncertain about the definition of old and I preferred not to reveal my ignorance any sooner than I had to. To understand the meaning of old, it helps to have a number. And wouldn't you know it—the onset of old age has been located anywhere between the ages of 40 and 85. What follows are examples of the broad range of chronological ages that have been used to identify the term old.

- At age 40 workers are old enough to be deemed in need of protection from age discrimination as defined by the 1967 Age Discrimination in Employment Act.
- At age 50 people become eligible for membership in AARP.
- At age 60 people are eligible to participate in activities at most senior centers.
- At age 62 residents can live in public housing for older adults and receive early Social Security retirement benefits.
- At age 67—for those born in 1960 or later—you can qualify for full Social Security benefits.

BOX 12.1 Aging and the International Cinema

An interesting analysis of 14 international feature-length films between 1989 and 2003 provides those interested in the field of cross-cultural aging with models of successful aging by older adults valued within their communities (Yahnke, 2005). Older people serve as role models and mentors for the young and middle-aged, and they apply experience and wisdom to the crises that they discover—and sometimes create. In general, old age in international cinema is viewed as a time of strength, and the old presented as an integral part of family and community.

I can personally recommend these films to you as an excellent way to sensitize yourself to cross-cultural aging. They highlight the hope, joy, and inspiration that can be found in old age. Old age role models in the American cinema have been increasing lately, and perhaps a comparable list of U.S. films can now be created.

- *Antonia's Line* (Holland, 1995)
- *Babette's Feast* (Denmark, 1989)
- *Central Station* (Brazil, 1998)
- *Cinema Paradiso* (Italy, 1990)
- *Eat Drink Man Woman* (Taiwan, 1994)
- *The King of Masks* (China, 1996)
- *Last Orders* (United Kingdom, 2001)
- *Minor Mishaps* (Denmark, 2002)
- *Shower* (China, 2000)
- *Since Otar Left ...* (France and Belgium, 2003)
- *Spring, Summer, Fall, Winter ... and Spring* (South Korea, 2003)
- *Tea with Mussolini* (United Kingdom and Italy, 1999)
- *Waking Ned Devine* (Ireland, 1998)
- *Yi Yi: A One and a Two* (Taiwan and Japan, 2000)
- *The Ballad of Narayama* (Japan, 1983)
- *Pushing Hands* (Taiwan, 1991)
- *Ikiru* (Japan, 1952)

- At age 70, you have exceeded the cutoff age for a population's "premature preventable mortality," a new metric for population health efforts (Jamison et al., 2024).
- At age 75 a patient is eligible for treatment at some geriatric primary care clinics.
- At age 80 or 85 about one third of people require assistance with mobility and activities of daily living.

Another way to think about chronology and aging is to ask people when someone is old. This was the strategy of a U.S. survey conducted by the National Council on Aging in 2000. The survey asked, "At what age is the average man or woman old?" The mean age, not surprisingly, was 65, but variation by the age of respondents was notable. Older respondents dated the start of old age to much older ages than younger respondents. For people aged 23 to 35, old age began at age 55. For people aged 75 to 85 it begins at age 80. Across all age groups, women dated the start of old age to older ages.

In a classroom exercise, students were asked that question. Students, aged 20 to 30, returned the age 65 benchmark quite reliably, with a standard deviation of 5. However, when posing the question in classrooms abroad, there were quite different answers.

Among Japanese students, it is 75. Among Israeli students, it is 70. In one classroom, a student insisted that people are never old whatever their age.

Despite this range, the more or less official chronological designation for old age in America is 65. This tradition began in Germany in 1884, when Chancellor Otto von Bismarck established age 70 as the standard retirement age, hoping, perhaps, that few if any would qualify for benefits. And few did. The qualifying age was eventually reduced to 65 in 1916. When Social Security was enacted in the United States in 1935, the practice of establishing 65 as the eligibility age continued, along with it being a de facto national definition of old age.

Gerontologists began to realize, however, that few meaningful statements can be made in general about those over age 65. They began to argue over the tendency to write about this age category as if older people were all the same when, in fact, the population has become increasingly diverse past this age marker.

Some gerontologists began to divide the older adult population into two groups for analysis, the *young old* and the *old old,* with age 75 as the dividing point at first, then age 80, and now it is not unusual to use age 85 as the transition point. Perhaps as the number of centenarians increases or when more of the baby boomers become of age, another dividing line will be added at age 100 in order to differentiate among the *young old, middle old,* and *old old.*

Dividing the older population into two or more categories is helpful for making policy decisions. Among those age 85 and older, about 96% have at least one chronic condition, disability, or functional limitation, versus 76% among those age 65 to 69. Of those aged 85 and older, about 50% have Alzheimer disease or its symptoms, versus 2% among those age 65 to 69. Among the noninstitutionalized, the average healthcare expenditures for those 85 and over are more than twice as high as for those age 65 to 69. The old old are considerably more physically, mentally, and financially vulnerable than the young old. And the old old is the fastest growing segment of the population.

Before the reader gets too carried away with the differences between the old old and the young old, we still cannot account for the considerable variability that remains at each chronological age. Some nonagenarians and centenarians are authoring books, recording and producing hit singles, completing marathons, and climbing mountains. Some sexagenarians are looking forward to becoming decreasingly active as they enter retirement.

Physically, there is no denying old age. Therefore, exercise, stay active, and make the most of it. As for the rest of old age, you are, or can be, a connoisseur of life. Make the most of that, too!

SUMMARY

Public policy needs to be responsive to the increasing diversity in America, with many cities and even states becoming "minority-majorities" (also referred to as "majority-minorities," you decide which sequence is preferable). No other country in the world has been so bold (despite its limited success) with attempts to integrate minorities and immigrants. Nonetheless, racial/ethnic discrimination in healthcare and in general has had a demonstrable negative effect on the health outcomes among African American, Latinx American, Asian American and Native Hawaiian/Pacific Islander, and American Indian and Alaska Native older adults.

Even though it is still a tremendous burden being an aging LGBTQ+ American, changes have been substantial and rapid in the United States. The legalization of gay marriage seemed to occur overnight, though it came after protracted struggle. Acceptance of LGBTQ+ rights has spread quickly throughout the country, though there remain stubborn pockets of resistance. Caitlyn Jenner, while making an ageist debut, has courageously furthered acceptance for transgender people.

The rural old are being left behind in the United States when it comes to healthcare services and other community resources, and their issues need to be addressed. The challenges of both rural and urban aging are global, both in developing and developed countries. China attempted to cut back on overpopulation and poverty, and wound up unintentionally diminishing both the number of family caregivers and the cultural value of respecting old age. The percentage of older adults in Japan has increased so rapidly that public policy and legislation continue to be challenged.

In general, though, aging throughout the world is being recognized as a challenge, and public policies and legislation are being developed and refined to meet the challenges that are accompanying it. Societies are rapidly aging, which is good news, as we all would like to live a long and fulfilling life.

REFERENCES

Only key references appear in the print edition. The full reference list can be accessed by visiting www.springerpub.com/courseconnect. See inside front cover and tear-out card for CourseConnect details.

Elwert, F., & Christakis, N. (2006). Widowhood and race. *American Sociological Review*, *71*, 16–41. https://doi.org/10.1177/000312240607100102

Falgas-Bague, I., Ramos, Z., del Cueto, P., Kim, E., Zhen-Duan, J., Wong, Y. J., Chieng, C. K., Frontera, W., & Alegría, M. (2021). Adaptation of an evidence-based intervention for disability prevention, implemented by Community Health Workers serving ethnic minority elders. *The American Journal of Geriatric Psychiatry*, *29*(3), 260–269. https://doi.org/10.1016/j.jagp.2020.07.014

Fredriksen-Goldsen, K. I., Kim, H. J., & Barkan, S. E. (2012). Disability among lesbian, gay, and bisexual adults. *American Journal of Public Health*, *102*, e16–e21. https://doi.org/10.2105/AJPH.2011.300379

Jamison, D. T., Summers, L. H., Chang, A. Y., Karlsson, O., Mao, W., Norheim, O. F., Ogbuoji, O., Schäferhoff, M., Watkins, D., Adeyi, O., Alleyne, G., Alwan, A., Anand, S., Belachew, R., Berkley, S. F., Bertozzi, S. M., Bolongaita, S., Bundy, D., Bustreo, F., … Yamey, G. (2024). Global health 2050: The path to halving premature death by mid-century. *Lancet (London, England)*. *404*(10462), 1561–1614. https://doi.org/10.1016/S0140-6736(24)01439-9

Smith, A. S., & Trevelyan, E. (2018). The older population in rural America: 2012–2016. *ACS-41, American Community Survey reports*. U.S. Census Bureau.

INDEX